D0882376

68W ADVANCED FIELD CRAFT
COMBAT MEDIC SKILLS

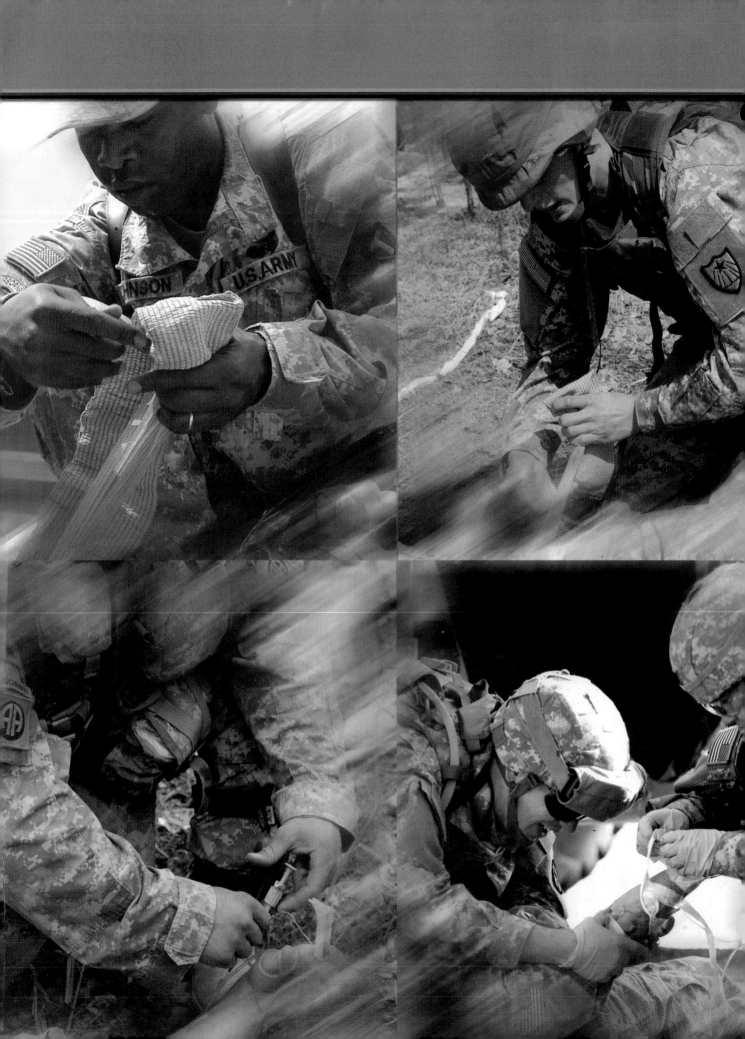

AAOS

68W ADVANCED FIELD CRAFT
COMBAT MEDIC SKILLS

Editor-in-Chief:
Casey Bond, MPAS, PA-C

Editors:
COL Patricia R. Hastings, DO, RN, MPH, NREMT, FACEP
Andrew N. Pollak, MD, FAAOS
Jennifer Kling, MFA

JONES AND BARTLETT PUBLISHERS

Sudbury, Massachusetts

BOSTON   TORONTO   LONDON   SINGAPORE

Jones and Bartlett Publishers

World Headquarters
40 Tall Pine Drive
Sudbury, MA 01776
978-443-5000
info@jbpub.com

Jones and Bartlett Publishers Canada
6339 Ormindale Way
Mississauga, ON L5V 1J2
Canada

Jones and Bartlett Publishers International
Barb House, Barb Mews
London W6 7PA
United Kingdom

AAOS
AMERICAN ACADEMY OF
ORTHOPAEDIC SURGEONS

Jones and Bartlett's books and products are available through most bookstores and online booksellers. To contact Jones and Bartlett Publishers directly, call 800-832-0034, fax 978-443-8000, or visit our website, www.jbpub.com.

Substantial discounts on bulk quantities of Jones and Bartlett's publications are available to corporations, professional associations, and other qualified organizations. For details and specific discount information, contact the special sales department at Jones and Bartlett via the above contact information or send an email to specialsales@jbpub.com.

Production Credits

Chief Executive Officer: Clayton Jones
Chief Operating Officer: Donald W. Jones, Jr
President, Higher Education and Professional Publishing:
 Robert Holland
V.P., Sales and Marketing: William J. Kane
V.P., Production and Design: Anne Spencer
V.P., Manufacturing and Inventory Control: Therese Connell
Publisher, Public Safety: Kimberly Brophy
Acquisitions Editor, EMS: Christine Emerton
Developmental Editor: Jennifer S. Kling
Associate Managing Editor: Amanda Green
Senior Production Editor: Susan Schultz
Production Assistant: Tina Chen

Photo Research Manager/Photographer: Kimberly Potvin
Director of Marketing: Alisha Weisman
Interior Design: Anne Spencer and Kristin Parker
Cover Design: Anne Spencer
Cover Images: (top left) Courtesy of Specialist Michael
 O'Neal/U.S. Army; (top right) Courtesy of Staff Sargeant
 Daniel Ewer, U.S. Army/U.S. Department of Defense; (bottom
 left) Courtesy of Staff Sergeant JoAnn S. Makinano, U.S. Air
 Force/U.S. Department of Defense; (bottom right) Courtesy
 of U.S. Department of Defense
Composition: Shepherd, Inc.
Text Printing and Binding: Courier Corporation
Cover Printing: Courier Corporation

ISBN: 978-0-7637-8659-5

Library of Congress Cataloging-in-Publication Data
68W advanced field craft : combat medic skills / editor, Casey Bond.
  p. ; cm.
 ISBN 978-0-7637-3564-7 (pbk.)
 1. Medicine, Military—Handbooks, manuals, etc. 2. United States. Army—Medical care—Handbooks, manuals, etc. I. Bond, Casey.
II. Title: Advanced field craft.
 [DNLM: 1. Emergency Treatment—methods. 2. Military Medicine—methods. 3. War. 4. Wounds and Injuries—nursing. WB 116
Z999 2009]
 RC971.A15 2009
 616.9'8023--dc22
 6048   2008047276
Printed in the United States of America
13 12 11 10 09   10 9 8 7 6 5 4 3 2

Brief Contents

Contents

Skill Drills

68W Advanced Field Craft: Combat Medic Skills

The combat medic of today is the most technically advanced ever produced by the United States Army. Such an advanced technician requires an advanced teaching and learning system. *68W Advanced Field Craft: Combat Medic Skills* is the first textbook designed to prepare the combat medic for today's challenges in the field.

The ability to save lives in war, conflicts, and humanitarian interventions requires a specific skill set. Today's combat medic must be an expert in emergency medical care, force health protection, limited primary care, evacuation, and warrior skills. *68W Advanced Field Craft: Combat Medic Skills* combines complete medical content with dynamic features to support instructors and to prepare combat medics for their missions.

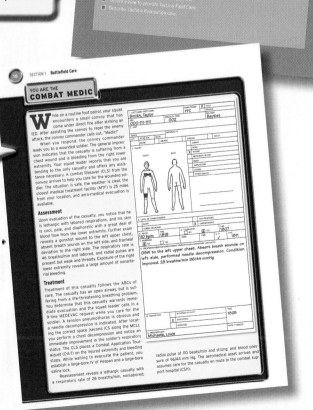

Objectives
Learning objectives are clearly presented for each chapter.

You Are the Combat Medic
Each chapter contains a case study that makes soldiers start to think about what they would do if they encounter a similar case on the battlefield. This feature is a valuable learning tool that encourages critical thinking skills.

SECTION 2 **Garrison Care**

Field Medical Care **TIPS**

Approximately 10% to 15% of people are sensitive to latex and have allergic reactions due to the powder in the latex glove. The most common reaction is contact dermatitis. Other symptoms include rash, itching, cracking, scaling, or weeping of the skin. An aerosol reaction (eg, itchy and red eyes, sneezing, runny or stuffed noses, itchy noses or palates) may occur when sensitive individuals are exposed to others who are wearing them.

Field Medical Care **TIPS**

All discarded materials are considered contaminated.

Field Medical Care Tips
Provide expert advice on how to handle emergencies on the battlefield.

the area with microorganisms that reside on the skin, hair, and clothing. All hair coverings should cover all hair on the head. The surgical mask should completely cover the mouth and the nose. Touch only the inside of the gown; the back of the gown is considered contaminated.

■ Infection Control

Standard Precautions

Standard precautions are a combination of universal precautions and **body substance isolation**. Universal precautions are designed to reduce the risk of transmission of bloodborne pathogens. Body substance isolation is designed to reduce the transmission of pathogens from moist body substances. Standard precautions apply to blood, all body fluids, secretions, excretions (except sweat), nonintact skin, and mucous membranes. They are designed to reduce the risk of transmission of microorganisms from both known and unknown sources of infection. Standard precautions consider all patients to be infected with bloodborne pathogens. You must use standard precautions in the care of all patients.

Wear gloves when in contact with blood, body fluids containing blood, secretions, excretions, nonintact skin, mucous membranes, or contaminated items. Change gloves after each contact with a patient. Wash your hands and skin surfaces immediately and thoroughly if you are contaminated with blood or body fluids, after each patient contact, and after removing gloves to prevent transfer of microorganisms between patients or between pati...

Wear a gown or apron when soiled. Wear a mask, eye protection while spraying of blood or body contaminated linens in a leak-proof...

Do not recap or break needles objects in a special, puncture-resi...

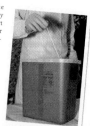 **FIGURE 19-6 ▶** . Use the needless system or safety syringes, if available. Report any exposure to blood or body fluids to your supervisor immediately.

Transmission-Based Precautions

Transmission-based precautions for treating patients with a suspected or known infectious disease are based on the disease's route of transmission. These precautions are designed to interrupt the transmission of pathogens. Airborne precautions are taken when tiny microorganisms from

FIGURE 19-6 Place needles and sharp objects in a special, puncture-resistant container after use.

evaporated droplets remain suspended in the air or are carried on dust particles and inhaled. Diseases transmitted this way include tuberculosis (TB), measles, and chickenpox. The patient may be placed in a private room that has monitored negative air flow pressure (air discharged outdoors or specially filtered before circulating to other areas). Doors to these rooms are to be kept closed. Wear a high-filtration particulate respirator when caring for TB patients **FIGURE 19-7 ▶** .

Droplet precautions are taken when microorganisms are propelled through the air from an infected person and depos-

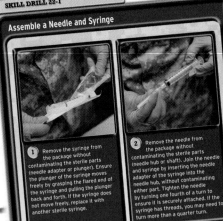

 SECTION 2 **Garrison Care**

SKILL DRILL 22-1

Assemble a Needle and Syringe

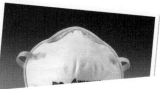

1 Remove the syringe from the package without contaminating the sterile parts (needle adapter or plunger). Ensure the plunger of the syringe moves freely by grasping the flared end of the syringe and pulling the plunger back and forth. If the syringe does not move freely, replace it with another sterile syringe.

2 Remove the needle from the package without contaminating the sterile parts (needle hub or shaft). Join the needle and syringe by inserting the needle adapter of the syringe into the needle hub, without contaminating either part. Tighten the needle by turning one fourth of a turn to ensure it is securely attached. If the syringe has threads, you may need to turn more than a quarter turn.

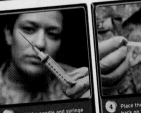

3 Hold the needle and syringe upright and remove the protective cover from the needle by pulling it straight off. Visually inspect the needle for burrs, barbs, damage, and contamination. If the needle has any defects or damage, replace the needle with another sterile needle.

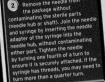

4 Place the protective cover back on the needle, being careful not to stick yourself or to contaminate the needle. Place the assembled needle and syringe on the work surface.

Skill Drills
Provide written step-by-step explanations and visual summaries of important skills and procedures.

number, the smaller the diameter (bore) of the needle. Small-bore needles are indicated for thin medications (watery medications) or slow infusion rates. Large-bore needles are indicated for thick medications or rapid infusion rates. Drawing medication from an ampule is covered in detail in Skill Drill 12-1 in Chapter 12, *Battlefield Medications*. Drawing medication from a stoppered vial that contains a prepared solution is covered in detail in Skill Drill 12-2 in Chapter 12.

Reconstitution of Powdered Medication

To reconstitute a powdered medication, follow the steps in **SKILL DRILL 22-2 ▶** .

1. Receive the doctor's orders (medication, route, dosage).
2. Select the correct medication from the storage area.
3. Peel back the protective plunger cap (**Step ①**).
4. Depress the top of the vial to dislodge the diluent into the powdered medication (**Step ②**).
5. Invert the vial several times until all of the powdered medication dissolved (**Step ③**).
6. Open an alcohol prep pad (**Step ④**).
7. Clean the stopper on vial with an alcohol pad (**Step ⑤**).
8. Insert the appropriate sized needle into the reconstituted medication. Wit... the predetermined medication amoun... the syringe (**Step** ...
9. Withdraw the nee... the vial and verify... correct dosage (**St**...

Aid Kit
End-of-chapter activities reinforce important concepts and improve soldiers' comprehension.

Ready for Review
Summarize chapter content in a comprehensive bulleted list.

Vital Vocabulary
Provide key terms and definitions from the chapter.

Combat Medic in Action
Promote critical thinking with case studies and multiple choice questions.

Aid Kit

Ready for Review

- Understanding the wound healing process and proper wound care management for a variety of wounds is essential knowledge basic to any health care setting.
- In a closed wound, soft tissues beneath the skin surface are damaged, but there is no break in the epidermis.
- An open wound is characterized by a disruption in the skin. Open wounds are potentially much more serious than closed wounds for two reasons: Open wounds are vulnerable to infection and they have a greater potential for serious blood loss.
- The types of wound healing are primary healing, secondary intention, and delayed primary closure (tertiary intention).
- Obtain the wound injury history from the patient.
- Always remember to manage the patient's airway, breathing, and circulation prior to applying wound care treatment.
- A drain is a device that is used to remove excess fluid from a wound or body part.
- The evaluation of wound healing is performed after each dressing change, application of heat and cold therapies, wound irrigation, or stress to the wound site.

Vital Vocabulary

abrasion An injury in which a portion of the body is denuded of epidermis by scraping or rubbing.

adhesion A band of scar tissue that binds together two anatomical surfaces normally separated.

adipose Referring to fat tissue.

amputation An injury in which part of the body is completely severed.

avulsion An injury that leaves a piece of skin or other tissue partially or completely torn away from the body.

cellulitis Infection of the skin characterized by heat, pain, redness, and edema.

closed (suction) drains Self-contained suction ... connect to drainage tubes with ...

closed wound ...

contusion A bruise; an injury that causes bleeding beneath the skin but does not break the skin.

deep fascia A dense layer of fibrous tissue below the subcutaneous tissue; composed of tough bands of tissue that ensheath muscles and other internal structures.

dehiscence Separation of a surgical incision or rupture of a wound closure.

delayed primary closure (tertiary intention) A combination of the primary and secondary intentions. The wound is initially cleaned, debrided, and irrigated, and then is observed for a period of time before closure.

dermis The inner layer of skin, containing hair follicle roots, glands, blood vessels, and nerves.

drain A device that is used to remove excess fluid from a wound or body part.

ecchymosis Extravasation of blood under the skin to produce a "black-and-blue" mark.

epidermis The outermost layer of the skin.

evisceration Protrusion of an internal organ through a wound or surgical incision.

exsanguination Excessive blood loss due to hemorrhage.

extravasation Passage or escape into the tissues, usually of blood, serum, or lymph.

exudate Fluid that has penetrated from blood vessels into the surrounding tissues resulting from inflammation.

hematoma A localized collection of blood in the soft tissues as a result of injury or a broken blood vessel.

Hemovac A drainage system used for larger amounts, up to 500 mL, of drainage.

homeostasis The tendency to constancy or stability in the body's internal environment.

incision A wound usually made deliberately, as in surgery; a clean cut, as opposed to a laceration.

integument The skin.

Jackson-Pratt ...

Penrose drain A soft tube that may be advanced or pulled out in stages as the wound heals from the inside out.

primary healing Wound closure immediately following the injury and prior to the formation of granulation tissue.

puncture wound A stab injury from a pointed object, such as a nail or a knife.

sanguineous Drainage that contains blood.

secondary intention A strategy of allowing a wound to heal on its own without surgical closure.

serosanguineous Drainage that contains serum and blood.

serous Clear, watery discharge that has been separated from its solid elements.

subcutaneous Beneath the skin.

tension lines The pattern of tautness of the skin, which is arranged over body structures and affects how well wounds heal.

COMBAT MEDIC in Action

You are the combat medic assisting at the Battalion Aid Station. You are changing the dressing on a patient confined to a hospital bed, who is healing from an open wound to the abdomen. Before receiving his wound, the patient had been on antibiotics for a prolonged period to clear up a stubborn sinus infection. You collect the proper equipment: clean gloves, gauze dressing, adhesive tape, a small basin, normal saline, a 60-mL syringe, and a waterproof pad.

After washing your hands and donning sterile gloves, you place the waterproof pad underneath the patient and you then gently loosen the adhesive tape around the wound. You

carefully remove the dressing, taking care not to damage the fragile skin underneath the dressing. When you reveal the wound, you find that the tissue is yellow.

1. Which known factors could be complicating the healing process in this patient?
   A. Prolonged antibiotic use
   B. Obesity
   C. Diabetes mellitus
   D. Age

2. Is the patient displaying any signs that you should bring to the attention of the MO?
   A. Yes, the open abdominal wound.
   B. Yes, the yellow tissue around the wound.
   C. No, this patient is healing nicely.
   D. No, you can handle this patient on your own.

3. Assessment of the wound includes the following four categories:
   A. Airway, breathing, circulation, exposure
   B. Pulse, capillary refill, skin color, skin temperature
   C. Color of the wound bed tissue, wound size, wound boundaries, drainage
   D. Drainage, skin color, pulse, skin temperature

4. The types of dressings used to care for a wound include:
   A. gauze dressings.
   B. transparent dressings.
   C. hydrocolloid dressings.
   D. all of the above.

5. Wound complications include:
   A. adhesion.
   B. cellulitis.
   C. compartment syndrome.
   D. all of the above.

Preface

THROUGHOUT HISTORY, during the course of conflict or during a humanitarian response, combat medics (68W) have brought back patients instead of victims, lessened hardship, and eased the transition of death. These soldiers understand the reality of war and disasters in ways that few people do, and yet they still respond. They are mastery-oriented and competency-based with a consistent capacity to achieve. Non-response is untenable in their values. Combat medics live the Army values every day and epitomize what is best in our Army.

Today's combat medic has been shaped over time by both visionaries and circumstance. The 68W is the embodiment of superior ability, competence, compassion, and discipline under any condition and at any time. Those visionaries include LTG James Peake and CSM James Aplin, the command team that designed the specialty; MG George Weightman, BG Daniel Perugini, CSM David Litteral, SGM Edward Norwood, CSM Michael Kelly, COL Alan Morgan, COL Patrick Wilson, and COL Fred Gerber, who made the vision a reality. Carrying the specialty into the future today are: MG Russell Czerw, CSM Riles, COL W John Luciano, LTC Paul Mayer, SGM Henry Myrick, Mr Don Parsons, Ms Meredith Hansen, MAJ Nancy Parson, LTC Peter Cuenca, MAJ Jimmie Cooper, and CSM(R) David Cahill, who, with the instructors at the Department of Combat Medic Training both past and present, prepare combat medics daily to "be there."

There are also many commanders and first sergeants who help combat medics to become soldiers, with all the heart that this entails. These include: LTC Brian Kueter, COL Bruce McVeigh, LTC John Lamoureux, CSM Abin, COL John Cook, COL Maureen Coleman, and COL Brad Freeman.

Very special thanks are also due to Mr Casey Bond, Ms Kimberly Brophy, and Ms Jennifer Kling for making this textbook a polished educational instrument.

Senator Daniel Inouye is an inspiration for his combat experience, his persistent support of International Humanitarian Law, and his support for medical training that better serves our nation in peace and, if necessary, in war.

This textbook was created by the instructors at the Department of Combat Medic Training, Army Medical Department Center and School at Fort Sam Houston, Texas. It was created to serve as a repository of the skills that the combat medic must learn to achieve entry level competence. Today's combat medic must be an expert in emergency medical care, force health protection, limited primary care, evacuation, and warrior skills. Similar to the *Combat Medic Field Manual*, this textbook recognizes the special needs of the combat medic. However, this textbook will and must change over time, as we acquire new lessons and learn better ways of saving lives.

Combat medic training has changed in the past decade. The lessons learned in previous conflicts and the requirements for Army transformation have been incorporated into current training. The combat medic of today is the most technically advanced conventional medic ever produced by the United States Army. The depth of understanding of anatomy and physiology and the sophistication of the skills that the combat medic must master requires an intense dedication to mission-craft.

The combat medic encompasses the best of the Army Medical Department. Whether required to work in austere environments or on a hospital ward, these soldiers have proven to be invaluable to their commanders. The combat medic is a highly trained force multiplier. Medics have earned the respect of the line throughout time. Today's combat medics are ready to earn their place in at home, in future conflicts, and in disasters. Theirs is a noble profession.

This historical reference and quote about the foundations for success of a country seems particularly relevant for combat medics. Sun Tzu, the ancient Chinese general, noted: "The art of war is of vital importance to the state. It is a matter of life and death, a road to either safety or ruin. Hence, under no circumstances, can it be neglected." Sun Tzu taught that this art was influenced by five factors and the outcome is determined by these factors:

Moral Law—the people are undismayed by danger, knowing their work is just.

Heaven—signifies night and day; cold and heat; times and seasons; and the ability to work under any circumstance.

Earth—includes distances, great and small; danger and security; terrain; and the capacity to overcome adversity.

Command—stands for the virtues of wisdom, sincerity, benevolence, and courage.

Method and Discipline—are the understanding of mission-craft and the determination to remain skilled and proficient.

If Sun Tzu were to examine the five factors in relation to the combat medic, he would conclude that any endeavor upon which the combat medic focuses upon will be successful.

Today's combat medics embody the best trained, qualified medics in the history of armed conflict. Dr Thomas Ditzler, noted psychologist and development anthropologist, who studies the characteristics of responders, related a method by which one is able to determine a person's or society's values. He said, "To find out what people really care about, watch them and see what they work for: friends, family, country; in the final analysis what we really care about may require hard work, but this work will be the central organizing principle of significance and consequence."

It is a sad truth that the work of the combat medic often takes place in a dangerous world. However, the Army Medical Department Center and School instructors and staff work hard to ensure that our combat medics can meet the challenges of this world.

As complicated as our life gets in the military, there are a few truths:

1. The combat medic only volunteers once, and in this commits an act of faith in self and country.

2. When medics go into harm's way, they show a faith in self, comrades, and the people they protect.

It is reassuring to know so many of our best are capable of committing acts of faith and do so willingly.

Past and present instructors of the Department of Combat Medic Training have authored this manual. We salute the combat medic and hope that this textbook will assist combat medics in understanding their profession.

"Soldier Medic/Warrior Spirit"

Dr Patricia R Hastings
Colonel, Medical Corps
Director, US Army EMS

Acknowledgments

■ Editor-in-Chief

Casey Bond, MPAS, PA-C
Program Director, Center for Pre-Deployment Medicine
Army Medical Department Center and School
Fort Sam Houston, Texas

■ Editors

Jennifer Kling, MFA

Patricia R. Hastings, DO, RN, MPH, NREMT, FACEP
Colonel, Medical Corps, US Army
Director, US Army EMS
Army Medical Department Center and School
Fort Sam Houston, Texas

■ Authors

Jeffery S. Cain, MD
Lieutenant Colonel, Medical Corps, US Army
Brooke Army Medical Center
Fort Sam Houston, Texas

Thomas F. Ditzler, PhD, MA, FRSPH, FRAI
Director of Research, Department of Psychiatry
Tripler Army Medical Center
Honolulu, Hawaii

Nadine A. Kahla, 68W48
Sergeant First Class, US Army
Combat Medic/68W Instructor/Writer
Department of Combat Medic Training
Army Medical Department Center and School
Fort Sam Houston, Texas

Paul T. Mayer, MD, MBA, FACEP
Lieutenant Colonel, Medical Corps, US Army
Director, Department of Combat Medic Training
Army Medical Department Center and School
Fort Sam Houston, Texas

John G. McManus, MD, MCR, FACEP, FAAEM
Lieutenant Colonel (Promotable), Medical Corps, US Army
Director, Center for Pre-Deployment Medicine
Army Medical Department Center and School
Fort Sam Houston, Texas

Donald L. Parsons, MPAS, PA-C
Deputy Director, Department of Combat Medic Training
Army Medical Department Center and School
Fort Sam Houston, Texas

Jason D. Reisler, 68W48
Sergeant First Class, US Army
Combat Medic/68W Instructor/Writer
Department of Combat Medic Training
Army Medical Department Center and School
Fort Sam Houston, Texas

Robert Thaxton, MD
Lieutenant Colonel, Medical Corps, US Air Force
Associate Program Director, SAUSHEC Emergency Medicine Residency
Brooke Army Medical Center
Fort Sam Houston, Texas

■ Contributing Authors

John A. DeArmond, NREMT-P
Senior Consultant, Emergency Management Resources
Half Moon Bay, California

Bob Elling, MPA, NREMT-P
Hudson Valley Community College
Andrew Jackson University
Colonie EMS Department
Times Union Center EMS
Colonie, New York

Robert Gurliacci, EMT-P
Paramedic Curriculum Chair
Westchester Community College
Valhalla, New York

Michael Hay, MHA, NREMT-P
EMS Program Manager
Reno Fire Department
Reno, Nevada

Brittany Ann Martinelli, MHSc, RRT-NPS, NREMT-P
Santa Fe Community College
Gainesville, Florida

Deborah L. Petty, BS, EMT-P I/C
Paramedic Training Officer
St. Charles County Ambulance District
St. Peters, Missouri

John J. Scotch II
Lieutenant, Fire Department of New York—EMS Academy
Bayside, New York

MSgt Michael G. Silver, NREMT-P
Medical NCO, 2nd CST(WMD)
Ballston Spa, New York

Scott A. Williams, BS, BA, NREMT-P, FP-C
Tulsa Life Flight
Tulsa, Oklahoma

Reviewers

Morris Beard, PA-C
Chief, Field Craft Branch
Department of Combat Medic Training
Army Medical Department Center and School
Fort Sam Houston, Texas

John Berg, PA-C
Captain, Specialty Corps, US Army
Officer in Charge, 68W Training Team 2
Department of Combat Medic Training
Army Medical Department Center and School
Fort Sam Houston, Texas

Paula Brady, EMT-I
Curriculum Development/Instructional Support
Department of Combat Medic Training
Army Medical Department Center and School
Fort Sam Houston, Texas

Jimmy Cooper, MD
Major, Medical Corps, US Army
Chief, Clinical Operations
Department of Combat Medic Training
Army Medical Department Center and School
Fort Sam Houston, Texas

Peter J. Cuenca, MD
Major (Promotable), Medical Corps, US Army
Chief, Academics
Department of Combat Medic Training
Army Medical Department Center and School
Fort Sam Houston, Texas

Armand A. Fermin, NREMT-B
Master Sergeant (Ret), US Army
Coordinator, Center for Pre-Deployment Medicine
Army Medical Department Center and School
Fort Sam Houston, Texas

Michael E. Franco, MSM, MPAS, PA-C
Major, Specialty Corps, US Army
Instructor/Training Coordinator
Department of Combat Medic Training
Army Medical Department Center and School
Fort Sam Houston, Texas

Meredith Hansen, MPH, PA-C
Chief, Curriculum Development
Department of Combat Medic Training
Army Medical Department Center and School
Fort Sam Houston, Texas

Kermit Huebner, MD, FACEP
Department of Emergency Medicine
Carl R. Darnell Army Medical Center
Fort Hood, Texas

David Kuhns, MD
Department of Emergency Medicine
Carl R. Darnell Army Medical Center
Fort Hood, Texas

Robert L. Mabrey, MD
Major, Medical Corps, US Army
Academic Course Director
Department of Combat Medic Training
Army Medical Department Center and School
Fort Sam Houston, Texas

Arnrae U. Moultrie, MPAS, PA-C
Captain, Specialty Corps, US Army
Officer in Charge, 68W Training Team 1
Department of Combat Medic Training
Army Medical Department Center and School
Fort Sam Houston, Texas

William Blair Pilgrim, 68W48
Sergeant First Class, US Army
NCOIC, US Army EMS
Army Medical Department Center and School
Fort Sam Houston, Texas

Andrew Pollak, MD, FAAOS
Medical Director, Baltimore County Fire Department
Associate Professor, University of Maryland School of Medicine
Baltimore, Maryland

Brian Savage, MPAS, PA-C
Captain, Specialty Corps, US Army
Officer in Charge, Situational Training Exercises
Department of Combat Medic Training
Army Medical Department Center and School
Fort Sam Houston, Texas

Charles Stanley, MPAS, PA-C
Captain, Specialty Corps, US Army
Officer in Charge, Situational Training Exercises
Department of Combat Medic Training
Army Medical Department Center and School
Fort Sam Houston, Texas

Patrick Williams, PA-C
Captain, Specialty Corps, US Army
Officer in Charge, Faculty Development
Department of Combat Medic Training
Army Medical Department Center and School
Fort Sam Houston, Texas

Photographic Contributors

We would like to thank Brian Slack and Kimberly Potvin, the photographers for the photo shoot at Fort Sam Houston. Thank you to SGT Charles Hall and Casey Bond for their technical expertise during the photo shoot. And finally, thank you to the outstanding models from the Fort Sam Houston Department of Combat Medic Training:

SGT Charles D. Hall
PV2 Philip Cormier
PV2 Monique Martinez
PV2 Diana Musgrove

PV2 Michael A. Randazzio
PV2 Bradley Van Meter
PV2 Sergiy Zadvornyy

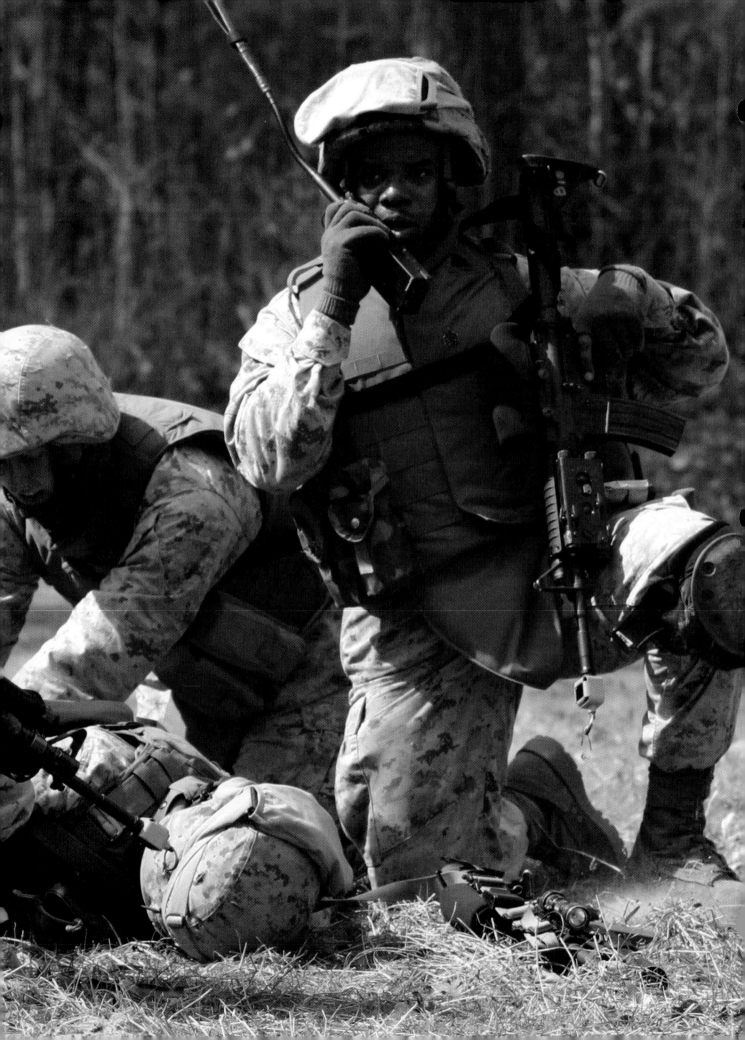

Battlefield Care

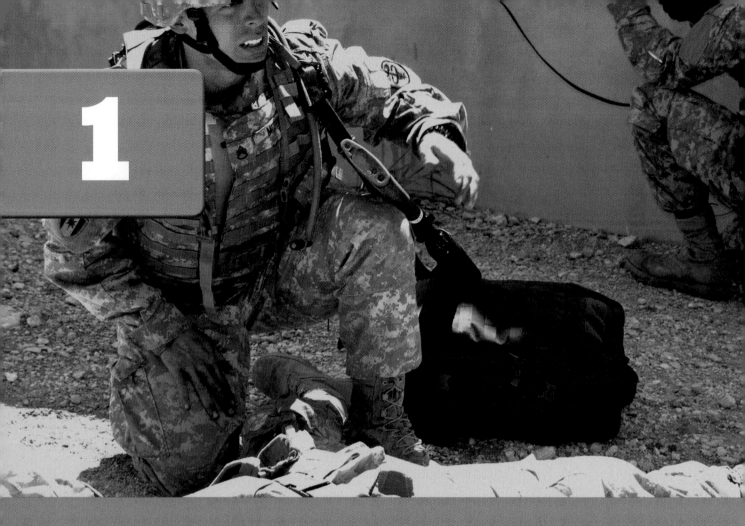

1

Introduction to Battlefield Medicine

Objectives

Knowledge Objectives

- ☐ Describe the principles of Tactical Combat Casualty Care (TC-3).
- ☐ List the stages of medical care in a tactical setting.
- ☐ Describe how to provide Care Under Fire.
- ☐ Describe how to provide Tactical Field Care.
- ☐ Describe Tactical Evacuation care.

Skills Objectives

- ☐ Apply a tourniquet to control bleeding.
- ☐ Perform a safe evacuation.

■ Introduction

Today, the United States is at war. As a combat medic, it is possible that you will be called on to deploy to a foreign country and provide medical care in a combat zone. You need to understand the differences between trauma management in the homeland and trauma management in a foreign country during wartime.

■ Overview of Tactical Combat Casualty Care

Medical training for combat medics is currently based on the principles for **emergency medical technicians (EMTs)**, basic life support (BLS), and advanced life support (ALS). These guidelines provide a standard systematic approach to the management of a trauma patient during a domestic emergency incident. This system works well in the civilian emergency medical services setting; however, some of these principles are not appropriate for the battlefield.

On the battlefield, the trauma patient is a wounded soldier or casualty. Most casualties in combat are the result of penetrating trauma, whereas blunt trauma is generally the chief cause in the civilian sector. Up to 90% of combat deaths occur on the battlefield before the casualty reaches a **medical treatment facility (MTF)**. There are additional differences in combat care; for example, the correct intervention must be performed at the correct time. A medically correct intervention performed at the wrong time can lead to additional casualties.

Caring for a casualty on the battlefield requires a different set of skills from a basic EMT. Factors such as enemy fire, medical equipment limitations, widely variable evacuation times, tactical considerations, and the unique problems encountered in transporting casualties must all be addressed. Enemy fire may prevent the treatment of casualties and may put you at risk while providing care. The only medical supplies you have on hand are those you carry with you in your medical aid bag, so providing proper care to a casualty can be challenging. In the civilian setting, evacuation can occur in under 25 minutes, but on the battlefield, it may be delayed for several hours. This widely variable evacuation time impacts the care you must provide to a casualty. Sometimes the mission takes precedence over medical care; tactical considerations always have to be weighed. Casualty transportation may or may not be available, because air superiority must be achieved before any air evacuation assets are deployed. The tactical situation dictates when or if casualty evacuation can occur. In addition, environmental factors may prevent evacuation assets from reaching your casualty. All of these factors affect the care you can provide the casualty.

■ Stages of Care

Tactical Combat Casualty Care (TC-3) has been approved by the American College of Surgeons and the National Association of EMTs. Casualty scenarios in combat usually entail a medical problem as well as a tactical problem. As combat medics, we want the best possible outcome for both the soldier and the mission. Good medicine can sometimes be bad tactics, and bad tactics can get soldiers killed and/or cause mission failure. The TC-3 approach recognizes an important principle: performing the correct intervention at the correct time in the continuum of battlefield care. The three goals of TC-3 are:

1. Treat the casualty.
2. Prevent additional casualties.
3. Complete the mission.

The management of casualties is divided into three distinct phases: Care Under Fire, Tactical Field Care, and Tactical Evacuation. **Care Under Fire** is the care rendered by you at the scene of the injury while you and the casualty are still under effective hostile fire. During this phase, the available medical equipment is limited to what is carried in your medical aid bag. **Tactical Field Care** is the care rendered by you once you and the casualty are no longer under effective hostile fire. It also applies to situations in which an injury has occurred, but there is no hostile fire. Available medical equipment is still limited to what was carried into the field by medical personnel. Time to evacuation to an MTF may vary considerably. **Tactical Evacuation** is the care rendered once the casualty has been picked up by an aircraft, vehicle, or boat. Additional medical personnel and equipment may have been prestaged and are available at this stage of casualty management.

■ Care Under Fire

Enemy Fire

When under enemy fire, there is very little time to provide comprehensive medical care to a casualty. Suppression of enemy fire and movement of the casualty to cover are paramount at this point in the operation. Most medical personnel carry small arms with which to defend themselves in the field. In unit operations, the additional firepower you provide may be essential in obtaining tactical fire superiority. The risk of injury to other personnel and additional injury to casualties will be reduced if immediate attention is directed to the suppression of hostile fire. You may initially need to assist in returning fire instead of stopping to care for the casualty. Remember, the best medicine on any battlefield is fire superiority. Casualties who are still able to fight should return fire. Casualties who are unable to fight should lay flat and motionless if no cover is available or move as quickly as possible to any nearby cover. You may be able to direct the casualty to provide self-aid for life-threatening hemorrhage, if he or she is able.

The tactical situation dictates when and how much care you can provide. When a MEDEVAC is requested, the tactical situation may not safely allow the air asset to respond.

Consider the following tragic situation. A wounded marine is down in the street. A colleague attempts to come to his rescue along with a second marine. Enemy fire continues in the area and the first rescuer is fatally wounded.

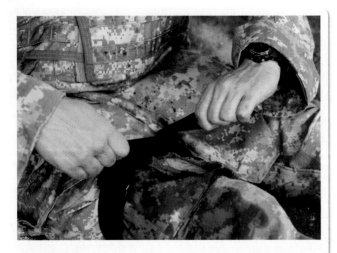

FIGURE 1-1 A tourniquet is the most reasonable initial choice to stop extremity bleeding if the casualty needs to be moved.

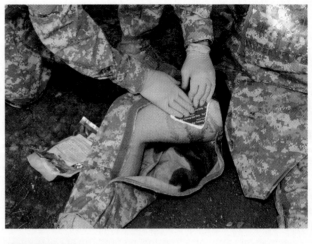

FIGURE 1-2 Hemostatic dressing.

The second rescuer returns behind cover. Eventually, after enemy fire is contained, the wounded marine is rescued but his initial rescuer dies from his wounds. When under enemy fire, you cannot afford to rush blindly into a danger area to rescue a fallen comrade; if you do, additional soldiers may be wounded or killed. Combat medical personnel are limited, and if injured, no others will be available until the time of evacuation during the Tactical Evacuation phase. Your first mission is to remain safe and able to provide care to casualties—do not become one yourself!

No immediate management of the airway should be anticipated at this time because of the need to move the casualty to cover as quickly as possible. There is little time and safety to adequately evaluate a casualty's airway and provide airway support while under fire and during movement to cover.

However, it is very important to stop major bleeding as quickly as possible. Injury to an artery or another major vessel may result in the very rapid onset of hypovolemic shock and **exsanguination** (total blood loss leading to death). Extremity hemorrhage is the leading cause of preventable combat death. Over 2,500 deaths occurred in Vietnam secondary to hemorrhage from extremity wounds; these casualties had no other injuries. These were preventable deaths.

If the casualty needs to be moved, a tourniquet that can be applied rapidly by the casualty, or his or her **battle buddy**, is the most reasonable initial choice to stop major extremity bleeding **FIGURE 1-1**. The new Combat Application Tourniquet (C-A-T) should be carried by every soldier. Tourniquets are appropriate in combat because direct pressure is hard to maintain during casualty transport under fire. Damage is rare if the tourniquet is left in place for less than 2 hours. Tourniquets are often left in place for several hours during surgical procedures. It is better to accept the small risk of damage to the limb than to watch a casualty bleed to death. Both you and the casualty are in grave danger while

a tourniquet is being applied during this phase, and non-life-threatening bleeding should be ignored until the Tactical Field Care phase.

Soldiers have died in combat with only a wound to the right knee area. In one incident, a combat medic was the first one killed on the mission. The remaining soldiers were either not trained in hemorrhage control or did not have the proper equipment. They made several attempts to control the bleeding but were unsuccessful and the combat medic died. In contrast, a soldier was saved when his battle buddies applied two effective improvised tourniquets to his legs, saving his life.

The need for immediate access to a tourniquet in such situations makes it clear that all soldiers on combat missions should have a suitable tourniquet readily available at a standard location on their battle gear and be trained in its use. To apply a Combat Application Tourniquet, follow the steps in **SKILL DRILL 1-1** :

1. Apply the tourniquet band above the bleeding wound (**Step ①**).
2. Adjust the friction adaptor buckle until the tourniquet is securely in place (**Step ②**).
3. Twist the windlass rod to provide direct pressure to the extremity; twist until the bleeding stops (**Step ③**).
4. Lock the windlass rod in place with the clip (**Step ④**).

For nonextremity wounds, the use of direct pressure with a hemostatic dressing is appropriate to control life-threatening hemorrhage **FIGURE 1-2** . Severe bleeding may occur with neck, axillary, or groin injuries. For these injuries, it may not be possible to effectively apply a tourniquet. Use of direct pressure and a hemostatic dressing may be required.

Penetrating neck injuries do not require c-spine immobilization. Other neck injuries such as falls over 15 feet, fast roping injuries, or motor vehicle collisions (MVCs) may

SKILL DRILL 1-1

Applying a Combat Application Tourniquet

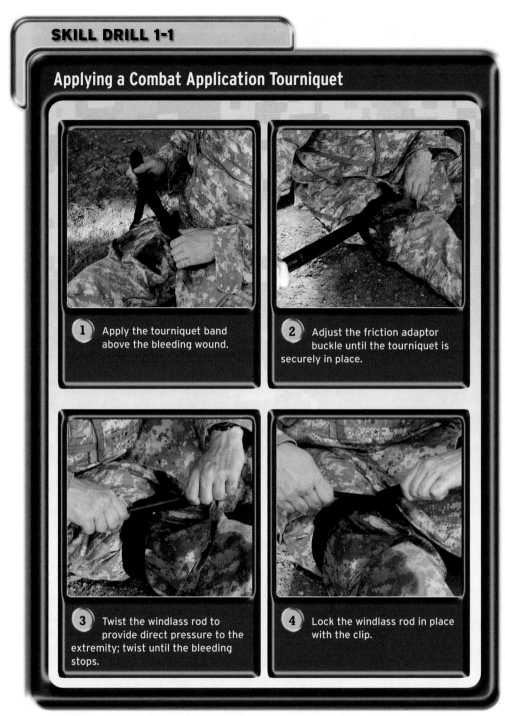

1. Apply the tourniquet band above the bleeding wound.

2. Adjust the friction adaptor buckle until the tourniquet is securely in place.

3. Twist the windlass rod to provide direct pressure to the extremity; twist until the bleeding stops.

4. Lock the windlass rod in place with the clip.

require c-spine immobilization unless the danger of hostile fire constitutes a greater threat. Adjustable rigid c-collars should be carried in your medical aid bag. If rigid c-collars are not available, a SAM splint can be used as a field-expedient c-collar.

Litters may not be available for movement of casualties. Consider alternate methods to move casualties, such as ponchos, pole-less litters, Sked or Talon II litters, discarded doors, dragging, or manual carries. Smoke and vehicles may act as screens to assist in casualty movement. There have been several instances of tanks being used as screens in Iraq to assist with the evacuation of casualties.

Performing a Safe Evacuation

To perform a safe evacuation during the Care Under Fire phase, follow the steps in **SKILL DRILL 1-2**:

1. Return fire as directed or required.
2. The casualty should also return fire if able.
3. Direct the casualty to cover and apply self-aid if able.
4. Try to keep the casualty from sustaining any additional wounds.
5. Stop any life-threatening hemorrhage with a tourniquet or hemostatic dressing, if applicable.

Field Medical Care TIPS

Do not attempt to salvage a casualty's rucksack unless it contains items critical to the mission.
Do take the casualty's weapon and ammunition, if possible, to prevent the enemy from using them against you.

Field Medical Care TIPS

Studies have shown that penetrating neck injuries occur in only 1.4% of those injured, so very few casualties could ever potentially benefit from c-spine immobilization.

■ Tactical Field Care

During the Tactical Field Care phase, you have more time to provide care and there is a reduced level of hazard from hostile fire. The time available to render care may be quite variable. In some cases, tactical field care may consist of rapid treatment of wounds with the expectation of a re-engagement of hostile fire at any moment. It is critical to avoid undertaking nonessential diagnostic and therapeutic measures.

At other times, care may be rendered once the mission has reached an anticipated evacuation point, without pursuit, and you are awaiting casualty evacuation. In this circumstance, there may be ample time to render whatever care is feasible in the field. The time prior to extraction may range from half an hour to many hours. Care must be taken to partition supplies and equipment in the event of prolonged evacuation times. Although you and the casualty are now in a somewhat less hazardous setting, this is still not the time or place for procedures that could be performed in a domestic emergency incident. Procedures such as diagnostic peritoneal lavage (inserting a catheter into the abdomen to determine if there is internal bleeding) and pericardiocentesis (inserting a needle into the pericardial sac of the heart to withdraw fluid) have no place in the combat setting. Initial evaluation should be directed to airway, breathing, and circulation.

If a victim of a blast or penetrating injury is found without a pulse, respirations, or other signs of life, do not attempt CPR. Attempts to resuscitate casualties in arrest have been found to be futile even in the domestic setting where the trauma patient is in close proximity to an emergency department. On the battlefield, the cost of attempting CPR on casualties with inevitably fatal injuries is additional lives lost. By attempting CPR, care is withheld from casualties with less severe injuries and you are exposed to hostile fire. Only in the case of nontraumatic disorders such as hypothermia, near-drowning, or electrocution should CPR be considered.

Casualties with an altered level of consciousness should be disarmed immediately, both weapons and grenades. This provides you with an additional safety measure, so when the casualty becomes more awake and alert, he or she does not mistake you for the enemy he or she was recently engaging.

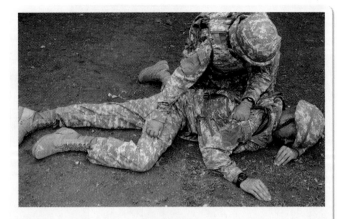

FIGURE 1-3 Many times positioning may be all a casualty needs to maintain a viable airway.

Field Medical Care TIPS

A casualty with maxillofacial trauma should never be evacuated on a litter lying supine.

Initial Assessment

During the Tactical Field Care phase, initial assessment consists of airway, breathing, and circulation. Due to the hazardous setting and time constraints, you must focus on assessing these three functions.

Airway

If the casualty is conscious and breathing well on his or her own, there should be no attempt at airway intervention. Allow a conscious casualty to assume any position that best protects the airway, including sitting up. Open the airway with a chin-lift or jaw-thrust maneuver without worrying about cervical spine immobilization. With unconscious casualties, insert a **nasopharyngeal airway (NPA)** or **Combitube** and place him or her in the recovery position **FIGURE 1-3 ▲**. This position will allow for drainage of blood and mucus that would otherwise be aspirated, and prevents the tongue from blocking the airway. Many times positioning alone may be all a casualty needs to maintain a viable airway.

An NPA has the advantage of being better tolerated than an **oropharyngeal airway (OPA)**, should the casualty subsequently regain consciousness, and is less easily dislodged during casualty transport. If the casualty needs a more advanced airway, the Combitube is the next recommended choice **FIGURE 1-4 ▶**.

In the domestic setting, the **endotracheal tube (ET)** traditionally is the gold standard for airway support; however, in combat, the ET has several disadvantages. Many combat med-

---

Field Medical Care TIPS

Soldiers with any altered level of consciousness should be disarmed immediately, to prevent unintentional discharge of weapons. The most common causes of altered mental status in combat are traumatic brain injury (open or closed), shock secondary to hypovolemia, pain caused by significant injuries, and pain medication.

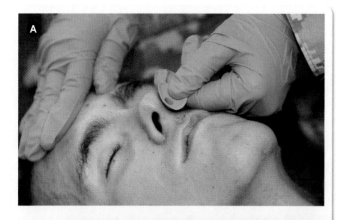

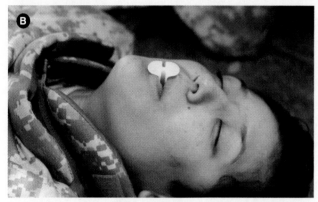

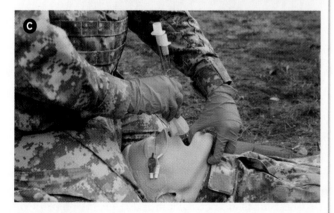

FIGURE 1-4 The airway of an unconscious casualty may be protected by a: **A.** nasopharyngeal airway, **B.** oropharyngeal airway, or **C.** Combitube.

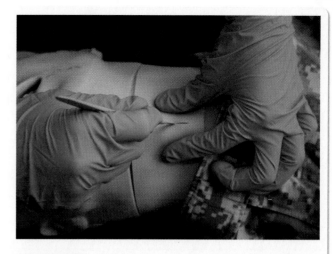

FIGURE 1-5 Make a vertical incision over the cricothyroid membrane to allow oxygen into the injured casualty's airway.

Field Medical Care TIPS

Supplemental oxygen is usually not available in the Tactical Field Care phase. Cylinders of compressed gas and the associated equipment for supplying the oxygen are too heavy to be feasible in the battlefield.

ics have never performed an endotracheal intubation on a live patient or even a cadaver. ET also entails the use of a white light on the battlefield, thus exposing you and the casualty to enemy fire. Finally, ET intubations are much less likely to be successful on the battlefield and may result in fatalities.

One study that examined first-time intubationists trained on manikins alone noted an initial success rate of only 42% in the ideal confines of the operating room with paralyzed patients. The Combitube is an effective airway designed for blind insertion. It is effective when placed in either the esophagus or the trachea. A study noted that it was successfully inserted 71% of the time for a first-line airway adjunct. That is why the Combitube is the gold standard for the battlefield.

If the casualty is unconscious and has an obstructed airway, and other airway techniques are not successful, you should perform a surgical **cricothyrotomy**. This may also be the airway of choice if maxillofacial injuries have disrupted the normal anatomy. This procedure has been reported safe and effective in trauma victims. Make a vertical incision over the **cricothyroid membrane** and insert an emergency catheter **FIGURE 1-5 ▲**. This opening allows oxygen into the casualty's airway.

Breathing

Attention should next be directed toward the casualty's breathing. If the casualty has a major traumatic defect of the chest wall, the wound should be covered with an occlusive bandage, such as a petrolatum gauze bandage and tape or an **emergency bandage** to hold it in place **FIGURE 1-6 ▶**. Soldiers with the **Improved First Aid Kit (IFAK)** can make an improvised occlusive bandage from the plastic wrapper on the emergency bandage **FIGURE 1-7 ▶**. Place the casualty in the sitting position. Apply an occlusive material to cover the defect and secure it in place on all four sides.

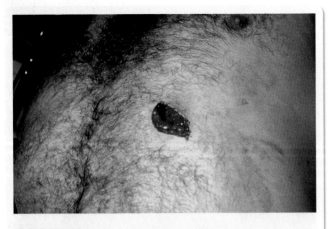

FIGURE 1-6   The classic sucking chest wound.

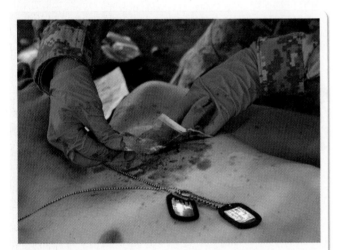

FIGURE 1-7   Soldiers with the IFAK can make an improvised occlusive bandage from the plastic wrapper on the emergency bandage.

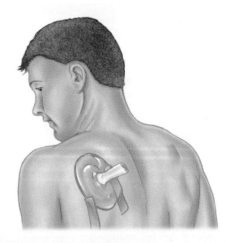

FIGURE 1-8   A casualty with an Asherman Chest Seal in place over his wound.

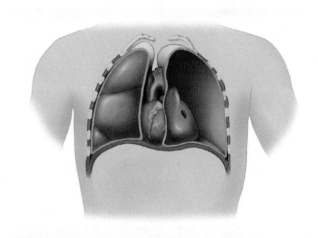

FIGURE 1-9   In a tension pneumothorax, air accumulates in the pleural space, eventually causing compression of the heart and great vessels.

An alternative is the **Asherman Chest Seal**, which has a one-way flutter valve that is appropriate for use with penetrating chest trauma   FIGURE 1-8 ▸ . Dry the chest wall completely of sweat and blood and apply **tincture of benzoin** to the area around the wound to assist the seal with sticking to the chest wall. If the casualty develops symptoms of a **tension pneumothorax**, it should be decompressed   FIGURE 1-9 ▸ . Chapter 5, *Injuries of the Thorax*, covers tension pneumothorax in detail.

Progressive respiratory distress, secondary to a unilateral penetrating chest trauma, should be considered to be a tension pneumothorax and decompressed with a 14-gauge needle. Chapter 5, *Injuries of the Thorax*, covers needle decompression in detail. The assessment in this setting should not rely on typical signs such as breath sounds, **tracheal shift**, and **hyperresonance** to percussion because these signs may not always be present. Even if they are, they may be exceedingly difficult to recognize on the battlefield. Any casualty with penetrating chest trauma will have some degree of **hemopneumothorax** as a result of the primary wound. The additional trauma caused by a **needle thoracostomy** is not

expected to worsen the casualty's condition if a tension pneumothorax is not present.

Chest tubes are not recommended in this phase of care because they are not needed to provide initial treatment for a tension pneumothorax. Also, chest tubes are more difficult and time consuming for inexperienced personnel to use, especially in the absence of adequate light. Chest tubes are more likely to cause additional tissue damage and subsequent infection than a less traumatic procedure. No documentation was found in the medical literature that demonstrates a benefit from tube thoracostomy performed by combat medics on the battlefield. Chest tube placement does not cause reinflation of the collapsed lung. In order for the lung to reinflate, you must have suction to create a negative pressure in the chest cavity or positive pressure ventilation to reinflate the lung from within.

Bleeding

Now address any significant bleeding sites not previously controlled. Only remove the absolute minimum of battle dress required to expose and treat injuries, because of both time constraints and the need to protect the casualty from environmental extremes.

As discussed previously, significant bleeding should be stopped as quickly as possible using a tourniquet. Once the tactical situation permits, consideration should be given to loosening the tourniquet and using direct pressure, a pressure dressing, or a hemostatic dressing to control any additional bleeding. Do not completely remove the tourniquet; just loosen it and leave in place.

If the tourniquet has been in place for more than 6 hours, then leave it alone. Tourniquets are very painful, so be prepared to manage your casualty's pain. If the casualty needs fluid resuscitation, do so before you loosen the tourniquet; also ensure there is a clinical response to the fluids. Do not periodically loosen the tourniquet to allow blood flow to the limb. This can be fatal. If you are unable to control bleeding with other means, retighten the tourniquet. Remember: it is better to sacrifice the limb than to allow the casualty to bleed to death.

If the bleeding does not stop or a tourniquet is not appropriate, use QuikClot Combat Gauze or WoundStat granules **FIGURE 1-10 ▾**. *Do not* apply these products near the casualty's eyes. Do not use these products on minor wounds. Use of these of these products for internal wounds is not yet recommended. After applying the product, you must apply pressure to the bleeding site for usually 2 to 8 minutes.

QuikClot Combat Gauze is applied as follows:

- Blot away excess blood, water, or dirt from the wound with a sterile gauze pad or the cleanest, driest product available.
- Tear open the QuikClot package.
- Place over or pack the dressing on the wound, which may require more than one QuikClot dressing.

- Apply direct, firm pressure to the wound using a sterile gauze bandage or the cleanest product available. Apply pressure for a minimum of 3 minutes or until the bleeding stops. Do not remove the QuikClot.
- Apply an absorbent dressing and a pressure bandage. If no pressure bandage is available, continue to apply direct pressure with your hands.
- Send the QuikClot packaging with the wound dressing to notify the medical team of its use.
- Note: Research is ongoing to evaluate the use of QuikClot for penetrating trauma; however, there are no current recommendations for this use.

WoundStat is applied as follows:

- Tear open the WoundStat pouch at the perforations.
- Empty the contents of the pouch (granules) directly into the wound.
- Firmly pack the WoundStat into all areas of the wound.
- Apply an absorbent dressing.
- Hold pressure for up to 3 minutes.
- If seepage occurs, perform additional packing of WoundStat.
- If bleeding continues, remove the bandage and add a second application.
- Place the WoundStat bag with the wound dressing to notify the medical team of its use.
- Hemostatic dressings should only be removed by qualified medical providers after evacuation to the next echelon of care.
- Note that new hemostatic agents are under study. The provider is responsible for knowledge related to each specific dressing. (Reference Arnaud F, et al. Comparative efficacy of granular and bagged formulas of the hemostatic agent QuikClot. *J Trauma* 2007;63(4):775–782.)

Intravenous Access

After controlling bleeding, intravenous access should be gained next. Chapter 13, *Intravenous Access*, covers this topic in complete detail. In the domestic setting, two large-bore

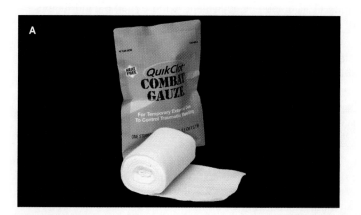
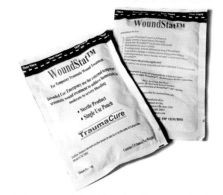

FIGURE 1-10   **A.** The QuikClot Combat Gauze can be packed directly into the wound like a gauze. **B.** WoundStat is applied directly into the wound.

(14- or 16-gauge) IVs are recommended, but the use of a single 18-gauge catheter is preferred on the battlefield because of the ease of starting. This also serves to ration supplies. Heparin or saline lock–type access tubing should be used unless the casualty needs immediate fluid resuscitation. Flushing the saline lock every 2 hours will usually suffice to keep it open without the need to use heparinized solution. Ensure that the IV is not started distal to a significant wound.

If you are unable to initiate a peripheral IV, consider starting a sternal **intraosseous (IO) infusion** to provide fluids. If you are unable to gain vascular access through a peripheral vein, there is an IO device available to gain access through the sternum. The FAST1 device is available and allows the puncture of the manubrium of the sternum and administration of fluids at rates similar to IVs. Chapter 12, *Battlefield Medications*, covers in detail how to perform an intraosseous infusion and how to perform the FAST1 procedure. Chapter 13, *Intravenous Access*, covers in detail how to initiate an IV.

Fluids

Chapter 13, *Intravenous Access*, covers the types of resuscitation fluids in detail. During the Tactical Field Care phase, the first consideration in selecting a resuscitation fluid is whether to use a crystalloid or colloid solution. **Crystalloids**

Algorithm for Fluid Resuscitation

Stethoscopes and blood pressure cuffs are rarely available or useful in the typically noisy and chaotic battlefield environment. A palpable radial pulse and normal mentation are adequate and tactically relevant resuscitation end points to either start or stop fluid resuscitation. Both can be adequately assessed in noisy and chaotic situations without mechanical devices. **TABLE 1-1 ▾** lists the treatment measures to take once you have assessed the casualty. Follow this algorithm for fluid resuscitation during the Tactical Field Care phase.

TABLE 1-1 Treatment Measures

Casualty's Condition	Treatment
Casualty has superficial wounds (> 50% injured)	No immediate IV fluids are needed; oral fluids should be encouraged.
Casualty is coherent and has a palpable radial pulse. • Significant extremity or truncal wound (neck, chest, abdomen, or pelvis) with or without obvious blood loss or hypotension.	Blood loss has likely stopped. Initiate a saline lock, hold fluids, and reevaluate as frequently as the situation allows.
Casualty is not coherent or has no radial pulse and there is significant blood loss from any wound. • Hypotensive casualty suffering from truncal injuries (lost a minimum of 1,500 mL of blood or 30% of circulating volume).	Stop the bleeding by whatever means available: tourniquet, direct pressure, hemostatic dressing, or hemostatic powder (QuikClot). After hemorrhage is controlled, start 500 mL of Hextend. If mental status improves and the radial pulse returns, maintain saline lock and hold fluids. If no response is seen, within 30 minutes give an additional 500 mL of Hextend and monitor vital signs. If no response is seen after 1,000 mL of Hextend, consider triaging supplies and giving attention to more salvageable casualties. (This amount is equivalent to more than 6 L of Ringer's lactate.)
Casualty has an uncontrolled hemorrhage (thoracic or intra-abdominal).	Requires rapid evacuation and surgical intervention. If this is not possible, determine the number of casualties versus the amount of available fluids. If supplies are limited or casualties are numerous, determine whether fluid resuscitation is recommended for this casualty.
Casualty is unconscious with a traumatic brain injury (TBI) and no peripheral pulse.	Resuscitate to restore the peripheral pulse.

Because of the need to conserve existing supplies, no casualty should receive more than 1,000 mL of Hextend. A number of studies involving uncontrolled hemorrhage models have clearly established that aggressive fluid resuscitation in the setting of unrepaired vascular injury is either of no benefit or results in an increase in blood loss and/or mortality when compared to no fluid resuscitation or hypotensive resuscitation. Several studies noted that only after uncontrolled hemorrhage was stopped did fluid resuscitation prove to be of benefit. You must stop the bleeding before you provide fluid resuscitation.

are fluids such as Ringer's lactate or normal saline, where sodium is the primary electrolyte. Sodium is needed to regulate the distribution of water throughout the body and is critical for cellular perfusion or balance. This fluid is often given to bring the body back into balance during shock. Because sodium eventually distributes throughout the entire extracellular space, most of the fluids in crystalloid solutions remain in the intravascular space for only a limited time.

<u>Colloids</u> (Hextend) solutions contain molecules (usually proteins) that are too large to pass out of the capillary membranes and therefore remain in the vascular compartment. Colloids draw fluid into the vascular compartments and work very well in reducing edema. These solutions are retained in the intravascular space for a much longer period than crystalloids. These fluids could cause dramatic fluid shifts and place the casualty in danger if they are not administered in a controlled manner.

Continuing the Tactical Field Care Phase

After ensuring that the casualty's airway, breathing, and circulation are stable, dress all wounds to prevent further contamination and help hemostasis. Emergency Trauma Dressings (HD/Israeli bandage) are ideal for this FIGURE 1-11 ▸ . Follow the manufacturer's instructions to apply Emergency Trauma Dressings to your casualty. Check for additional exit wounds because the high-velocity projectiles from modern assault rifles may tumble and take erratic courses when traveling through tissues, often leading to exit wound sites that are remote from the entry wound.

Only remove enough clothing to expose and treat wounds. Care must be taken to protect the casualty from hypothermia. Casualties who are hypovolemic become hypothermic quite rapidly if they are traveling in an evacuation asset and are not protected from the wind coming in the doors of the aircraft, regardless of the ambient temperature FIGURE 1-12 ▸ . Protect the casualty by wrapping him or her in a protective wrap like the Blizzard Rescue Wrap, which utilizes a cellular technology that traps air and allows the body heat to maintain body temperature. Ensure that the casualty's head is covered FIGURE 1-13 ▸ .

FIGURE 1-14 ▸ shows some new technologies to help keep casualties warm. When exposed to air, the Ready Heat

Blanket warms to between 110°F and 118°F and, in conjunction with the Blizzard Survival Blanket, provides excellent protection from hypothermia. This equipment should be applied before the casualty is transported to the MTF.

There are some field-expedient ways to warm IV fluids and to help prevent hypothermia. These methods help ensure the IV fluids have been prewarmed prior to administration. The use of heaters on either side of an IV bag or a blood box with a hole cut in it and a lightbulb to provide heat helps to warm IV fluids. This helps to prevent hypothermia from developing in casualties who have become hypovolemic; regardless of ambient temperature.

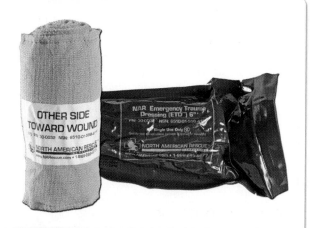

FIGURE 1-11 Emergency Trauma Dressings are ideal for quickly dressing wounds on the battlefield.

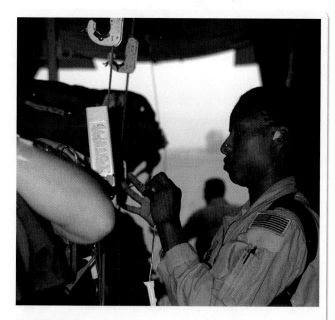

FIGURE 1-12 The open doors of the aircraft can cause hypothermia in casualties.

Monitoring

Pulse oximetry may be available to assist with clinical assessment of your casualty ▐ **FIGURE 1-15 ▶** ▐. However, these readings could be misleading with a casualty in shock or in severe hypothermia. Never solely rely on technology when monitoring your casualty. Use all of the assessment techniques available to you.

Pain Control

Pain control is the next step in the Tactical Field Care phase. Medication administration is covered in detail in Chapter 12, *Battlefield Medications*. If the casualty is able to fight, then administer 15 mg meloxicam (Mobic) orally initially with two 650-mg doses of acetaminophen (bi-layered Tylenol caplets) every 8 hours. Along with an antibiotic, this makes up the **Combat Pill Pack**.

If the casualty is unable to fight, administer by IV 5 mg of morphine every 10 minutes until adequate pain control is achieved. If a saline lock is used, it should be flushed with 5 mL of saline after the morphine administration. Ensure some visible indication of time and the amount of morphine given

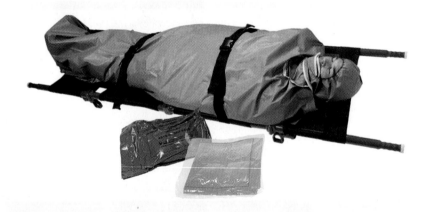

FIGURE 1-13 Ensure that the casualty is thoroughly protected from the elements.

Field Medical Care TIPS

Intranasal ketamine is being developed for noninjectable pain control.

---

and document on the casualty's **field medical card (FMC)** ▐ **FIGURE 1-16 ▶** ▐.

Combat medics who administer morphine should also be trained in its side effects and in the use of naloxone (Narcan). Naloxone is given in the event of severe side effects, particularly respiratory depression. Twenty-five milligrams of promethazine (Phenergan) may be given by IV or IM to combat the nausea and vomiting associated with morphine administration. Morphine administration is covered in detail in Chapter 12, *Battlefield Medications*.

Currently, pain relief can be attained by the use of fentanyl transmucosal lozenges. These sucker-like lozenges can be placed between the cheek and gum and are absorbed through the oral mucosa and swallowed. These lozenges provide pain relief similar to 10 mg of morphine. This method allows for narcotic pain relief to be delivered to casualties without the need for IV access ▐ **FIGURE 1-17 ▶** ▐. Administer one 400-mcg lozenge orally initially. Taping the lozenge stick to the casualty's finger is an added safety measure. Reassess the casualty's condition in 15 minutes. Add a second lozenge in the other cheek if necessary. Monitor the casualty for respiratory depression after administering this medication.

Antibiotics should be considered for all battlefield wounds because these wounds are prone to infection. Infection is a late cause of morbidity and mortality in wounds sustained on the battlefield. In soldiers who are awake and alert, 400 mg

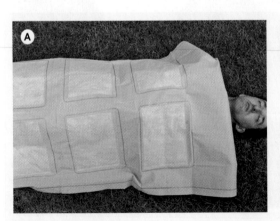
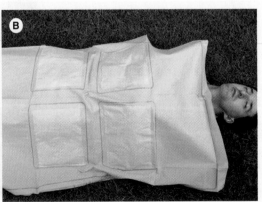
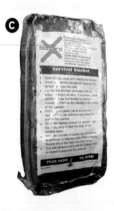

FIGURE 1-14 New technologies have been developed to keep casualties safe from hypothermia. **A.** The six-cell Ready Heat Blanket. **B.** The four-cell Ready Heat Blanket. **C.** The Blizzard Survival Blanket.

of moxifloxacin given orally every day is an acceptable regimen. Each soldier is issued this medication prior to deployment. In unconscious casualties, administer 2 g of cefotetan (Cefotan) by IV or IM, which may be repeated at 12-hour intervals until evacuation. An additional injectable antibiotic, Ertapenem (1 g), may be used IV or IM. The IV route may not be pushed; it must be administered over 30 minutes. When giving it IM, it must be mixed with 3.2 mL of 1% lidocaine and used within 1 hour. The administration of antibiotics is covered in detail in Chapter 12, *Battlefield Medications*.

Combat is a frightening experience, especially if wounded. Reassurance to the casualty can be simply telling them that you are there and are going to take care of them. This can be as effective as morphine in relieving anxiety. Also explain the care that you are providing.

Documentation

Documentation is a critical step in the Tactical Field Care phase. Document clinical assessments, treatment rendered, and changes in the casualty's status. This documentation should be forwarded with the casualty to the next level of care. If this form is not available, use 3″ white tape on the casualty's chest and a Sharpie pen to document care.

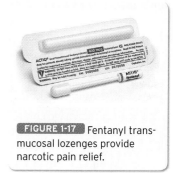

FIGURE 1-17 Fentanyl transmucosal lozenges provide narcotic pain relief.

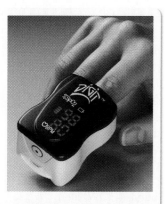

FIGURE 1-15 Pulse oximetry may be available as an adjunct to clinical monitoring.

	NECK/BACK INJURY	
	X BURN	
	AMPUTATION	
	STRESS	
	OTHER (Specify)	

4. LEVEL OF CONSCIOUSNESS

ALERT		**X** PAIN RESPONSE
VERBAL RESPONSE		UNRESPONSIVE

5. PULSE **100** TIME **1415** 6. TOURNIQUET **X** NO ☐ YES TIME

7. MORPHINE ☐ NO **X** YES DOSE **10 mg** TIME **1420** 8. IV **LR** TIME **1419**

9. TREATMENT/OBSERVATIONS/CURRENT MEDICATION/ALLERGIES/NBC (ANTIDOTE)

FIGURE 1-16 On the casualty's FMC, note the amount of morphine given.

■ Tactical Evacuation

At some point in the operation, the casualty will be evacuated; however, evacuation time may vary greatly, from minutes to hours to days. A multitude of factors affect the ability to evacuate a casualty, including availability of **evacuation assets** (aircraft or vehicles), weather, tactical situation, and mission.

The best arrangement in the evacuation asset is a two-person team composed of an aviation medic who is familiar with that particular airframe and a physician or physician's assistant with as much recent trauma or critical care experience as possible. Although there may be times when more than two people would be useful, two is the most reasonable number because of space constraints within the evacuation asset and a limited number of specialized medical personnel in the theater.

Only minor differences exist between the care provided in the Tactical Evacuation phase and the Tactical Field Care phase. Additional medical personnel may accompany the casualty and assist you on the ground. This may be important for the following reasons:

- You may be among the casualties.
- You may be dehydrated, hypothermic, or otherwise debilitated.
- The casualty's medical equipment may need to be prepared prior to evacuation.
- There may be multiple casualties that exceed your capability to care for them simultaneously.

Additional medical equipment can be brought with the evacuation asset to augment the equipment you already have. Oxygen should be available during this phase, thanks to the evacuation asset's ability to transport heavier pieces of medical equipment. Resupply may also be accomplished at this

Field Medical Care TIPS

For personnel with allergies to fluoroquinolones or cephalosporins, consider other broad-spectrum antibiotics in the planning (predeployment) phase.

Field Medical Care TIPS

Perform routine checks on your equipment. Blood pressure cuffs can dry rot in excessive heat. Dry rot causes the tubing to become cracked and inoperable.

time. In the evacuation asset, electronic monitoring systems capable of providing blood pressure, heart rate, pulse oximetry, and a **capnographer** are available and may be beneficial for air medical transport care. Thermal Angel fluid warming devices can help prepare IV fluids for casualties to prevent hypothermia. Finally, pneumatic antishock garments (PASGs) may be available to help stabilize pelvic fractures and can assist with hemorrhage control. All of these devices, while too large or heavy for you to carry, may easily be transported in the evacuation asset.

An IV rate of 250 mL per hour of Ringer's lactate for casualties not in shock helps to reverse mild dehydration and prepare the casualty for possible general anesthesia once arriving at the MTF. Ringer's lactate may be used for fluid resuscitation because there are no restrictions on weight in the Tactical Evacuation phase and sustained intravascular volume expansion is less critical. Administration of blood products may also be a possibility in some cases during this phase.

Combat Medical Aid Bag

It is critical that you become familiar with your medical equipment and aid bag as soon as you arrive to your unit. If you do not know where your equipment is in your combat medical aid bag, you will waste valuable time digging around and tossing items aside to locate what you are looking for.

Each body system has specific equipment associated with it. It is best to plan each combat medical aid bag around what equipment you will be carrying and devise a load plan around the equipment. All equipment must be inspected for cleanliness or sterility (if necessary), function, and contamination

prior to packing. **TABLE 1-2 ▸** lists the equipment placement for the combat medical aid bag.

Summary

Medical care during combat operations differs significantly from the care provided in the civilian community. New concepts in hemorrhage control, fluid resuscitation, analgesia, and antibiotic therapy are important steps in providing the best possible care for our combat soldiers. These timely interventions will be the mainstay in decreasing the number of combat fatalities on the battlefield.

During ground combat, casualties die from:
- Penetrating head trauma (31%)
- Surgically uncorrectable torso trauma (25%)
- Potentially correctable surgical trauma (10%)
- Exsanguination from extremity wounds (9%)
- Mutilating blast trauma (7%)
- Tension pneumothorax (5%)
- Airway problems (1%)
- The final 12% died of wounds (DOW) after evacuation to an MTF, mostly due to infections and complications of shock.

There are three categories of casualties on the battlefield:
- Soldiers who will do well regardless of what we do for them
- Soldiers who will die regardless of what we do for them
- Soldiers who will die if we do not do something for them now (7% to 15% of all casualties)

Remember the two actions that you can take to save lives:
- Stop bleeding by using a tourniquet.
- Relieve a tension pneumothorax.

TABLE 1-2 Combat Medical Aid Bag

Location	Equipment	Location	Equipment

Internal flap	• Two 14-gauge 3.25" needle/catheters
	• Two 28F nasopharyngeal airways with Surgilube packets
	• One penlight
	• One pair trauma shears/bandage scissors
	• Eight tongue depressors wrapped together with tape to use as an improvised tourniquet
		Main compartment	• Two SAM splints
			• One bag-valve-mask device for ventilation (when available)
			• Four intravenous kits—comprised of the following:
			  – One IV tubing set
			  – One 250-cc normal saline IV bag
			  – One Tegaderm dressing
			  – Two alcohol prep pads
			  – Two 18-gauge IV catheters
			  – One saline lock device
			  – Two constricting bands

Top left pocket	• Eight pairs properly fitting gloves	Left internal compartment	• Two 6" Ace wraps • Two 4" Ace wraps • Four Kerlix/compressed gauze • One 3" roll surgical tape • Four 6" emergency trauma bandages/dressings
Top right pocket	• Ten 2" x 2" sterile gauze • Ten alcohol prep pads • One roll 1" surgical tape		
Middle left pocket	• One vial 0.9% normal saline • Four 5-cc syringes • Two 18-gauge needles • Two 25-gauge needles • Two Surgilube packets	Right internal compartment	• Two Asherman Chest Seals • Two Vaseline/petrolatum gauze dressings • Eight muslin bandages (cravats) • Four sterile 4" x 4" gauze dressings • One 11" x 8" large abdominal dressing • Two 7" x 8" small abdominal dressings • One casualty blanket
Middle right pocket	• One blood pressure cuff with case		
Bottom large compartment	• One stethoscope • Pulse oximeter (if available) • Minor surgical set (if available)		

YOU ARE THE
COMBAT MEDIC

While on a routine foot patrol, your squad encounters a small convoy that has come under direct fire after striking an IED. After assisting the convoy to repel the enemy attack, the convoy commander calls out, "Medic!"

When you respond, the convoy commander leads you to a wounded soldier. The general impression indicates that the casualty is suffering from a chest wound and is bleeding from the right lower extremity. Your squad leader reports that you are tending to the only casualty and offers any assistance necessary. A combat lifesaver (CLS) from the convoy arrives to help you care for the wounded soldier. The situation is safe, the weather is clear, the closest medical treatment facility (MTF) is 25 miles from your location, and aero-medical evacuation is available.

Assessment

Upon evaluation of the casualty, you notice that he is lethargic with labored respirations, and his skin is cool, pale, and diaphoretic with a great deal of blood flow from the lower extremity. Further exam reveals a gunshot wound to the left upper chest, absent breath sounds on the left side, and tracheal deviation to the right side. The respiratory rate is 46 breaths/min and labored, and radial pulses are present but weak and thready. Exposure of the right lower extremity reveals a large amount of nonarterial bleeding.

Treatment

Treatment of this casualty follows the ABCs of care. The casualty has an open airway, but is suffering from a life-threatening breathing problem. You determine that this casualty warrants immediate evacuation and the squad leader calls in a 9-line MEDEVAC request while you care for the soldier. A tension pneumothorax is obvious and a needle decompression is indicated. After locating the correct space (second ICS along the MCL), you perform a chest decompression and notice an immediate improvement in the soldier's respiratory status. The CLS places a Combat Application Tourniquet (C-A-T) on the injured extremity and bleeding stops. While waiting to evacuate the patient, you establish a large-bore IV of Hespan and a large-bore saline lock.

Reassessment reveals a lethargic casualty with a respiratory rate of 28 breaths/min, nonlabored;

radial pulse of 110 beats/min and strong; and blood pressure of 96/44 mm Hg. The aeromedical asset arrives and assumes care for the casualty en route to the combat support hospital (CSH).

1. LAST NAME, FIRST NAME				RANK/GRADE	X	MALE
Smith, Taylor				PFC		FEMALE
SSN		SPECIALTY CODE			RELIGION	
000-111-1111		002			Baptist	

2. UNIT

FORCE					NATIONALITY	
A/T	AF/A	N/M	MC/M			
	BC/BC		NBI/BNC		DISEASE	PSYCH

3. INJURY		
		AIRWAY
FRONT BACK		HEAD
	X	WOUND
		NECK/BACK INJURY
		BURN
		AMPUTATION
		STRESS
		OTHER (Specify)

4. LEVEL OF CONSCIOUSNESS			
ALERT		PAIN RESPONSE	
VERBAL RESPONSE	X	UNRESPONSIVE	

5. PULSE	TIME	6. TOURNIQUET		TIME
110 bpm	1819	☐ NO ☒ YES		1807

7. MORPHINE		DOSE	TIME	8. IV	TIME
☒ NO ☐ YES				✓	1811

9. TREATMENT/OBSERVATIONS/CURRENT MEDICATION/ALLERGIES/NBC (ANTIDOTE)

GSW to the left upper chest. Absent breath sounds on left side, performed needle decompression. Condition improved. 28 breaths/min 96/44 mmHg

10. DISPOSITION		RETURNED TO DUTY	TIME
	X	EVACUATED	1825
		DECEASED	

11. PROVIDER/UNIT	DATE (YYMMDD)
Michaels, Louis	

Aid Kit

Ready for Review

- Caring for a casualty on the battlefield requires a different set of skills from those of a basic EMT. Factors such as enemy fire, medical equipment limitations, widely variable evacuation times, tactical considerations, and the unique problems encountered in transporting casualties must all be addressed.

- The TC-3 approach recognizes an important principle—performing the correct intervention at the correct time in the continuum of battlefield care. A medically correct intervention performed at the wrong time in combat may lead to further casualties.

- The best medicine on any battlefield is fire superiority.

- During the Tactical Field Care phase, you have more time to provide care and there is a reduced level of hazard from hostile fire.

- At some point in the operation, the casualty will be scheduled for evacuation; however, evacuation time may vary greatly, from minutes to hours to days.

Vital Vocabulary

Asherman Chest Seal A commercial occlusive bandage used to close open chest wounds.

battle buddy A soldier's fighting buddy.

capnographer Device that attaches in between the endotracheal tube and bag-valve-mask device; contains colorimetric paper, which should turn yellow during exhalation, indicating proper tube placement.

Care Under Fire Phase of care when the medic and casualty are under enemy fire.

colloids Solutions that contain proteins that are too large to pass out of the capillary membranes and therefore remain in the vascular compartment.

Combat Pill Pack Small pack of pain control medications and an antibiotic tablet that can be self-administered by the injured soldier.

Combitube Commercial supraglottic airway used to maintain a casualty's airway.

cricothyroid membrane A thin, superficial membrane located between the thyroid and cricoid cartilages that is relatively avascular and contains few nerves; the site for emergency surgical access to the airway.

cricothyrotomy Surgical procedure to provide an emergency airway by opening the cricothyroid membrane.

crystalloids Solutions of dissolved crystals (salt or sugar) in water.

emergency bandage Commercial bandage used as a pressure bandage to control hemorrhage.

emergency medical technician (EMT) An EMS professional who is trained and licensed by the state to provide emergency medical care in the field.

endotracheal tube (ET) A tube designed to be placed into the trachea for the purpose of airway management.

evacuation asset Usually either an air or a ground ambulance, but it may be a vehicle of opportunity to evacuate casualties to a medical treatment facility.

exsanguination Total blood loss leading to death.

field medical card (FMC) Form used to record medical information on patient care in the field.

hemopneumothorax An injury to the chest cavity causing blood and air to collect in the chest cavity.

hyperresonance A high-pitched sound heard when percussing the chest of a casualty with a tension pneumothorax.

Improved First Aid Kit (IFAK) New first aid kit carried by every soldier in the Army.

intraosseous (IO) infusion A technique of administering fluids, blood and blood products, and medications into the intraosseous space of a long bone.

medical treatment facility (MTF) A medical facility used for treatment of casualties; varies in size from a battalion aid station to a combat support hospital.

nasopharyngeal airway (NPA) An airway adjunct inserted into the nostril of a casualty who is not able to maintain a viable airway.

needle thoracostomy The introduction of a needle catheter unit into the chest cavity to remove air under pressure.

oropharyngeal airway (OPA) An airway adjunct inserted into the mouth to keep the tongue from blocking the upper airway.

Tactical Combat Casualty Care (TC-3) Principles of care used when providing care to casualties in a tactical or combat environment.

Tactical Evacuation Phase of care when the casualty is being evacuated.

Tactical Field Care Phase of care that begins when the casualty and combat medic are no longer under hostile fire; the phase when most medical care is provided.

tension pneumothorax Accumulation of air under pressure in the chest cavity, usually secondary to a penetrating chest wound; can be rapidly fatal if not treated.

tincture of benzoin A liquid that, when applied to skin, becomes very sticky and helps hold bandages and dressings in place.

tracheal shift A deviation of the trachea from its normal anatomic position; usually associated with tension pneumothorax.

COMBAT MEDIC in Action

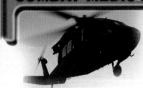

While providing medical support on a medium-sized convoy, the lead vehicle comes under attack. After a short firefight the scene is now safe to perform medical treatment. The weather is clear and the temperature is warm. While approaching the lead vehicle you notice that three occupants have been ejected. The convoy commander states that only three soldiers were in the vehicle. Upon assessment of the scene, you notice that Casualty 1 has severe second- and third-degree burns to the face and chest. Casualty 2 has an open fracture to the right humerus. Casualty 3 has a small-caliber gunshot wound to the abdomen.

1. Which casualty is the most critical based on what you have assessed so far?
   A. Casualty 1
   B. Casualty 2
   C. Casualty 3

2. The CSH is approximately 15 minutes from your location by ground; it will take a MEDEVAC aircraft 30 minutes to reach your location. How will you choose to evacuate the casualties?
   A. Wait on scene for the helicopter.
   B. Load the casualties onto a vehicle and evacuate by ground.
   C. Wait for the CSH to send assistance.
   D. Evacuate the casualties to a battalion aid station 30 minutes from your present location.

3. Casualty 2 is complaining of severe pain secondary to her open fracture. After splinting the injury, you obtain a set of vital signs: blood pressure is 126/78 mm Hg; pulse is 126 beats/min, strong and regular; and respirations are 22 breaths/min nonlabored. Would you give this casualty pain medication?
   A. No, the patient will be going into surgery and can have no medication.
   B. Yes, supply the patient with a fentanyl lozenge attached to a tongue depressor, allowing the patient to self-medicate.
   C. Yes, administer medication for pain relief.
   D. No, it is only a short ride to the CSH.

4. During transport, Casualty 3 complains of severe shortness of breath. Upon evaluation, you notice that he is cool and diaphoretic with tracheal deviation to the left side. Lung sounds are absent on the right and an occlusive dressing was placed on the wound by a CLS. Upending a flap on the occlusive dressing provides no relief for the casualty. How would you care for this casualty?
   A. Do nothing, it is a short ride to the CSH.
   B. Keep venting the occlusive dressing.
   C. Perform a chest decompression on the right side.
   D. Perform a chest decompression on the left side.

5. Casualty 1 is unresponsive to all stimuli. How would you want to maintain the airway?
   A. Insert an oral airway and use a bag-valve-mask (BVM).
   B. Insert an endotracheal tube.
   C. Perform a surgical cricothyrotomy.
   D. Do nothing, it is a short ride to the CSH.

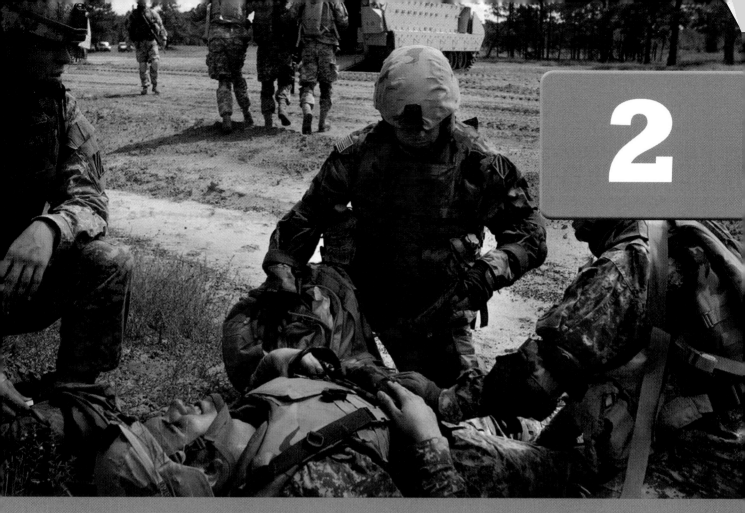

2

Casualty Assessment

Objectives

Knowledge Objectives

- [ ] Determine the threats in the area near the casualty during the situational assessment.
- [ ] Perform an initial casualty assessment.
- [ ] Identify immediate life-threatening injuries.
- [ ] Perform an additional casualty assessment.
- [ ] Obtain a SAMPLE history.

Skills Objectives

- [ ] Perform a situational assessment.
- [ ] Perform an initial assessment.
- [ ] Perform a rapid trauma survey.
- [ ] Perform an additional assessment on a casualty.

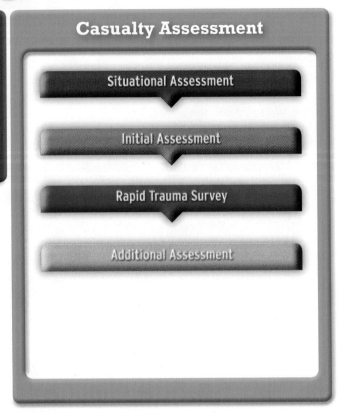

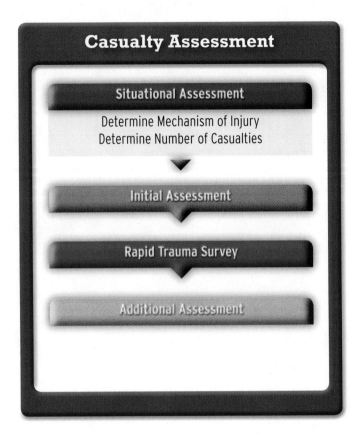

■ Introduction

On the battlefield, rapid systematic assessment of a casualty increases the likelihood that life-threatening injuries are identified and prioritized. If life-threatening injuries are identified during the assessment, lifesaving treatment and interventions can be initiated immediately.

This chapter provides a clear and comprehensive approach to casualty assessment. The chapter is divided into four sections. Every section is color coded and numbered for easy reference. The Casualty Assessment Flowchart, which provides a quick visual reference, is repeated at every section to show you at a glance where you are in the casualty assessment process.

Casualty Assessment

Casualty assessment is the cornerstone of battlefield care. The very basis of casualty care is centered on a solid, systematic approach to assessing the casualty. The casualty assessment process includes the following components:

- Perform a situational assessment.
- Perform an initial assessment.
- Perform a rapid trauma survey.
- Perform an additional assessment.

■ Situational Assessment

The combat medic **situational assessment** differs from the civilian scene size-up in that it centers around an awareness of the tactical situation and current hostilities in order to safely and effectively render care. You perform a situational assessment by examining the battlefield and determining zones of fire during engagement. You should determine routes of access to the casualty and egress with the casualty to ensure safety. Remember, additional casualties can occur at any time, and these additional casualties change the demands on your services and resources.

Body Substance Isolation

The best way to reduce your risk of exposure is to follow **body substance isolation (BSI)** precautions. The concept of BSI assumes that all body fluids present a possible risk for infection. Protective gloves are *always* indicated.

Scene Safety

Scene safety is focused on ensuring your safety, the casualties' safety, and your comrades' safety. If at any time the scene becomes unsafe, you must leave the area. You cannot help your casualty if you become injured. Situations can change and become threatening without being noticed once you concentrate your attention on casualty assessment and care.

Look for the following possible dangers in an area:

- Effective hostile fire
- No cover and concealment
- Leaking gasoline or diesel fuel

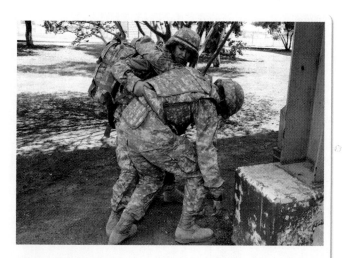

FIGURE 2-1 If the casualty can move, exit the area quickly, maintaining a low profile.

- Downed electrical lines
- Hostile bystanders with the potential for violence
- Fire or smoke
- Possible hazardous or toxic materials
- Secondary incendiary devices at an improvised explosive device (IED) site

During the scene safety assessment, consider care under fire. Anticipate the care you will offer at the casualty's side and what effect the care being given will have on drawing fire, such as movement, noise, or light. Determine what care is best offered at the casualty's side and what is best given after movement to safety. Do not offer extensive assessment and care until you can move the casualty to cover or at least concealment.

As you enter a fire zone, recognize hazards, seek cover and concealment, and carefully scan the area for potential dangers:

- Survey the area for small arms fire.
- Review the area for fire or explosive devices.
- Determine whether there is a threat from chemical or biological agents.
- Survey the building's structure for stability.

Remove the casualty to a safe area, if necessary, prior to assessment or treatment. Getting the casualty to cover (or concealment) may entail moving the casualty. Tell the casualty to move as quickly as possible to cover while maintaining a low profile **FIGURE 2-1 ▲**. If the casualty is unable to move, you may need to assist him or her using manual evacuation. The risk in moving the casualty is the possibility of aggravating existing injuries, but the benefit of protection outweighs the risk.

You should never hesitate to move a casualty who is exposed to fire. Each situation is different. You must evaluate the pros and cons of movement. If the casualty is not currently receiving fire and a c-spine injury is likely, you may elect to delay movement until it can be done safely. Ideally, choose a technique that is least likely to aggravate the casualty's injuries.

Request covering fire to reduce the risk to you and the casualty during movement to and from the casualty's location. Be sure that the location you are moving to can provide optimum cover and concealment. Plan your evacuation route prior to exposing yourself to hostile fire.

Consider the limitations a nuclear, biologic, and chemical (NBC) environment might place on your ability to effectively care for a casualty. For example, during a chemical attack, you may not be able to remove the casualty's chemical, biological, radiological, nuclear, explosive (CBRNE) gear due to the risk of life-threatening contamination. Any wounds or injuries will need to remain hidden beneath the gear until you and the casualty can be evacuated and decontaminated.

Determine the Mechanism of Injury

The **mechanism of injury (MOI)** is how the casualty became injured. Determining the MOI will help you find hidden injuries and should be your first clue of a potentially critically injured casualty. With a traumatic injury, the body has been exposed to some force or energy that has resulted in a temporary injury, permanent damage, or even death. You can learn a great deal about that force by simply determining the MOI.

Our body is structured to be protected, but certain areas of the body are more easily injured than others. Although protected by the skull, the vertebrae, and several layers of soft tissues, the brain and the spinal cord are easy to injure. Even small insults to the eye may result in serious injury. Body armor and eye protection are designed to assist in this protection. The bones and certain organs are stronger and can absorb small insults without sustaining serious injury.

Three factors can be used to determine the MOI as a guideline to predicting the potential for a serious injury: the amount of force, the length of time the force was applied, and the areas of the body insulted. Also keep in mind two principles of physics. The first principle states that force travels in a straight line until acted on by an outside force. The outside force takes the form of automobiles, the ground, or even body organs impacting internal body structures. It's not the fall that hurts . . . it's the sudden stop. The second principle of physics states that energy cannot be created or destroyed but can change form. When force or energy comes into contact with the body, it continues until it is forced to deviate. In other words, energy impacts a body structure. It is at that point that energy translates into bodily injury such as fractures or injury to internal organs.

On the battlefield, the most common mechanisms of injury are:

- Burns
- Ballistics
- Falls
- NBC weapons
- Blasts

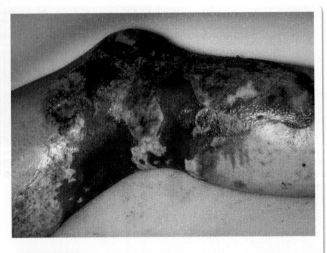

FIGURE 2-2 Burns are most often caused by explosions.

Burns

On the battlefield, burns are most often caused by explosions **FIGURE 2-2 ▲**. The casualty may also have been thrown some distance from the original spot of the incident. The casualty may have associated internal injuries, fractures, or spinal injuries as well as external burns.

Ballistic Injuries

Ballistic injuries are covered in detail in Chapter 11, *Ballistic and Blast Injuries*. Ballistic injuries present most commonly as entrance and exit wounds **FIGURE 2-3 ▼**. These injuries can also include embolisms, fractures, lacerations, and perforations.

Falls

In falls, the amount of force that is applied to the body depends on the distance fallen, the type of surface the casualty lands on, and the area of the body that impacts first. Any casualty who has fallen more than three times his or her own height should be considered at risk for multiple injuries.

Nuclear, Biologic, and Chemical (NBC) Weapons

Nonconventional incidents are covered in depth in Chapters 31 to 34. Your first priority is your own safety. Ensure that you are wearing all CBRNE gear before performing a situational assessment. In addition to the specific injuries that nonconventional weapons will produce, the casualty may be suffering from blast injuries such as fractures and lacerations.

Blast Injuries

Blast injuries are covered in detail in Chapter 11, *Ballistic and Blast Injuries*. In addition to burns, the casualty may experience the following injuries after an explosion:

- Blast injury
- Cavitation
- Crush injury
- Embolism
- Fractures
- Lacerations
- Perforations

Determine the Number of Casualties

After determining the MOI, determine the number of casualties and request additional help, if available and if necessary. Information on the additional help available can be obtained from situational reports and evacuation requests. Determining the number of casualties is critical for your estimate of the need for additional resources and equipment.

The number of casualties determines how and where you treat. Keep in mind these considerations:

- Care of casualties under fire
- A mass casualty situation
- Management of time, equipment, and supplies for casualty treatment

Triage is the process of sorting casualties and is covered in detail in Chapter 14, *Triage*. Once triage has been accomplished, you can begin to establish treatment and transport priorities. Always call for additional resources as soon as possible. By nature, you are less likely to request help after

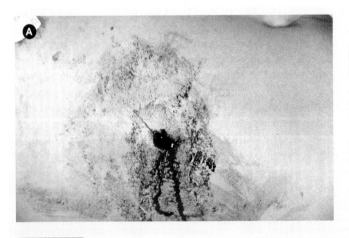
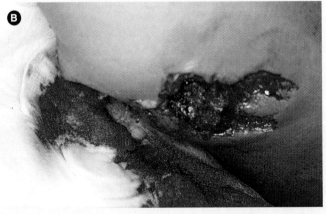

FIGURE 2-3 Ballistic injuries present most commonly as (**A**) entrance and (**B**) exit wounds.

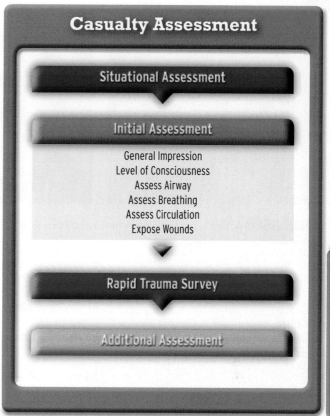

you begin casualty care, particularly if c-spine stabilization is required. Also consider whether any other equipment is needed (ie, airway adjuncts, oxygen, KED, etc.).

You should request assistance in movement and treatment prior to attempting to move the casualty. Direct **combat lifesavers (CLS)** to provide treatment. Combat lifesavers are nonmedical personnel organic to the unit, who have been trained in bandaging, splinting, and IV initiation. CLS can be utilized and directed once hostilities have ceased. Assign individuals to perform self-aid or buddy aid as needed.

Steps of a Complete Situational Assessment

To perform a complete situational assessment, follow the steps in **SKILL DRILL 2-1**:

1. Determine the BSI precautions that need to be taken.
2. Determine scene safety.
3. Determine the mechanism of injury.
4. Determine the casualty count.
5. Determine the need for additional personnel or resources.
6. Determine if any special equipment is needed.

■ Initial Assessment

The purpose of the initial assessment is to prioritize the casualty and to determine the existence of immediate life-threatening conditions. Do not interrupt the initial assessment except for airway obstruction or cardiac arrest.

General Impression

The general impression is important, because it helps you to determine the potential for life-threatening conditions. To help form a general impression, observe the position and appearance of the casualty. The casualty's posture can relay additional information about the MOI. The accessibility of the casualty is also a factor to consider at this point in the process.

When observing the appearance of the casualty, note the following items:

- Age, sex, and approximate weight
- Obvious major injuries
- Obvious major bleeding
- Apparent level of consciousness
- Emotional state
- Activity level
- If the casualty is a female, consider pregnancy

After making your observations, begin to establish priorities of care and establish c-spine control, if needed.

Level of Consciousness

Evaluating a casualty's mental status is important because it reflects the functioning of the brain. Mental status and level of

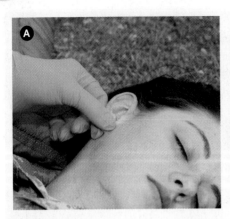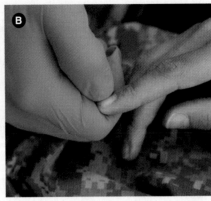

FIGURE 2-4 **A.** Gently but firmly pinch the casualty's earlobe. **B.** Gently but firmly press down on the casualty's fingernail beds.

consciousness can be evaluated in just a few seconds by using two tests: responsiveness and orientation. To test for **responsiveness**, assess how a casualty responds to external stimuli, including verbal stimuli (sound) and painful stimuli (touch, such as pinching the casualty's earlobe). Responsiveness can be evaluated by using the **AVPU scale**:

- **Alert:** The casualty's eyes open spontaneously as you approach, and the casualty is aware of and responsive to the environment. The casualty follows commands (such as squeezing your finger when told).
- **Responsive to verbal stimuli:** The casualty's eyes do not open spontaneously, but open to verbal stimuli, and the casualty is able to respond in some way when spoken to.
- **Responsive to pain:** The casualty does not respond to your questions but may respond to painful stimuli by moaning, pushing your hand away, or withdrawing from the pain. This response is tested by firmly pinching the casualty's earlobe and fingernail beds **FIGURE 2-4 ▲** .
- **Unresponsive:** The casualty does not respond to any stimuli.

For a casualty who is alert or responding to verbal stimuli, you should next evaluate orientation. **Orientation** tests assess mental status by checking the casualty's memory of person, place, time, and event. These questions evaluate long-term memory (name and place), intermediate-term memory (place and time), and short-term memory (event). If the casualty answers these questions appropriately, the casualty is alert and fully oriented. If a casualty is not able to answer one or more of your questions appropriately, the casualty is considered disoriented. Loss of intermediate- and long-term memory (person and place) is thought to be related to more severe problems than loss of short-term memory.

A casualty who is less than alert and fully oriented is considered to have an **altered mental status**. A level of consciousness less than fully alert requires a search for the cause during the rapid trauma survey.

Assess the Airway

If the casualty is unable to speak or is unconscious, evaluate the airway further. If you identify an airway problem, stop the assessment process and open the airway using the head tilt–chin lift or jaw thrust, as appropriate. The immediate assessment of the patency of a casualty's airway is paramount in an unresponsive casualty or one with a decreased level of consciousness. If it is open, continue your assessment. If the airway is not clear, use an appropriate method to clear it. Attempt to ventilate the casualty. If you are unsuccessful, reposition the head and attempt to ventilate again. Observe the casualty for obvious obstruction. Suction, if needed, using a suction machine or a bulb syringe. Consider foreign body airway management techniques.

Airway obstruction in an unresponsive casualty is most commonly due to relaxation of the tongue, which falls back and occludes the posterior pharynx; a nasopharyngeal or oropharyngeal airway can make the casualty's airway patent. If these do not open the casualty's airway, consider a Combi-tube, which will be discussed in detail in Chapter 3, *Airway Management*. The last treatment option is a needle cricothyrotomy, which is also discussed in detail in Chapter 3.

Assess Breathing

As you observe the casualty's breathing, use the look, listen, and feel technique to evaluate the adequacy of an unresponsive casualty's breathing. Also assess the amount of work it takes for the casualty to breathe. Shallow respirations can be identified by minimal and/or rapid rise and fall of the chest. Deep respirations can be observed as a larger expansion of the chest and at a slower rate. Does the casualty have to use accessory muscles to breathe? If so, this is a sign of labored breathing.

Assist with ventilation if inadequate breathing is present. Full and regular breaths indicate normal respiration. Labored, shallow, irregular, or absent breaths indicate abnormal respiration. Also note the rate and quality of the casualty's breathing.

If breathing is absent, then ventilate twice and check the casualty's pulse to determine whether CPR is required. Provide positive pressure ventilation at 12 to 15 breaths/min with 15 L/min of supplemental oxygen. If the casualty's breathing rate is greater than 12 breaths/min, then assist ventilation by bag-valve-mask (BVM) device at 12 to 15 breaths/min with 15 L/min of supplemental oxygen. If there is a low tidal volume, then assist ventilation by BVM at 12 to 15 breaths/min with 15 L/min of supplemental oxygen. If breathing is labored, give oxygen by nonrebreathing mask at 15 L/min. If breathing is normal or rapid, the casualty should receive supplemental high-flow oxygen.

In the battlefield, the ventilation rate is 12 to 15 breaths/min instead of 10 to 12 breaths/min. This is due to the casualty being without oxygen for an extended period of time.

The increase in ventilation rate also allows for mask leak that can average up to 40%.

Here are some specific treatment actions for certain airway sounds:

- **Snoring:** Perform a jaw thrust.
- **Gurgling:** Provide suction.
- **Stridor:** Consider a Combitube.
- **Silence:** Assess the airway for a foreign body obstruction.

Assess Circulation

Circulation is evaluated by assessing the presence and quality of the pulse, evaluating skin condition, and identifying external bleeding. Palpate the carotid and radial pulse. Also, reassess whether breathing is adequate enough to support oxygenation.

If the radial pulse is present, note the rate and the quality. If **bradycardia** is present, consider spinal shock or head injury. If **tachycardia** is present, attempt to calm the casualty to reduce the pulse rate and consider shock. If the radial pulse is absent, check the carotid pulse.

If the carotid pulse is present, note the rate and quality. If the pulse is less than 60 beats/min, consider spinal shock or head injury. If the pulse is greater than 120 beats/min, consider shock. If the carotid pulse is absent, provide CPR, BVM, and defibrillation as appropriate.

Remember, in a combat situation CPR is **METT-T** (mission, enemy, terrain, troops and equipment, time available) depending on personnel resources, supplies, and number of casualties. Only if METT-T allows and you have few or minimal casualties, enough time, and the assets needed, would you provide medical support to the expectant casualty and start CPR.

Next, assess the skin for color, condition, and temperature. Inspect the skin for:

- Cyanosis
- Diaphoresis
- Temperature
- Pallor
- Flush

If the casualty's skin is pale, cool, and clammy, consider shock. If cyanosis is present, reconsider inserting a Combitube and recheck oxygen, if applicable.

Next, assess for major bleeding. Controlling bleeding is covered in depth in Chapter 4, *Controlling Bleeding and Hypovolemic Shock*. If there is major bleeding, stop it by using:

- Direct pressure and elevation
- Pressure dressing
- Pressure points
- Tourniquet
- Pneumatic antishock garment (PASG)

Expose Wounds

Remove all equipment and clothing (except in an NBC environment or field of fire) from the area around the casualty's wounds. Identify any additional life-threatening injuries. In some instances, blood loss can be very rapid and can quickly result in shock and even death. Therefore, this step demands your immediate attention as soon as the casualty's airway is secured and breathing is stabilized. Signs of blood loss include active bleeding from wounds and/or evidence of bleeding such as blood on the clothes or near the casualty. When you evaluate an unresponsive casualty, perform a blood sweep by running your gloved hands from head to toe, pausing periodically to see whether your gloves are bloody.

The method you use to control external bleeding differs based on your tactical situation. Point of injury care involves the tourniquet initially; tactical field care involves the use of bandages and direct pressure, along with elevating the extremity if bleeding is from the arms or legs. When direct pressure and elevation are not successful, you may apply pressure directly over arterial pressure points. See Chapter 4, *Controlling Bleeding and Hypovolemic Shock*, for detailed information on controlling bleeding in a casualty.

Steps of the Initial Assessment

To perform a complete initial assessment, follow the steps in **SKILL DRILL 2-2 ▶**:

1. Determine whether c-spine immobilization is necessary (**Step 1**).
2. Obtain a general impression of the casualty (**Step 2**).
3. Assess the level of consciousness (**Step 3**).
4. Assess the airway (**Step 4**).
5. Assess the breathing rate and quality (**Step 5**).
6. Perform the appropriate airway and ventilation interventions (**Step 6**).
7. Assess the pulses (**Step 7**).
8. Assess the skin (**Step 8**).
9. Assess for bleeding (**Step 9**).

Initial Assessment

SKILL DRILL 2-2

Perform an Initial Assessment

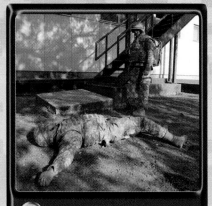

1 Determine whether c-spine immobilization is necessary.

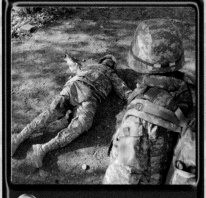

2 Obtain a general impression of the casualty.

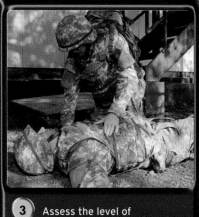

3 Assess the level of consciousness.

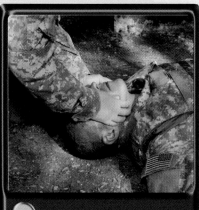

4 Assess the airway.

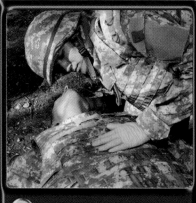

5 Assess the breathing rate and quality.

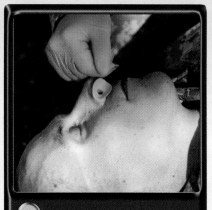

6 Perform the appropriate airway and ventilation interventions.

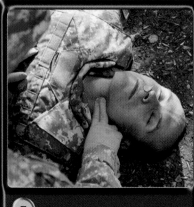

7 Assess the pulses.

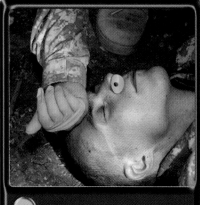

8 Assess the skin.

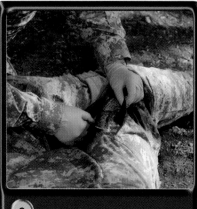

9 Assess for bleeding.

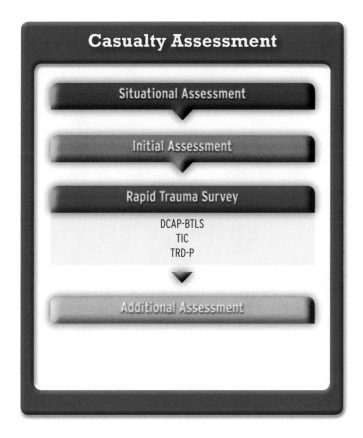

Casualty Assessment

Situational Assessment

↓

Initial Assessment

↓

Rapid Trauma Survey

DCAP-BTLS
TIC
TRD-P

↓

Additional Assessment

Field Medical Care **TIPS**

Always assume a spinal injury in any casualty who has a significant MOI. If mission allows, package up the casualty with regards to the potential spinal injury. Be sure to expose wounds and/or suspected areas of the casualty so you can completely assess and treat the casualty.

- Control major external bleeding.
- Seal sucking chest wounds.
- Stabilize flail chest.
- Decompress tension pneumothorax.
- Stabilize impaled objects.

The rapid trauma survey is used to find possible injuries to the body. The rapid trauma survey is indicated for any casualty with a significant MOI or abnormal findings in the initial assessment and for all unresponsive casualties. The general process is to do a rapid head to toe inspection and palpation of the entire body, looking and feeling for **DCAP-BTLS**:

- Deformities
- Contusions
- Abrasions
- Punctures/Penetrations
- Burns
- Tenderness
- Lacerations
- Swelling

■ Rapid Trauma Survey

The **rapid trauma survey** is a brief exam done to find all life-threatening injuries. A more thorough detailed exam follows later, if time permits. No splinting is done during the rapid trauma survey except for anatomically splinting the casualty to a backboard **FIGURE 2-5 ▾**. In fact, other than administering high-flow oxygen and providing spinal immobilization, only a few procedures are done on the battlefield:

- Provide initial airway management.
- Assist ventilation.
- Begin CPR if METT-T allows.

Head

Inspect the head for DCAP-BTLS, obvious hemorrhage, and major facial injuries. Look for abnormalities of the head. Palpate the head for deformities, tenderness, or crepitus. **Crepitus** is a grinding sensation that is often felt or heard when two ends of a broken bone rub together.

A more detailed exam of these areas should include a check of the head, face, scalp, ears, eyes, nose, and mouth for fluids, abrasions, lacerations, and contusions. Examine the eyes and eyelids, checking for swelling; nodules; discharge; and color of the lids, sclera, and conjunctiva (such as redness or jaundice). Use a penlight to check whether the pupils are equal and reactive to light. Also check for foreign objects and/or blood in the anterior chamber of the eye. Look for bruising or discoloration around the eyes (**raccoon eyes**) and behind the ears (**Battle's sign**); these signs may be associated with head trauma.

Look for swelling, fluid drainage, and crusting of secretions or blood around the ears and nose. Palpate the face, scalp, eyes, ears, and nose for

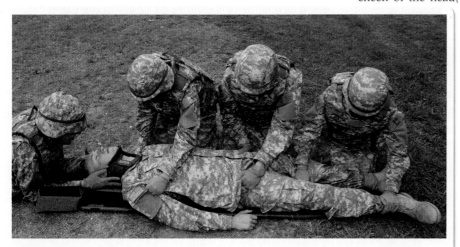

FIGURE 2-5 No splinting is done during the rapid trauma survey except for anatomically splinting the casualty to a backboard.

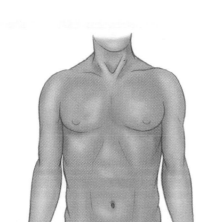

FIGURE 2-6 Retraction at the suprasternal notch on inspiration is an indication that you should reconsider other airway adjuncts.

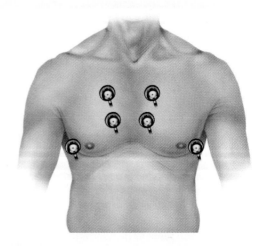

FIGURE 2-7 Auscultate only the bilateral apices at the midclavicular line and bilateral bases using midaxillary lines for presence and equality of breath sounds.

tenderness, altered sensation, deformity, and instability. Tenderness or abnormal movement of bones often signals a serious injury and may cause upper airway obstruction. Look and feel inside the mouth for loose or broken teeth or a foreign object because they may block the airway. You should also look for lacerations, swelling, and bleeding around and in the casualty's mouth. Note any discoloration in the mouth and the tongue such as pallor or cyanosis. Pallor suggests blood loss or hypoperfusion, and cyanosis suggests inadequate oxygenation.

Neck

Inspect the neck for DCAP-BTLS. Check the neck for signs of trauma, swelling, or bleeding. Feel the skin of the neck for air underneath the skin, known as **subcutaneous emphysema**, and for abnormal lumps or masses. Retraction at the **suprasternal notch** on inspiration, swelling, and bruising are indicators that you should reconsider other airway adjuncts **FIGURE 2-6 ▲**. Deviation of the trachea from the midline indicates that you should consider **tension pneumothorax**. Chapter 3, *Airway Management*, discusses the treatment of tension pneumothorax in detail. Jugular vein distension indicates that you should consider **cardiac tamponade** or tension pneumothorax. The use of accessory muscles during breathing is another indication that the casualty is not getting enough oxygen and needs assistance breathing.

Palpate the front and back of the neck for tenderness, instability, crepitus, and cervical spine step-off or deformity. Auscultate for air sounds in the trachea indicating stridor, gurgling, and snoring. After the examination of the neck, apply the cervical collar.

Chest

Inspect the chest for DCAP-BTLS. Check for paradoxical motion/flail chest and stabilize if indicated. Check for retraction of intercostal spaces. Palpate the chest for tenderness,

instability, and crepitus. Inspect the vertebrae and ribs for symmetry and tenderness. Look for abnormal breathing signs, including **retractions** (when the skin pulls in around the ribs during inspiration) or **paradoxical motion** (when one section falls on inspiration while the remainder of the chest rises). Perform an anterior-to-posterior compression of the thorax as well as a lateral-to-lateral compression of the thorax. Palpate the clavicles and the costochondral junction.

Auscultate the chest for lung and heart sounds. Auscultate only the bilateral apices at the midclavicular line and bilateral bases using midaxillary lines for presence and equality of breath sounds **FIGURE 2-7 ▲**. Absent or unequal breath sounds in the left or right bases of the lungs require percussion. Auscultate for heart sounds briefly at the lower left sternal border or apex for baseline heart sounds.

Next, percuss the chest for abnormal lung sounds. If you find dullness, this indicates fluid in the lung; however, no immediate interventions should be performed. Hyperresonance is the collection of air or gas in the pleural spaces causing the lung to collapse. It also can indicate pneumothorax. It may be the result of an open chest wound that permits the entrance of air or may occur spontaneously without apparent cause.

Tension pneumothorax must be considered if some or all of the following signs are present:

- Decreased or absent breath sounds
- Decreased level of consciousness
- Absent radial pulses
- Cyanosis
- Jugular vein distension
- Tracheal deviation from midline
- Decreasing bag compliance

With tension pneumothorax, the conservative management is oxygen, positive pressure ventilation, and rapid transport. The indications for performing emergency needle decompression are the presence of a tension pneumothorax with decompensation as evidenced by more than one of the following:

- Respiratory distress and cyanosis
- Loss of the radial pulse (late shock)
- Decreasing level of consciousness

Abdomen

Inspect the abdomen for DCAP-BTLS. Palpate the abdomen firmly for **tenderness, rigidity, distension, and pulsating masses (TRD-P)**. Visually inspect the abdomen for bruising or other discoloration, bleeding, swelling, masses, and **aortic pulsations**. Palpate all four quadrants, beginning with the quadrant that is farthest from any pain, if present. Use the terms "firm," "soft," "tender," or "distended" (swollen) to report your abdominal exam findings. If the·casualty is conscious and alert, ask him or her to describe the pain. Do not palpate obvious soft-tissue injuries, and be careful not to palpate too hard.

Pelvis

Inspect the pelvis for DCAP-BTLS. Abnormal signs include incontinence and **priapism**, an abnormal, continuing erection of the penis caused by spinal trauma. Signs of obvious injury, bleeding, or deformity indicate the need for rapid evacuation because injuries to the pelvis and abdomen may result in severe internal bleeding.

Palpate for **tenderness, instability, and crepitus (TIC)** by gently pushing down on the symphysis and gently pushing in on iliac crests. If the casualty denies pain, gently press inward and downward on the pelvic bones. Do not rock the pelvis because this motion may move an unstable spine. Use the heel of your hand to press down gently over the pubic symphysis to check for stability. If you feel any deformities or crepitus or the casualty reports pain or tenderness to palpation, there may be a severe injury. If the pelvis is unstable or is painful to palpation, do not log roll the casualty when placing him or her onto the backboard. Instead, use an orthopaedic (scoop) litter to place the casualty onto a backboard, if available; if no scoop litter is available, stabilize the pelvis manually during transfers.

Extremities

Examine the lower and then the upper extremities. Inspect the extremities for DCAP-BTLS. Look for lacerations, **ecchymosis**, swelling, obvious injuries, and bleeding. Ask the casualty about tenderness or pain. Palpate the extremities for TIC.

Assess the extremities for **pulse, motor function, and sensory function (PMS)** in each extremity:

- **Pulse:** Evaluate the pulse sites. Assess the dorsalis pedis pulse in the lower extremities. Assess the radial pulse in the upper extremities.
- **Motor function:** Assess the strength and gross motor skills in each extremity. Ask the alert casualty to wiggle fingers or toes. An inability to move a single

extremity can be the result of a bone, muscle, or nerve injury. Inability to move several extremities may be a sign of a brain abnormality or spinal cord injury. Verify that spinal precautions are in place.
- **Sensory function:** Assess for impaired sensation in each extremity. Evaluate normal feeling in the extremity by asking the casualty to close his or her eyes. Gently squeeze or pinch a finger or toe, and ask the casualty to identify what you are doing. The inability to feel sensation in an extremity may indicate a local nerve injury. The inability to feel in several extremities may be a sign of spinal cord injury. Recheck to be sure that you have begun and/or are maintaining spinal immobilization. Log roll and place the casualty on a backboard at this time. Pelvic instability or bilateral femur fractures indicate the use of a scoop litter when available.

Back

When placing the casualty onto a backboard, it is particularly important that you check the back as you log roll. Inspect for DCAP-BTLS, rectal bleeding, discoloration, or open wounds, and palpate for tenderness or deformity. Ensure that you keep the spine in line at all times as you log roll the patient onto his or her side. Carefully palpate the spine from the neck to the pelvis with the other hand, examining for tenderness or deformity, and look for obvious injuries, including bruising and bleeding. Palpate the thorax and lumbar areas for TIC or step-offs.

Steps for Rapid Trauma Assessment

To perform a complete rapid trauma assessment, follow the steps in **SKILL DRILL 2-3 ▶**:

1. Inspect and palpate the scalp and ears. Inspect the eyes. Inspect and palpate the face, nasal, and oral areas (**Step ①**).
2. Inspect and palpate the neck. Assess for tracheal deviation (**Step ②**).
3. Inspect the chest. Palpate the chest. Auscultate the chest (**Step ③**).
4. Assess the heart for baseline heart sounds (apex or left lower sternal border) (**Step ④**).
5. Inspect the abdomen. Palpate the abdomen (**Step ⑤**).
6. Inspect the pelvis. Palpate the pelvis (**Step ⑥**).
7. Inspect the lower extremities. Palpate the lower extremities. Check the pulses. Assess sensory and motor activity (**Step ⑦**).
8. Inspect the upper extremities. Palpate the upper extremities. Check the pulses. Assess sensation and motor activity (**Step ⑧**).
9. Inspect and palpate the thoracic spine. Inspect and palpate the lumbar spine (**Step ⑨**).

Perform a Rapid Trauma Survey

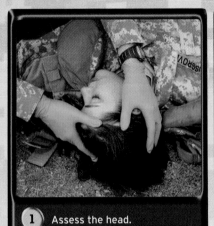

1 Assess the head.

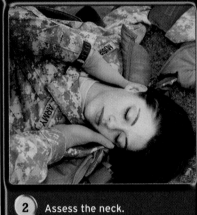

2 Assess the neck.

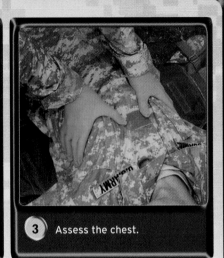

3 Assess the chest.

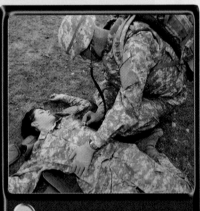

4 Assess the heart for baseline heart sounds.

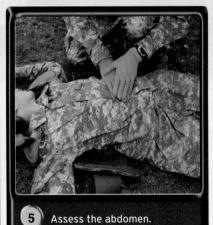

5 Assess the abdomen.

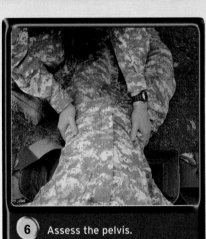

6 Assess the pelvis.

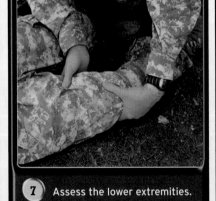

7 Assess the lower extremities.

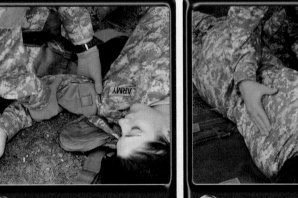

8 Assess the upper extremities.

9 Assess the back.

Rapid Trauma Survey

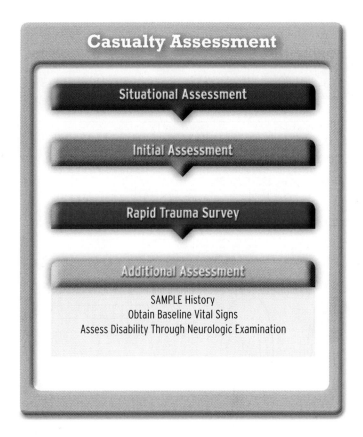

Casualty Assessment

Situational Assessment

Initial Assessment

Rapid Trauma Survey

Additional Assessment

SAMPLE History
Obtain Baseline Vital Signs
Assess Disability Through Neurologic Examination

■ Additional Assessment

After you have completed the rapid trauma assessment, it is time to obtain a **SAMPLE history**, obtain baseline vital signs, and assess for disability through a neurologic examination.

Obtain a SAMPLE History

Remember that the mnemonic SAMPLE includes the following elements:

- **Signs and symptoms:** A sign is objective, something you see, hear, feel, or smell when examining a casualty (eg, sweaty skin, gait changes, unequal pupils). A symptom is subjective, something the casualty tells you about (eg, chest pain, nausea, and dizziness).
- **Allergies:** Primarily to medications, but also environmental allergies. Check the casualty's ID tag to see if a red allergy tag is affixed.
- **Medications:** These include prescribed medications, over-the-counter medications, and recreational drug usage.
- **Past medical history:** Prior injuries/complications/ medical conditions.
- **Last oral intake:** The time and content of the most recent intake.
- **Events preceding the incident:** "What were you doing at the time of injury?"

Obtain Baseline Vital Signs

Obtain the baseline vital signs at this point. The baseline vital signs provide useful information about the overall functions of the casualty's heart and lungs. They also provide a starting point by which you begin to trend and monitor the casualty. **Trending** is the process of determining, following several sets of baseline vital signs, whether a severely injured casualty's condition has stabilized or is deteriorating.

Assess Disability

Do a brief neurologic examination if the casualty has any alterations in his or her mental status. Assess the **pupils for equality and reactivity to light (PERL)**. Determine a **Glasgow Coma Scale (GCS)** score. Assess the patient for signs of cerebral herniation:

- Unconsciousness
- Dilated pupils
- Bradycardia
- Body posturing
- Hypertension

Perform a Complete Additional Assessment

To perform a complete additional assessment, follow the steps in **SKILL DRILL 2-4**:

1. Obtain a SAMPLE history.
2. Obtain the baseline vital signs.
3. Assess disability, PERL, and GCS score. Assess for signs of herniation, unconsciousness, dilated pupils, posturing, or hypertension.

■ Summary

It is essential to assess casualties in a systematic way that allows for quickly finding and treating immediate threats to life. This search is called the casualty assessment. By forming a general assessment; determining mental status; evaluating airway, breathing, and circulation; and determining the casualty's priority, you can find and correct the problems that could otherwise end a casualty's life in just a few minutes.

YOU ARE THE
COMBAT MEDIC

While driving back from the combat support hospital (CSH), your vehicle encounters a group of soldiers who have been ambushed. Gunfire is still present. After a short while, air support arrives and neutralizes the threat. After a quick situational assessment of the area, you determine that there is one casualty who requires your assistance. The casualty was involved in refueling operations when the attack occurred, and was thrown 25′ secondary to an explosion that occurred during the sniper attack. The weather is clear and the nearest CSH or other higher level medical care is more than 60 miles away. Aeromedical assets are available.

Assessment

Upon initial assessment, the casualty is alert and very anxious, speaking in three- or four-word bursts, and in a great deal of pain. The casualty is suffering from second- and third-degree burns to the torso, face, and both upper extremities. Additionally, the impact of the explosion caused the casualty to suffer an open fracture to the right tibia/fibula region. There is no bleeding.

Treatment

After initial airway management, it is important to realize that prompt evacuation is necessary due to possible swelling from the facial and torso burns. If the airway becomes totally occluded, surgical cricothyrotomy may be necessary. The fueling site commander calls in a 9-line MEDEVAC request while you care for the casualty.

After the initial cooling of the site, a dry sterile dressing should be applied. Care should be given to manage the casualty's body temperature. Intravenous therapy should be initiated with Ringer's lactate with the largest bore possible. The casualty's vital signs support medication, so you should administer morphine sulfate via slow IV. Consideration should also be given to the administration of promethazine (Phenergan) to suppress nausea and vomiting. While awaiting the aeromedical evacuation assets, a combat lifesaver on scene applies a splint to the injured extremity. Reassessment reveals a less anxious casualty after receiving 10 mg of intravenous morphine. Vital signs are blood pressure 112/64 mm Hg; pulse 100 beats/min, strong and regular; and respiratory rate of 22 breaths/min, nonlabored. The casualty is loaded onto the aircraft and transported to the CSH for treatment.

1. LAST NAME, FIRST NAME		RANK/GRADE	X	MALE
Doe, John		2LT/01		FEMALE
SSN	SPECIALTY CODE		RELIGION	
000-000-0000			Bapt	

2. UNIT
553 Am Company 125 5/S BN

FORCE				NATIONALITY	
A/T	AF/A	N/M	MC/M	US	
	BC/BC		NBI/BNC	DISEASE	PSYCH

3. INJURY

					X	AIRWAY
						HEAD
FRONT			BACK			WOUND
						NECK/BACK INJURY
					X	BURN
						AMPUTATION
						STRESS
						OTHER (Specify)

4. LEVEL OF CONSCIOUSNESS

X	ALERT		PAIN RESPONSE
	VERBAL RESPONSE		UNRESPONSIVE

5. PULSE	TIME	6. TOURNIQUET		TIME
100	1515	X NO ☐ YES		

7. MORPHINE		DOSE	TIME	8. IV	TIME
☐ NO X YES		10 mg	1510	LR	1507

9. TREATMENT/OBSERVATIONS/CURRENT MEDICATION/ALLERGIES/NBC (ANTIDOTE)

2″/3″ burns over 40% BSA. Open Fx Ⓡ lower extremity. Clean dry dsg to burns. IV LR 18 g Ⓛ hand. 10 mg MS. Pain relieved. Splint to Ⓡ lower extremity. Evac to CSH by "Dustoff" 067.

10. DISPOSITION	RETURNED TO DUTY		TIME
	X EVACUATED		1530
	DECEASED		

11. PROVIDER/UNIT	DATE (YYMMDD)
Jl. Watts 68 W 3 ACR Med Trp	090610

Ready for Review

- On the battlefield, rapid systematic assessment of a casualty increases the likelihood that life-threatening injuries are identified and prioritized.

- The combat medic situational assessment differs from the civilian scene size-up in that it centers around an awareness of the tactical situation and current hostilities in order to safely and effectively render care.

- The purpose of the initial assessment is to prioritize the casualty and to determine the existence of immediate life-threatening conditions. Do not interrupt the initial assessment except for airway obstruction or cardiac arrest.

- The rapid trauma survey is a brief exam done to find all life-threatening injuries. A more thorough detailed exam follows later, if time permits.

- After you have completed the rapid trauma assessment, it is time to obtain a SAMPLE history, obtain baseline vital signs, and assess for disability through a neurologic examination.

Vital Vocabulary

altered mental status A change in the way a casualty thinks and behaves that may signal damage in the central nervous system.

aortic pulsations Pulsations of the aorta.

AVPU scale A method of assessing a casualty's level of consciousness by determining whether a casualty is Awake and alert, responsive to Verbal stimuli or Pain, or Unresponsive; used principally in the initial assessment.

Battle's sign Bruising behind an ear.

body substance isolation (BSI) An infection control concept and practice that assumes that all body fluids are potentially infectious.

bradycardia A slow heart rate, less than 60 beats/min.

cardiac tamponade A life-threatening state of cardiac compression that develops as a result of a large pericardial effusion.

combat lifesavers (CLS) Nonmedical personnel in the unit who have been trained in bandaging, splinting, and IV initiation.

crepitus A grating or grinding sensation caused by fractured bone ends or joints rubbing together; also air bubbles under the skin that produce a crackling sound or crinkly feeling.

DCAP-BTLS Mnemonic standing for Deformities, Contusions, Abrasions, Penetrations, Burns, Tenderness, Lacerations, and Swelling.

ecchymosis Bruising or discoloration associated with bleeding within or under the skin.

Glasgow Coma Scale (GCS) A widely accepted method of assessing level of consciousness that is based on three independent measurements: eye opening, verbal response, and motor response.

mechanism of injury (MOI) The way in which traumatic injuries occur; the forces that act on the body to cause damage.

METT-T Mnemonic standing for Mission, Enemy, Terrain, Troops and equipment, and Time available.

orientation The mental status of a casualty as measured by memory of casualty: name, place (current location), time (current year, month, and approximate date), and event (what happened).

paradoxical motion The motion of the chest wall that is detached in a flail chest; the motion is exactly the opposite of normal motion during breathing: in during inhalation, out during exhalation.

PMS Mnemonic standing for pulse, motor function, sensory function.

priapism An abnormal, continuing erection of the penis caused by spinal trauma.

pupils for equality and reactivity to light (PERL) An assessment tool which measures the casualty's level of consciousness.

raccoon eyes Bruising under the eyes that may indicate skull fracture.

rapid trauma survey A brief exam done to find all life-threatening injuries.

responsiveness The way in which a casualty responds to external stimuli, including verbal stimuli (sound), tactile stimuli (touch), and painful stimuli.

retractions Movements in which the skin pulls in around the ribs during inspiration.

SAMPLE history A key brief history of a casualty's condition to determine Signs and symptoms, Allergies, Medications, Pertinent past history, Last oral intake, and Events leading to injury.

situational assessment Centers around an awareness of the tactical situation and current hostilities in order to safely and effectively render care to the casualty.

subcutaneous emphysema The presence of air in soft tissues, causing a characteristic crackling sensation on palpation.

suprasternal notch Found on the neck, where the sternum and clavicle meet.

tachycardia A rapid heart rate, more than 100 beats/min.

tension pneumothorax An accumulation of air or gas in the pleural cavity that progressively increases the pressure in the chest, with potentially fatal results.

TIC Mnemonic standing for Tenderness, Instability, and Crepitus.

trending Process of determining, following several sets of baseline vital signs, whether a severely injured casualty's condition has stabilized or is deteriorating.

TRD-P Mnemonic standing for Tenderness, Rigidity, Distension, and Pulsating masses.

COMBAT MEDIC *in Action*

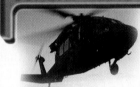

While sitting in line for Internet access, the garrison comes under mortar attack. After the attack is over, you begin to search for casualties. Your situational assessment reveals four casualties. Casualty 1 has an open fracture to the right tibia/fibula. Casualty 2 has some shrapnel embedded in his upper torso, but is alert and oriented without complaint at this time. Casualty 3 was standing by a fuel can. The can exploded and Casualty 3 has second- to third-degree burns to 95% of his body and is pulseless and apneic. Casualty 4 complains of ringing in her ears from the explosion.

1. Which casualty is the most urgent at this time?
   A. Casualty 1
   B. Casualty 2
   C. Casualty 3
   D. Casualty 4

2. Which casualty is least urgent at this time?
   A. Casualty 1
   B. Casualty 2
   C. Casualty 3
   D. Casualty 4

3. Aero-medical evacuation is not available. A ground ambulance will transport three casualties on litters. In which order will the three casualties be placed in the ambulance?
   A. 1,2,4
   B. 4,1,2
   C. 2,1,4
   D. 4,2,1

4. After the three casualties are loaded onto the ground ambulance and the ambulance has departed, the base commander discovers two additional casualties who were missed during the situational assessment. Casualty 1 has an obvious closed fracture to the left radius. Casualty 2 is lethargic, arousable only to pain, and has visible raccoon eye. Which casualty is more critical at this time?
   A. Casualty 1
   B. Casualty 2

5. Aero-medical evacuation is now available. How will you call for this assistance?
   A. Utilizing a 9-line MEDEVAC request
   B. Using a cell phone
   C. Sending a runner to the CSH

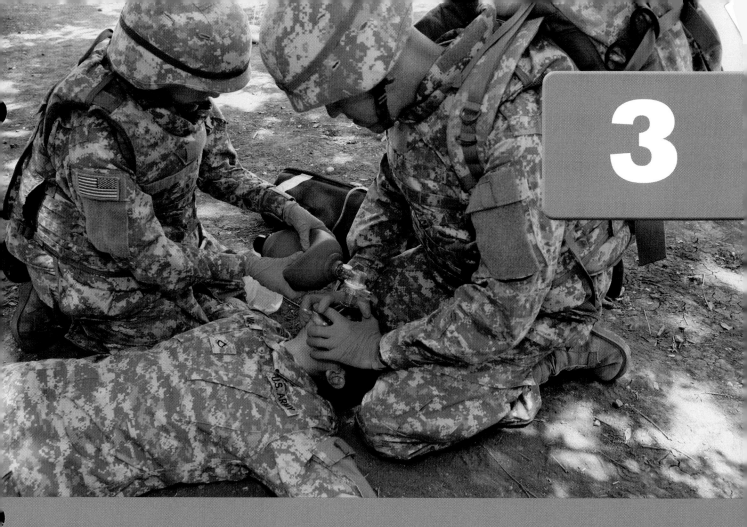

3

Airway Management

Objectives

Knowledge Objectives

- [ ] Describe the anatomy and physiology of the airway.
- [ ] Identify the signs of inadequate breathing.
- [ ] Identify the sources for airway obstruction.
- [ ] Differentiate between mild and severe airway obstruction.
- [ ] Identify the techniques for providing care to a casualty with an obstructed airway.
- [ ] Identify the indications for a nasopharyngeal airway adjunct.
- [ ] Identify the indications for an oropharyngeal airway (J tube) adjunct.
- [ ] Identify the indications for an emergency cricothyrotomy.
- [ ] Identify the indications for suctioning.

Skills Objectives

- [ ] Manage an airway obstruction.
- [ ] Perform the head tilt–chin lift maneuver.
- [ ] Perform the jaw-thrust maneuver.
- [ ] Insert a nasopharyngeal airway.
- [ ] Insert an oropharyngeal airway (J tube).
- [ ] Insert a Combitube.
- [ ] Insert a KING LT-D.
- [ ] Perform an emergency cricothyrotomy.
- [ ] Perform mouth-to-mask ventilation.
- [ ] Perform one-person bag-valve-mask device ventilation.
- [ ] Perform two-person bag-valve-mask device ventilation.
- [ ] Perform oropharyngeal and nasopharyngeal suctioning.

■ Introduction

One of the most critical skills you must have is airway management. Without proper airway management techniques and oxygen administration, your casualty may die needlessly. You must be able to choose and effectively use the proper equipment for administering oxygen. Establishment of a functional airway is your first priority in an emergency lifesaving trauma situation.

■ Respiratory System Anatomy and Physiology Review

Anatomy of the Upper Airway

The **upper airway** consists of all anatomic airway structures above the level of the vocal cords. Its major functions are to warm, filter, and humidify air as it enters the body through the nose and mouth. The first portion of the upper airway, the **pharynx** (throat), is a muscular tube that extends from the nose and mouth to the level of the esophagus and trachea. The pharynx is composed of the nasopharynx, oropharynx, and laryngopharynx (also called the hypopharynx). The laryngopharynx is the lowest portion of the pharynx; it opens into the larynx anteriorly and the esophagus posteriorly **FIGURE 3-1 ▾** .

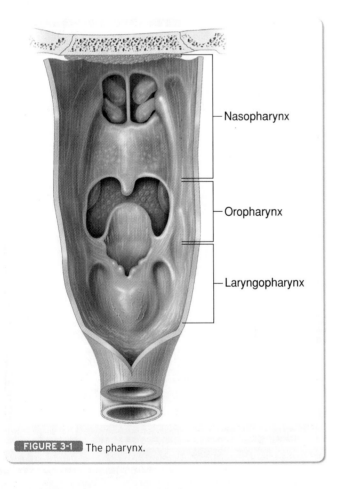

Nasopharynx

Oropharynx

Laryngopharynx

FIGURE 3-1 The pharynx.

Nasopharynx

On inhalation, air normally enters the body through the nose and passes into the **nasopharynx**, which is formed by the union of the facial bones. The orientation of the nasal floor is toward the ear, not the eye.

The entire nasal cavity is lined with a ciliated mucous membrane that keeps contaminants such as dust and other small particles out of the respiratory tract. In illness, the body produces additional mucus to trap potentially infectious agents. This mucous membrane is extremely delicate and has a rich blood supply. Any trauma to the nasal passages, such as improper or overly aggressive placement of airway devices, may result in profuse bleeding from the posterior nasal cavity. Bleeding from this area cannot be controlled by direct pressure.

Three bony shelves, called **turbinates**, protrude from the lateral walls of the nasal cavity and extend into the nasal passageway, parallel to the nasal floor. The turbinates serve to increase the surface area of the nasal mucosa, thereby improving the processes of warming, filtering, and humidification of inhaled air.

The nasopharynx is divided into two passages by the **nasal septum**, a rigid partition composed of bone and cartilage. Normally, the nasal septum is in the midline of the nose. In some people the septum may be deviated to one side or the other—a condition that becomes important when inserting a nasal airway.

The **sinuses** are cavities formed by the cranial bones. Fractures of these bones may cause cerebrospinal fluid (CSF) to leak from the nose or the ears. The sinuses prevent contaminants from entering the respiratory tract and act as tributaries for fluid to and from the eustachian tubes and tear ducts. When excessive bacteria enter the sinuses, for example, they may result in an infection.

Oropharynx

The **oropharynx** forms the bottom portion of the oral cavity, which is bordered by the hard and soft palates, the cheeks, and the tongue **FIGURE 3-2 ▸** . The 32 adult teeth are embedded in the gums so that significant force is required to dislodge them. However, trauma of lesser severity may result in fracture or avulsion of the teeth, potentially obstructing the upper airway or causing **aspiration** of tooth fragments into the lungs.

The tongue is a large muscle attached to the mandible and the **hyoid bone**—a small, horseshoe-shaped bone to which the jaw, tongue, epiglottis, and thyroid cartilage attach. The tongue is the most common cause of upper airway obstruction, especially in casualties with altered mental status.

The **palate** forms the roof of the mouth and separates the oropharynx and nasopharynx. The anterior portion is the hard palate and the posterior portion, beyond the teeth, is the soft palate. The **adenoids**, which are located on the posterior nasopharyngeal wall, are lymphatic tissue that filters bacteria. The **tonsils**, which are also made of lymphatic tissue, are located in the posterior pharynx and help to trap bacteria. The adenoids and tonsils often become swollen and infected;

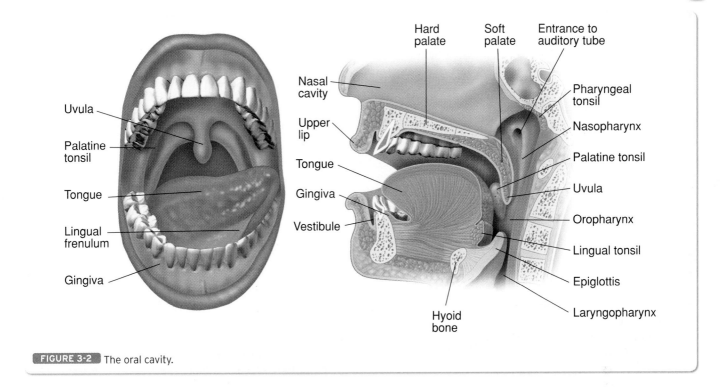

FIGURE 3-2 The oral cavity.

they may be surgically removed if they become chronically inflamed or are otherwise problematic.

The **uvula**, a soft-tissue structure that resembles a punching bag, is located in the posterior aspect of the oral cavity, at the base of the tongue.

The superior border of the glottic opening is the **epiglottis**. This leaf-shaped cartilaginous flap prevents food and liquid from entering the larynx during swallowing. When swallowing begins, the laryngeal muscles contract to cause downward movement of the epiglottis and upward movement of the glottis. Combined with closure of the vocal cords, these actions cover the glottic opening, preventing aspiration during eating or drinking.

The **vallecula** is an anatomic space, or "pocket," located between the base of the tongue and the epiglottis. It is an important landmark for endotracheal intubation.

Larynx

The **larynx** is a complex structure formed by many independent cartilaginous structures **FIGURE 3-3 ▸**. It marks where the upper airway ends and the lower airway begins.

The **thyroid cartilage**, the main supporting cartilage of the larynx, is a shield-shaped structure formed by two plates that join in a "V" shape anteriorly to form the laryngeal prominence known as the Adam's apple. The thyroid cartilage is suspended in place by the thyroid ligament and is directly anterior to the glottic opening.

The **cricoid cartilage**, or cricoid ring, lies inferiorly to the thyroid cartilage; it forms the lowest portion of the larynx. The cricoid cartilage is the first ring of the trachea and the only upper airway structure that forms a complete ring.

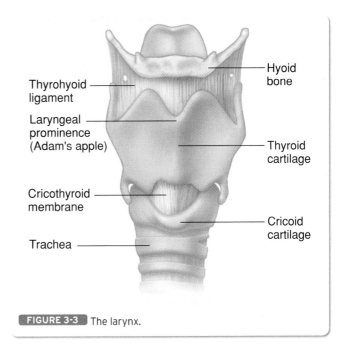

FIGURE 3-3 The larynx.

Between the thyroid and cricoid cartilages is the **cricothyroid membrane**. This thin, superficial membrane is relatively avascular and contains few nerves. The cricothyroid membrane is a site for emergency surgical and nonsurgical access to the airway (cricothyrotomy). Because it is bordered laterally and inferiorly by the highly vascular thyroid gland, you must locate the anatomic landmarks carefully when accessing the airway via this site.

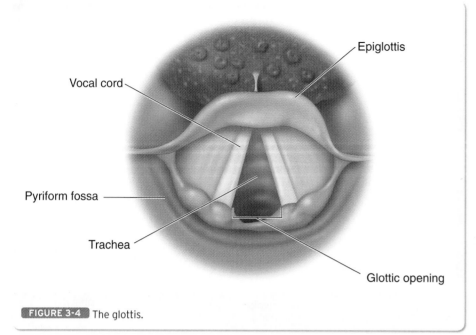

FIGURE 3-4 The glottis.

Other structures of the upper airway include the carotid arteries and jugular veins, the branches of which cross and lie closely alongside the trachea.

The **glottis**, also called the glottic opening, is the space in between the vocal cords and the narrowest portion of the adult's airway **FIGURE 3-4 ▲**. Airway patency in this area is heavily dependent on adequate muscle tone. The lateral borders of the glottis are the **vocal cords**. At rest, these white bands of tough tissue are partially separated (ie, the glottis is partially open). During forceful inhalation, the vocal cords open widely to provide minimum resistance to air flow.

The **arytenoid cartilages** are pyramid-like cartilaginous structures that form the posterior attachment of the vocal cords; they are valuable guides for endotracheal intubation. As the arytenoid cartilages pivot, the vocal cords open and close, which regulates the passage of air through the larynx and controls the production of sound; hence, the larynx is sometimes called the "voice box."

The **pyriform fossae** are two pockets of tissue on the lateral borders of the larynx. Airway devices are occasionally inadvertently inserted into these pockets, resulting in a tenting of the skin under the jaw.

When the airway is stimulated (eg, during aspiration of foreign material), defensive reflexes cause a **laryngospasm**—spasmodic closure of the vocal cords—which seals off the airway. This reflex normally lasts a few seconds. Persistent laryngospasm can threaten the airway by preventing ventilation altogether.

Anatomy of the Lower Airway

The function of the lower airway is to exchange oxygen and carbon dioxide. Externally, it extends from the fourth cervical vertebra to the xiphoid process. Internally, it spans the glottis to the pulmonary capillary membrane.

The **trachea**, or windpipe, is the conduit for all entry into the lungs. This tubular structure is approximately 10 to 12 cm in length and consists of a series of C-shaped cartilaginous rings. The trachea begins immediately below the cricoid cartilage and descends anteriorly down the midline of the neck and chest to the level of the fifth or sixth thoracic vertebra. It divides into the right and left mainstem bronchi at the level of the **carina**. These bronchi are lined with mucus-producing cells that, when stimulated, result in bronchodilation.

The right bronchus is somewhat shorter and straighter than the left bronchus. An endotracheal tube that is inserted too far will often come to lie in the right mainstem bronchus.

All of the blood vessels and the bronchi enter each lung at the **hilum**. The lungs consist of the entire mass of tissue that includes the smaller bronchi, bronchioles, and alveoli **FIGURE 3-5 ▶**. In total, the lungs can hold approximately 6 L of air.

The right lung has three lobes and the left lung has two lobes. These lobes are all made of parenchymal tissue. The lungs are covered with a thin, slippery outer lining called the **visceral pleura**. The **parietal pleura** lines the inside of the thoracic cavity. A small amount of fluid is found between the pleurae, which decreases friction during breathing. The **mediastinum** is the region between the lungs that contains the heart, great blood vessels, esophagus, trachea, and lymph nodes.

Upon entering the lungs, each bronchus divides into increasingly smaller bronchi, which in turn subdivide into **bronchioles**. The bronchioles, which are made of smooth muscle, dilate or constrict in response to various stimuli. The smaller bronchioles branch into alveolar ducts that end at the alveolar sacs.

The balloon-like clusters of single-layer air sacs known as **alveoli** are the functional site for the exchange of oxygen and carbon dioxide. This exchange occurs by simple diffusion between the alveoli and the pulmonary capillaries. Alveoli increase the surface area of the lungs. When they expand during deep inhalation, they become even thinner, facilitating diffusion.

The alveoli are lined with a proteinaceous substance called **surfactant**, which decreases surface tension on the alveolar walls and keeps them expanded. If the amount of pulmonary surfactant is decreased or the alveoli are not inflated, they will collapse.

Ventilation

Ventilation is the process of moving air into and out of the lungs. If a casualty is not breathing or is breathing inadequately, he or she no longer has an effective mechanism to intake oxygen and eliminate carbon dioxide. Ensuring adequate ventilation is one of the highest priorities in treating any casualty.

Ventilation consists of two phases:

- **Inspiration** (inhalation) is the process of moving air into the lungs.
- **Expiration** (exhalation) is the process of moving air out of the lungs.

The Mechanics of Ventilation

Ventilation is accomplished through pressure changes in the lungs, which in turn are brought about by contraction and relaxation of the intercostal muscles and diaphragm. The **diaphragm**, which is the major muscle of breathing, is the anatomic point of separation between the thoracic cavity and the abdominal cavity.

Inhalation is an active process that is initiated by contraction of the respiratory muscles. As the diaphragm contracts, it descends and flattens out, increasing the vertical dimensions of the thorax. At the same time, the intercostal muscles contract, causing the ribs and sternum to move upward and outward, increasing the horizontal dimensions of the chest cavity. The effect is to increase the volume of the chest. The lungs, being highly elastic and "glued" via the visceral pleura to the chest wall, undergo a comparable increase in volume. The air in the lungs now suddenly occupies a larger space, so the pressure within the lungs drops rapidly. As the air pressure inside the chest falls below that in the outside atmosphere, air begins to flow from the region of higher pressure (outside the body) to the region of lower pressure (the lungs)—a process called **negative-pressure ventilation**. When the pressures inside and outside the lungs are equalized, inhalation stops. Oxygen and carbon dioxide are then able to diffuse across the alveolar–capillary membrane in the lungs.

In contrast to inhalation, exhalation is a passive process. At the end of inhalation, the respiratory muscles relax. The natural elasticity (recoil) of the lungs passively exhales the air. **FIGURE 3-6 ▾** illustrates the processes of inhalation and exhalation.

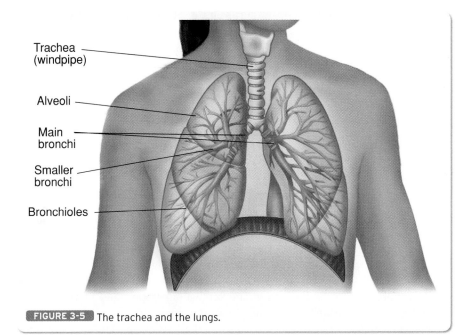

FIGURE 3-5 The trachea and the lungs.

- Trachea (windpipe)
- Alveoli
- Main bronchi
- Smaller bronchi
- Bronchioles

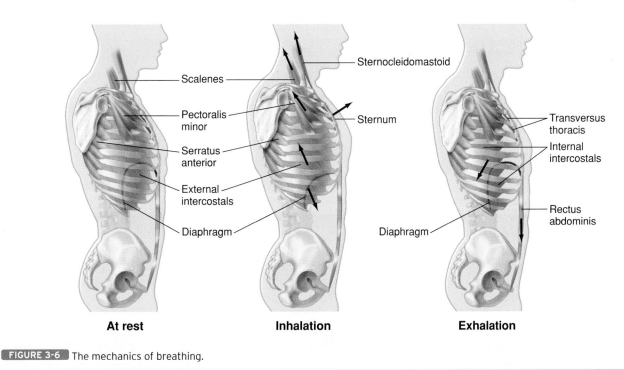

FIGURE 3-6 The mechanics of breathing.

At rest

Inhalation

Exhalation

- Scalenes
- Pectoralis minor
- Serratus anterior
- External intercostals
- Diaphragm
- Sternocleidomastoid
- Sternum
- Transversus thoracis
- Internal intercostals
- Rectus abdominis
- Diaphragm

Respiration

Respiration is defined as the exchange of gases between a living organism and its environment. The major gases of respiration are oxygen and carbon dioxide.

There are two types of respiration: external and internal. External (or pulmonary) respiration is the exchange of gases between the lungs and the blood cells in the pulmonary capillaries. Internal (or cellular) respiration is the exchange of gases between the blood cells and tissues.

The gas exchange during respiration occurs by a process of **diffusion**, in which a gas moves from an area of higher concentration to an area of lower concentration. Oxygen and carbon dioxide dissolve in water and pass through the alveolar membrane by diffusion.

Dissolved oxygen crosses the pulmonary capillary membrane and binds to the hemoglobin of the red blood cells. Without hemoglobin, there is no transport of oxygen. This is why replacing large amounts of lost blood with the standard intravenous fluids will be less effective in resuscitation. Isotonic crystalloid solutions lack the hemoglobin necessary for transport of oxygen. Approximately 97% of the total oxygen (O_2) is bound to hemoglobin; the remainder is dissolved in the plasma. A pulse oximeter reads the percentage of hemoglobin that is saturated, which is normally greater than 98% (SaO_2). The remaining oxygen that is dissolved in the plasma makes up the partial pressure of oxygen, also called the PaO_2 or PO_2.

Carbon dioxide (CO_2) is a by-product of cellular respiration. The majority of CO_2 is transported in the blood in the form of bicarbonate ions, with about 33% bound to the hemoglobin. As O_2 crosses from the alveoli into the blood, CO_2 diffuses from the blood into the alveoli. The CO_2 dissolved in the plasma makes up the partial pressure of CO_2, also called the $PaCO_2$ or PCO_2.

Carbon dioxide levels in the blood fluctuate in relation to changes in breathing. **Hypoventilation** causes carbon dioxide to build up because the slow respiratory rate does not allow for removal of enough carbon dioxide. Conversely, **hyperventilation** rids the body of excessive amounts of carbon dioxide. Because carbon dioxide adds to our total acid-base balance and our stimulus to breathe, it is imperative to closely control carbon dioxide levels in the blood.

The **total lung capacity** is the volume of gas contained in the lung at the end of maximal inhalation, about 4,000 to 6,000 cc. Although a small amount of gas exchange occurs in the alveolar ducts and terminal bronchioles, most of the gas exchange occurs in the alveoli. **Tidal volume** is the volume of gas inhaled or exhaled during the normal respiratory cycle, about 500 cc. **Dead air space** is the amount of air that remains in the upper air passages where it is unavailable for

TABLE 3-1 Respiratory Rates	
Adult	12–20/min
Child	20–40/min
Infant	> 40/min

gas exchanges, about 150 cc. **Alveolar air** is the amount of air that reaches the alveoli and participates in gas exchange with capillary blood, about 350 cc.

Respiratory Rates

The **respiratory rate** is the number of times a person breathes in 1 minute **TABLE 3-1 ▲**. The neural control of breathing originates in the brain and brain stem. Respirations increase or decrease based on the body's need at any given time. As body temperature rises, respirations increase in response to the increased metabolic activity. Certain medications cause the respiratory rate to increase or decrease, depending on their physiologic action. Pain and strong emotions can also increase respirations. **Hypoxia**, which is a powerful stimulus to breathe, increases respirations in an effort to bring in more oxygen. Respirations decrease as metabolism slows, such as during sleep.

■ Airway Management Review

The objective of airway maintenance is to immediately establish and maintain a **patent** (open) airway. First determine whether the casualty is breathing. Consider artificial ventilation to provide supplemental oxygenation. Ventilation skills are covered in detail later in this chapter. Recognizing the need for oxygen and ventilation support and properly establishing and maintaining an open airway are skills that are sometimes neglected on the battlefield. The casualty must have an open airway to survive.

Note any modified forms of respiration. Protective reflexes of the airway include coughing, sneezing, and gagging. Coughing is the forceful exhalation of a large volume of air from the lungs. Sneezing clears the nasopharynx and is often caused by an irritant, such as dust. The **gag reflex** is a spastic pharyngeal and esophageal reflex caused by a stimulus of the posterior pharynx to prevent foreign objects from entering the trachea.

Sighing, hiccupping, and grunting are other modified forms of respiration. Sighing is a slow, deep inspiration followed by a prolonged expiration. Sighing hyperinflates the lungs and re-expands the lung areas. The average person normally sighs about once per minute. Hiccupping is the intermittent spastic closure of the glottis and is caused by spasm of the diaphragm. Grunting is an indication of respiratory distress.

Inadequate ventilation is a reduction of either the rate or volume of inhalation. The casualty's respiratory rate may be rapid, but the depth of breathing is so shallow that little air exchange takes place. A state of decreased ventilation may be brought on by depressed respiratory function, fractured ribs, drug overdose, spinal injury, or head injury.

Hyperventilation is an increase in the number of respirations per minute above the normal range for a given age group.

Hypoventilation is a decrease in the number of respirations per minute that falls below the normal range for a given age group. **Compliance** is the ability of the lungs and chest wall to expand and contract in response to the application of force. For example, the chest wall and lungs of children may have a higher degree of compliance compared to those of an adult.

■ Assess for Airway Obstruction

The airway connects the body to the life-giving oxygen in the atmosphere. If it becomes obstructed, this lifeline is cut and the casualty dies—often within minutes. You must recognize the signs of an obstructed airway and immediately take corrective action.

Causes of Airway Obstruction

In an adult, sudden foreign body airway obstruction usually occurs during a meal. A significant number of people die from foreign body airway obstructions each year, often as the result of choking on a piece of food. A foreign body may cause a mild or severe airway obstruction, depending on the size of the object and its location in the airway. Signs may include choking, gagging, stridor, dyspnea, **aphonia** (inability to speak), and **dysphonia** (difficulty speaking). Treatment for the casualty depends on whether he or she is effectively moving air. Techniques for foreign body airway obstruction removal are covered in detail later in this chapter.

A multitude of other conditions can cause an airway obstruction, including the tongue, laryngeal edema, laryngeal spasm (laryngospasm), trauma, and aspiration. In the unconscious casualty, the jaw relaxes and the tongue tends to fall back against the posterior wall of the pharynx, closing off the airway. A casualty with mild obstruction from the tongue will have snoring respirations; a casualty whose airway is severely obstructed will have no respirations. Fortunately, obstruction of the airway by the tongue is simple to correct using a manual maneuver (eg, head tilt–chin lift, jaw-thrust).

With trauma inflicted during combat, the airway may be obstructed by loose teeth, facial bone fractures, tissue, clotted blood, or a neck wound. In addition, penetrating or blunt trauma may obstruct the airway by fracturing or displacing the larynx, allowing the vocal cords to collapse into the tracheal lumen. If an obstruction, such as teeth or vomitus, is allowed to enter the lungs, the result can be increased interstitial fluid and pulmonary edema in the casualty. The end result can be severe damage to the alveoli, thus causing hypoxemia. In addition to obstructing the airway, aspiration destroys delicate bronchiolar tissue, introduces pathogens into the lungs, and decreases the casualty's ability to ventilate (or be ventilated). Suction should be readily available for any casualty who is unable to maintain his or her own airway. Always assume that the casualty has a full stomach.

A laryngeal spasm (laryngospasm) results in spasmodic closure of the vocal cords, completely occluding the airway. The causes of laryngeal spasm include anaphylaxis; epiglottitis; inhalation of superheated air, smoke, or toxic substances; or aspiration. It is often caused by trauma during an overly aggressive intubation attempt or immediately upon **extubation**, especially when the casualty is semiconscious.

Laryngeal edema causes the glottic opening to become extremely narrow or totally closed. Conditions that commonly cause this problem include epiglottitis, anaphylaxis, or inhalation injury (eg, burns to the upper airway).

Airway obstructions caused by laryngeal spasm or edema may be relieved by aggressive ventilation to force air past the narrowed airway or a forceful upward pull of the jaw in an attempt to reposition the airway. In certain cases, muscle relaxant medications may be effective in relieving laryngeal spasm. Do not let your guard down after the laryngospasm appears to have resolved; resolution of the crisis does not mean that laryngospasm will not recur.

Airway patency depends on good muscle tone to keep the trachea open. Fracture of the larynx increases airway resistance by decreasing airway size secondary to decreased muscle tone, laryngeal edema, and ventilatory effort. Endotracheal intubation or other aggressive airway techniques may be required to maintain a patent airway.

Recognition of an Airway Obstruction

A foreign body lodged in the upper airway can cause a mild (partial) or severe (complete) airway obstruction. A rapid but careful assessment is required to determine the seriousness of the obstruction, because the differences in managing mild versus severe cases are significant.

A casualty with a mild airway obstruction is conscious and able to exchange air, but may show varying degrees of respiratory distress. The casualty will usually have noisy respirations and may be coughing. He or she may wheeze between coughs but does not become cyanotic. *Patients with a mild airway obstruction should be left alone! A forceful cough is the most effective means of dislodging the obstruction.* Attempts to manually remove the object could force it farther down into the airway and cause a severe obstruction. Closely monitor the casualty's condition and be prepared to intervene if you see signs of worsening airway obstruction.

A casualty with a severe airway obstruction typically experiences a sudden inability to breathe, talk, or cough—classically during a meal. The casualty may grasp at his or her throat (universal sign of choking), begin to turn cyanotic, and make frantic, exaggerated attempts to move air. Casualties with a severe airway obstruction have a weak, ineffective, or absent cough and are in marked respiratory distress; weak inspiratory stridor and cyanosis are often present.

Emergency Medical Care for Foreign Body Airway Obstruction

If the casualty with a suspected airway obstruction is conscious, ask, "Are you choking?" If the casualty nods "yes," begin treatment immediately. If the obstruction is not promptly cleared, the amount of oxygen in the blood will decrease dramatically, resulting in severe hypoxia and death.

Manage any unresponsive casualty as if he or she has a compromised airway. Open and maintain the airway with the appropriate manual maneuver, assess for breathing, and provide artificial ventilation if necessary.

If, after opening the airway, you are unable to ventilate the casualty (no chest rise and fall) or you feel resistance when ventilating (poor lung compliance), reopen the airway and again attempt to ventilate the casualty. **Lung compliance** is the ability of the alveoli to expand when air is drawn into the lungs during either negative-pressure ventilation or positive-pressure ventilation. Poor lung compliance is characterized by increased resistance during ventilation attempts.

If large pieces of vomitus, mucus, or blood clots are found in the airway, sweep them forward and out of the mouth with your gloved index finger. *Blind finger sweeps of the mouth are not recommended and may cause further harm; only attempt to remove foreign bodies that you can see and easily retrieve.* After the casualty's airway is open, insert your index finger down along the inside of the casualty's cheek and into his or her throat at the base of the tongue, then try to hook the foreign body to dislodge it and maneuver it into the mouth. Take care not to force the foreign body deeper into the airway. Do *not* blindly insert any object other than your finger into the casualty's mouth to remove a foreign body, because an instrument jammed into the throat can damage the delicate structures of the pharynx and compound the obstruction with hemorrhage. Suctioning should be used to clear the airway of secretions as needed. Suctioning is covered in detail later in this chapter.

The steps for managing an airway obstruction in a conscious casualty are listed here and shown in **SKILL DRILL 3-1 ▶**:

1. Determine whether the casualty is choking by asking, "Are you choking?" If the casualty nods "yes," then help is needed (**Step ①**).
2. Perform the Heimlich maneuver until the object is expelled or the casualty becomes unconscious.
3. Stand behind the casualty and wrap your arms around his or her waist. Use chest thrusts in place of abdominal thrusts if the casualty is pregnant or obese.
4. Place a fist thumb-side toward the abdomen, midway between the xiphisternal notch and navel (**Step ②**).
5. Grasp the properly positioned fist with your other hand and apply pressure inward and up toward the casualty's head. Deliver as many abdominal thrusts as needed until the object is expelled or the casualty becomes unconscious (**Step ③**).
6. For an unconscious casualty, place him or her in a supine position. Kneel and straddle the casualty at the thigh level, facing his or her chest. Deliver five abdominal thrusts (**Step ④**).
7. Perform finger sweeps and suctioning if necessary (**Step ⑤**).

The **Heimlich maneuver** (abdominal thrusts) is the most effective method of dislodging and forcing an object out of the airway. It aims to create an artificial cough by forcing residual air out of the casualty's lungs, thereby expelling the object. You should perform the Heimlich maneuver on any casualty with a severe airway obstruction until the obstructing object is expelled or until the casualty becomes unconscious. If the conscious casualty with a severe airway obstruction is in the advanced stages of pregnancy or is morbidly obese, perform chest thrusts instead of abdominal thrusts.

■ Establish an Airway

Perform Manual Maneuvers

Sometimes the simplest, most low-tech techniques are the fastest and most effective way to open a casualty's airway. In the unresponsive casualty, the most common cause of airway obstruction is the casualty's tongue **FIGURE 3-7 ▾**. To correct this problem, manually maneuver the patient's head to propel the tongue forward and open the airway. Techniques used to accomplish this include the head tilt–chin lift maneuver and the jaw-thrust maneuver.

Head Tilt–Chin Lift Maneuver

Opening the airway to relieve an obstruction can often be done quickly and easily by simply tilting the casualty's head back and lifting the chin. This **head tilt–chin lift maneuver** is the preferred technique for opening the airway of a casualty who has not sustained trauma. Occasionally, this simple maneuver is all that is required for the casualty to resume breathing. Following are some considerations when using the head tilt–chin lift maneuver:

- **Indications:** An unresponsive casualty, no mechanism for cervical spine injury, or unable to protect his or her own airway.
- **Contraindications:** A responsive casualty or a possible cervical spine injury.

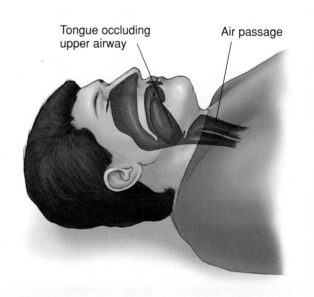

FIGURE 3-7 When the tongue falls back and occludes the posterior pharynx, it may obstruct the airway.

Tongue occluding upper airway

Air passage

SKILL DRILL 3-1

Managing an Airway Obstruction

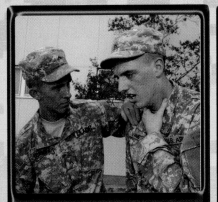

1 Determine whether the casualty is choking by asking, "Are you choking?" If the casualty nods "yes," then help is needed.

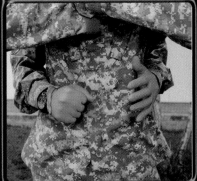

2 Stand behind the casualty and wrap your arms around his or her waist. Place a fist thumb-side toward the abdomen, midway between the xiphisternal notch and navel.

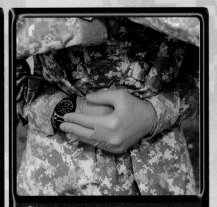

3 Grasp the properly positioned fist with your other hand and apply pressure inward and up towards the casualty's head. Deliver as many abdominal thrusts as needed until the object is expelled or the casualty becomes unconscious.

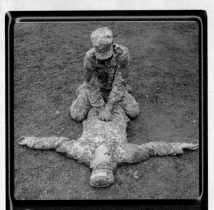

4 For an unconscious casualty, place him or her in a supine position. Kneel and straddle the casualty at the thigh level, facing his or her chest. Deliver five abdominal thrusts.

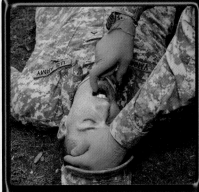

5 Perform finger sweeps and suctioning if necessary.

- **Advantages:** No equipment is required, and the technique is simple, safe, and noninvasive.
- **Disadvantages:** It is hazardous to casualties with spinal injury and does not protect from aspiration.

Perform the head tilt–chin lift maneuver in the following manner **SKILL DRILL 3-2 ▸**:

1. With the casualty in a supine position, position yourself beside the casualty's head (**Step ①**).

2. Place your hand that is closest to the casualty's head on his or her forehead (**Step ②**).

3. Place the tips of two fingers of your other hand under the lower jaw near the bony part of the chin (**Step ③**). Do not compress the soft tissue under the chin, because this may block the airway.

4. Simultaneously, apply backward and downward pressure to the casualty's forehead and lift the jaw straight up (**Step ④**). Do not use your thumb to lift the chin. Lift so that the teeth are nearly brought together, but avoid closing the mouth completely.

Jaw-Thrust Maneuver

If you suspect that the casualty has experienced a cervical spine injury, open the airway with the <u>jaw-thrust maneuver</u>. In this technique, you open the airway by placing your fingers behind the angle of the jaw and lifting the jaw forward. The jaw is displaced forward at the mandibular angle. You can easily seal a mask around the casualty's nose and mouth while performing this maneuver. Following are some considerations when using the jaw-thrust maneuver:

- **Indications:** An unconscious casualty, possible cervical spine injury, or unable to protect his or her own airway.
- **Contraindications:** Conscious casualty or resistance to opening the mouth.
- **Advantages:** May be used in a casualty with a cervical spine injury, may use with cervical collar in place, and does not require special equipment.
- **Disadvantages:** Cannot maintain if the casualty becomes conscious or combative, difficult to maintain

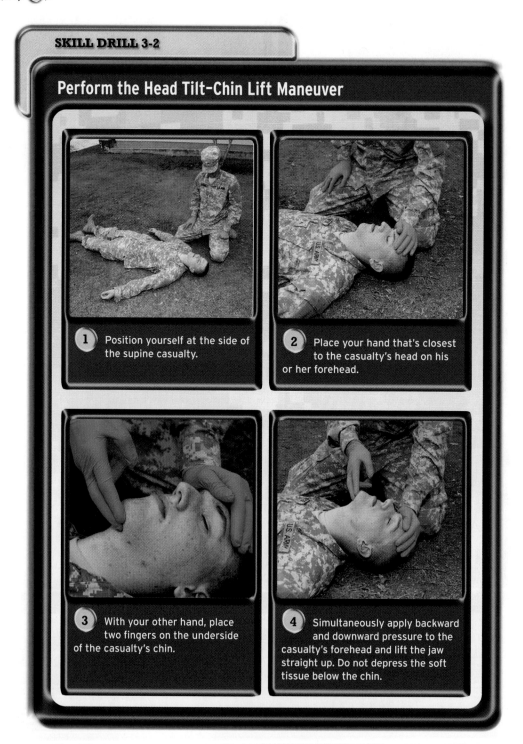

SKILL DRILL 3-2

Perform the Head Tilt-Chin Lift Maneuver

1 Position yourself at the side of the supine casualty.

2 Place your hand that's closest to the casualty's head on his or her forehead.

3 With your other hand, place two fingers on the underside of the casualty's chin.

4 Simultaneously apply backward and downward pressure to the casualty's forehead and lift the jaw straight up. Do not depress the soft tissue below the chin.

for an extended period of time, very difficult to use in conjunction with bag-valve-mask (BVM) ventilation, thumb must remain in place to maintain jaw displacement, requires second rescuer for BVM ventilation, and does not protect against aspiration.

Perform the jaw-thrust maneuver in the following manner **SKILL DRILL 3-3 ▼** :

1. Position yourself at the top of the casualty's head (**Step ①**).

2. Place the meaty portion of the base of your thumbs on the zygomatic arches and hook the tips of your index fingers under the angle of the mandible, in the indent below each ear (**Step ②**).

3. While holding the casualty's head in a neutral inline position, displace the jaw upward and open the casualty's mouth with the tips of your thumbs (**Step ③**).

Airway Adjuncts

If the casualty is semiconscious or unconscious, an artificial airway may be needed to help maintain an open air passage. *An artificial airway is not a substitute for proper head positioning.* Even after an airway adjunct has been inserted, the appropriate manual position of the head must be maintained.

Nasopharyngeal Airway

The **nasopharyngeal airway (NPA)** is a 6″ long, soft rubber tube that is inserted through the nose into the posterior pharynx behind the tongue, thereby allowing passage of air from the nose to the lower airway. The purpose of the NPA is to maintain an artificial airway for oxygen therapy or airway management when suctioning is necessary. The NPA is much better tolerated than an oral airway in conscious or semiconscious casualties who have an intact gag reflex **FIGURE 3-8 ▼** .

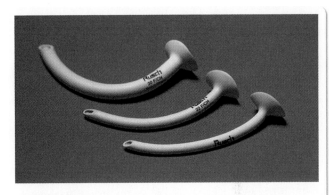

FIGURE 3-8 An NPA is better tolerated by casualties who have an intact gag reflex.

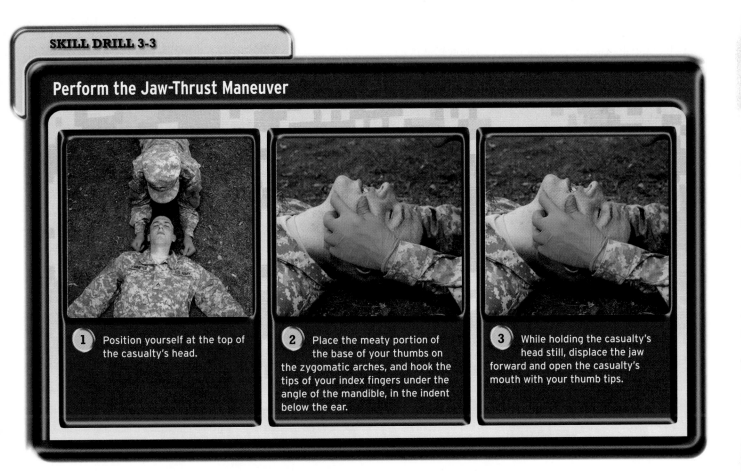

SKILL DRILL 3-3

Perform the Jaw-Thrust Maneuver

① Position yourself at the top of the casualty's head.

② Place the meaty portion of the base of your thumbs on the zygomatic arches, and hook the tips of your index fingers under the angle of the mandible, in the indent below the ear.

③ While holding the casualty's head still, displace the jaw forward and open the casualty's mouth with your thumb tips.

Do not use this device when the casualty has experienced trauma to the nose, you have reason to suspect a skull fracture (eg, cerebrospinal fluid [CSF] leaking from the nose), the roof of the mouth is fractured, or brain matter is exposed. Inserting the NPA in such cases may cause it to enter the brain through the hole caused by the fracture.

The nasopharyngeal airway must be inserted gently to avoid precipitating epistaxis (nosebleed). Lubricate the airway generously with a water-soluble jelly, preferably one that contains local anesthetic, and slide the NPA gently, tip downward, into one nostril. *Do not try to force it.* If you meet resistance, try to pass the airway down the other nostril. Following are considerations when using an NPA:

- **Indications:** Conscious or semiconscious casualty, casualty with an intact gag reflex, mouth injuries (broken teeth, massive oral tissue damage), seizure, casualty who may have clenched teeth due to seizing.
- **Contraindications:** Any evidence of head injury; roof of mouth fracture; exposed brain matter; CSF draining from nose, mouth, or ears.
- **Complications:** Minor tissue trauma (nosebleeds). This is not an indication to remove the airway. In some casualties, a nasal airway will trigger the gag reflex.

As an alternative, the proper size of the NPA can be determined by measuring from the tip of the nostril to the angle of the jaw rather than the earlobe. If the NPA is too long, it may obstruct the casualty's airway. If the casualty becomes intolerant of the NPA, gently remove it from the nasal passage. Although the NPA is not as likely to cause vomiting as the oropharyngeal airway, you should have suction readily available if possible.

Most nasopharyngeal airways are made to fit the right nostril. If you have to insert it into the left nostril, turn the airway upside down so that the bevel remains toward the septum. Then insert it straight back until you reach the posterior pharynx. Turn the NPA 180° until it lies behind the tongue. The steps for inserting an NPA are listed here and shown in **SKILL DRILL 3-4 ▶**:

1. Place the casualty on a firm surface in the supine position with the c-spine stabilized (**Step ①**).
2. Before inserting the NPA, make sure you have selected the proper size. Measure the distance from the tip of the nostril to the earlobe. In almost all individuals, one nostril is larger than the other. The diameter should be roughly equal to the casualty's little finger (**Step ②**).
3. After lubricating the NPA with a water-soluble gel, place the NPA in the larger nostril, with the curvature of the device following the curve of the floor of the nose and the bevel facing the septum (**Step ③**).
4. Place the bevel toward the septum and insert it gently along the nasal floor, parallel to the mouth. *Do not force the airway* (**Step ④**).

5. If resistance is met, do not continue. Stop, remove the NPA, relubricate, and try the other nostril. If resistance is still met, check for the proper size or use an alternate artificial airway method.
6. When completely inserted, the flange should rest against the nostril. The distal end of the airway will open into the posterior pharynx.
7. Administer oxygen therapy and ventilate the casualty at this time if necessary. Follow local protocol (**Step ⑤**).
8. To remove the NPA, pull out with a steady motion along the curvature of the nasal cavity (**Step ⑥**).

Oropharyngeal Airway

The **oropharyngeal airway (OPA)** (or J tube) is a curved, hard plastic device that fits over the back of the tongue with the tip in the posterior pharynx **FIGURE 3-9 ▾**. It is designed to hold the tongue away from the back of the throat, thereby preventing an airway obstruction in a casualty without a gag reflex. It also allows for drainage and/or suction of secretions, thereby preventing aspiration.

An OPA should be inserted promptly in an unresponsive casualty—breathing or not—who has no gag reflex. Because its distal end sits in the back of the throat, this device will stimulate gagging and retching in a conscious or semiconscious casualty. For that reason, the OPA should be used only in a deeply unconscious, unresponsive casualty without a gag reflex. To assess a casualty's gag reflex, use the **eyelash reflex**. If the casualty's lower eyelid contracts when you gently stroke the upper eyelashes, the casualty probably has an intact gag reflex. If the casualty gags during insertion of the OPA, remove the device immediately and be prepared to suction the oropharynx. Following are some considerations when using an OPA:

- **Indications:** Utilized for the unconscious casualty without a gag reflex.
- **Contraindications:** Conscious casualties, casualties with a gag reflex present.

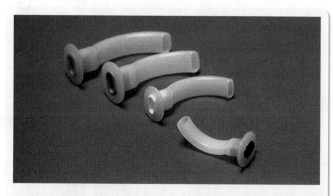

FIGURE 3-9 An OPA is used for unconscious patients who have no gag reflex. It keeps the tongue from blocking the airway.

The OPA can induce vomiting and aspiration when the gag reflex is present. If the OPA is improperly sized or is inserted incorrectly, it could actually push the tongue back into the pharynx, creating an airway obstruction. Rough insertion of the OPA can injure the hard palate, resulting in oral bleeding and creating a risk of vomiting or aspiration. Prior to inserting an OPA, suction the oropharynx as needed to ensure that the mouth is clear of blood or other fluids.

SKILL DRILL 3-4

Inserting a Nasopharyngeal Airway

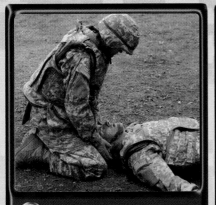

1 Place the casualty on a firm surface in the supine position with the c-spine stabilized.

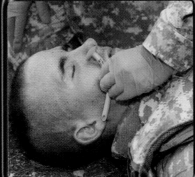

2 Before inserting the NPA, make sure you have selected the proper size. Measure the distance from the tip of the nostril to the earlobe. In almost all individuals, one nostril is larger than the other. The diameter should be roughly equal to the casualty's little finger.

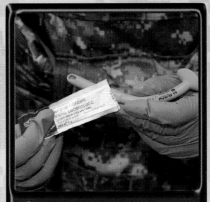

3 After lubricating the NPA with a water-soluble gel, place in the larger nostril, with the curvature of the device following the curve of the floor of the nose and the bevel facing the septum.

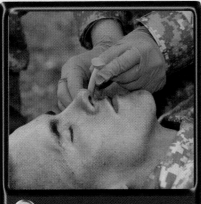

4 Place the bevel toward the septum and insert it gently along the nasal floor, parallel to the mouth. *Do not force the airway.*

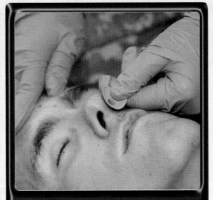

5 When completely inserted, the flange should rest against the nostril. The distal end of the airway will open into the posterior pharynx. Administer oxygen therapy and ventilate the casualty at this time if necessary. Follow local protocol.

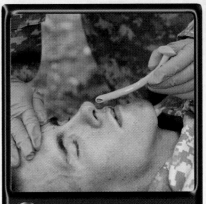

6 To remove the NPA, pull out with a steady motion along the curvature of the nasal cavity.

The steps for inserting an OPA (J tube) are listed here and shown in **SKILL DRILL 3-5 ▸**:

1. Select the proper size airway by measuring from the casualty's earlobe to the corner of his or her mouth or from the center of the casualty's mouth to the angle of the lower jawbone (**Step ①**).

2. Place the casualty on a flat surface in a supine position.

3. Open the airway using the appropriate maneuver. Use the head tilt–chin lift maneuver for a casualty with no risk of spinal injury. Use the jaw-thrust maneuver for a casualty with a possible spinal injury (**Step ②**).

4. Maintain the casualty's airway by utilizing manual techniques and/or mechanical devices.

5. With your nondominant hand, use the cross-finger technique to open the casualty's mouth (**Step ③**).

6. Visualize inside the mouth, and suction if necessary. Do *not* use the OPA until you have cleared the mouth of fluids, foreign materials, loose teeth, and debris.

7. Holding the OPA in your dominant hand, position the correct size airway so that the tip is pointing toward the roof of the casualty's mouth (**Step ④**).

8. Insert the OPA into the casualty's mouth by sliding the tip along the roof past the uvula or until resistance is met by the soft palate (**Step ⑤**).

9. Gently rotate the airway 180 degrees, so the tip is positioned behind the back of the tongue (**Step ⑥**).

10. The flange of the airway should rest against the casualty's lips.

11. If the J tube is too large for the casualty (more than a quarter of its length protruding from the casualty's lips), remove it and choose the proper size to prevent occlusion of the airway.

12. Administer oxygen and ventilate as necessary, in accordance with local standard procedures.

13. Monitor the casualty closely. If the casualty gags or regains consciousness, remove the airway immediately.

14. Remove the airway by pulling it out in line with the natural curvature of the mouth. *Do not* rotate (**Step ⑦**).

15. Vomiting may occur once the airway is removed. Have a suction device ready when removing the airway adjunct.

■ Advanced Airway Management

Combitube

The **Combitube** is an esophageal-tracheal double-lumen airway. It is considered to be an intermediate airway whose abilities lie between airway adjuncts (oropharyngeal and nasopharyngeal) and endotracheal intubation. The Combitube is designed to provide a patent airway for arrested casualties and

can be blindly inserted. It has been used successfully in casualties with difficult airways secondary to severe facial burns, trauma, upper airway bleeding, and vomiting where there was an inability to visualize the vocal cords. It can be used in casualties whose cervical spine has been immobilized with a rigid cervical collar, though placement may be more difficult. Ventilation does not seem to be affected by the rigid cervical collar if the Combitube can be placed. The double-lumen design allows for effective ventilations to be provided regardless of whether the tube is placed in the trachea or esophagus. The Combitube comes in two sizes: 37F and 41F.

The indications for inserting a Combitube include adult casualties in respiratory or cardiac arrest. The contraindications include an intact gag reflex, people under 5′ tall, casualties with known esophageal disease, and ingestion of a caustic substance (acid or lye). The side effects and complications include an increased incidence of sore throat, dysphagia, and upper airway hematoma when compared to endotracheal intubation. Esophageal rupture is a rare complication, but has been reported.

Complications may be partially preventable by avoiding overinflation of the distal and proximal cuffs. Always take appropriate body substance isolation (BSI) precautions, including facial protection, because vomiting can occur through the no. 2 tube if the initial placement is in the casualty's esophagus.

To insert a Combitube, follow the steps in **SKILL DRILL 3-6 ▸**:

1. Inspect the casualty's upper airway for visible airway obstructions (**Step ①**).

2. Hyperventilate the casualty for 30 seconds (**Step ②**).

3. Position the casualty's head in a neutral position (**Step ③**).

4. Test both cuffs (white and blue) for leaks by inflating with 15 mL (white) or 100 mL (blue) of air (**Step ④**).

5. Insert the Combitube in the same direction as the natural curvature of the pharynx.

6. Grasp the tongue and lower jaw between your thumb and index fingers and lift upward (jaw-lift maneuver).

7. Insert the Combitube gently but firmly until the black rings on the tube are positioned between the casualty's teeth (**Step ⑤**).

8. Inflate the no. 1 (blue) balloon with 100 mL of air using a 100-mL syringe. Inflate the no. 2 (white) balloon with 15 mL of air using a 20-mL syringe (**Step ⑥**).

9. Ventilate through the no. 1 (blue) tube. If auscultation of breath sounds is positive and auscultation of gastric sounds is negative, continue ventilations.

10. If auscultation of breath sounds is negative and gastric **insufflation** (inhaling oxygen into the body cavity) is positive, immediately begin ventilations through the shorter (white) connecting tube no. 2. Confirm tracheal ventilation of breath sounds and absence of gastric insufflation (**Step ⑦**).

Insert an Oropharyngeal Airway (J Tube)

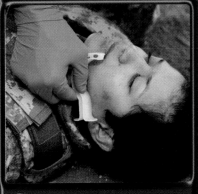

1 Select the proper size airway by measuring from the casualty's earlobe to the corner of his or her mouth or from the center of the casualty's mouth to the angle of the lower jawbone.

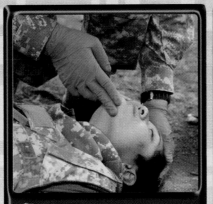

2 Place the casualty on a flat surface in a supine position. Open the airway using the appropriate maneuver. Maintain the casualty's airway.

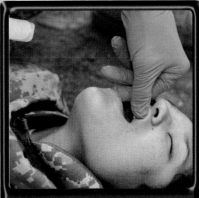

3 With your nondominant hand, use the cross-finger technique to open the casualty's mouth.

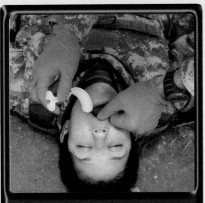

4 Visualize inside the mouth, and suction if necessary. Holding the OPA in your dominant hand, position the correct size airway so that the tip is pointing toward the roof of the casualty's mouth.

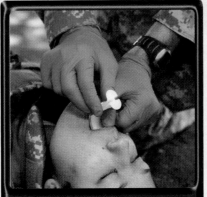

5 Insert the oral airway into the casualty's mouth by sliding the tip along the roof past the uvula or until resistance is met by the soft palate.

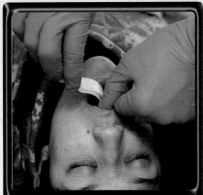

6 Gently rotate the airway 180°, so the tip is positioned behind the back of the tongue.

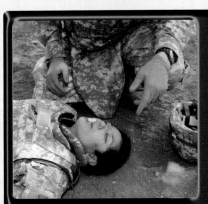

7 The flange of the airway should rest against the casualty's lips. Administer oxygen and ventilate as necessary. Remove the airway by pulling it out in line with the natural curvature of the mouth. *Do not* rotate.

11. If auscultation of breath sounds and auscultation of gastric insufflation are negative, the Combitube may have been advanced too far into the pharynx. Deflate the no. 1 balloon/cuff and move the Combitube approximately 2 to 3 cm out of the casualty's mouth (**Step 8**).

12. Re-inflate the no. 1 balloon with 100 mL of air and ventilate through the longer no. 1 connecting tube. If auscultation of breath sounds is positive and auscultation of gastric insufflation is negative, continue ventilations.

13. If breath sounds are still absent, immediately deflate both cuffs and extubate the casualty. Insert an oropharyngeal or a nasopharyngeal airway and hyperventilate the casualty with a BVM device (**Step 9**).

Once successfully inserted, the Combitube should not be removed unless either the tube placement can no longer be determined, the casualty can no longer tolerate the tube (begins to gag), or there is a palpable pulse and the casualty starts breathing on his or her own. Make certain that a physician or physician's assistant (PA) is present to place an endotracheal tube. Have suction equipment ready. Log roll the casualty to the side and deflate the pharyngeal cuff using the no. 1 pilot balloon. Deflate the distal cuff using the no. 2 pilot balloon and gently remove the Combitube while suctioning the airway.

The **KING LT-D** is a new addition to the advanced airways used in the battlefield. The KING LT-D is designed to keep the casualty's airway patent and to assist in providing supplemental ventilation. The KING LT-D comes in three sizes which are dependent upon the casualty's height.

To insert a KING LT-D, follow the steps in **SKILL DRILL 3-7 ▶**:

1. Select the proper KING LT-D based upon the casualty's height.

2. Position the casualty's airway using the appropriate maneuver.

3. Test the cuffs of the KING LT-D. If the cuffs inflate properly, then lubricate the tip (**Step 1**).

4. Lift the casualty's chin and insert the tip of the KING LT-D into the corner of the casualty's mouth (**Step 2**).

5. Ensure that the tube is behind the base of the tongue, and then rotate the tube (**Step 3**).

6. The base of the tube should align with the casualty's teeth.

7. Inflate the cuffs according to the size of the KING LT-D (**Step 4**).

8. Attach a bag-valve-mask device to the KING LT-D and ventilate the casualty (**Step 5**).

9. To remove the KING LT-D, deflate the cuffs and gently extract the KING LT-D from the airway (**Step 6**).

Emergency Cricothyrotomy

The inability to intubate the trachea with a Combitube or an ET is an indication for creating a surgical airway in a casualty. Additional indications are severe maxillofacial injury, airway

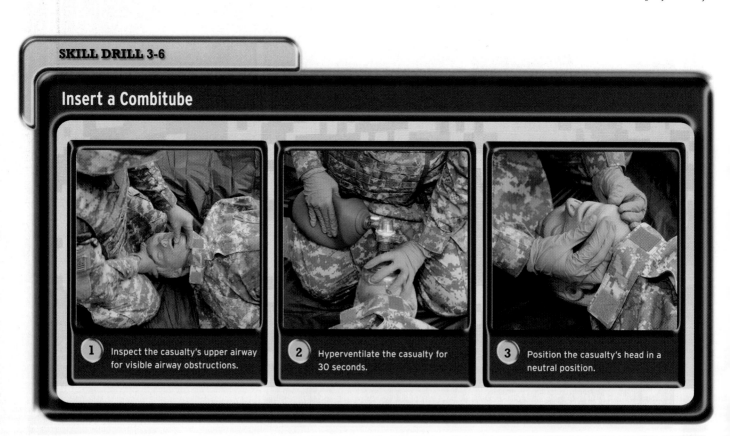

SKILL DRILL 3-6

Insert a Combitube

1 Inspect the casualty's upper airway for visible airway obstructions.

2 Hyperventilate the casualty for 30 seconds.

3 Position the casualty's head in a neutral position.

Insert a Combitube (*continued*)

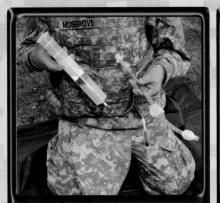

4 Test both cuffs (white and blue) for leaks by inflating with 15 mL (white) or 100 mL (blue) of air.

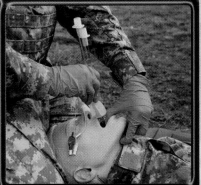

5 Insert the Combitube in the same direction as the natural curvature of the pharynx. Grasp the tongue and lower jaw between your thumb and index fingers and lift upward (jaw-lift maneuver). Insert the Combitube gently but firmly until the black rings on the tube are positioned between the casualty's teeth.

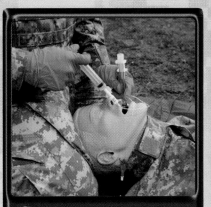

6 Inflate the no. 1 (blue) balloon with 100 mL of air using a 100-mL syringe. Inflate the no. 2 (white) balloon with 15 mL of air using a 20-mL syringe.

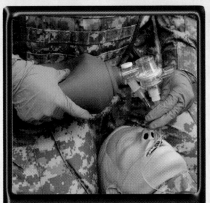

7 Ventilate through the no. 1 (blue) tube. If auscultation of breath sounds is positive and auscultation of gastric sounds is negative, continue ventilations. If auscultation of breath sounds is negative and gastric insufflation is positive, immediately begin ventilations through the shorter (white) connecting tube no. 2. Confirm tracheal ventilation of breath sounds and absence of gastric insufflation.

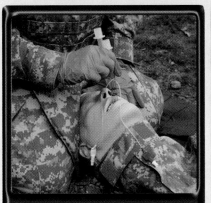

8 If auscultation of breath sounds and auscultation of gastric insufflation are negative, the Combitube may have been advanced too far into the pharynx. Deflate the no. 1 balloon/cuff and move the Combitube approximately 2 to 3 cm out of the casualty's mouth.

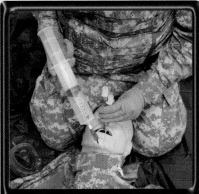

9 Re-inflate the no. 1 balloon with 100 mL of air and ventilate through the longer no. 1 connecting tube. If auscultation of breath sounds is positive and auscultation of gastric insufflation is negative, continue ventilations. If breath sounds are still absent, immediately deflate both cuffs and extubate the casualty. Insert an oropharyngeal or a nasopharyngeal airway and hyperventilate the casualty with a BVM device.

SKILL DRILL 3-7

Insert a KING LT-D

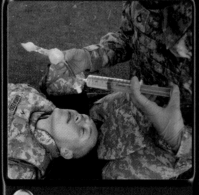

1 Select the proper KING LT-D based upon the casualty's height. Position the casualty's airway using the appropriate maneuver. Test the cuffs of the KING LT-D. If the cuff inflates properly, then lubricate the tip.

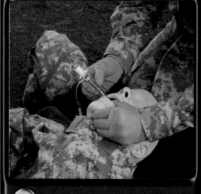

2 Lift the casualty's chin and insert the tip of the KING LT-D into the corner of the casualty's mouth.

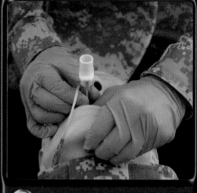

3 Ensure that the tube is behind the base of the tongue, and then rotate the tube.

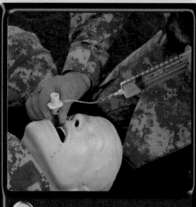

4 The base of the tube should align with the casualty's teeth. Inflate the cuffs according to the size of the KING LT-D.

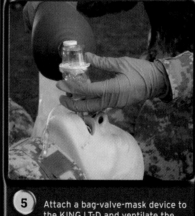

5 Attach a bag-valve-mask device to the KING LT-D and ventilate the casualty.

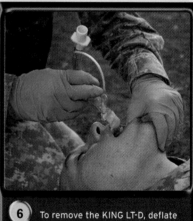

6 To remove the KING LT-D, deflate the cuffs and gently extract the KING LT-D from the airway.

obstruction, and structural deformities of the airway. When maxillofacial, cervical spine, head, or soft-tissue injuries are present, several factors may prevent intubation. These factors include gross distortion of structures, airway obstruction, massive emesis, and significant hemorrhage. In such casualties, emergency (surgical) cricothyrotomy is an excellent way to obtain definitive control of the airway. The complications of an emergency cricothyrotomy include incorrect tube placement, blood aspiration, esophageal laceration, hematoma, laceration of the trachea, vocal cord paralysis, and hoarseness.

To perform an emergency cricothyrotomy, follow the steps in **SKILL DRILL 3-8 ▸**.

1. Gather the equipment that you will need to perform the procedure: a #10 or #11 scalpel or knife blade and an airway tube (a #6 or #7 ET with cuff, cannula, or a noncollapsible tube).

2. Put on gloves.

3. Place the casualty in a supine position and hyperextend the casualty's neck.

4. Place a blanket or a rolled up poncho under the casualty's neck or between the shoulder blades to keep the casualty's airway straight (**Step** ①).

5. Locate the cricothyroid membrane. Place a finger on the thyroid cartilage and slide the finger down to the cricoid cartilage.

6. Palpate for the V notch (**Step** ②).

7. Slide the index finger down into the depression between the thyroid and cricoid cartilage.

8. Raise the skin to form a tent-like appearance over the cricothyroid space, using the index finger and thumb (**Step** ③).

9. Stabilize and clean the area (**Step** ④).

10. With a blade, make a 1½″ vertical incision through the raised skin to the cricothyroid space. Do not cut the cricothyroid membrane with this incision (**Step** ⑤).

11. Open the incision with hemostats to visualize the cricothyroid membrane and the cricothyroid space (**Step** ⑥).

12. Have a combat lifesaver (CLS) stabilize the larynx with one hand. While keeping the incision open with the hemostats, cut or poke through the cricothyroid membrane. If using a #10 or a knife blade, then make a ½″ horizontal incision through the elastic tissue of the cricothyroid membrane. If using a #11 scalpel, poke through the cricothyroid membrane (**Step** ⑦).

13. Use the other end of the scalpel to make a blunt dissection (**Step** ⑧).

14. Use a hook to stabilize the opening (**Step** ⑨).

15. Insert the end of the ET or cannula between edges of the the incision. The tube should be in the trachea and directed toward the lungs (**Step** ⑩).

16. Inflate the cuff with 5 to 10 cc of air. Do not advance the tube more than 2″ to 3″ (**Step** ⑪).

17. Check for air exchange and placement of the tube. Listen and feel for air passing in and out of the tube. Look for bilateral rise and fall of the chest.

18. Connect a BVM device to the tube or have a CLS perform mouth-to-tube respirations.

19. As the CLS pumps or blows air into the tube, auscultate the abdomen and both lung fields while observing for bilateral rise and fall of the chest. If there are bilateral breath sounds and bilateral rise and fall of the chest, the tube is in place and can be secured (**Step** ⑫).

20. Incorrect tube placement calls for correction. Either:
    a. Deflate the cuff, retract the tube 1″ to 2″, and recheck the placement.
    b. Remove the tube, reinsert, and recheck the placement (**Step** ⑬).

21. If the tube is placed correctly and the casualty is still not breathing, direct the CLS to perform rescue breathing.
    a. Connect the tube to a BVM device and oxygen if available and have the casualty ventilated.
    b. If no BVM device is available, the CLS should perform mouth-to-tube breathing.
    c. Once rescue breathing has started, secure the tube (**Step** ⑭).

22. Suction the tube as necessary.
    a. Insert the suction catheter 4″ to 5″ into the tube. Apply suction only while withdrawing the catheter.
    b. Apply 1 cc of saline into the airway to loosen any secretions and to help suctioning.

23. Apply a dressing to further protect the tube and the incision by either:
    a. Cut two 4″ × 4″ or 4″ × 8″ gauze pads halfway through. Place them on opposite sides of the tube so that the tube comes up through the cut and the gauze overlaps. Tape securely.
    b. Apply a sterile dressing under the casualty's tube by making a V-shaped fold in a 4″ × 8″ gauze pad and placing it under the edge of the cannula to prevent irritation to the casualty. Tape securely.

24. Monitor respirations. Reassess the air exchange and placement every time that the casualty is moved. Assist in ventilations if the respiration rate falls below 12 breaths/min or rises above 20 breaths/min (**Step** ⑮).

■ Ventilation

If a casualty is found with inadequate breathing or is apneic, you must provide ventilation through mouth-to-mask ventilation or with a **bag-valve-mask (BVM) device**. To perform mouth-to-mask (mouth-to-mouth) ventilation, follow the steps in **SKILL DRILL 3-9 ▶**:

1. Position yourself at the casualty's head and open the airway using the head tilt–chin lift technique. If trauma is suspected, open using the jaw-thrust technique instead (**Step** ①).

2. Connect oxygen to the inlet on the face mask. Oxygen should run at 15 L/min (**Step** ②).

3. Position the mask on the casualty's face so that the apex is over the bridge of his or her nose and the base is between the lower lip and the prominence of the chin (**Step** ③).

4. Hold the mask firmly in place while maintaining the proper head tilt (**Step** ④).

Perform an Emergency Cricothyrotomy

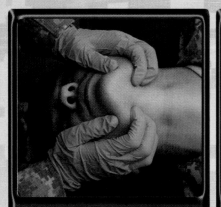

1 Gather the equipment. Put on gloves. Place the casualty in a supine position and hyperextend the casualty's neck. Place a blanket or a rolled up poncho under the casualty's neck or between the shoulder blades to keep the casualty's airway straight.

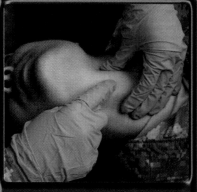

2 Locate the cricothyroid membrane. Place a finger on the thyroid cartilage and slide the finger down to the cricoid cartilage. Palpate for the V notch.

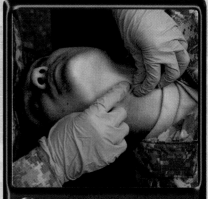

3 Slide the index finger down into the depression between the thyroid and cricoid cartilage. Raise the skin to form a tent-like appearance over the cricothyroid space, using the index finger and thumb.

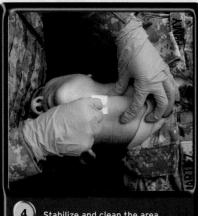

4 Stabilize and clean the area.

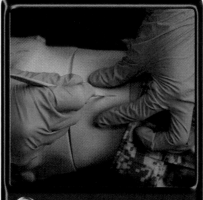

5 With a blade, make a 1½″ vertical incision through the raised skin to the cricothyroid space. Do not cut the cricothyroid membrane with this incision.

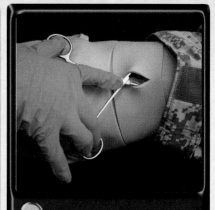

6 Open the incision with hemostats to visualize the cricothyroid membrane and the cricothyroid space.

SKILL DRILL 3-8

Perform an Emergency Cricothyrotomy (*continued*)

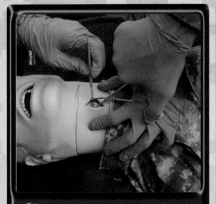

7 Have a combat lifesaver (CLS) stabilize the larynx with one hand. While keeping the incision open with the hemostats, cut or poke through the cricothyroid membrane. If using a #10 or a knife blade, then make a ½″ horizontal incision through the elastic tissue of the cricothyroid membrane. If using a #11 scalpel, poke through the cricothyroid membrane.

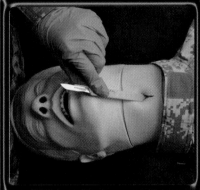

8 Use the other end of the scalpel to make a blunt dissection.

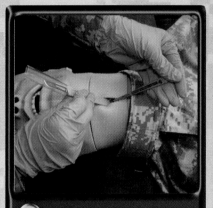

9 Use a hook to stabilize the opening.

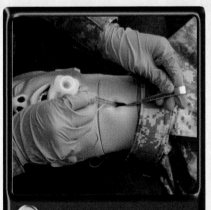

10 Insert the end of the ET or cannula between the incision. The tube should be in the trachea and directed toward the lungs.

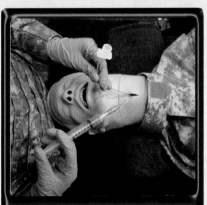

11 Inflate the cuff with 5 to 10 cc of air. Do not advance the tube more than 2″ to 3″.

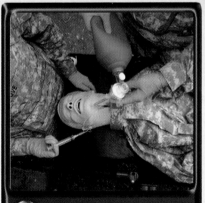

12 Check for air exchange and placement of the tube. Connect a BVM device to the tube or have a CLS perform mouth-to-tube respirations. As the CLS pumps or blows air into the tube, auscultate the abdomen and both lung fields while observing the chest. If there are bilateral breath sounds and bilateral rise and fall of the chest, the tube is in place and can be secured.

Perform an Emergency Cricothyrotomy (*continued*)

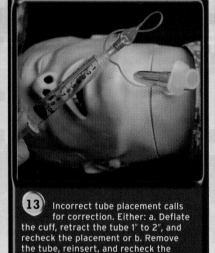

13 Incorrect tube placement calls for correction. Either: a. Deflate the cuff, retract the tube 1" to 2", and recheck the placement or b. Remove the tube, reinsert, and recheck the placement.

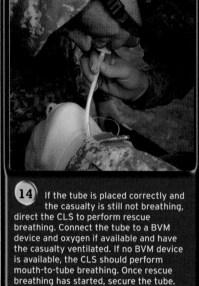

14 If the tube is placed correctly and the casualty is still not breathing, direct the CLS to perform rescue breathing. Connect the tube to a BVM device and oxygen if available and have the casualty ventilated. If no BVM device is available, the CLS should perform mouth-to-tube breathing. Once rescue breathing has started, secure the tube.

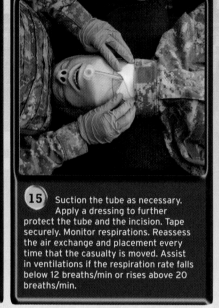

15 Suction the tube as necessary. Apply a dressing to further protect the tube and the incision. Tape securely. Monitor respirations. Reassess the air exchange and placement every time that the casualty is moved. Assist in ventilations if the respiration rate falls below 12 breaths/min or rises above 20 breaths/min.

5. Take a deep breath and exhale into the mask port (**Step 5**).

6. Remove your mouth from the port and allow for passive exhalation (**Step 6**).

To provide ventilation using the one-person BVM device technique, follow the steps in **SKILL DRILL 3-10**:

1. Position yourself at the casualty's head and establish an open airway using the head tilt–chin lift technique. If trauma is suspected, open using the jaw-thrust technique instead.

2. Select the correct size mask.

3. Form a "C" around the ventilation port with your thumb and index finger, and use your middle and ring fingers to lift up on the jaw.

4. With your other hand, squeeze the bag once every 4 to 5 seconds.

5. Release pressure on the bag and let the casualty exhale passively.

6. Observe for gastric distension, changes in compliance of bag with ventilation, and improvement or deterioration of ventilation status.

To provide ventilation using the two-person BVM device technique, follow the steps in **SKILL DRILL 3-11 ▸**:

1. Position yourself at the casualty's head and establish an open airway using the head tilt–chin lift technique. If trauma is suspected, open the casualty's airway using the jaw-thrust technique instead (**Step 1**).

2. Select the correct mask size.

3. Kneel at the casualty's head. Place your thumbs over the nose portion of the mask and place your index and middle fingers over the portion of the mask that covers the mouth (**Step 2**).

4. Use your ring and little fingers to bring the jaw upward, toward the mask.

5. The second rescuer should squeeze the bag once every 5 seconds (with the two-hand technique) to ventilate the casualty (**Step 3**).

■ Suction the Airway

The purpose of suctioning is to keep the casualty's airway clear of all foreign matter (eg, blood, saliva, vomitus, and debris), which could be aspirated into the trachea or

SKILL DRILL 3-9

Mouth-to-Mask Ventilation

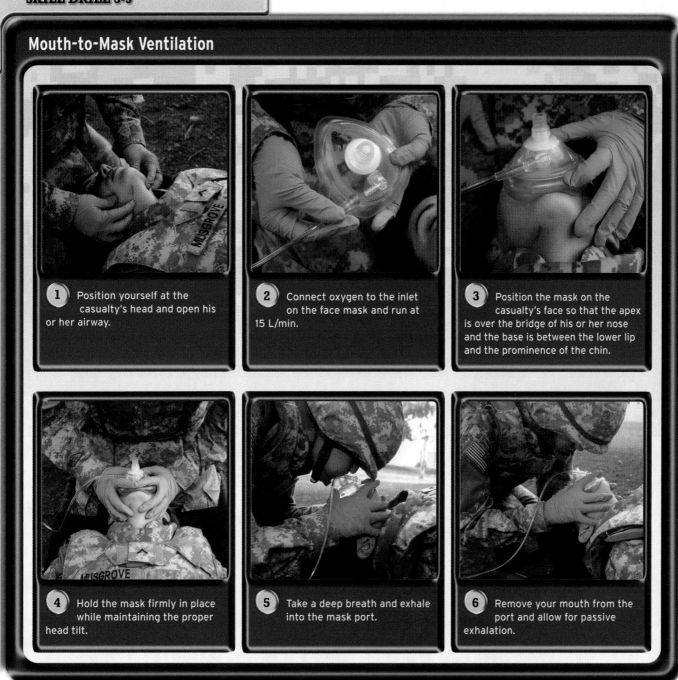

1 Position yourself at the casualty's head and open his or her airway.

2 Connect oxygen to the inlet on the face mask and run at 15 L/min.

3 Position the mask on the casualty's face so that the apex is over the bridge of his or her nose and the base is between the lower lip and the prominence of the chin.

4 Hold the mask firmly in place while maintaining the proper head tilt.

5 Take a deep breath and exhale into the mask port.

6 Remove your mouth from the port and allow for passive exhalation.

the lungs. When the casualty's mouth or throat becomes filled with vomitus, blood, or secretions, a suction apparatus enables you to remove the liquid material quickly and efficiently, thereby allowing you to ventilate the casualty. Ventilating a casualty with secretions in his or her mouth will force material into the lungs, resulting in an upper airway obstruction or aspiration. If you hear gurgling, the casualty needs suctioning!

The indications for suctioning include:

- Casualties who have a decreased level of consciousness and are unable to clear their own airway
- Casualties who cannot clear their airway because of excessive amounts of foreign matter

You can use a flexible suction catheter, which is a sterile tube used for oropharyngeal or nasopharyngeal suctioning of fluids or small foreign particles. Suction catheters are sized in French (F) gauge. The Yankaeur (rigid) suction tip (tonsil tip) is used for oropharyngeal suction only. It is not necessary to measure, just keep sight of the tip when inserting it. The large-bore opening of the Yankaeur suction tip is the preferred method of removing large particles of foreign material. It comes in only one size.

To perform oropharyngeal and nasopharyngeal suctioning on a casualty, follow the steps in **SKILL DRILL 3-12 ▸**:

1. Preoxygenate the casualty for 1 to 2 minutes to increase the oxygen saturation in the blood. This reduces the risk of causing hypoxemia.

2. Position the casualty properly. For a nontrauma and conscious casualty, position yourself at the casualty's head and turn his or her head to the side. For a trauma and unconscious casualty, position yourself at the casualty's head and maintain spinal alignment while log rolling the casualty toward you.

3. Select and measure the suction catheter. Measure the catheter from the corner of the mouth to the earlobe.

4. Consider the route: oropharyngeal or nasopharyngeal.

5. Check the suctioning unit and equipment (**Step ①**).

6. Ensure that a power source is available and the unit is functioning before beginning the procedure.

7. Cover the proximal port with your thumb and set the suction vacuum at 100 to 120 mm Hg for an adult or a child and 60 to 100 mm Hg for an infant (**Step ②**).

8. Release your thumb from the port before inserting it; do not suction on the way in.

9. To perform oropharyngeal suctioning, open the casualty's mouth using the cross-finger technique and clear the mouth of any visible fluids or obstructions with a gloved finger (**Step ③**).

10. If you are using a Yankaeur (rigid) tip, insert it with the convex (bulging out) side against the roof of the mouth and stop at the beginning of the pharynx.

11. If you are using a flexible suction catheter, insert the catheter up to the base of the tongue.

12. To perform nasopharyngeal suctioning, insert the catheter gently into one nostril and then the other.

13. Cover the proximal port to begin suctioning.

14. Suction as you slowly withdraw, moving the tip from side to side.

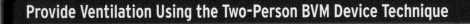

SKILL DRILL 3-11

Provide Ventilation Using the Two-Person BVM Device Technique

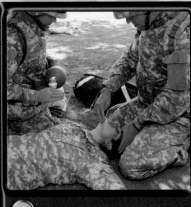

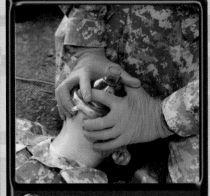

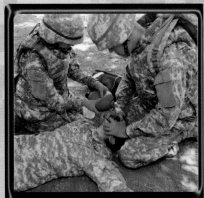

① Position yourself at the casualty's head and establish an open airway.

② Select the correct mask size. Kneel at the patient's head. Place your thumbs over the nose portion of the mask and place your index and middle fingers over the portion of the mask that covers the mouth. Use your ring and little fingers to bring the jaw upward, toward the mask.

③ The second rescuer should squeeze the bag once every 5 seconds (with the two-hand technique) to ventilate the casualty.

15. Suction for 15 seconds or less.

16. Reoxygenate the casualty after suctioning (Step ④).

17. Observe the casualty for hypoxemia, color change, increased or decreased pulse rate, or a change in breathing.

■ Summary

It is critical to know how to use and maintain oxygen delivery equipment. Resuscitation measures should never be delayed in order to locate, retrieve, or set up oxygen delivery devices. Having your equipment ready, being properly trained on oxygen administration procedures, and having efficient skills in airway management will improve the casualty's respiratory status, thereby, increasing the casualty's chance for survival.

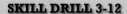

SKILL DRILL 3-12

Perform Oropharyngeal and Nasopharyngeal Suctioning

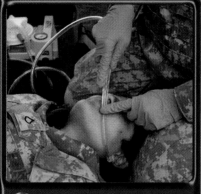

1 Preoxygenate the casualty. Position the casualty properly. Select and measure the suction catheter. Check the suctioning unit and equipment.

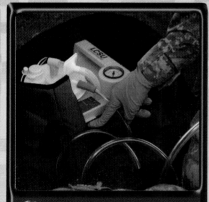

2 Ensure that a power source is available and the unit is functioning before beginning the procedure. Cover the proximal port with your thumb and set the suction vacuum.

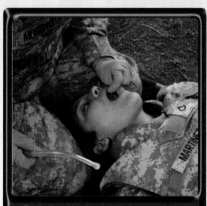

3 Release your thumb from the port before inserting it; do not suction on the way in. To perform oropharyngeal suctioning, open the casualty's mouth using the cross-finger technique and clear the mouth of any visible fluids or obstructions with a gloved finger. To perform nasopharyngeal suctioning, insert the catheter gently into one nostril and then the other.

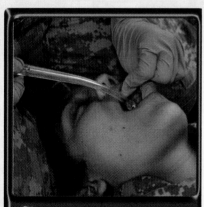

4 If you are using a Yankaeur (rigid) tip, insert it with the convex (bulging out) side against the roof of the mouth and stop at the beginning of the pharynx. If you are using a flexible suction catheter, insert the catheter up to the base of the tongue. Cover the proximal port to begin suctioning. Suction as you slowly withdraw, moving the tip from side to side. Suction for 15 seconds or less. Reoxygenate the casualty after suctioning.

YOU ARE THE
COMBAT MEDIC

While on patrol, a member of your unit suffers a gunshot wound to the face. You find your casualty lying face up on the ground with an obvious airway emergency.

Assessment

Your casualty is unconscious and unresponsive with snoring, stridorous respirations at 10 breaths/min. If you do not take care of the airway, this casualty will die from hypoxia.

Treatment

Because there is massive facial damage due to the gunshot wound, you cannot insert a NPA, OPA, Combitube, or KING LT-D. In order to create a patent airway in this casualty, you must perform an emergency cricothyrotomy. Using a #10 blade, you make a 1½" vertical incision, open the incision with hemostats, and then make a ½" horizontal incision in the casualty's cricothyroid membrane. After using the other end of the scalpel to make a blunt dissection, you insert an ET and inflate the cuff. There is bilateral rise and fall of the casualty's chest, so you have a combat lifesaver (CLS) attach a BVM device to the ET and provide ventilations.

You make the determination that this casualty warrants immediate evacuation and the platoon commander calls for immediate 9-line MEDEVAC evacuation. Now that the casualty has been ventilated, you suction the ET to ensure that the airway is patent. Then you apply a sterile dressing under the casualty's tube by making a V-shaped fold in a 4" × 8" gauze pad and placing it under the edge of the cannula to prevent irritation to the casualty and tape securely. The casualty's respirations improve to 19 breaths/min as the transport arrives.

1. LAST NAME, FIRST NAME		RANK/GRADE		X	MALE
Addison, Craig		SGT			FEMALE
SSN	SPECIALTY CODE			RELIGION	
000-111-0000	ØZ			Baptist	

2. UNIT

FORCE				NATIONALITY	
A/T	AF/A	N/M	MC/M		
	BC/BC		NBI/BNC	DISEASE	PSYCH

3. INJURY			
		X	AIRWAY
			HEAD
FRONT	BACK	X	WOUND
			NECK/BACK INJURY
			BURN
			AMPUTATION
			STRESS
			OTHER (Specify)

4. LEVEL OF CONSCIOUSNESS			
ALERT			PAIN RESPONSE
VERBAL RESPONSE		X	UNRESPONSIVE

5. PULSE	TIME	6. TOURNIQUET			TIME
40 bpm	0450	X NO		YES	

7. MORPHINE		DOSE	TIME	8. IV	TIME
X NO	YES			—	

9. TREATMENT/OBSERVATIONS/CURRENT MEDICATION/ALLERGIES/NBC (ANTIDOTE)

Gunshot wound to the face. Performed emergency cricothyrotomy to establish airway. Airway improved. Breathing went from 10 breaths/min to 19 breaths/min.

10. DISPOSITION	RETURNED TO DUTY		TIME
	X EVACUATED		0500
	DECEASED		

11. PROVIDER/UNIT	DATE (YYMMDD)
Sydney, Phil	

Ready for Review

- One of the most critical skills that you must know is airway management. Without proper airway management techniques and oxygen administration, your casualty may die needlessly.

- The objective of airway management is to immediately establish and maintain a patent (open) airway.

- The airway connects the body to the life-giving oxygen in the atmosphere. If it becomes obstructed, this lifeline is cut and the casualty dies—often within minutes.

- Sometimes the simplest, most low-tech techniques are the fastest and most effective way to open a casualty's airway.

- Orotracheal intubation is the placement of an endotracheal tube (ET) orally, through the vocal cords and into the trachea.

- If a casualty is found with inadequate breathing or is apneic, you must provide ventilation through mouth-to-mask ventilation or with a bag-valve-mask (BVM) device.

- The purpose of suctioning is to keep the casualty's airway clear of all foreign matter (eg, blood, saliva, vomitus, and debris), which could be aspirated into the trachea or the lungs.

Vital Vocabulary

adenoids Lymphatic tissues located on the posterior nasopharyngeal wall that filter bacteria.

alveolar air The amount of air that reaches the alveoli and participates in gas exchange with capillary blood, about 350 cc.

alveoli Balloon-like clusters of single-layer air sacs that are the functional site for the exchange of oxygen and carbon dioxide in the lungs.

aphonia Inability to speak.

arytenoid cartilages Pyramid-like cartilaginous structures that form the posterior attachment of the vocal cords.

aspiration Entry of fluids or solids into the trachea, bronchi, and lungs.

bag-valve-mask (BVM) device Manual ventilation device that consists of a bag, mask, reservoir, and oxygen inlet; capable of delivering up to 100% oxygen.

bronchioles Subdivision of the smaller bronchi in the lungs; made of smooth muscle; dilate or constrict in response to various stimuli.

carina Point at which the trachea bifurcates (divides) into the left and right mainstem bronchi.

Combitube Multilumen airway device that consists of a single tube with two lumens, two balloons, and two ventilation ports; an alternative device if endotracheal intubation is not possible or has failed.

compliance The ability of the lungs and chest wall to expand and contract in response to the application of force.

cricoid cartilage Forms the lowest portion of the larynx; also referred to as the cricoid ring; it is the first ring of the trachea and the only upper airway structure that forms a complete ring.

cricothyroid membrane A thin, superficial membrane located between the thyroid and cricoid cartilages that is relatively avascular and contains few nerves; the site for emergency surgical and nonsurgical access to the airway.

dead air space Any portion of the airway that does not contain air and cannot participate in gas exchange.

diaphragm The major muscle of breathing. It is the anatomic point of separation between the thoracic cavity and the abdominal cavity.

diffusion Movement of a gas from an area of higher concentration to an area of lower concentration.

dysphonia Difficulty speaking.

endotracheal tube (ET) Tube that is inserted into the trachea; equipped with a distal cuff, a proximal inflation port, a 15/22-mm adapter, and cm markings on the side.

epiglottis Leaf-shaped cartilaginous structure that closes over the trachea during swallowing.

expiration Passive movement of air out of the lungs; also called exhalation.

extubation The process of removing the tube from an intubated patient.

eyelash reflex Contraction of the patient's lower eyelid when upper eyelashes are stroked; fairly reliable indicator of the presence or absence of an intact gag reflex.

gag reflex Automatic reaction when something touches an area deep in the oral cavity; helps protect the lower airway from aspiration.

glottis The space in between the vocal cords that is the narrowest portion of the adult's airway; also called the glottic opening.

head tilt–chin lift maneuver Manual airway maneuver that involves tilting the head back while lifting up on the chin; used to open the airway of a semiconscious or unconscious nontrauma patient.

Heimlich maneuver Abdominal thrusts performed to relieve a foreign body airway obstruction.

hilum Point of entry of all of the blood vessels and the bronchi into each lung.

hyoid bone A small, horseshoe-shaped bone to which the jaw, tongue, epiglottis, and thyroid cartilage attach.

hyperventilation Occurs when CO_2 elimination exceeds CO_2 production; also the increase in the number of respirations per minute above the normal range.

hypoventilation Occurs when CO_2 production exceeds the body's ability to eliminate it by ventilation; also the decrease in the number of respirations per minute that falls below the normal range.

hypoxia A lack of oxygen to the body's cells and tissues.

inspiration The active process of moving air into the lungs; also called inhalation.

insufflation Inhaling oxygen into the body cavity.

jaw-thrust maneuver Manual airway maneuver that involves stabilizing the patient's head and thrusting the jaw forward; the preferred method of opening the airway of a semiconscious or unconscious trauma patient.

KING LT-D A disposable supraglottic airway used as an alternative to tracheal intubation or mask ventilation.

laryngospasm Spasmodic closure of the vocal cords.

larynx A complex structure formed by many independent cartilaginous structures that all work together; where the upper airway ends and the lower airway begins.

lung compliance The ability of the alveoli to expand when air is drawn into the lungs during either negative-pressure ventilation or positive-pressure ventilation.

mediastinum The region between the lungs that contains the heart, great blood vessels, esophagus, trachea, and lymph nodes.

nasal septum A rigid partition composed of bone and cartilage; divides the nasopharynx into two passages.

nasopharyngeal airway (NPA) A soft rubber tube about 6" long that is inserted through the nose into the posterior pharynx behind the tongue, thereby allowing passage of air from the nose to the lower airway.

nasopharynx The nasal cavity; formed by the union of the facial bones.

negative-pressure ventilation Drawing of air into the lungs; airflow from a region of higher pressure (outside the body) to a region of lower pressure (the lungs); occurs during normal (unassisted) breathing.

oropharyngeal airway (OPA) A hard plastic device that is curved in such a way that it fits over the back of the tongue with the tip in the posterior pharynx.

oropharynx Forms the posterior portion of the oral cavity, which is bordered superiorly by the hard and soft palates, laterally by the cheeks, and inferiorly by the tongue.

palate Forms the roof of the mouth and separates the oropharynx and nasopharynx.

parietal pleura Thin membrane that lines the chest cavity.

patent Open.

pharynx Throat.

positive-pressure ventilation Forcing of air into the lungs.

pyriform fossae Two pockets of tissue on the lateral borders of the larynx.

respiration The exchange of gases between a living organism and its environment.

respiratory rate The number of times a casualty breathes in 1 minute.

sinuses Cavities formed by the cranial bones that trap contaminants from entering the respiratory tract and act as tributaries for fluid to and from the eustachian tubes and tear ducts.

surfactant A proteinaceous substance that lines the alveoli; decreases alveolar surface tension and keeps the alveoli expanded.

thyroid cartilage The main supporting cartilage of the larynx; a shield-shaped structure formed by two plates that join in a V shape anteriorly to form the laryngeal prominence known as the Adam's apple.

tidal volume A measure of the depth of breathing; the volume of air that is inhaled or exhaled during a single respiratory cycle.

tonsils Lymphatic tissues located in the posterior pharynx; they help to trap bacteria.

total lung capacity The total volume of air that the lungs can hold; approximately 6 L in the average adult male.

trachea The conduit for all entry into the lungs; a tubular structure that is approximately 10 to 12 cm in length and is composed of a series of C-shaped cartilaginous rings; also called the windpipe.

turbinates Three bony shelves that protrude from the lateral walls of the nasal cavity and extend into the nasal passageway, parallel to the nasal floor; serve to increase the surface area of the nasal mucosa, thereby improving the processes of warming, filtering, and humidification of inhaled air.

upper airway All anatomic airway structures above the level of the vocal cords.

uvula A soft-tissue structure that resembles a punching bag; located in the posterior aspect of the oral cavity, at the base of the tongue.

vallecula An anatomic space, or "pocket," located between the base of the tongue and the epiglottis; an important anatomic landmark for endotracheal intubation.

ventilation The process of moving air into and out of the lungs.

visceral pleura The thin membrane that lines the lungs.

vocal cords White bands of tough tissue that are the lateral borders of the glottis.

COMBAT MEDIC in Action

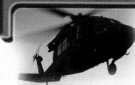

While on a mission in a rural village, you hear a loud bang. You are taken to a casualty and he appears to be unconscious and unresponsive. For now, the perimeter is safe and there is only one casualty. The general impression indicates that the casualty is suffering from burns to the face. He is covered in soot and you note stridorous respirations. You decide to insert an oropharyngeal airway. You measure the device, open the airway, and gently, without pushing the tongue back into the pharynx, you insert the device upside down and rotate it into place. You prepare your casualty for evacuation.

1. Oropharyngeal airways are hard plastic tubes designed to:
   A. prevent the tongue from obstructing the glottis.
   B. facilitate oral suctioning.
   C. facilitate oral tracheal intubation.
   D. guarantee that the airway will remain open.

2. Which of the following signs or conditions may indicate that a casualty has an inhalation injury?
   A. Hoarseness
   B. Peripheral edema
   C. Pain or paresthesia
   D. Skin sloughing on the anterior chest

3. One major disadvantage of using the nasopharyngeal airway is:
   A. you cannot suction through them.
   B. they do not provide a secured airway.
   C. they cannot be used on a conscious patient.
   D. they can only be used on an unconscious patient.

4. To measure an OPA, you measure:
   A. from the corner of the mouth to the casualty's earlobe.
   B. the length of the casualty's hand.
   C. the length of the casualty's nose.
   D. from the corner of the mouth to the casualty's jaw.

5. An additional name for an OPA is:
   A. a hard tube.
   B. an ET.
   C. a J tube.
   D. a curved tube.

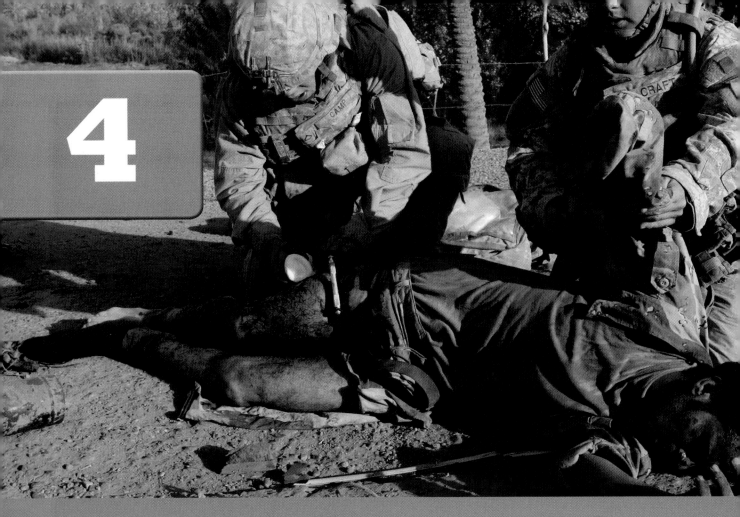

4

Controlling Bleeding and Hypovolemic Shock

Objectives

Knowledge Objectives

- ☐ Describe the anatomy and physiology of the cardiovascular system.
- ☐ Identify the signs and symptoms of hemorrhage.
- ☐ Identify the signs and symptoms of hypovolemic shock.
- ☐ Describe the treatment measures for hemorrhage.
- ☐ Describe the treatment measures for hypovolemic shock.

Skills Objectives

- ☐ Control bleeding by applying a tourniquet.
- ☐ Initiate treatment for hypovolemic shock.

■ Introduction

As a combat medic, you will provide medical care in a variety of situations; the methods you will use to control hemorrhage in your casualties will depend on the circumstances on the battlefield. Control of bleeding in a civilian environment is vastly different from the control of bleeding on the battlefield. This chapter concentrates on the methods for the battlefield. Your ability to successfully control bleeding under extreme circumstances will save lives.

Basic lifesaving steps for the combat medic include clearing the airway, restoring breathing, stopping the bleeding, protecting the wound, and treating/preventing shock. These are the ABC measures that apply to all injuries. Certain types of wounds and burns will require special precautions and procedures when applying these measures. This chapter provides specific information on controlling bleeding. When properly applied, these techniques will save lives.

Bleeding is the most common cause of shock. In this chapter, **shock** describes a state of collapse and failure of the cardiovascular system in which blood circulation slows and eventually ceases. Shock is actually a normal compensatory mechanism used by the body to maintain systolic blood pressure (BP) and brain perfusion during times of distress. If not treated promptly, shock will injure the body's vital organs and ultimately lead to death. Your early and rapid actions can help significantly reduce the morbidity and mortality rates from bleeding and shock.

■ Anatomy and Physiology of the Cardiovascular System Review

The cardiovascular system is designed to carry out one crucial job: keep the blood flowing between the lungs and the peripheral tissues. In the lungs, blood dumps the gaseous waste products of metabolism—chiefly carbon dioxide—and picks up life-giving oxygen. In the peripheral tissues, the process is reversed: Blood unloads oxygen and picks up wastes. If blood flow were to stop or slow significantly, the results would be catastrophic. The cells of the brain, heart, and other organs of the body would have nowhere to eliminate their wastes and would rapidly be engulfed by the toxic by-products of their own metabolism. Oxygen delivery to the tissues would also be disrupted. For a few minutes, the cells could switch to an emergency metabolic system—one that does not require oxygen (anaerobic metabolism), but that form of metabolism produces even more acids and toxic wastes. Within a few minutes of circulatory failure, cells throughout the body would begin to suffocate and die, leading to the state known as shock.

To keep the blood moving continuously through the body, the circulatory system requires three intact components **FIGURE 4-1 ▶**:

- **A functioning pump:** The heart
- **Adequate fluid volume:** The blood and body fluids
- **An intact system of tubing capable of reflex adjustments (constriction and dilation) in response to changes in pump output and fluid volume:** The blood vessels

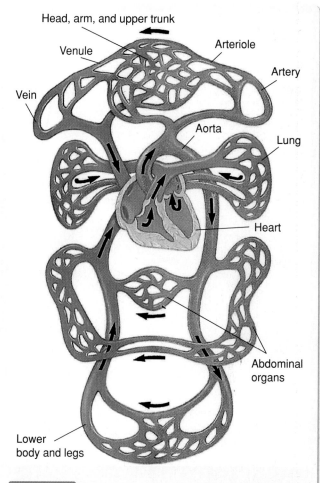

FIGURE 4-1 The circulatory system requires three intact components: the heart, the blood and body fluids, and the blood vessels.

All three components must interact effectively to maintain life. If any one becomes damaged or is deficient, the whole system is in jeopardy.

Structures of the Heart

The **heart** is a muscular, cone-shaped organ whose function is to pump blood throughout the body. Located behind the sternum, the heart is about the size of a closed fist—roughly 5″ long, 3″ wide, and 2½″ thick. It weighs 10 to 12 oz in men and 8 to 10 oz in women. Roughly two thirds of the heart lies in the left part of the **mediastinum**, the area between the lungs that also contains the great vessels.

The human heart consists of four chambers: two atria (upper chambers) and two ventricles (lower chambers). The right atrium receives oxygen-poor blood (deoxygenated) from the body and upon contraction sends it to the right ventricle.

The right ventricle receives blood from the right atrium and pumps the blood out to the lungs via the pulmonary arteries. The left atrium receives oxygen-rich (oxygenated) blood from the lungs. When the left atrium contracts, it sends blood to the left ventricle.

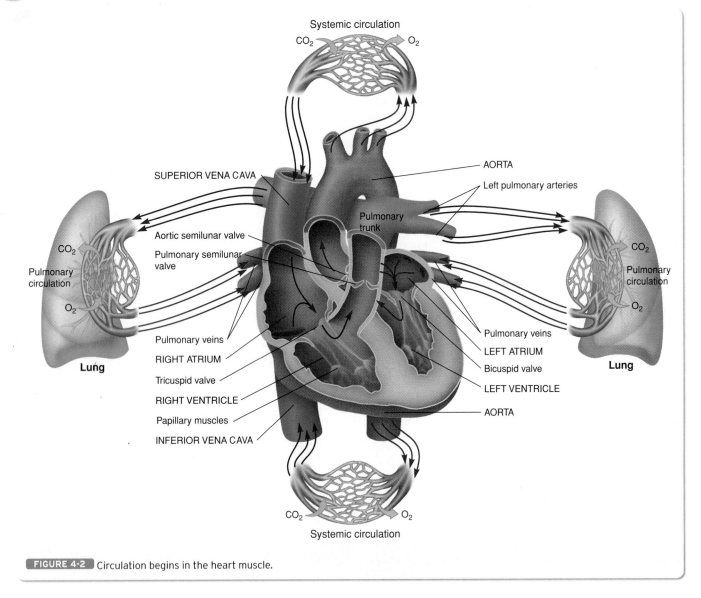

FIGURE 4-2 Circulation begins in the heart muscle.

The left ventricle pumps blood into the aorta for distribution to the entire body. The left ventricle is the most muscular and strongest chamber of the heart.

The upper and lower portions of the heart are separated by the atrioventricular valves, which prevent backward flow of blood. The semilunar valves, which serve a similar function, are located between the ventricles and the arteries into which they pump blood. Blood enters the right atrium via the superior and inferior venae cavae and the **coronary sinus**, which consists of veins that collect blood returning from the walls of the heart. Blood from four **pulmonary veins** enters the left atrium.

Blood Flow Within the Heart

Two large veins, the **superior vena cava** and the **inferior vena cava**, return deoxygenated blood from the body to the right atrium **FIGURE 4-2 ▲**. Blood from the upper part of the body returns to the heart through the superior vena cava; blood from the lower part of the body returns through the

inferior vena cava (the larger of the two veins). From the right atrium, blood passes through the tricuspid valve into the right ventricle. The right ventricle then pumps the blood through the pulmonic valve into the **pulmonary artery** and then to the lungs.

In the lungs, oxygen is returned to the blood and carbon dioxide and other waste products are removed from it. The freshly oxygenated blood returns to the left atrium through the pulmonary veins. Blood then flows through the mitral valve into the left ventricle, which pumps the oxygenated blood through the aortic valve, into the **aorta** (the body's largest artery), and then to the entire body.

Major Arteries and Veins

Arteries carry blood away from the heart **FIGURE 4-3 ▶**. Arterial blood is oxygenated except for that in the pulmonary artery, which carries oxygen-poor blood from the right ventricle to the lungs. The coronary arteries arise from the base of the aorta and supply blood to the heart muscle. The aorta

Major Arteries

Major Veins

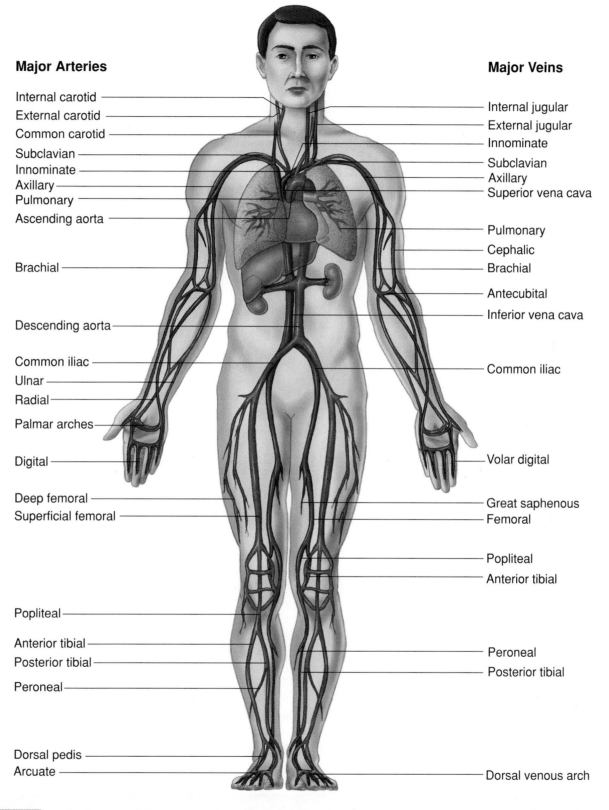

Internal carotid

External carotid

Common carotid

Subclavian

Innominate

Axillary

Pulmonary

Ascending aorta

Brachial

Descending aorta

Common iliac

Ulnar

Radial

Palmar arches

Digital

Deep femoral

Superficial femoral

Popliteal

Anterior tibial

Posterior tibial

Peroneal

Dorsal pedis

Arcuate

Internal jugular

External jugular

Innominate

Subclavian

Axillary

Superior vena cava

Pulmonary

Cephalic

Brachial

Antecubital

Inferior vena cava

Common iliac

Volar digital

Great saphenous

Femoral

Popliteal

Anterior tibial

Peroneal

Posterior tibial

Dorsal venous arch

FIGURE 4-3   The major veins and arteries of the human body.

proceeds superiorly from the left ventricle, curves to the left, then travels along the spine inferiorly, splitting at the level of the umbilicus to form the right and left iliac arteries. As the iliac arteries reach the thighs, the arteries are called the femoral arteries. The right and left pulmonary arteries carry oxygen-poor blood to the lungs. The carotid arteries arise from the aorta bilaterally and travel through the neck to supply blood to the head and brain. The external and internal carotid arteries split superiorly in the neck.

The largest arteries of the lower extremities split into the superficial and deep femoral arteries bilaterally. The brachial arteries are bilateral, and are the continuance of the subclavian artery in the upper arm to the elbow. The brachial artery splits at the level of the elbow to form the radial and ulnar arteries, two large arteries in each forearm. The posterior tibial artery is found at the posterior aspect of the medial malleolus. The dorsalis pedis artery is located at the top of the foot. An **arteriole** is the smallest branch of an artery. **Capillaries** are tiny blood vessels arising from the arterioles; they are found throughout the body. This is where oxygen (O_2) and carbon dioxide (CO_2) are exchanged, nutrients are delivered to the tissues, and waste products are removed.

A **venule** is the smallest branch of a vein. **Veins** carry blood from the capillaries back to the heart. Important veins include the venae cavae (the superior vena cava and the inferior vena cava), and the pulmonary vein. The venae cavae return blood to the right atrium. The superior vena cava (SVC) drains blood mostly from the upper extremities and the head. The inferior vena cava (IVC) drains blood received from the thorax, abdomen, pelvis, and lower extremities. The pulmonary vein carries oxygenated blood from the lungs to the left atrium of the heart.

Blood and Its Components

Blood consists of plasma and formed elements or cells that are suspended in the plasma. These cells include red blood cells (RBCs), white blood cells (WBCs), and platelets. The purpose of blood is to carry oxygen and nutrients to the tissues and cellular waste products away from the tissues. In addition, the formed elements serve as the mainstay of numerous other body functions, such as fighting infections and controlling bleeding.

Plasma is a watery, straw-colored fluid that accounts for more than half of the total blood volume. It consists of 92% water and 8% dissolved substances such as chemicals, minerals, and nutrients. It transports proteins, hormones, blood cell components, glucose, and other substances to various tissues, organs, and other targets in the body. It also transports waste to be excreted by the body via the lungs, liver, or kidneys. Water enters the plasma from the digestive tract, from fluids between cells, and as a by-product of metabolism.

The **red blood cells (erythrocytes)** are the most numerous of the formed elements. Their primary function is to carry oxygen to the tissues and carbon dioxide away from the tissues. Erythrocytes are unable to move on their own; instead, the flowing plasma passively propels them to their destinations. RBCs contain **hemoglobin**, a protein that gives them their reddish color. Hemoglobin binds oxygen that is absorbed in the lungs and transports it to the tissues where it is needed.

Several types of **white blood cells (leukocytes)** exist, each of which has a different function. The primary function of all white blood cells is to fight infection. White blood cells are involved in destroying microorganisms. Antibodies to fight infection may be produced, or leukocytes may directly attack and kill bacterial invaders.

Platelets (thrombocytes) are small cells in the blood that are essential for clot formation. The blood clotting (coagulation) process is a complex series of events involving platelets, clotting proteins in the plasma (clotting factors), other proteins, and calcium. During coagulation, platelets aggregate in a clump and form much of the foundation of a blood clot. Clotting proteins produced by the liver solidify the remainder of the clot, which eventually includes red and white blood cells.

Perfusion

Perfusion is the circulation of blood within an organ or tissue in adequate amounts to meet the cells' current needs for oxygen, nutrients, and waste removal. Blood must pass through the cardiovascular system at a speed that is fast enough to maintain adequate circulation throughout the body, yet slow enough to allow each cell time to exchange oxygen and nutrients for carbon dioxide and other waste products. Although some tissues, such as the lungs and kidneys, never rest and require a constant blood supply, most tissues require circulating blood only intermittently, but especially when they are active. Muscles, for example, are at rest and require a minimal blood supply when you sleep. In contrast, during exercise, muscles need a large blood supply. As another example, the gastrointestinal (GI) tract requires a high flow of blood after a meal. After digestion is completed, it can do quite well with a small fraction of that flow.

The autonomic nervous system monitors the body's needs from moment to moment, adjusting the blood flow as required. During emergencies, it automatically redirects blood away from other organs and toward the heart, brain, lungs, and kidneys. Thus, the cardiovascular system is dynamic, constantly adapting to changing conditions. Sometimes, however, it fails to provide sufficient circulation for every body part to perform its function, resulting in hypoperfusion or shock.

The heart requires constant perfusion, or it will not function properly. The brain and spinal cord cannot go for more than 4 to 6 minutes without perfusion, or the nerve cells will be permanently damaged—recall that cells of the central nervous system do not have the capacity to regenerate. The kidneys will be damaged after 45 minutes of inadequate perfusion. Skeletal muscles demonstrate difficulty tolerating more than 2 hours of inadequate perfusion. The GI tract can exist with limited (but not absent) perfusion for several hours. These times are based on a normal body temperature (98.6°F

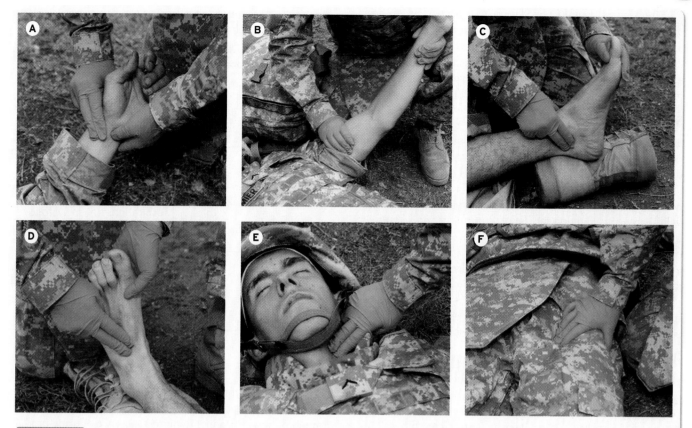

FIGURE 4-4 The locations for assessing a casualty's pulse. **A.** Radial pulse. **B.** Brachial pulse. **C.** Posterior tibial pulse. **D.** Dorsalis pedis (pedal) pulse. **E.** Carotid pulse. **F.** Femoral pulse.

[37.0°C]). An organ or tissue that is considerably colder is better able to resist damage from hypoperfusion because of the slowing of the body's metabolism.

The pulse forms when the left ventricle contracts, sending a wave of blood through the arterial system. The locations for assessing a casualty's pulse are **FIGURE 4-4 ▲** :

- Radial pulse
- Brachial pulse
- Posterior tibial pulse
- Dorsalis pedis (pedal) pulse
- Carotid pulse
- Femoral pulse

Blood pressure is the force blood exerts against the walls of blood vessels. Systolic pressure is created in the arteries by blood when the left ventricle contracts. It is reported first, in units of mm Hg (millimeters of mercury). The normal systolic range in adults is 90 to 145. Diastolic pressure measures what remains in the arteries when the left ventricle of the heart is relaxed and refilling. It is reported second. The normal diastolic range in adults is 60 to 85 mm Hg.

Stethoscopes and blood pressure cuffs are rarely available or effective to the combat medic in the typically noisy and chaotic battlefield environment. A palpable radial pulse and normal mentation (mental activity) may be the best indicators of the need to initiate fluid therapy.

■ Identify Hemorrhage and Hypovolemic Shock

<u>Hemorrhage</u> (bleeding) is the escape of blood and plasma from capillaries, veins, and arteries. The average adult body contains approximately 5 to 6 L of blood and can normally lose 1 to 2 pints of blood (the usual amount given by donors, about one fourth of an IV bag) without any harmful effects. The severity of hemorrhage depends on the amount of blood lost in relation to the physical size of the casualty. The amount of visible blood is often not a good way to judge the severity of an injury; for example, serious injuries, such as open femur fractures, do not bleed heavily externally whereas relatively minor injuries, such as a scalp laceration, will bleed profusely.

Internal bleeding can result in severe blood loss with resultant shock (hypoperfusion) and subsequent death. Suspicion and severity of internal bleeding should be based on the mechanism of injury (MOI). Although not usually visible, internal bleeding can result in serious blood loss. A casualty with internal bleeding can develop shock before you realize the extent of the casualty's injuries.

The casualty's baseline medical condition has a great effect on the severity of shock. High-risk casualties include multiple trauma casualties, pregnant women, the elderly, and casualties with chronic medical conditions and taking multiple medications.

Traumatized, painful, swollen, and deformed extremities, or long bone fractures may also lead to serious internal blood loss. A fractured humerus or tibia may be associated with the loss of up to 750 mL of blood. A femur fracture is commonly associated with a loss of 1,500 mL, and several liters of blood may accumulate in the pelvis from a pelvic fracture.

Sources of Bleeding and Characteristics

Arterial bleeding is rapid, profuse, and pulsating with the blood escaping in spurts synchronized with the pulse. It is usually bright red because it is rich in oxygen.

This type of bleeding is the least frequent, but it is the most serious form of hemorrhage encountered on the battlefield. Early consideration for use of a tourniquet on a severely bleeding extremity in the tactical environment is the standard of care. As per Tactical Combat Casualty Care (TC-3), early use of *temporary* tourniquets will greatly decrease the mortality of severely injured casualties.

Venous bleeding is a steady flow. It is usually dark red or maroon in color because it is oxygen-poor. Capillary bleeding is slow and oozing. It often clots spontaneously.

Hypovolemic Shock

Hypovolemic shock is a state of inadequate tissue perfusion, with markedly decreased blood flow, oxygen delivery, and glucose supply to vital tissues and organs. In hypovolemic shock, the body's compensatory mechanisms redistribute blood flow to the three vital organs: the kidneys, heart, and brain. Hypovolemic shock can be due to blood loss (hemorrhagic) or less often to fluid loss. For many casualties in hypovolemic shock, the cause will be immediately apparent (eg, obvious bleeding or severe diarrhea). Internal hemorrhage may not be so obvious. Any injured casualty who has cool, clammy skin and is tachycardic (pulse > 100 beats/min) is in hypovolemic shock until proven otherwise.

Almost all casualties with multiple injuries will have a degree of hypovolemia. **Hypovolemia** occurs when there is a large drop in body fluids, such as following a severe burn, severe vomiting, and/or diarrhea. Severe internal bleeding occurs in injuries caused by a violent force (blunt force injury); puncture wounds (knife), and fractures. The clinical signs of acute hemorrhage with hypovolemic shock are listed in **TABLE 4-1 ▸** .

Another common sign of hypovolemic shock is cool, clammy, and pale skin caused by the constriction of peripheral blood vessels (cool), activation of sweat glands (clammy), and cellular ischemia (pale). Cyanosis is another sign; it is a bluish tinge of the nailbeds, lips, and earlobes.

A rapid, weak, and thready pulse is another sign. The rapid heart rate is a compensatory mechanism where the body attempts to increase cardiac output, which increases oxygen supply to tissue. The weak and thready pulse is caused by a narrowing pulse pressure due to a fall in systolic blood pressure and a rise in diastolic blood pressure (secondary to vasoconstriction).

In later stages of hypovolemic shock, the pulses may be imperceptible. Shallow, rapid breathing and grunting may

TABLE 4-1 Clinical Signs of Acute Hemorrhage With Hypovolemic Shock

Class	% Blood Loss	Clinical Signs
I	< 750 mL (15%)	Slight increase in heart rate; no change in blood pressure or respiratory rate
II	750 to 1,500 mL (15% to 30%)	Increased heart rate and respirations; increased diastolic blood pressure, anxiety, fright, or hostility
III	1,500 to 2,000 mL (30% to 40%)	Increased heart rate and respirations; fall in systolic blood pressure; significant altered mental status
IV	> 2,000 mL (> 40%)	Severe tachycardia; severe lowering of systolic blood pressure; cold and pale skin; severely altered mental status

be heard. Body temperature may be subnormal due to a depressed heat-regulating mechanism. **Oliguria** (diminished urine production) leading to **anuria** (absence of urine production) are additional signs of hypovolemic shock. This occurs due to the body's effort to salvage the two primary organs—the brain and the heart (shunting of blood away from the renal arteries in an attempt to provide increased perfusion of the heart, lungs, and brain). As shock worsens, listlessness, stupor, and loss of consciousness occur. Other symptoms include **polydipsia** (excessive thirst).

Internal signs of hemorrhage with hypovolemic shock may include the above findings, plus:

- Bruising, which indicates bleeding into the skin (soft tissues)
- Tenderness or rigidity of the abdomen or pelvis
- **Hemoptysis** (coughing up blood)
- Vomiting blood the color of coffee grounds or bright red (**hematemesis**); the blood may be mixed with food
- Passing of feces with a black, tarry appearance (**melena**) or the passing of bright red blood through the rectum

Hemorrhage

As stated before, hemorrhage simply means bleeding. Bleeding can range from a nick to a capillary while shaving, to a severely spurting artery from a deep slash with a knife, to a ruptured spleen from striking the steering column during a car crash. External bleeding (visible hemorrhage) can usually be easily controlled by using direct pressure or a pressure bandage. Internal bleeding (hemorrhage that is not visible) is usually not controlled until a surgeon locates the source and sutures it closed. Because internal bleeding is not as obvious, you must rely on signs and symptoms to determine the extent and severity of the hemorrhage.

External Hemorrhage
External bleeding is usually due to a break in the skin. External bleeding includes lacerations, puncture wounds, amputation, abrasions, and incisions. Its extent or severity is often a function of the type of wound and the types of blood vessels that have been injured. Bleeding from a capillary usually oozes, bleeding from a vein flows, and bleeding from an artery spurts.

These descriptions are not infallible. For example, considerable oozing from capillaries is possible when a casualty gets a very large abrasion (such as road rash). Likewise, varicose veins in the leg can produce copious bleeding.

Arteries may spurt initially, but as the casualty's BP decreases, often the blood simply flows. In addition, an artery that is incised directly across or in a transverse manner will often recoil and attempt to slow its own bleeding. By contrast, if the artery is cut on a bias, it does not recoil and continues to bleed.

Some injuries that you might expect to be accompanied by considerable external bleeding do not always have serious hemorrhaging. For example, a person who falls off the platform at the train station and is run over by a train may have amputations of one or more extremities, yet experience little bleeding because the wound was cauterized by the heat of the train's wheels on the rail. Conversely, a person who pulled over on the shoulder of the road and was removing the jack from his car's trunk when another motorist slammed into the rear of the car, pinning him between the two vehicles, may have severely crushed legs. In such a case, bleeding may be severe, with the only effective means of bleeding control being two tourniquets.

Internal Hemorrhage
Internal bleeding as a result of trauma may appear in any portion of the body. A fracture of a small bone (such as humerus, ankle, or tibia) produces a somewhat controlled environment in which a relatively small amount of bleeding can occur. By contrast, bleeding into the trunk (that is, thorax, abdomen, or pelvis), because of its much larger space, tends to be severe and uncontrolled. Nontraumatic internal hemorrhage usually occurs in cases of GI bleeding from the upper or lower GI tract, ruptured ectopic pregnancies, ruptured aneurysms, or other conditions.

Any internal bleeding must be treated promptly. The signs of internal hemorrhage (such as discoloration or hematoma) do not always develop quickly, so you must rely on other signs and symptoms and an evaluation of the MOI (fall, blast injury, penetrating trauma) to make this diagnosis. Pay close attention to casualty complaints of pain or tenderness, development of tachycardia, and pallor. In addition to evaluating the MOI, be alert for the development of shock when you suspect internal bleeding.

Management of a casualty with internal hemorrhaging focuses on the treatment of shock. Eventually, the casualty will likely need a surgical procedure to stop the bleeding.

Controlled Versus Uncontrolled Hemorrhage
Bleeding that you can control (such as external bleeding that responds to direct pressure) and bleeding that you cannot control (such as a bleeding peptic ulcer) are serious emergencies. As a consequence, the initial assessment of the casualty includes a search for life-threatening bleeding. If found, the hemorrhage must be controlled; if the hemorrhage cannot be controlled on the battlefield, all of your efforts should concentrate on attempting to control the bleeding as you await evacuation.

Most external bleeding can be managed with direct pressure, although arterial bleeding may take five or more minutes of direct pressure to form a clot. (Remember this if you accidentally cannulate the brachial artery instead of the vein in the arm!) Military experience has shown that the use of pressure points is not as effective as previously thought and is difficult to manage while trying to rapidly evacuate a person from the battlefield. For this reason, most military medical training calls for use of a tourniquet for external bleeding to an extremity that cannot be controlled with direct pressure and a pressure bandage.

Field Medical Care TIPS

Consider bleeding to be serious if any of the following conditions are present:
- A significant MOI, especially when the MOI suggests that severe forces affected the abdomen or chest
- Poor general appearance of the casualty
- Signs and symptoms of shock
- Significant amount of blood loss
- Rapid blood loss
- Uncontrollable bleeding

Physiologic Response to Hemorrhage
Typically, bleeding from an open artery is bright red (because of the high oxygen content) and spurts in time with the pulse. The pressure that causes the blood to spurt also makes this type of bleeding difficult to control. As the amount of blood circulating in the body drops, so does the casualty's BP and, eventually, the arterial spurting.

Blood from an open vein is much darker (low oxygen content) and flows steadily. Because it is under less pressure, most venous blood does not spurt and is easier to manage. Bleeding from damaged capillary vessels is dark red and oozes from a wound steadily but slowly. Venous and capillary bleeding is more likely to clot spontaneously than arterial bleeding.

On its own, bleeding tends to stop rather quickly, within about 10 minutes, in response to internal clotting mechanisms and exposure to air. When vessels are lacerated, blood flows rapidly from the open vessel. The open ends of the vessel then begin to narrow (vasoconstrict), which reduces the amount of bleeding. Platelets aggregate at the site, plugging the hole and sealing the injured portions of the vessel, a process called **hemostasis**. Bleeding will not stop if a clot does not form, unless the injured vessel is completely cut off from the main blood supply. Direct contact with body tissues and fluids or the external environment commonly triggers the blood's clotting factors.

Despite the efficiency of this system, it may fail in certain situations. A number of medications, including anticoagulants such as aspirin and prescription blood thinners, interfere with normal clotting. With a severe injury, the damage to the vessel may be so extensive that a clot cannot completely block the hole. Sometimes, only part of the vessel wall is cut, preventing it from constricting. In these cases, bleeding will continue unless it is stopped by external means. In a case involving acute blood loss, the casualty might die before the body's hemostatic defenses of vasoconstriction and clotting can help.

■ Hemorrhage Treatment

Direct pressure is the quickest method to control bleeding. Keep in mind that in a tactical environment, the use of temporary tourniquets is the treatment of choice for controlling rapid or massive bleeding on the battlefield. The application of combat application tourniquets is covered in detail in Chapter 1, *Introduction to Battlefield Medicine*. Application of a standard tourniquet is covered later in this chapter.

To control bleeding through direct pressure, first completely expose the wound.

Place a sterile dressing on the wound and apply pressure with your hand until the bleeding has stopped. Use a bandage or cravat to tie a knot over or tape directly over the sterile dressing covering the wound. Ensure that the bandage is only tight enough to control the bleeding. If the bleeding is not controlled, apply another dressing over the first or apply direct pressure with your hand over the wound. The casualty or another soldier can assist you in applying direct pressure FIGURE 4-5 ▼ .

Elevate an injured arm or leg above the level of the heart. Elevation should be used in conjunction with direct pressure. Do not elevate an extremity if you suspect a fracture until it has been properly splinted and you are certain that elevation will not cause further injury. Use a stable object to maintain elevation, such as a rucksack; placing the extremity on an unstable object may cause further injury.

If the bleeding is not controlled with direct pressure and a field dressing, you may need to apply a pressure dressing to control bleeding. Place a roll of Kerlix, an Ace wrap, or a cravat over the previous dressing directly over the wound. (You may use anything to apply extra pressure over the wound, even a rock.) Place an additional dressing, roller gauze, Ace wrap, cravat, or other material over the pressure device and wrap this additional dressing over the wound and previous dressing. This will assist in applying increased pressure to control the bleeding. Secure the pressure dressing in place so it will not slip. The Emergency (Israeli) bandage is used very effectively as a pressure dressing and can easily control severe hemorrhage.

Pressure points are used in cases of severe bleeding when direct pressure and elevation are not effective in controlling the bleeding. Applying pressure to the appropriate pressure point may control arterial bleeding. Pressure points are the areas of the body where the blood flow can be controlled by pressing the artery against an underlying bone. Pressure is applied with the fingers, thumb, or heel of the hand.

The pressure points most often used include:

- **Arm (brachial):** Used to control severe bleeding of the lower part of the arm and elbow. Located above the elbow on the inside of the arm in the groove between the muscles. Using your fingers or thumb, apply pressure to the inside of the arm over the bone FIGURE 4-6 ▼ .
- **Groin (femoral) area:** Used to control severe bleeding of the thigh and lower leg. Located on the front, center part of the crease in the groin FIGURE 4-7 ▶ .

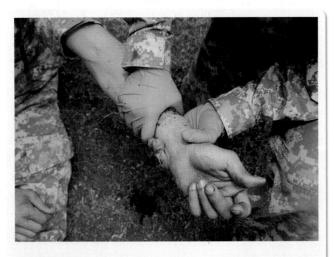

FIGURE 4-5 Try to control bleeding first through direct pressure.

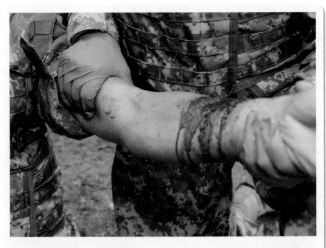

FIGURE 4-6 The brachial pressure point is used to control bleeding of the lower part of the arm and elbow.

To apply pressure to the casualty's pressure points, position the casualty on his or her back, kneeling on the opposite side from the wounded extremity. Place the heel of your hand directly on the pressure point and lean forward to apply pressure. If the bleeding is not controlled, it may be necessary to press directly over the artery with the flat surface of your fingertips; apply additional pressure on the fingertips with the heel of your other hand.

Splinting or immobilization is an effective means of controlling bleeding. Broken bone fragments may continue to grate on blood vessels and increase bleeding if they are not immobilized; muscular activity can also increase the rate of blood flow. Pneumatic (air) splints may be used to apply direct circumferential pressure over an extremity, compressing the extremity, its soft tissues, and the bleeding vessels. Splinting using a pneumatic splint gives a double benefit: splinting and direct pressure.

Principles of Tourniquet Use

In a combat scenario under enemy fire, a tourniquet is the initial choice to stop major extremity hemorrhage. Although many civilian prehospital texts and other authorities discourage the use of tourniquets, tourniquets are appropriate and lifesaving in combat. Direct pressure and pressure points are impossible to maintain during casualty transport when under effective fire. Tissue and nerve damage is rare if the tourniquet is left in place for less than 2 hours.

During orthopaedic surgery, surgeons routinely apply tourniquets to reduce bleeding, and leave them in place for 2 hours, without any adverse effects to the limb. Longer tourniquet times are possible without injury, but the longer a tourniquet is left in place, the more likely ischemia or nerve damage will occur. With massive hemorrhage and amputations, it

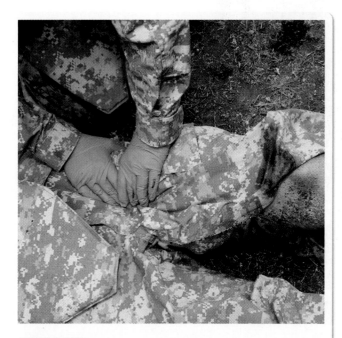

The femoral pressure point is used to control severe bleeding of the thigh and lower leg.

is better to accept the small risk of tissue and nerve damage than lose a casualty to blood loss and hypovolemic shock.

Direct pressure, elevation, pressure dressings, or pressure points will not control some bleeding; prompt application of a tourniquet may be life saving. If the nature of the wound is such that direct pressure or pressure points will not be effective, go directly to a tourniquet. Traumatic amputation of an extremity is one of those situations. Forceful, arterial bleeding from an extremity wound may require early use of a tourniquet. In this case, do not waste time attempting a pressure dressing.

To be effective in saving a life, the decision to apply a tourniquet needs to be made very quickly (seconds, not minutes), and the application needs to be equally fast (seconds, not minutes). A tourniquet ideally is 1″ to 2″ in width; this width decreases the amount of nerve and tissue damage occurring under the tourniquet. If this width is not available, use any equipment that will create an effective tourniquet.

Standard Tourniquet Procedure

To apply a standard tourniquet, follow the steps in **SKILL DRILL 4-1 ▸** :

1. Place the tourniquet between the heart and the wound, leaving at least 2″ of uninjured skin between the tourniquet and the wound. Do not apply the cravat directly over the wound unless you have no other choice. Do not apply a tourniquet over a joint. If you do not have a cravat, use a belt, rope, a strap from load bearing equipment/load carrying equipment (LBE/LCE), roller gauze, a torn battle dress uniform (BDU) sleeve, a BP cuff (pumped up to at least 200 mm Hg), or any other material that is immediately available (**Step ①**).

2. Place a roll or pad over the artery to be compressed.

3. Wrap the tourniquet around the extremity, and tie a half-knot (overhand) anteriorly over the padding. Do not apply the knot directly over the wound unless you have no other choice (**Step ②**).

4. After tying the half-knot, place a stick or similar object (windlass) on the half-knot, tie a square knot, and start twisting. Twisting will tighten the bandage; keep twisting until the bleeding stops. Tourniquets should be tightened to eliminate the distal pulse. If a stick is not available, use a tent peg or bayonet scabbard; use whatever materials you may have at hand (**Step ③**).

5. Secure the windlass in place so it doesn't unwind, and transport the victim as quickly as possible to a medical treatment facility (MTF). Use additional bandaging if necessary. Tourniquet sites should be exposed during the Tactical Field Care phase (**Step ④**).

6. If time allows, using a marker, make a "T" on the casualty's forehead. You can also mark a "T" and the time that you applied the tourniquet. Place the time and date the tourniquet was applied on a field medical card (FMC) attached to the casualty.

SKILL DRILL 4-1

Applying a Standard Tourniquet

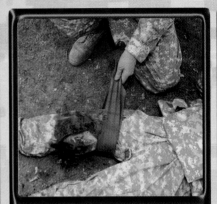

1 Place the tourniquet between the heart and the wound, leaving at least 2" of uninjured skin between the tourniquet and the wound. Do not apply the cravat directly over the wound unless you have no other choice. If you don't have a cravat, use any other material that is immediately available.

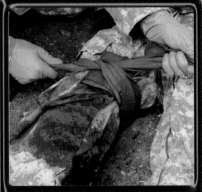

2 Place a roll or pad over the artery to be compressed. Wrap the tourniquet around the extremity, and tie a half-knot (overhand) anteriorly over the padding. Do not apply the knot directly over the wound unless you have no other choice.

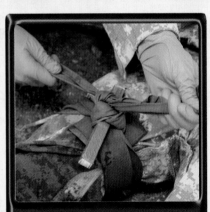

3 After tying the half-knot, place a stick or similar object (windlass) on the half-knot, tie a square knot, and start twisting. Twisting will tighten the bandage; keep twisting until the bleeding stops. Tighten until the distal pulse is eliminated in the wounded extremity. If a stick is not available, use whatever materials you may have at hand.

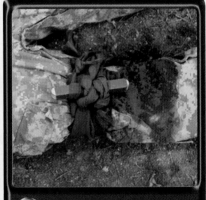

4 Secure the windlass in place so it doesn't unwind, and transport the victim as quickly as possible. Use additional bandaging if necessary. Avoid covering the tourniquet.

Tourniquet removal should not be attempted if the anticipated evacuation time is less than 2 hours.

Amputation Care

In the case of complete amputation, apply a dressing to cover the end of the stump. Often blood vessels collapse or retract, limiting the bleeding from the wound site. Control bleeding by tourniquet. When possible, wrap the amputated part in a dry sterile dressing.

To preserve amputated parts, rinse the amputated part free of debris with saline, if available. Wrap the part loosely in saline-moistened sterile gauze, and seal the amputated part inside a plastic bag or wrap in a cravat. The amputated part should then be placed in another container containing ice. Keep cool, but do not allow it to freeze. To avoid further injury to the amputated part:

- Never warm an amputated part.
- Never place an amputated part in water.
- Never place an amputated part directly in contact with ice.
- Never use dry ice to cool an amputated part.

■ Treatment for Hypovolemic Shock

Treatment Goals

The goal of treating hypovolemic shock is to increase tissue perfusion and oxygenation status. Treatment is directed at providing adequate oxygenation and ventilation, stopping the bleeding, and maintaining circulation with the replacement of appropriate fluids.

Treatment Steps

To treat hypovolemic shock, follow the steps in **SKILL DRILL 4-2** :

1. Ensure an open airway using the head tilt–chin lift or jaw-thrust maneuver.

2. Provide ventilatory support, if required, by providing oxygen at 15 L/min by nonrebreathing mask as soon as possible.

3. Control external bleeding through direct pressure, pressure points, splinting, or a tourniquet.

4. If it is possible and you have assistance, control breathing and bleeding simultaneously. However, on the battlefield, control bleeding first. A tourniquet may be your first choice.

5. Circulation can be maintained through IV fluid administration, which is covered in detail in Chapter 13, *Intravenous Access*.

6. Obtain a set of baseline vital signs and a brief neurologic examination that determines level of consciousness (AVPU), eye motion, and pupillary response.

7. Position the casualty and expose the hemorrhage sites. Place the casualty so the head is lower than the feet if possible (except in head or suspected neck injuries and suspected respiratory compromise); elevate the legs 6″ to 12″ (Trendelenberg position). If the casualty is vomiting or bleeding around the mouth, place the

Field Medical Care TIPS

CELOX (pronounced *cell-locks*) is the newest generation of emergency hemostatic agents. CELOX quickly controls even the most severe arterial bleeding. Just pour granules in, pack, and apply pressure. CELOX and CELOX ACS are awaiting FDA approval. CELOX works in hypothermic conditions and clots heparinized blood. CELOX is safe to use on the entire body including head, neck, and chest wounds. CELOX can be used instantly and without hesitation as a fast, safe, and simple emergency treatment for serious bleeding.

casualty on his or her side (recumbent) or back with the head turned to the side (except in the case of head or suspected spinal injuries). When exposing the casualty, look for associated injuries (eg, gunshot wounds with an entrance injury usually have an exit injury).

8. Attempt to maintain normal body temperature, to prevent hypothermia and minimize the effects of shock. Wrap the casualty in a blanket or poncho liner, if available.

9. Perform the neurologic examination and measure the vital signs every 5 minutes.

10. Transport the casualty to the nearest MTF as soon as possible.

■ Summary

As a combat medic, knowledge of the principles and techniques of controlling hemorrhage, by direct pressure or the judicious use of a tourniquet, can save soldiers' lives on the battlefield. Keep in mind that in a tactical environment, the use of temporary tourniquets is the treatment of choice for controlling rapid or massive extremity bleeding on the battlefield.

YOU ARE THE
COMBAT MEDIC

While on patrol, your squad enters the courtyard of a house and begins taking fire from a second story balcony. Your exposed position allows the enemy to use small arms and hand grenades against your team. Due to effective leadership and teamwork, your squad quickly gains fire supremacy and neutralizes the threat. Once a cease-fire has been called, you hear someone shout, "Medic!" As you run across the courtyard, you see a soldier lying on the ground holding a bloody hand over his left eye with a large amount of blood flowing from his left upper arm. The squad leader tells you that two enemy combatants are dead on the balcony, the situation is secure, and that you are treating the only casualty. The closest MTF is 40 miles away.

Assessment

Upon evaluation of the casualty, you notice he is anxious, complaining of pain to his left eye, and an inability to see. He appears to be unaware of the injury to his arm. You notice his respirations are increased and his skin is cool, pale, and diaphoretic. Since he is speaking to you without difficulty, you determine his airway to be intact and proceed to remove his body armor and expose his chest. Seeing no signs of chest trauma, with equal, bilateral chest expansion and no accessory muscle use, you focus your attention on his face and arm. There is blood flowing from a 1 cm laceration above his left eyebrow and pooling in his left eye. You also note a large amount of dark red, maroon-colored blood flowing heavily from his left upper arm and no apparent other bleeding. The casualty's radial pulses are present, but weak and rapid bilaterally.

Treatment

Treatment of this casualty follows the ABCs of care. His airway is open and breathing is adequate. Although he is distracted by the minor laceration to his eyebrow, his more threatening problem is the significant venous bleeding in his left upper extremity. Because you are not under direct fire and have assistance, you decide not to use a tourniquet yet. You expose the left upper arm completely and notice multiple deep lacerations of varying lengths most likely caused by shrapnel from one of the grenades. Using a sterile dressing to apply direct pressure, you instruct a combat lifesaver (CLS) to assist you by maintaining the direct pressure while you prepare a pressure bandage. Once the pressure bandage is applied, you instruct the CLS to apply pressure to the

brachial artery pressure point. The bleeding now seems to be controlled and you instruct the squad leader to call for aeromedical evacuation.

Recognizing the need for IV fluid administration, you decide to defer it for the moment and obtain a baseline set of vital signs: blood pressure 100/50 mm Hg, heart rate 30 beats/min weak and regular, respirations 22 breaths/min nonlabored. During your rapid trauma survey, you find no other significant injuries and decide to clean and bandage his left eye. When you reassess the bleeding in his arm, you find that it has completely stopped. As a perimeter and nearby landing zone are established, you decide to use the time waiting for the evacuation to obtain IV access and begin fluid administration. You also elevate the casualty's legs by placing them on top of a rucksack and cover him with a poncho liner to treat him for shock. The aero-medical evacuation team arrives and assumes care for the casualty as they transport him to the MTF.

---

1. LAST NAME, FIRST NAME		RANK/GRADE	X	MALE
Gomez, Robert		SGT/E5		FEMALE
SSN	SPECIALTY CODE			RELIGION
555-000-1234	00A			Catholic

2. UNIT

FORCE				NATIONALITY			
A/T	AF/A	N/M	MC/M				
	BC/BC		NBI/BNC		DISEASE		PSYCH

3. INJURY

AIRWAY	
HEAD	
X WOUND	
NECK/BACK INJURY	
BURN	
AMPUTATION	
STRESS	
OTHER (Specify)	

FRONT   BACK

4. LEVEL OF CONSCIOUSNESS

X	ALERT		PAIN RESPONSE
	VERBAL RESPONSE		UNRESPONSIVE

5. PULSE	TIME	6. TOURNIQUET		TIME
130	2141	X NO ☐ YES		

7. MORPHINE		DOSE	TIME	8. IV	TIME
X NO ☐ YES				X	2150

9. TREATMENT/OBSERVATIONS/CURRENT MEDICATION/ALLERGIES/NBC (ANTIDOTE)

Clean & bandage LW over eye. Obtained IV access at 2150 to restore fluid.

10. DISPOSITION		RETURNED TO DUTY		TIME
	X	EVACUATED		
		DECEASED		

11. PROVIDER/UNIT	DATE (YYMMDD)
Smith, Jason	

Ready for Review

- Control of bleeding in a civilian environment is vastly different from the control of bleeding on the battlefield.
- Bleeding is the most common cause of shock.
- Internal bleeding can result in severe blood loss with resultant shock (hypoperfusion) and subsequent death.
- The goal of treating hypovolemic shock is to increase tissue perfusion and oxygenation status.
- Treatment is directed at providing adequate oxygenation and ventilation, stopping the bleeding, and maintaining circulation with the replacement of appropriate fluids.

Vital Vocabulary

anuria Absence of urine production.

aorta The principal artery leaving the left side of the heart and carrying freshly oxygenated blood to the body.

arteries The blood vessels that carry blood away from the heart.

arteriole The smallest branch of an artery leading to the vast network of capillaries.

blood The fluid tissue that is pumped by the heart through the arteries, veins, and capillaries; consists of plasma and formed elements or cells, such as red blood cells, white blood cells, and platelets.

capillary The fine end-divisions of the arterial system that allow contact between cells of the body tissues and the plasma and red blood cells.

coronary sinus Veins that collect blood that is returning from the walls of the heart.

heart A hollow muscular organ that receives blood from the veins and propels it into the arteries.

hematemesis Vomiting up blood.

hemoglobin An iron-containing pigment found in red blood cells; carries 97% of oxygen.

hemoptysis Coughing up blood.

hemorrhage The escape of blood and plasma from capillaries, veins, and arteries; bleeding.

hemostasis Control of bleeding by formation of a blood clot.

hypovolemia A large drop in body fluids.

hypovolemic shock A condition that occurs when the circulating blood volume is inadequate to deliver adequate oxygen and nutrients to the body.

inferior vena cava One of the two largest veins in the body; carries blood from the lower extremities and the pelvic and abdominal organs into the heart.

mediastinum The space between the lungs, in the center of the chest, that contains the heart, trachea, mainstem bronchi, part of the esophagus, and large blood vessels.

melena Passing of feces with a black, tarry appearance.

oliguria Diminished urine production.

perfusion The circulation of blood within an organ or tissue in adequate amounts to meet the cells' current needs.

plasma A sticky, yellow fluid that carries the blood cells and nutrients and transports cellular waste material to the organs of excretion.

platelets (thrombocytes) Tiny, disk-shaped elements that are much smaller than the cells; they are essential in the initial formation of a blood clot, the mechanism that stops bleeding.

polydipsia Excessive thirst.

pulmonary artery The major artery leading from the right ventricle of the heart to the lungs; it carries oxygen-poor blood.

pulmonary veins The four veins that return oxygenated blood from the lungs to the left atrium of the heart.

red blood cells (erythrocytes) Cells that carry oxygen to the body's tissues.

shock An abnormal state associated with inadequate oxygen and nutrient delivery to the metabolic apparatus of the cell.

superior vena cava One of the two largest veins in the body; carries blood from the upper extremities, head, neck, and chest into the heart.

veins The blood vessels that transport blood back to the heart.

venule The smallest branch of a vein.

white blood cells (leukocytes) Blood cells that play a role in the body's immune defense mechanisms against infection.

COMBAT MEDIC in Action

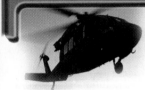

While on a routine mounted patrol in an urban area, the lead vehicle is struck by an IED and the patrol comes under direct small arms fire. As the firefight continues, you are called to treat the casualties who have now been removed from the vehicle. Casualty 1 is highly anxious with a complete amputation below the left knee. His respirations are rapid and he has a rapid, bounding radial pulse. Casualty 2 seems unusually calm with a large laceration to the left upper arm and a heavy flow of maroon blood. His respirations are rapid and his radial pulse is rapid and weak.

1. Which casualty is the most critical based on what you have assessed so far?
   A. Casualty 1
   B. Casualty 2
   C. Neither is critical
   D. Both

2. Based on the above information, how much of his blood supply has Casualty 1 lost?
   A. Less than 15%
   B. 15%-30%
   C. 30%-40%
   D. 100%

3. Which casualty would receive a tourniquet?
   A. Casualty 1 only
   B. Casualty 2 only
   C. Both
   D. Neither

4. If Casualty 1 were to suddenly become calm or lethargic, that might be a sign of:
   A. improvement. His anxiety has been relieved.
   B. decline. He is decompensating.
   C. acceptance of his injury and deformity.
   D. this is not a sign.

5. To care for Casualty 1's amputated extremity, you should
   1. Apply a dressing to cover the end of the stump.
   2. Rinse the amputated part free of debris with saline.
   3. Wrap the part loosely in saline-moistened sterile gauze.
   4. Place the amputated part directly on ice for transport with the casualty.
   5. Seal the amputated part in a plastic bag or wrap in a cravat.
   6. Submerse the amputated part in water if ice is unavailable.
      A. 1,2,3,4,5
      B. 1,2,3,5,6
      C. 1,2,3,5
      D. All of the above

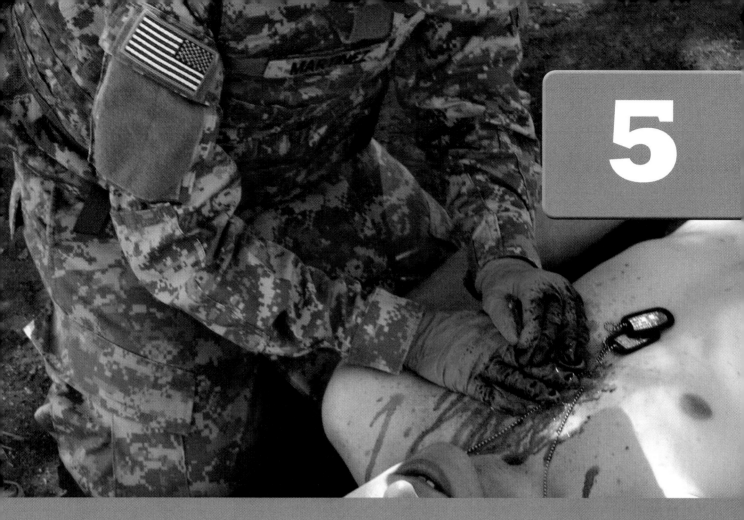

5

Injuries of the Thorax

Objectives

Knowledge Objectives

☐ Describe the anatomy and physiology of the thorax.

☐ Describe which thoracic injuries are associated with penetrating or blunt trauma.

☐ Identify immediate life-threatening thoracic injuries.

☐ Identify the signs and symptoms of a chest injury.

☐ Identify the steps to take to ensure that thoracic injuries do not become life-threatening.

Skills Objectives

☐ Perform an emergency needle decompression on the battlefield.

■ Introduction

Knowledge of the anatomy of the thoracic cavity is essential when managing chest trauma. You must recognize the signs and symptoms of major thoracic injuries and provide appropriate care. Open chest injuries can be the result of a motor vehicle accident, bullet, missile wound, fall, or blow. These injuries are serious and, unless treated rapidly and correctly, can result in significant mortality.

Thoracic trauma is not uniquely a disease of modern society. For as long as humans have been capable of falling or injuring one another, damage to the thoracic cavity has been a significant concern FIGURE 5-1 ▾ . Given the specific organs that are housed within the thoracic cavity, it is not surprising that these injuries can be so deadly. In addition, the mechanism producing these injuries often involves a great deal of force transmitted to the body.

■ Anatomy and Physiology of the Thorax

The **thorax** consists of a bony cage overlying some of the most vital organs in the human body. The dimensions of the thorax are defined posteriorly by the thoracic vertebrae and ribs, inferiorly by the diaphragm, anteriorly and laterally by the ribs, and superiorly by the **thoracic inlet** FIGURE 5-2 ▸ .

The dimensions of this area of the body are of great importance in the rapid trauma survey of the casualty. Although the thoracic cavity extends to the 12th rib posteriorly, the diaphragm inserts into the anterior thoracic cage just below the fourth or fifth rib. With the movement of the diaphragm during respiration, the size and dimensions of the thoracic cavity will vary FIGURE 5-3 ▸ , which could, in turn, affect the organs or cavities (thoracic versus abdominal) in a blunt or penetrating injury.

The bony structures of the thorax include the sternum, clavicle, scapula, thoracic vertebrae, and 12 pairs of ribs. The **sternum** consists of three separate portions: the superior **manubrium**, the central sternal body, and the inferior **xyphoid process**. The space superior to the manubrium is termed the **suprasternal notch**; the junction of the manubrium and sternal body is referred to as the **angle of Louis**.

The **clavicle** is an elongated, S-shaped bone that connects to the manubrium medially and overlies the first rib as it proceeds laterally toward the shoulder. Beneath the clavicle lies the subclavian artery and vein. Laterally, the clavicle connects to the acromion process of the **scapula**, the triangular bone that overlies the posterior aspect of the upper thoracic cage.

Each of the 12 matched pairs of ribs attach posteriorly to the 12 thoracic vertebrae FIGURE 5-4 ▸ . Anteriorly, the first

Field Medical Care TIPS

Thoracic injuries, whether severe or seemingly minor, often give rise to elusive findings that are overshadowed by associated injuries.

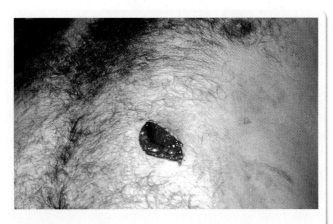

FIGURE 5-1 Thoracic trauma is a significant concern in casualty management.

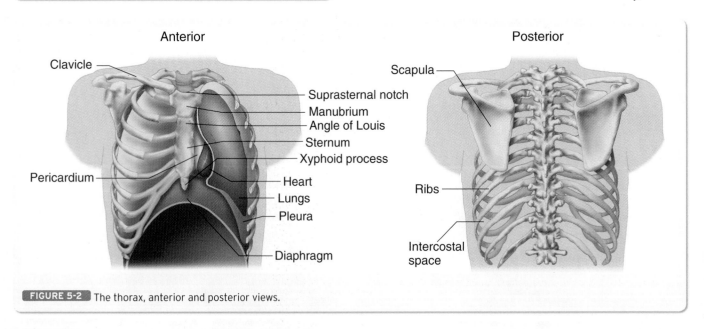

FIGURE 5-2 The thorax, anterior and posterior views.

seven pairs of ribs attach directly to the sternum via the costal cartilage. The costal cartilage then continues inferiorly from the seventh ribs and provides an indirect connection between the anterior portions of the 8th, 9th, and 10th ribs and the sternum. The 11th and 12th ribs have no anterior connection and, therefore, are known as the "floating ribs."

Between each rib lies an **intercostal space**. These spaces are numbered according to the rib superior to the space (ie, the space between the second and third ribs is the second intercostal space). These spaces house the intercostal muscles and the **neurovascular bundle**, which consists of an artery, vein, and nerve.

The central region of the thorax is the **mediastinum**, which contains the heart, great vessels, esophagus, lymphatic channels, trachea, mainstem bronchi, and paired vagus and phrenic nerves. The heart resides within a tough fibrous sac called the **pericardium**. Much like the pleura, the pericardium has two surfaces—the inner visceral layer, which adheres to the heart and forms the epicardium, and the outer parietal layer, which comprises the sac itself. The pericardium that covers the inferior aspect of the heart is directly attached to the diaphragm. The heart is positioned so that the most anterior portion is the right ventricle, which has relatively thin chamber walls. The pressure within the right ventricle is approximately one fourth of the pressure within the left ventricle. Most of the heart is protected anteriorly by the sternum. With each beat, the apex of the heart can be felt in the fifth intercostal space along the midclavicular line, a phenomenon known as cardiac impulse. The average cardiac output for an adult (heart rate times the stroke volume) is $70 \times 70 = 4{,}900$ mL/min, though it varies depending on the size of the individual.

The aorta is the largest artery in the body. As it exits the left ventricle, it ascends toward the right shoulder before turning to the left and proceeding inferiorly toward the abdomen. This artery has three points of attachment. These attachments represent sites of potential injury when the vessel is subject to significant shearing forces such as those seen during sudden deceleration mechanisms like a motor vehicle accident (MVA).

The lungs occupy most of the space within the thoracic cavity. Like the pericardium, the lungs are lined with a dual layer of connective tissue known as the **pleura**. The parietal pleura lines the interior of each side of the thoracic cavity. The visceral pleura lines the exterior of each lung.

A small amount of viscous fluid separates the two layers of pleura. This fluid allows the two layers of connective tissue to move against each other without friction or pain. It creates a surface tension that holds the layers together, thereby keeping the lung from collapsing away from the thoracic cage

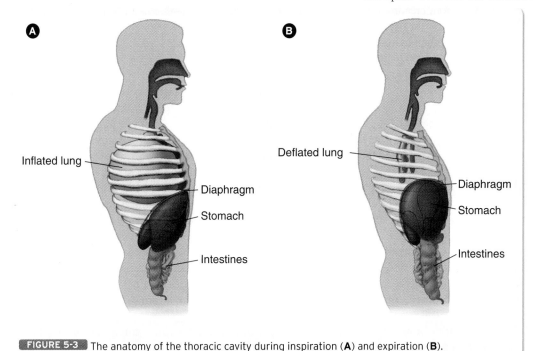

FIGURE 5-3 The anatomy of the thoracic cavity during inspiration (**A**) and expiration (**B**).

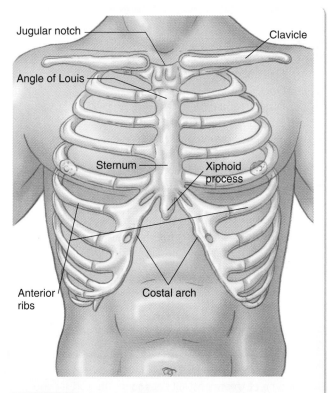

FIGURE 5-4 The organs within the thoracic cavity are protected by the ribs, which are connected in the back by the vertebrae and in the front, through the costal cartilages, to the sternum.

on exhalation. If this space becomes filled with air, blood, or other fluids, the surface tension is lost and the lung collapses.

The **diaphragm**, the primary muscle of breathing, forms a barrier between the thoracic and abdominal cavities. It works in conjunction with the intercostal muscles to increase the size of the thoracic cavity during inspiration, creating the negative pressure that pulls air in via the trachea. In times of distress, this breathing effort can be aided by other accessory muscles of the thoracic cavity.

The upper abdominal organs are also protected by the lower rib cage. These organs include:

- Spleen
- Kidneys
- Liver
- Stomach
- Pancreas

Physiology

The primary physiologic functions of the thorax and its contents are to maintain oxygenation and ventilation and (via the heart) to maintain circulation. The process of breathing includes both the delivery of oxygen to the body and the elimination of carbon dioxide from the body. Intercostal muscles between the adjacent ribs function as secondary muscles of respiration. As the diaphragm and the chest wall relax, positive pressure is created within the thorax. The air from which oxygen has been absorbed and into which carbon dioxide has been diffused is then exhaled. With each subsequent respiration (inhalation and exhalation), the process is repeated.

Proper functioning of the heart is essential to the delivery of blood to the body's tissues. As blood returns from the body via the inferior and superior venae cavae, it's pumped from the right side of the heart to the lungs, where the processes of oxygenation and ventilation take place. As oxygenated blood returns from the lungs, it enters the left side of the heart and is then pumped out to the body.

The ability to pump blood depends on having a functional pump (the heart), an adequate volume of blood to be pumped, and an appropriate amount of resistance to the pumping mechanism—properties that collectively determine the cardiac output. **Cardiac output** is the volume of blood delivered to the body in 1 minute. The volume is identified by counting the number of times the heart beats per minute (heart rate) and determining the amount of blood delivered to the body with each beat (stroke volume). Thus, cardiac output equals the heart rate (beats/min) multiplied by the stroke volume (mL of blood per beat). Any injury that limits the heart's pumping ability, the delivery of blood to the heart, the blood's ability to leave the heart, or the heart rate will affect cardiac output.

■ Assessment of Thoracic Trauma

Mechanism of Injury

The first step in assessing a thoracic injury is to determine the mechanism of injury (MOI). Thoracic injuries may be the result of penetrating objects or blunt trauma. Penetrating

Field Medical Care **TIPS**

A penetrating thoracic wound at the fourth intercostal space (level of the nipples) or lower should be assumed to be an abdominal injury as well as a thoracic injury (because the diaphragm is higher in expiration).

injuries may be caused by gunshot or stab wounds; in both cases, the forces of the injury occur over a small area. Unlike a stab wound, the trajectory of a bullet can be unpredictable, and all thoracic and abdominal structures are at risk.

Blunt trauma injuries may be caused when the force is distributed over a larger area. Visceral injuries may occur from deceleration (sudden stops, MVAs, airplane crashes), compression (crush injuries), bursting (traumatic rupture of the aorta, falls from great height), and shearing forces (MVAs).

The next step is to assess the casualty. Identify the casualty's signs and symptoms. Assess the casualty's responsiveness by using the AVPU scale (alert, responsive to verbal stimuli, responsive to pain, and unresponsive). Ensure that airway, breathing, and circulation are all intact before moving ahead in your assessment.

Next, perform a rapid trauma survey according to the protocols presented in Chapter 2, *Casualty Assessment*. Signs indicative of chest injury may include:

- Shock
- Cyanosis
- Hemoptysis (coughing up blood)
- Chest wall contusion
- Flail chest
- Open wounds
- Distended neck veins
- Tracheal deviation
- Subcutaneous emphysema (presence of air in subcutaneous tissue)

Next, move on to the additional assessment. Assess the baseline vital signs of the casualty. Assess the casualty's:

- **Pulse.**
- **Blood pressure.** (This might not be possible when providing care under fire. Use palpable pressure

Field Medical Care **TIPS**

When assessing the casualty and providing treatment, the type of treatment will depend on the setting you are in. Treatment of thoracic injuries in a combat environment may differ from the treatment provided in a civilian setting.

assessment until further security is provided.) Assess the casualty for hypertension or hypotension.

- **Respiratory rate and effort.** Assess for tachypnea (rapid respiratory rate) or bradypnea (slow respiratory rate). Watch for labored breathing, retractions (utilizing accessory muscles to assist breathing), and evidence of respiratory distress.

Assess the casualty's skin. Look for **diaphoresis** (excessive secretion of sweat), **pallor** (absence of color), cyanosis, open wounds, and ecchymosis. Assess the casualty's neck, looking at the position of the trachea. Also assess for subcutaneous emphysema, jugular venous distension, and penetrating wounds. Assess the chest for contusions, tenderness, asymmetry, open wounds or impaled objects, crepitation, paradoxical movement (opposite from the rest of the chest), and lung sounds. Check for absent or decreased lung sounds, unilateral lung sounds, or bilateral lung sounds, as well as bowel sounds in the lung area. Use percussion to assess the lung sounds. Hyperresonance indicates pneumothorax or tension pneumothorax. Hyporesonance indicates hemothorax. Assess the heart sounds; signs of thoracic injury include muffled or distant heart sounds.

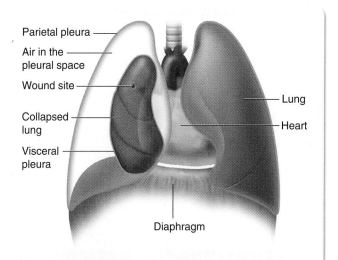

FIGURE 5-5 Pneumothorax occurs when air leaks into the space between the pleural surfaces from an opening in the chest wall or the surface of the lung. The lung collapses as air fills the pleural space.

■ Immediate Life-Threatening Thoracic Injuries

There are a select few injuries that you must be able to identify and treat during your assessment of the casualty's breathing—namely, open pneumothorax, tension pneumothorax, and flail chest. These injuries, if missed, may claim the casualty's life.

Simple Pneumothorax

Simple pneumothorax is caused by a blunt or penetrating trauma or by fractured ribs. Occasionally a simple pneumothorax occurs for no apparent reason (spontaneous), usually seen in tall slender males who are smokers. In this condition, air enters through a hole in the chest wall or the surface of the lungs as the casualty attempts to breathe, causing the lung on that side to collapse **FIGURE 5-5**.

The presentation and physical findings in a casualty with a pneumothorax depend on the size of the pneumothorax and the degree of resulting pulmonary compromise. With a small pneumothorax, the casualty may complain only of mild dyspnea and pleuritic chest pain on the affected side. The diagnosis is based on pleuritic chest pain, dyspnea, decreased or absent breath sounds on the affected side, and hypertympany to percussion on the affected side.

As the pneumothorax increases in size, the degree of compromise likewise increases. Casualties with larger pneumothoraces will complain of increasing dyspnea and demonstrate signs of more serious respiratory compromise and hypoxia: agitation, altered mental status, tachypnea, tachycardia, cyanosis, and even absent breath sounds on the affected side.

Oxygen aids the casualty in overcoming any degree of hypoxia that may exist. The most critical intervention for these casualties is repeated assessments to ensure that the

injury has not progressed to a tension pneumothorax. Most pneumothoraces result from a small pulmonary injury that seals itself off, preventing further air loss. For those that do progress, however, rapid recognition and management of this condition can be lifesaving.

Management begins with ensuring the airway. Administer oxygen at 15 liters per minute (L/min), if available. Insert a large-bore IV catheter and treat for shock. Initiate cardiac monitoring, if available, and evacuate the casualty to the nearest medical treatment facility (MTF). Chest tube insertion can take place under the direction of a physician or physician's assistant.

Open Pneumothorax

An **open pneumothorax** is caused by penetrating thoracic injury and may present as a sucking chest wound. Air does not enter the lung, oxygenation of the blood is reduced, ventilation is impaired, and hypoxia results, just as in a closed or simple pneumothorax.

When you assess the airway, exposure of the chest will reveal a chest wall defect or impaled object. If air is being drawn into the chest by the negative inspiratory pressure, a "sucking chest wound" may be noted **FIGURE 5-6**. If air is being forced out of the chest with the positive pressure of expiration, the result may be a bubbling wound. The movement of air in and out of the open wound may also lead to dissection of that air within the subcutaneous tissue, resulting in subcutaneous emphysema.

With any injury that has the potential to violate the integrity of the thoracic cavity, your assessment should focus on evaluating the casualty for the presence of a pneumothorax. Due to the decreased ability to oxygenate and ventilate, the casualty will experience tachycardia, tachypnea, and restlessness. These symptoms may be simply a manifestation of

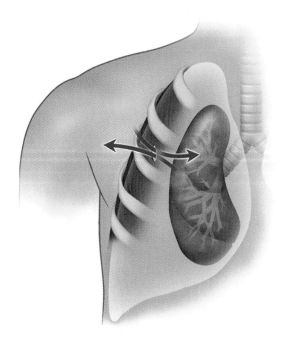

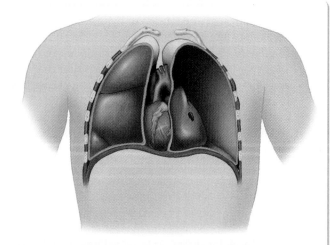

FIGURE 5-7 In a tension pneumothorax, air accumulates in the pleural space, eventually causing compression of the heart and great vessels.

FIGURE 5-6 With a sucking chest wound, air passes from the outside into the pleural space and back out with each breath, creating a sucking sound. The defect does not need to be large to compromise ventilation.

the pain from the injury, but other findings may confirm an underlying pneumothorax.

As the air within the interpleural space (the pneumothorax) increases, the casualty's breath sounds will diminish on the affected side. Because this expanding volume consists of air, percussion of the chest will aid in the assessment by demonstrating a hyperresonant sound. These physical findings should confirm your suspicion of a pneumothorax although they may be very difficult to appreciate on the battlefield.

Management of this injury begins by ensuring an airway. Quickly close the chest wall defect with an occlusive dressing. Close both the entrance and exit wounds (if present). Tape all four sides of the occlusive dressing to ensure a proper seal and to avoid the dressing becoming loose during transport of the casualty, per the Tactical Combat Casualty Care (TC-3) doctrine. Occlusive dressings may cause the casualty to develop a tension pneumothorax, so continuously monitor the casualty for progressive respiratory difficulty and treat for tension pneumothorax per the tenets of TC-3. Administer oxygen at 15 L/min, if available. Assess the casualty for evi-

dence of shock per the tenets of TC-3 and initiate IV therapy per fluid resuscitation guidelines. The Algorithm for Fluid Resuscitation is in Chapter 1, *Introduction to Battlefield Medicine*. Initiate cardiac monitoring, if available, and transport the casualty to the nearest MTF.

Tension Pneumothorax

Tension pneumothorax occurs when a one-way valve is created from either penetrating or blunt trauma **FIGURE 5-7 ▲**. It may also occur with the application of an occlusive dressing on an open chest wound when air cannot leave the plural space and pressure develops. This causes further collapse of the affected lung, pushing the mediastinum in the opposite direction as pressure increases, which may compromise the good lung, major vessels, and heart.

Clinical signs include:
- Anxiety, apprehension, and agitation
- Diminished or absent breath sounds
- Increasing dyspnea; may have hypertympany to percussion
- Tachypnea
- Hyperresonance to percussion on the affected side
- Hypotension and cold clammy skin, as the casualty begins to rapidly deteriorate
- Distended neck veins and cyanosis
- Tracheal deviation away from the side of the tension pneumothorax (late finding)

The development of decreased lung compliance in an intubated casualty should alert you to the possibility of tension pneumothorax. Tracheal deviation is a late finding and its absence does not rule out the presence of a tension pneumothorax. Remember that any casualty with unilateral chest trauma with progressive respiratory distress should be evaluated for the development of a tension pneumothorax. The

Field Medical Care TIPS

If possible, consider using the Asherman Chest Seal. This is a circular dressing with adhesive on one side to adhere to the chest wall, designed with a built-in one-way valve to prevent tension pneumothorax.

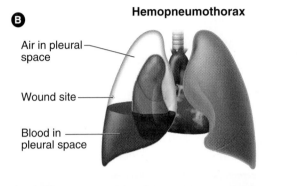

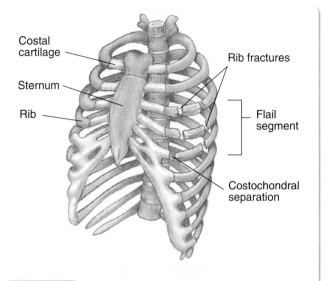

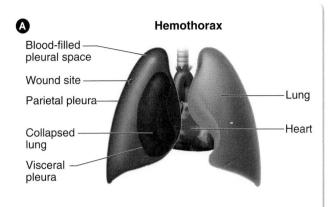

Hemothorax

Blood-filled pleural space

Wound site

Parietal pleura

Collapsed lung

Visceral pleura

Lung

Heart

B

Hemopneumothorax

Air in pleural space

Wound site

Blood in pleural space

FIGURE 5-8 **A.** A hemothorax is a collection of blood in the pleural space produced by bleeding within the chest. **B.** In a hemopneumothorax, both air and blood are present.

Costal cartilage

Sternum

Rib

Rib fractures

Flail segment

Costochondral separation

FIGURE 5-9 In flail chest injuries, two or more adjacent ribs are fractured in two or more places. A flail segment will move paradoxically when the casualty breathes.

above findings may be difficult to assess in a combat situation; you must be alert to this problem with penetrating chest trauma. The initial management of a pneumothorax secondary to penetrating chest trauma is an occlusive dressing. Establish an open airway, and administer oxygen at 15 L/min, if available if tension pneumothorax is suspected. Decompress the affected side of the chest with needle decompression, which is covered in detail later in this chapter.

Massive Hemothorax

Massive hemothorax is defined as 1,500 cc of blood loss into the thoracic cavity or 200 mL/h of drainage from a chest tube **FIGURE 5-8**. Physical assessment of the massive hemothorax will reveal signs of both ventilatory insufficiency (hypoxia, agitation, anxiety, tachypnea, dyspnea) and hypovolemic shock (tachycardia, hypotension, pale and clammy skin). The physical findings that help to differentiate this hemothorax from other injuries include the lack of jugular vein distension, the lack of tracheal deviation, possible bloody sputum (hemoptysis), and dullness that may be noted on percussion of the affected side of the chest. Additional signs and symptoms include:

- Hypotension from blood loss or compression of the heart or a great vessel
- Neck veins usually flat secondary to profound hypovolemia, but could be distended due to mediastinal compression

- Dullness to percussion on the affected side and decreased breath sounds
- Anxiety and/or confusion secondary to hypovolemia or hypoxia

Management begins by ensuring the casualty's airway. Administer oxygen at 15 L/min, if available. Rapidly transport to the appropriate echelon of care because this injury requires surgical management. Carefully replace the fluid volume with IV fluids in accordance with the tenets of TC-3. Maintain the blood pressure (BP) just high enough to preserve a peripheral pulse (radial pulse equal to a BP of 80 mm Hg, systolic). If the blood pressure is elevated beyond that, the increased pressure can increase the bleeding into the chest. Closely observe for possible development of a tension pneumothorax, which would require a needle decompression.

Flail Chest

Flail chest occurs when three or more adjacent ribs are fractured in at least two places **FIGURE 5-9**. The result is a segment of chest wall that is not in continuity with the thorax. The flail segment moves with paradoxical (opposite) motion relative to the rest of the chest wall.

The force necessary to produce this injury also frequently bruises the underlying lung tissue, and this pulmonary contusion will also contribute to hypoxia. The casualty is also at risk for development of hemothorax or pneumothorax and may be in marked respiratory distress.

Pain from the chest wall injury exacerbates the already impaired respirations from the paradoxical motion and the underlying lung contusion. Chest wall palpation may reveal crepitus in addition to the abnormal respiratory motion.

Rapid trauma survey is the key to identifying a casualty with a flail segment. Beginning with general inspection of the chest, you will note evidence of soft-tissue injury to the chest. On further examination, you may observe paradoxical chest wall movement, although the casualty's efforts to splint the injury may prevent its visibility. On palpation, crepitus and tenderness may be noted at the site, and dissection of air into the tissues should raise your suspicion for this injury and an underlying pneumothorax. As the injury begins to affect the casualty's physiology, the expected signs and symptoms of hypoxia, hypercarbia, and pain will become apparent. The casualty would be expected to have one or more of the following associated findings: complaints of pain, tenderness on palpation, splinting, shallow breathing, agitation/anxiety (hypoxia) or lethargy (hypercarbia), tachycardia, and cyanosis.

Management of this injury begins by ensuring the airway. Administer oxygen at 15 L/min, if available. Assist with ventilation. Pneumothorax is commonly associated with a flail chest, and needle decompression may be needed to relieve tension pneumothorax. Establish an IV. You may need to limit fluids, because fluid overload may worsen hypoxemia. Initiate manual pressure to stabilize the flail segment, and then use bulky dressing taped to the chest wall. This is usually not accomplished until the casualty is stabilized on a long spine board (if available). Do not transport the casualty with the injured side up. This further inhibits expansion of the chest and causes increased **atelectasis** (collapse of some of the alveoli) of the injured lung. Initiate cardiac monitoring because associated myocardial trauma is frequent. On the battlefield, IV morphine is the appropriate pain medication. Watch for respiratory depression with morphine administration. Transport the casualty to the nearest MTF.

Pulmonary Contusion

Pulmonary contusion is a common chest injury produced by blunt trauma FIGURE 5-10 ▾ . This bruising of the lung can produce marked hypoxemia secondary to bleeding into the alveoli and interstitium of the lung. Pulmonary contusion is the most common potentially lethal chest injury. Hypoxia and carbon dioxide retention lead to respiratory distress, dyspnea, tachypnea, agitation, and restlessness. Due to the capillary injury and the hemorrhage into the pulmonary parenchyma, the casualty may present with hemoptysis (coughing up blood). Evidence of overlying injury may include contusions, tenderness, crepitus, or paradoxical motion. Auscultation may reveal wheezes, crackles or rales, or diminished lung sounds in the affected area.

Management of this injury consists of oxygen administration at 15 L/min, if available. Insert a large-bore IV and administer only enough fluids for maintenance. Casualties with contused lungs do not tolerate excess IV fluids. Perform cardiac monitoring, and transport the casualty to the nearest MTF.

Myocardial Contusion

Myocardial contusion is a potentially lethal injury resulting from blunt chest injury. Blunt injury to the anterior chest is transmitted via the sternum to the heart, and may cause valvular rupture, cardiac rupture, or pericardial tamponade; however, myocardial contusion is the most common injury. On the battlefield, a casualty with significant chest trauma is assumed to have a myocardial contusion. This bruising is the same injury as a myocardial infarction and may present with similar signs and symptoms. Sharp, retrosternal chest pain is the most common complaint among casualties with myocardial contusion. Inspection of the area may reveal soft-tissue or bony injury in the area.

Additional signs and symptoms include dysrhythmias and cardiogenic shock (rare).

Management of this injury consists of oxygen administration at 15 L/min, if available. Establish a large-bore IV line to keep vein open (TKO). These casualties do not need large volumes of fluids. Perform cardiac monitoring, and transport the casualty to the nearest MTF.

Cardiac Tamponade

Cardiac tamponade occurs usually from a penetrating injury. The pericardial sac is an inelastic membrane surrounding the heart FIGURE 5-11 ▸ . When blood rapidly collects between the heart and the pericardium from a cardiac injury, the ventricles of the heart will be compressed, which prevents the ventricles from filling. A small amount of pericardial blood (< 100 mL) can compromise cardiac filling. Common, but not always present, signs and symptoms include:

- Hypotension (narrow pulse pressure)
- Muffled heart sounds
- Distended neck veins
- Beck's triad, which consists of all of the above

Management of this injury begins by ensuring the airway and administering oxygen at 15 L/min, if available. Initiate an IV bolus of electrolyte solution (500 to 1,000 mL). This may increase the filling of the heart and increase cardiac output. Only give enough fluid to maintain a peripheral pulse (BP at 80 to 90 mm Hg). Remember that a radial pulse equals a BP of 80 mm Hg, systolic. Cardiac tamponade is rapidly fatal and

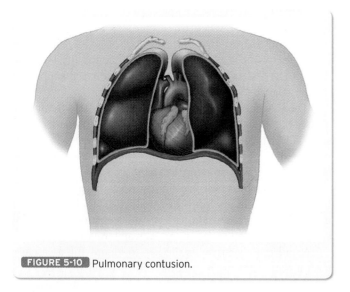

FIGURE 5-10 Pulmonary contusion.

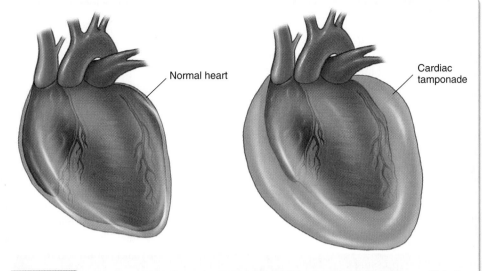

FIGURE 5-11 Cardiac tamponade is a potentially fatal condition in which fluid builds up within the pericardial sac, compressing the heart's chambers and dramatically impairing its ability to pump blood.

cannot be readily treated in the battlefield by a combat medic but may be treated by a physician or physician's assistant. Initiate cardiac monitoring, and evacuate the casualty to the nearest MTF immediately.

■ Identify Thoracic Injuries

Simple Rib Fracture

Simple rib fractures are the most frequent injury to the chest (most commonly seen in the lateral aspect of ribs three to eight). Pain may prohibit the casualty from breathing adequately. On palpation, the area of rib fracture may be unstable and will be tender. Simple rib fractures are rarely life-threatening in adults. Of greater importance is the evaluation and recognition of associated injuries to underlying structures, which may be life-threatening. Fractures of the lower ribs can be associated with liver, kidney, or spleen injuries.

Management begins with the administration of oxygen at 15 L/min, if available. Monitor for pneumothorax, hemothorax, or other associated injuries. Encourage the casualty to breathe deeply; this will help to prevent atelectasis and pneumonia. Provide pain management. Evacuate the casualty to the nearest MTF for monitoring and further treatment.

Diaphragmatic Tears

Diaphragmatic tears can result from a severe blow to the abdomen. A sudden increase in intra-abdominal pressure can tear the diaphragm and allow herniation of the abdominal organs into the thoracic cavity. This injury occurs more commonly on the left side of the body because the liver helps protect the diaphragm on the right side. Large radial tears in the diaphragm result from blunt trauma; penetrating trauma may also produce small holes. Marked respiratory distress is caused from herniation of abdominal contents into the thoracic cavity. Diminished breath sounds and, infre-

quently, bowel sounds may be heard when the casualty's chest is auscultated.

Management begins by ensuring the casualty's airway. Administer oxygen at 15 L/min, if available. Insert a large-bore IV and treat for shock. Transport the casualty to the appropriate echelon of care.

Traumatic Asphyxia

Traumatic asphyxia results from severe compression injury to the chest. Sudden compression of the heart and mediastinum transmits the force to the capillaries of the neck and head. Casualties appear similar to those suffering from strangulation with cyanosis and swelling of the head and neck. The lips and tongue may be swollen and conjunctival hemorrhage may be evident. The skin below the level of the crush injury will remain pink unless there are other associated injuries. Management includes ensuring an airway. Insert a large-bore IV and treat for shock. Treat any other injuries, and transport the casualty to the nearest MTF.

Impalement Injuries

Impalement injuries are caused by a penetrating object. *Do not* remove the object because it may be preventing severe hemorrhage. Management begins with ensuring the airway and administering oxygen at 15 L/min, if available. Stabilize the impaled object. Insert a large-bore IV and treat for shock. Transport the casualty to the nearest MTF.

Tracheal or Bronchial Tree Injury

Tracheal or bronchial tree injury results from a penetrating or blunt trauma. Penetrating upper airway injuries frequently have associated major vascular injuries and extensive tissue destruction. A blunt injury may present with subtle findings. It can also rupture the trachea or mainstem bronchus near the carina. Presenting signs include:

- Dyspnea
- Hemoptysis
- Subcutaneous emphysema of the chest, neck, or face
- Associated pneumothorax or hemothorax

Management begins with the establishment of an airway. In these casualties, this may be difficult due to altered anatomy and even a surgical airway may not be helpful. Administer oxygen at 15 L/min, if available. Insert a large-bore IV and treat for shock. Observe for signs of a pneumothorax or hemothorax. Tracheobronchial injuries require significant force to occur, so be alert for other injuries. Transport the casualty to the nearest MTF.

■ Treatment of Tension Pneumothorax

A tension pneumothorax is a life-threatening condition that results from continued air accumulation within the intrapleural space. Air may enter the pleural space from an open thoracic injury, an injury to the lung parenchyma due to blunt trauma (the most common cause of tension pneumothorax), barotrauma due to positive-pressure ventilation, or tracheobronchial injuries due to shearing forces.

An injury to the lung can cause a one-way valve to develop, allowing air to move into the pleural space but not to exit from it. As it continues to accumulate, the air exerts increasing pressure against the surrounding tissues. This growing pressure compresses the involved lung, diminishing its ability to oxygenate blood or eliminate carbon dioxide from the blood. Eventually, the lung will both collapse and push toward the mediastinum, shifting the mediastinum away from the injured side.

This pressure increase may even exceed the pressure within the major venous structures, decreasing venous return to the heart, diminishing preload, and eventually resulting in a shock state. As venous return decreases, the casualty's body attempts to compensate by increasing the heart rate in an attempt to maintain cardiac output.

To manage this life-threatening injury, you may need to perform a needle chest decompression. This procedure is applicable to the rapidly deteriorating casualty with a life-threatening tension pneumothorax, as evidenced by the following signs and symptoms:

- Respiratory distress, anxiety, agitation, and tachypnea
- Decreasing level of consciousness
- Loss of peripheral pulse
- Hyperresonance on percussion of the chest on the affected side
- Jugular venous distension and cyanosis
- Tracheal deviation (late finding, the absence of which does not preclude a tension pneumothorax from existing)

The accumulation of air within the pleural space decreases the lung volume and diminishes the breath sounds on the affected side when you auscultate the chest. Because air causes the loss of breath sounds on that side, the chest will be resonant (like a bell) when percussed, as opposed to the dull sensation expected with fluid or blood.

Due to the injury and the collapsing lung, a patient with a tension pneumothorax often complains of pleuritic chest pain and dyspnea. The resulting hypoxia may cause the casualty to become anxious, tachycardic, tachypneic, and even cyanotic.

Immediate relief of the elevated pressures must be accomplished through a **needle decompression**, also referred to as a needle thoracentesis or needle thoracostomy. The steps for performing a needle decompression are described in **SKILL DRILL 5-1 ▶**.

1. Assess the casualty to ensure that the presentation matches that of a tension pneumothorax.
2. Administer high-flow oxygen and ventilatory assistance.

3. Determine whether the indications for emergency decompression are present (**Step ①**).
4. Identify the second intercostal space on the anterior chest at the midclavicular line on the same side as the pneumothorax (**Step ②**).
5. Quickly prepare the area with an antiseptic. Use a catheter that is long enough to enter the pleural space. Ensure that the maximum catheter length is 3.25″ (**Step ③**).
6. Remove the plastic cap from a 3.25″ large-bore catheter. Insert the needle into the skin over the superior border of the third rib, midclavicular line, and direct it into the intercostal space at a 90° angle to the third rib. The needle entry into the chest should not be medial to the nipple line. The needle should be directed straight posteriorly and not toward the heart (**Step ④**).
7. As the needle enters the pleural space, there will be a pop and hiss of air. Continue to advance the needle to the hub (**Step ⑤**).
8. Remove the needle and leave the catheter in place.
9. Stabilize the catheter hub to the chest with tape. Leave the plastic catheter in place until it is replaced by a chest tube at the MTF. Intubate the casualty if indicated. Monitor the casualty for reoccurrence of pneumothorax (**Step ⑥**).

Complications of this procedure include:

- Laceration of the intercostal vessels may cause hemorrhage. The intercostal artery and vein run along the inferior margin of each rib. Poor needle placement can lacerate one of these vessels.
- Creation of a pneumothorax may occur if not already present. If your assessment was incorrect, you may create a pneumothorax when you insert the needle into the chest.
- Risk of infection is a consideration. Adequate skin preparation with an antiseptic will usually prevent this.
- Intercostal nerve/artery injury is possible if the needle is placed beneath the rib accidentally. A tube thoracostomy should be accomplished by a physician's assistant or doctor ASAP, because the needle may be inadequate to continuously decompress the chest if a major bronchus is ruptured.

■ Summary

In multiple trauma casualties, chest injuries are common and many times are considered life-threatening. You must have the ability to identify the injury while performing the rapid trauma survey and appropriately treat the injury to salvage the casualty.

There are a select few injuries that you must be able to identify and treat during your assessment of the casualty's breathing—namely, open pneumothorax, tension pneumothorax, and flail chest. These injuries, if missed, may claim the casualty's life.

SKILL DRILL 5-1

Emergency Needle Decompression

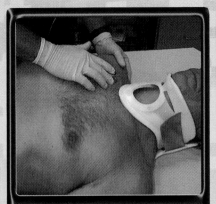

1 Assess the casualty. Administer high-flow oxygen and ventilatory assistance. Determine whether the indications for emergency decompression are present.

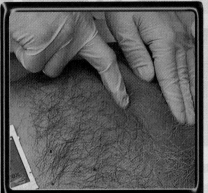

2 Identify the second intercostal space on the anterior chest at the midclavicular line on the same side as the pneumothorax.

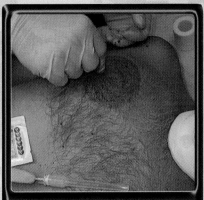

3 Quickly prepare the area with an antiseptic. Use a catheter that is long enough to enter the pleural space. Ensure that the maximum catheter length is 3.25″.

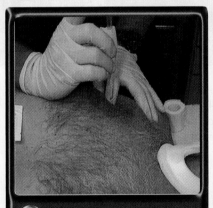

4 Remove the plastic cap from a 3.25″ large-bore catheter. Insert the needle into the skin over the superior border of the third rib, midclavicular line, and direct it into the intercostal space at a 90° angle to the third rib. The needle entry into the chest should not be medial to the nipple line. The needle should be directed straight posteriorly and not toward the heart.

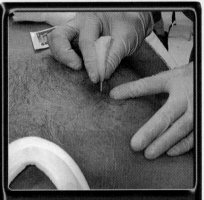

5 As the needle enters the pleural space, there will be a pop and hiss of air. Continue to advance the needle to the hub.

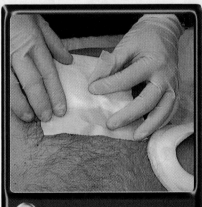

6 Remove the needle and leave the catheter in place. Stabilize the catheter hub to the chest with tape. Leave the plastic catheter in place until it is replaced by a chest tube at the MTF. Intubate the casualty if indicated. Monitor the casualty for reoccurrence of pneumothorax.

YOU ARE THE
COMBAT MEDIC

While on patrol, you witness a vehicle driven by a military contractor skid off the road and hit a low brick wall. You and a combat life saver (CLS) approach the scene with caution. Once you determine that the scene is safe, you approach the vehicle to begin your situational assessment. The mechanism of injury is clear, trauma caused by a motor vehicle crash. There are two casualties in the vehicle. The driver can speak and says that he is all right, just a bit sore. The other military contractor is in the back seat of the vehicle. He is not wearing a seatbelt.

Assessment

You immediately begin your initial assessment of this casualty. Due to the mechanism of injury, you instruct the CLS to apply c-spine control. The casualty does not respond to your voice or to a gentle pinch to his earlobe. You insert an orophayngeal airway before extracting the casualty. Once the casualty is extracted, you and the CLS assist ventilations with a bag-valve-mask device at 15 L/min. His pulse rate is 128 beats/min and his skin is cool, pale, and diaphoretic. There is no bleeding.

Treatment

As you perform the rapid trauma survey, you find that his neck reveals jugular vein distension. After determining that the casualty has a tension pneumothorax, you perform a needle decompression. You hear a rapid rush of air as the catheter enters the thoracic cavity. You stabilize the catheter with tape and prepare the casualty for evacuation to the Medical Treatment Facility (MTF). A helicopter evacuates the casualty to the nearest MTF, where a chest tube will be inserted to stabilize his breathing.

---

1. LAST NAME, FIRST NAME Dupre, Gene | RANK/GRADE | ✓ MALE
| | | FEMALE
SSN 000-111-2222 | SPECIALTY CODE | RELIGION Catholic
2. UNIT

FORCE | | | | NATIONALITY
A/T | AF/A | N/M | MC/M |
| BC/BC | | NBI/BNC | | DISEASE | | PSYCH

3. INJURY | X | AIRWAY
FRONT   BACK | | HEAD
| | WOUND
| | NECK/BACK INJURY
| | BURN
| | AMPUTATION
| | STRESS
| | OTHER (Specify)

Trauma to chest

4. LEVEL OF CONSCIOUSNESS
ALERT | | PAIN RESPONSE
VERBAL RESPONSE | X | UNRESPONSIVE

5. PULSE 128 bpm | **TIME** 0820 | **6. TOURNIQUET** [X] NO [ ] YES | TIME
7. MORPHINE [X] NO [ ] YES | DOSE | TIME | **8. IV** | TIME

9. TREATMENT/OBSERVATIONS/CURRENT MEDICATION/ALLERGIES/NBC (ANTIDOTE)
Found jugular vein distension during rapid trauma survey & assessed a tension pneumothorax. Performed a needle decompression & inserted opa.

10. DISPOSITION | RETURNED TO DUTY | TIME
| X | EVACUATED
| | DECEASED
11. PROVIDER/UNIT Deforge, Michael | DATE (YYMMDD)

Ready for Review

- Open chest injuries can be the result of a motor vehicle accident, bullet, missile wound, fall, or blow.
- These injuries are serious and, unless treated rapidly and correctly, can result in substantial mortality.
- The first step in assessing a thoracic injury is to determine the mechanism of injury (MOI).
- Thoracic injuries may be the result of penetrating objects or blunt trauma.
- A tension pneumothorax is a life-threatening condition that results from continued air accumulation within the intrapleural space.

Vital Vocabulary

angle of Louis Prominence on the sternum that lies opposite the second intercostal space.

atelectasis Alveolar collapse that prevents use of that portion of the lung for ventilation and oxygenation.

cardiac output The volume of blood delivered to the body in 1 minute.

cardiac tamponade Accumulation of excess fluid or blood in the pericardial sac to the extent that it interferes with cardiac function.

clavicle An S-shaped bone, also called the collarbone, that articulates medially with the sternum and laterally with the shoulder.

diaphoresis Excessive secretion of sweat.

diaphragm Large skeletal muscle that plays a major role in breathing and separates the chest cavity from the abdominal cavity.

flail chest An injury that involves two or more adjacent ribs fractured in two or more places, allowing the segment between the fractures to move independently of the rest of the thoracic cage.

intercostal space The space between two ribs, named according to the number of the rib above it, that contains the intercostal muscles and neurovascular bundle.

manubrium The superior segment of the sternum; its lower border defines the angle of Louis.

mediastinum Space within the chest that contains the heart, major blood vessels, vagus nerve, trachea, and esophagus; located between the two lungs.

myocardial contusion Blunt force injury to the heart that results in capillary damage, interstitial bleeding, and cellular damage in the area.

needle decompression Also referred to as a needle thoracotomy or needle thoracentesis, this procedure introduces a needle or angiocath into the pleural space in an attempt to relieve a tension pneumothorax.

neurovascular bundle A closely placed grouping of an artery, a vein, and a nerve that lies beneath the inferior edge of a rib.

open pneumothorax The result of a defect in the chest wall that allows air to enter the thoracic space.

pallor Absence of color.

pericardium Double-layered sac containing the heart and the origins of the superior vena cava, inferior vena cava, and pulmonary artery.

pleura Membrane lining the outer surface of the lungs (visceral pleura), the inner surface of the chest wall, and the thoracic surface of the diaphragm (parietal pleura).

pulmonary contusion Injury to the lung parenchyma that results in capillary hemorrhage into the tissue.

scapula A large, flat, triangular bone along the posterior thorax that articulates with the clavicle and humerus.

sternum Also known as the breastbone, this bony structure along the midline of the thorax provides a point of anterior attachment for the thoracic cage.

suprasternal notch The indentation formed by the superior border of the manubrium and the clavicles, often used as a landmark for procedures such as subclavian vein access.

tension pneumothorax A life-threatening collection of air within the pleural space; the volume and pressure have both collapsed the involved lung and caused a shift of the mediastinal structures to the opposite side.

thoracic inlet The superior aspect of the thoracic cavity, this ring-like opening is created by the first vertebra, the first rib, the clavicles, and the manubrium.

thorax The part of the body between the neck and the diaphragm, encased by the ribs.

xyphoid process An inferior segment of the sternum often used as a landmark for CPR.

COMBAT MEDIC *in Action*

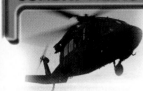

While on patrol, a member of your team slips on a staircase and falls about 20'. The casualty complains of chest pain and shortness of breath. Your CLS applies c-spine control while you perform your initial assessment. While exposing the casualty to assess for wounds, you notice some bruising to his upper back that extends into his left flank area.

1. Because this casualty is complaining of shortness of breath and chest pain, you should suspect which of the following injuries?

   A. Tension pneumothorax
   B. Flail chest
   C. Pulmonary contusion
   D. All of the above

2. All of the following are classic signs of a tension pneumothorax, EXCEPT:

   A. distended neck veins.
   B. tachypnea.
   C. penetrating chest wound.
   D. a patent airway.

3. Treatment of a tension pneumothorax begins with:

   A. splinting.
   B. applying a tourniquet.
   C. providing oxygen at 15 L/min.
   D. performing a needle decompression.

4. The signs of a massive hemothorax include:

   A. bloody sputum.
   B. lack of jugular vein distension.
   C. none of the above.
   D. all of the above.

5. Upon further examination of this casualty, you observe that part of his chest does not move when he inhales. This is a sign of:

   A. flail chest.
   B. massive hemothorax.
   C. tension pneauthorax.
   D. open pneumothorax.

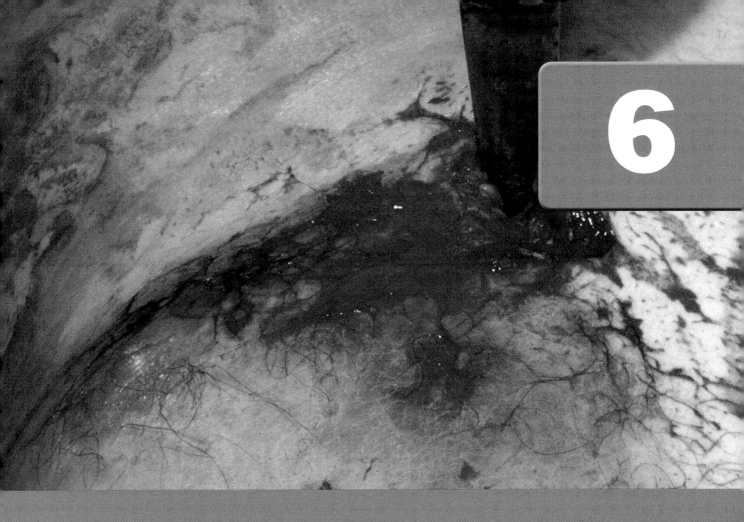

6

Abdominal Injuries

Objectives

Knowledge Objectives

☐ Describe the anatomy and physiology of the abdomen.

☐ Identify the organs in each abdominal quadrant.

☐ Differentiate between blunt and penetrating injuries.

☐ Describe what to look for when palpating the abdomen.

☐ Identify how to treat injuries of the abdomen.

■ Introduction

Abdominal injuries are difficult to evaluate in the Medical Treatment Facility (MTF) and even more so on the battlefield. Immediate surgical intervention is needed for penetrating abdominal injuries. Blunt injuries may be more subtle in their presentation, but may be just as deadly. Whether the result of penetrating or blunt trauma, abdominal injury presents two life-threatening dangers: infection and hemorrhage. With prompt recognition and immediate intervention, you will sustain the casualty until the casualty can get to a definitive treatment facility where he or she can receive the required lifesaving surgical intervention.

Uncontrolled hemorrhage has immediate consequences to life; thus, you must be alert to the danger of early shock in casualties with abdominal injury. Infection can be just as fatal, but with prompt recognition of abdominal injury and rapid evacuation of the casualty, field intervention will not be required. In this chapter, you will gain an understanding of the anatomy of the abdomen and the types of injuries you may encounter. You will learn the principles of abdominal injury assessment and casualty stabilization at the appropriate echelon of care.

■ Anatomy and Physiology Review of the Abdomen

The abdominal cavity is below (inferior to) the diaphragm FIGURE 6-1 ▾ . Its boundaries include the anterior abdominal wall, pelvic bones, spinal column, and the muscles of the abdomen and flanks. The cavity is divided into three spaces or into quadrants. The **thoracic abdomen** is below the diaphragm but enclosed by the lower ribs. It contains the liver, gallbladder, spleen, stomach, and transverse colon. The **true abdomen** contains the small intestines, bladder, and in females the uterus, fallopian tubes, and ovaries. The **retroperitoneal abdomen** lies behind the thoracic and true abdomen and contains the kidneys, ureters, pancreas, posterior duodenum, ascending and descending colon, abdominal aorta, and inferior vena cava. Because of its location away from the anterior surface of the body, retroperitoneal injuries are difficult to recognize and evaluate. Hemorrhage in the true abdomen may cause distension, but hemorrhage severe enough to cause shock may occur in the retroperitoneal space without evident distension.

Quadrants

To describe a location in the abdomen, or a source of pain found when conducting your assessment, the quadrant system is generally used FIGURE 6-2 ▸ . If you were to place a large imaginary "+" sign with the center directly on the umbilicus (navel), the vertical axis extending from the symphysis pubis to the xiphoid process, and the horizontal axis extending to both flanks, this would create four quadrants. These four regions are as follows: the right upper quadrant (RUQ), the right lower quadrant (RLQ), the left lower quadrant (LLQ), and the left upper quadrant (LUQ).

The organs found in the right upper quadrant (RUQ) are:

- Liver (solid organ at risk for hemorrhage)
- Gallbladder
- Portion of colon (hepatic flexure of colon)

The organs in the left upper quadrant (LUQ) are:

- Stomach
- Spleen (solid organ at risk for hemorrhage)
- Portion of colon (splenic flexure of colon)

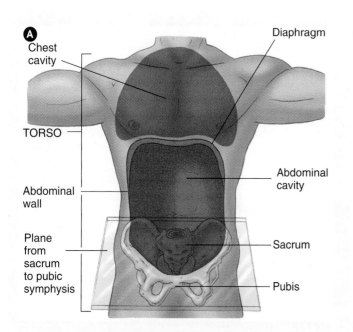

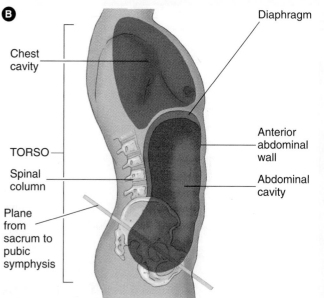

FIGURE 6-1   The abdominal cavity is below the diaphragm. Its boundaries include the anterior abdominal wall, pelvic bones, spinal column, and muscles of the abdomen and flanks. **A.** Anterior view. **B.** Lateral view.

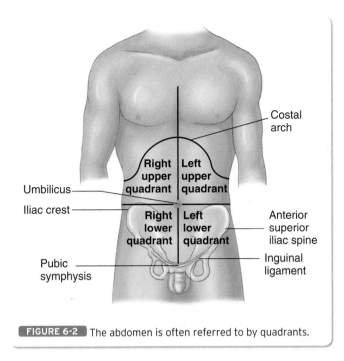

FIGURE 6-2 The abdomen is often referred to by quadrants.

The organs found in the right lower quadrant (RLQ) are:

- Large intestine (cecum)
- Appendix
- Small intestine
- Portion of the bladder, uterus, right fallopian tube, and right ovary

The organs found in the left lower quadrant (LLQ) are:

- Small intestine
- Large intestine (sigmoid colon)
- Portion of the bladder, uterus, left fallopian tube, and left ovary

Abdominal Organs

The abdomen contains many organs, including those that belong to the digestive system. The liver is a solid organ that is the largest organ in the abdomen. It lies in the right upper quadrant, superior and anterior to the gallbladder and the hepatic and cystic ducts. Among its many functions, the liver detoxifies the blood and produces bile (which is necessary to break down ingested fats) that drains into the small intestine.

Like the liver, the spleen is a solid organ. This highly vascular organ lies in the left upper quadrant and is partially protected by the left lower rib cage. It functions to clear bloodborne bacteria.

The gallbladder is a saclike organ located on the lower surface of the liver that acts as a reservoir for bile, one of the digestive enzymes produced by the liver. The liver continually secretes bile, and the gallbladder stores it until it is released through the cystic duct during the digestive process.

The pancreas is an organ in the middle of the abdomen. It secretes enzymes into the bowel that aid in digestion. The pancreas also secretes the hormone insulin, which is responsible for helping glucose enter the cells.

The stomach lies in the left upper quadrant. The esophagus passes through the diaphragm and opens into the stomach. The stomach secretes acid that assists in the digestive process.

The small and large intestines run from the end of the stomach to the anus. Intestines digest and absorb water and nutrients. Their contents pass through the stomach, and move through a circumferential muscle at the end of the stomach that acts as a valve between the stomach and the duodenum. Finally, stool passes through the rectum and out of the body through the anus.

The retroperitoneum contains organs of the urinary system. The kidneys filter blood and excrete body wastes in the form of urine. The urinary bladder is a hollow, muscular sac situated in the pelvis along the midline that stores urine until it is excreted. The ureters are a pair of thick-walled, hollow tubes that carry urine from the kidneys to the urinary bladder.

The abdomen also contains organs of the reproductive system. The female reproductive system contains the uterus, a pear-shaped organ located in the midline of the lower abdomen that allows the implantation, growth, and nourishment of a fetus during pregnancy. The female reproductive system also contains the ovaries (the female reproductive organs), located one on each side of the lower abdominal quadrants. The ovaries produce the precursors to mature eggs, and produce hormones that regulate female reproductive function.

The male reproductive system includes the penis, the male external reproductive organ, as well as the testes, also known as the testicles. The testes produce sperm and secrete male hormones such as testosterone. The scrotum is the pouch of skin and muscle that contains the testes.

Last but not least, the abdomen contains the diaphragm—the dome-shaped muscle that separates the thoracic cavity from the abdominal cavity. It curves from its point of attachment in the flanks at the 12th rib and peaks in the center at the fourth intercostal space.

Physiology Review

Abdominal injury may be caused by blunt (most common) or penetrating trauma (gunshot wounds or stab wounds). Multiple organ injury is common. The places where enough blood can be lost to cause shock include the thorax, abdomen, retroperitoneal space (including the pelvis), and muscle compartments of the proximal lower extremities **FIGURE 6-3 ▶**. Because the abdomen and retroperitoneal space can accommodate large amounts of blood, the bleeding may produce few signs and symptoms of the trauma. Even the casualty's baseline vital signs and a rapid trauma survey may not indicate the bleeding.

The organs that are most frequently injured after a blunt trauma are the spleen, followed by the liver. Because of its size, the liver is the most frequently injured organ in penetrating trauma. Solid organs, such as the liver or spleen, can easily be crushed by external blunt trauma. They both have a

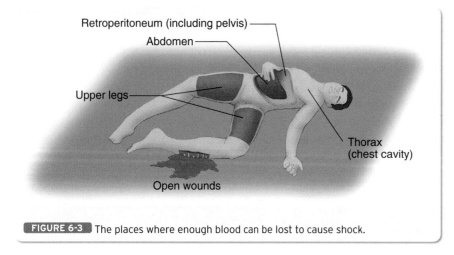

Retroperitoneum (including pelvis)
Abdomen
Upper legs
Thorax (chest cavity)
Open wounds

FIGURE 6-3 The places where enough blood can be lost to cause shock.

large blood supply and can bleed profusely. If a casualty has unexplained symptoms of shock, suspect abdominal trauma.

Hollow organs are more resilient to blunt trauma and less likely to be injured by trauma unless they are full. When a hollow organ is full, it is likely to be injured and can burst in the same way a chemical cold pack breaks when you apply pressure to the outer bag. The danger of bursting hollow organs is that they hold toxins (such as urine, bile, stomach acids, or stool) that can spill out into the abdominal cavity. This spillage can cause **peritonitis**, an inflammation of the lining of the abdomen. Peritonitis is a life-threatening condition. Shock can also occur with abdominal injuries.

■ Mechanism of Injury

The index of suspicion is the primary factor in assessing abdominal trauma. It is not an accurate diagnosis of the injury, but rather the determination that an abdominal injury does exist. A high index of suspicion is often based on the mechanism of injury (MOI) and your visual assessment. The major cause of morbidity and mortality in abdominal trauma is the delay in determining whether an injury exists and the resulting delay in treatment.

Did the casualty fall from a significant height or did a vehicle strike the casualty? Was there an explosion that threw the casualty against immobile objects or transmitted blast pressure to organs inside the abdomen? Keep in mind that due to overpressure, hollow organs can rupture with no apparent external injury.

If conscious, question the casualty to determine whether a weapon was used. Bystanders may be useful. Determine:

- Type of weapon used (ie, firearm, knife, etc.)
- Distance from weapon
- Blunt mechanisms
- High probability of accompanying injuries to other parts of the body

The abdominal injury may be from:

- Direct compression of the abdomen
- Solid organs being fractured (liver, spleen)
- "Blowout" of hollow organs (blast injuries in confined spaces)
- Deceleration—tearing of organs or their blood vessels (shearing)

These injuries are easily missed because the casualty may have little or no pain with minimal external evidence of injury. Casualties with lower rib fractures frequently have severe intra-abdominal injuries without significant abdominal pain. Pain from the fractured ribs may overshadow the abdominal pain. Be aware that any injury at the level of the fourth intercostal space (ICS) may result in thoracic trauma as well as abdominal injury.

Blunt Trauma

Blunt trauma to the abdomen results from compression or deceleration forces and can often lead to a **closed abdominal injury**—one in which soft-tissue damage occurs inside the body, but the skin remains intact. When assessing the abdominal cavity in a casualty who has received blunt trauma, consider three common mechanisms of injury: shearing, crushing, and compression.

In the rapid deceleration of a casualty during a motor vehicle crash or fall from a height, a shearing force can be created as the internal organs continue their forward motion. This will cause hollow, solid, and visceral organs and vascular structures to tear, especially at their points of attachment to the abdominal wall. Organs that shear or tear would include the liver, kidneys, small and large intestines, and spleen. In motor vehicle collisions, this MOI has been described as the third collision (for example, first the car into the wall, then the casualty into the steering column, and third the internal organs into the casualty's inner rib cage).

Crush injuries are the result of external factors at the time of impact; they differ from deceleration injuries occurring before impact. When abdominal contents are crushed between the anterior abdominal wall and the spinal column (or other structures in the rear), crushing occurs. Solid organs like the kidneys, liver, and spleen are at the greatest risk of injury from this mechanism. Direct application of crushing forces to the abdomen would come from things like the dashboard or the front hood of a car (in a vehicle collision) or from falling objects.

The last MOI to consider is compression injury resulting from a direct blow or external compression from a fixed object (such as a lap belt). These compression forces will deform hollow organs, increasing the pressure within the abdominal cavity. This dramatic change in abdominal pressure can cause a rupture of the small intestine or diaphragm. Rupture of organs can lead to uncontrollable hemorrhage and peritonitis.

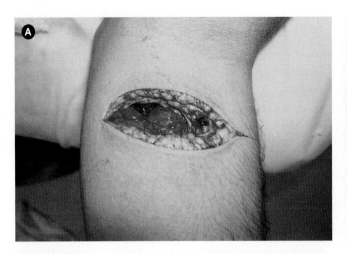

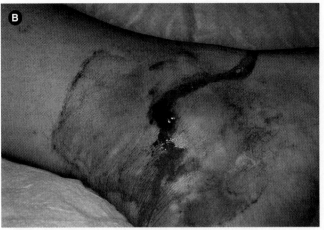

FIGURE 6-4 The velocity delivered during penetrating trauma is typically divided into three levels. **A.** Low velocity. **B.** Medium velocity.

Penetrating Trauma

<u>Penetrating trauma</u> results from gunshot or stab wounds. Penetrating trauma causes an **open abdominal injury**—one in which a break in the surface of the skin or mucous membrane exposes deeper tissue to potential contamination. In general, gunshot wounds cause more injury than stab wounds because bullets travel deeper into the body and have more kinetic energy. Gunshot wounds most commonly involve injury to the small bowel, colon, liver, and vascular structures; the extent of injury is less predictable than for an injury caused by stab wounds because gunshot wounds depend mostly on the characteristics of the weapon and the bullet. In penetrating trauma from stab wounds, the liver, small bowel, diaphragm, and colon are the organs most frequently injured.

The extent of damage from a penetrating injury is often a function of the energy that has been imparted to the body. The permanent injury as well as the temporary injury from the track of the projectile can be considerable with high-velocity penetrations. The velocity delivered during penetrating trauma is typically divided into three levels. Low velocity, such as from a knife, bayonet, or ice pick; medium velocity, such as from a handgun, 9-mm gun, or shotgun fired at a distance; and high velocity, such as from a high-powered sporting rifle or military assault rifles (M-16, AK-47) **FIGURE 6-4 ▲**. The trajectory or direction the projectile traveled and the distance it had to travel, as well as the profile of the bullet, can contribute considerably to the extent of the injury.

Ballistics affect abdominal trauma greatly. Shrapnel wounds may be low, medium, or high velocity depending on the distance of the casualty from the blast. Consider the trajectory and distance of the bullet. The bullet may pass through numerous structures in various body locations. (Penetrating trauma in the gluteal area is associated with significant intra-abdominal trauma in up to 50% of the cases.)

With stab wounds, the casualty may not initially appear to be in shock unless the knife penetrates a major vessel or organ (liver or spleen). Life-threatening peritonitis can develop within a few hours. The path of the penetrating object may not be apparent from the wound location. The path also depends on whether the casualty was inhaling or exhaling during the injury. This could cause the injury to be an abdominal, a lung, or a heart injury. The diaphragm rises to the level of the fourth ICS posteriorly during exhalation. A stab wound to the chest may also penetrate the abdomen. You must be aware of the possibility of intra-abdominal bleeding with hypovolemic (hemorrhagic) shock. Remember, never remove an impaled object!

Falls From Heights

The position or orientation of the body at the moment of impact will help determine the types of injuries sustained and their survivability. The surface onto which the casualty has fallen, and the degree to which that surface can deform under the force of the falling body (plasticity), can help in dissipating the forces of sudden deceleration.

Blast Injuries

Blast injuries, particularly those from weapons designed specifically for antipersonnel effects (such as mines or grenades) can generate fragments traveling at velocities of 4,500 feet per second. This is nearly double the velocity of a projectile from a high-speed rifle. Any energy transmitted from a blast fragment will cause extensive and disruptive damage to tissue **FIGURE 6-5 ▶**. Casualties who are injured in explosions may be injured by any of four different mechanisms. The primary blast injury is caused by the pressure wave. The secondary blast injury is caused by debris or fragments from the explosion. The tertiary blast injury is produced when a casualty is propelled through the air and strikes another object. There are also injuries called miscellaneous blast injuries that include burns and respiratory injuries from hot gases or chemicals.

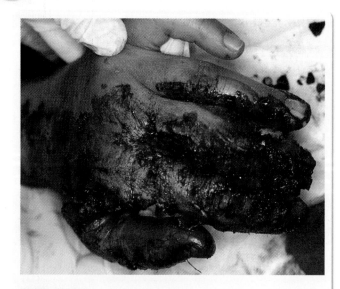

FIGURE 6-5 Any energy transmitted from a blast fragment will cause extensive and disruptive damage to tissue.

■ Care

Rapid Trauma Survey

Perform an initial assessment on the casualty to ensure airway patency, adequate breathing, and circulation (ABCs) prior to assessing the abdomen. During the rapid trauma survey, inspect for:

- Abrasions
- Contusions
- External blood loss
- Wounds
- Impaled objects
- Evisceration

Carefully log roll the casualty to inspect the posterior for exit wounds or contusions. Bruising of the flank and posterior may be an indication of significant trauma or internal hemorrhage. Then palpate for tenderness, guarding/rigidity, pelvic instability (which indicates a possible pelvic fracture), and distension. Avoid deep palpation because this may aggravate an existing injury.

Auscultation is not very useful with abdominal trauma and should not be performed; little is gained and critical time is lost by this examination technique.

Ensure you perform an evaluation of the chest cavity as well as the abdomen, as discussed in detail in Chapter 5, *Injuries of the Thorax*. Perform an examination of the perineum, rectum, and vagina. Examine for contusions, scrotal hematoma, lacerations, and urethral and rectal bleeding. Blood at the urethral meatus is a positive finding for urethral trauma, which should alert you to trauma involving the genitourinary system.

Severe hemorrhage may be associated with distension, tenderness, or tenseness. Tenderness may not be a reliable indicator if the casualty presents with an altered mental status or spinal injury at or above the level of the abdomen.

The diaphragm is the only muscle sheet separating the chest from the abdomen, so injury to both is common. Abdominal injuries may present with shoulder pain. Left posterior shoulder pain indicates injury to the spleen and right posterior shoulder pain indicates injury to the liver. Free blood in the abdomen causes irritation of the phrenic nerve that runs along the bottom of the diaphragm and causes the referred pain to the respective shoulder. Absence of signs and/or symptoms does not rule out abdominal injuries. Assess for shock.

General Care

To provide general emergency medical care for the abdominal injury, first ensure an open airway. Provide supplemental oxygen by nonrebreather mask at 15 L/min, if available. Assess the casualty for fluid resuscitation, keeping in mind the tenets of Tactical Combat Casualty Care (TC-3), covered in detail in Chapter 1, *Introduction to Battlefield Medicine*. Initiate a large-bore IV and treat for shock. If you suspect that the casualty may still be actively hemorrhaging, then the casualty requires expedient evacuation to a surgical facility for hemorrhage control. If the casualty is unable to be evacuated, be cautious with fluid resuscitation.

Penetrating Abdominal Wounds

In penetrating abdominal wounds, administer intravenous antibiotics if the evacuation is delayed 3 hours or more. Ensure that you flush the saline lock after administration. If the casualty is conscious, he or she may have been issued an oral antibiotic if the evacuation was delayed 3 hours or more. Casualties with allergies to antibiotics may need other medications to control infection; be familiar with your soldiers. Penetrating abdominal wounds should never be probed with fingers or instruments.

Abdominal Injuries Without Eviscerations

Expose the wound area, control the hemorrhage, and prevent further contamination to the wound. Apply a dry sterile dressing to the wound and bandage it securely in place. Keep the casualty calm.

Abdominal Injuries With Eviscerations

Do not touch or attempt to push abdominal contents protruding from a wound back into the abdominal cavity. Cover any organ or viscera protruding from a wound with a saline- or water-moistened gauze. You may also use occlusive material, plastic, or even aluminum foil. Remember, intestines may become irreversibly damaged if they are allowed to dry.

Field Medical Care TIPS

There has been controversy over the administration of oral antibiotics to casualties with penetrating abdominal wounds. If possible, utilize the IV or IM route; however, oral antibiotics can be utilized if this is the best route of administration available.

Impaled Objects

Do not remove a foreign object that is impaled in the abdomen. Stabilize the object in place with bulky dressings. Expose the wound area, and control the hemorrhage according to the procedures in Chapter 4, *Controlling Bleeding and Hypovolemic Shock*. Give the casualty nothing by mouth (NPO)—no food or anything to drink—except medications such as antibiotics or narcotic pain medications when no other route of administration is available. Initiate a large-bore IV and treat for shock per TC-3 protocol.

If evacuation is prolonged over 3 hours, then give antibiotics per local protocol. Transport to an MTF with a surgical capability.

■ Summary

Uncontrolled hemorrhage and time are the enemies of the abdominal trauma casualty and have immediate consequences to life. You must be alert to the dangers associated with the failure to promptly recognize abdominal injury and the early onset of shock in these casualties. As you've seen, early recognition, rapid evacuation, and stabilization at the appropriate echelon of care are the key to survival for casualties with abdominal injury.

YOU ARE THE
COMBAT MEDIC

Upon your arrival, you find controlled chaos with what appears to a significant and aggressive attack within a housing encampment. You approach a row of housing trailers noting major damage to the structures. You make your way into a pancaked structure and follow the voice of a woman.

Upon gaining entry, you find a 25-year-old female contractor holding her stomach. As you and a combat lifesaver (CLS) gain complete access to the casualty, you begin to assess her. You note that she has sustained inhalation burns, but is moving air with no upper airway noise. Her peripheral pulses are absent then present. You do not visualize any immediate life-threatening injuries.

Assessment

The casualty states that upon the impact of the mortar, she was thrown forward into and against her living room furniture. She denies loss of consciousness or shortness of breath. She does complain of severe abdominal pain and is guarding the midsection of her stomach. You establish that she is currently stable but her condition is highly suspicious because she is guarding her abdomen.

You and the CLS clear an area for her to lay down while waiting for extraction. You palpate and inspect her four abdominal quadrants and find bruising just below the xyphoid process extending to just above the umbilicus. You also find tenderness and guarding at the midline. She states that when you palpate, she feels a tearing and burning sensation that radiates to her back. You feel a pulsating mass along the same area. The remainder of her assessment reveals only paradoxical pulses and an elevated respiratory rate.

1. LAST NAME, FIRST NAME	RANK/GRADE		MALE	
Smith, Sara		✓	FEMALE	
SSN 000-555-1111	SPECIALTY CODE		RELIGION	

2. UNIT

FORCE				NATIONALITY		
A/T	AF/A	N/M	MC/M			
	BC/BC		NBI/BNC		DISEASE	PSYCH

3. INJURY		
		AIRWAY
		HEAD
FRONT BACK	X	WOUND
		NECK/BACK INJURY
		BURN
		AMPUTATION
		STRESS
		OTHER (Specify)

Trauma to abdomen

_____

4. LEVEL OF CONSCIOUSNESS		
X	ALERT	PAIN RESPONSE
	VERBAL RESPONSE	UNRESPONSIVE

5. PULSE	TIME	6. TOURNIQUET		TIME
		X NO	☐ YES	

7. MORPHINE		DOSE	TIME	8. IV	TIME
X NO	☐ YES				

9. TREATMENT/OBSERVATIONS/CURRENT MEDICATION/ALLERGIES/NBC (ANTIDOTE)

Guarding and tenderness at the midline. Palpate a pulsating mass at midline.

10. DISPOSITION	RETURNED TO DUTY		TIME
	X EVACUATED		
	DECEASED		

11. PROVIDER/UNIT	DATE (YYMMDD)
Wilson, Kevin	

Ready for Review

- Abdominal injuries are difficult to evaluate in the MTF and even more so on the battlefield.
- Immediate surgical intervention is needed for penetrating abdominal injuries.
- Blunt injuries may be more subtle in their presentation than penetrating injuries, but may be just as deadly.
- Whether the result of penetrating or blunt trauma, abdominal injury presents two life-threatening dangers: infection and hemorrhage.
- The index of suspicion is the primary factor in assessing abdominal trauma.
- A high index of suspicion is often based on the mechanism of injury (MOI) and your visual assessment.
- To provide general emergency medical care for the abdominal injury, first ensure an open airway, and then assess the casualty for fluid resuscitation.
- If you suspect that the casualty may still be actively hemorrhaging, then the casualty requires expedient evacuation to a surgical facility for hemorrhage control.
- If the casualty is unable to be evacuated, be cautious with fluid resuscitation.

Vital Vocabulary

blunt trauma Injury resulting from compression or deceleration forces, potentially crushing an organ or causing it to rupture.

closed abdominal injury An injury in which there is soft-tissue damage inside the body, but the skin remains intact.

open abdominal injury An injury in which there is a break in the surface of the skin or mucous membrane, exposing deeper tissue to potential contamination.

penetrating trauma An injury in which the skin is broken; direct contact results in laceration of the structure.

peritonitis Inflammation of the lining around the abdominal cavity (peritoneum) that results from either blood or hollow organ contents spilling into the abdominal cavity.

retroperitoneal abdomen Area that lies behind the thoracic and true abdomen and contains the kidneys, ureters, pancreas, posterior duodenum, ascending and descending colon, abdominal aorta, and inferior vena cava.

thoracic abdomen Area below the diaphragm but enclosed by the lower ribs.

true abdomen Area that contains the small intestine, bladder, and in females the uterus, fallopian tubes, and ovaries.

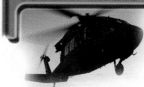

COMBAT MEDIC in Action

A motor vehicle collision occurs at an intersection. After determining that the scene is safe, you find two vehicles, one of which is broadsided on the driver's side. The driver is still in the vehicle. You notice that the damage to the driver's side is significant. The driver is responsive and alert. She is complaining of pain in the left upper quadrant of her abdomen, just below her rib cage. Her vital signs are 20 breaths/min and pulse at 130 beats/min. The c-spine is stabilized and she is extricated. You perform a complete assessment. Everything is unremarkable except that she has pain on palpation to her upper quadrant and pain in her left shoulder. Her abdomen is soft, and she is not guarding it.

1. Which are the solid organs of the abdomen?
   A. Liver, spleen, kidneys, and pancreas
   B. Liver, spleen, and pancreas
   C. Large intestine, small intestine, stomach
   D. Liver, spleen, kidneys, and intestines

2. The abdominal cavity is lined with a membrane called the:
   A. retroperitoneal space.
   B. pylorus.
   C. peritoneum.
   D. stomach.

3. The spleen is a highly vascular organ that lies in which quadrant?
   A. Right upper
   B. Left lower
   C. Left upper
   D. Right lower

4. Rupture of an organ can lead to hemorrhage and:
   A. tension pneumothorax.
   B. internal bleeding.
   C. blunt trauma.
   D. penetrating trauma.

5. True or false? Casualties without abdominal pain or abnormal vital signs are unlikely to have serious intrabdominal injuries.
   A. True
   B. False

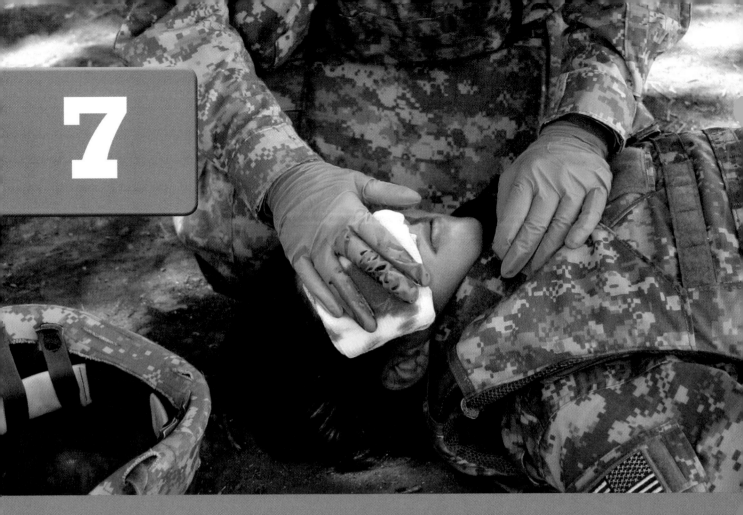

7

Head Injuries

Objectives

Knowledge Objectives

- [ ] Describe the anatomy and physiology of the head.
- [ ] Identify the basic management techniques for a head injury.
- [ ] List the signs of intracranial pressure of the brain.
- [ ] Identify the possible injuries of the head and brain.
- [ ] Identify the signs and symptoms of ocular injuries.
- [ ] Describe how to care for ocular injuries.

Skills Objectives

- [ ] Perform an upper eyelid eversion.
- [ ] Perform eye irrigation.
- [ ] Perform the visual acuity test.
- [ ] Bandage an impaled object in the eye.
- [ ] Instill eye drops.
- [ ] Instill eye ointment.

■ Introduction

On the battlefield, the structures that regulate the senses are extremely important for a casualty's survival. Delicate structures such as the eye demand diligent care when injured or damaged. Additionally, when soft-tissue injuries are caused by either blunt or penetrating trauma, underlying structures such as the cranium, brain, trachea, neck vessels, and cervical spine may also be damaged. Whether on the battlefield or in garrison operations, the potential exists for you to encounter a casualty with an injury to the eye or surrounding soft tissues.

You must be familiar with the anatomy, physiology, signs and symptoms, and treatment of ocular injuries to avoid significant and/or permanent disability to the casualty's vision. A comprehensive knowledge of the basic anatomy and physiology of the head, brain, and spinal column is necessary to manage the head-injured casualty effectively. In warfare, the types of injuries sustained are a direct result of the types of weapons being used. With today's increase in use of improvised explosive devices (IEDs), rocket-propelled grenades, and motor vehicle accidents, there is an increase in head injuries. Many head injuries are being missed or overlooked because they are secondary injuries. Primary injuries are usually obvious and therefore treated expeditiously, but secondary injuries are harder to identify and are often missed because of more obvious injuries. To help identify secondary head injuries, the MACE assessment tool has been adopted.

■ Anatomy and Physiology of the Head

The Scalp

The brain—the most important organ in the body—requires maximum protection from injury. The human body ensures that it receives this protection by housing the brain within several layers of soft and hard wrappings. Starting from the outside and proceeding inward toward the brain, the first protective layer is the scalp, which consists of the following layers, given in descending order:

- Skin with hair.
- Subcutaneous tissue, which contains major scalp veins that bleed profusely when lacerated.
- Loose connective tissue (alveolar tissue), which is easily stripped from the layer beneath in scalping injuries. The looseness of the alveolar layer also provides room for blood to accumulate between the scalp and skull bone after blunt trauma.

The scalp bleeds freely when lacerated and prolonged hemorrhage may lead to significant blood loss.

The Skull

At the top of the axial skeleton is the **skull** (cranium), which consists of 28 bones. The skull encloses and protects brain tissue. It is divided into two large structures: the cranium and the face **FIGURE 7-1 ▾**. The mandible (lower jaw), the only movable facial bone, is connected to the cranium by the temporomandibular joint in front of each ear. The other bones of the anterior cranium that connect to facial bones are the maxillae (fused bones of the upper jaw), zygomatic bones (cheekbones), and nasal bone (provides some of the structure of the nose).

The **foramen magnum** is the primary opening through which pressure on the brain can be released. It is a circular opening located at the base of the skull through which the spinal cord passes.

The orbits enclose and protect the eyes. In addition to the eyeball and the muscles that move it, the orbit contains blood vessels, nerves, and fat. A blow to the eye may result in a fracture of the orbital floor because the bone is extremely thin and breaks easily. A blowout fracture **FIGURE 7-2 ▸** results in transmission of forces away from the eyeball itself to the bone. Blood and fat then leak into the maxillary sinus.

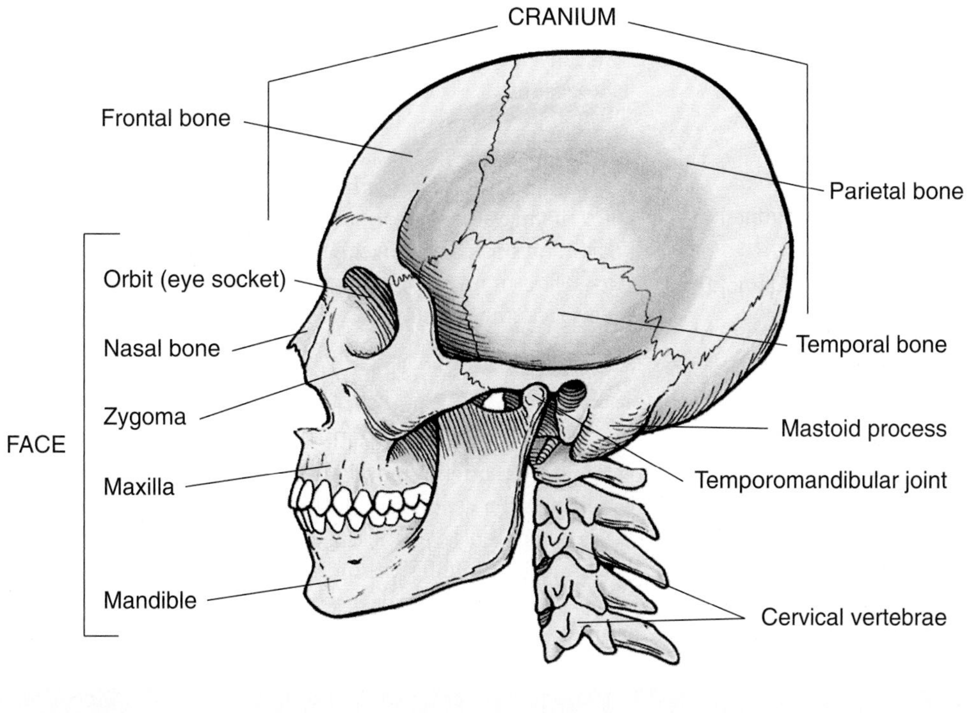

FIGURE 7-1   The skull has two large structures: the cranium and the face.

The nose is one of the two primary entry points for use as an airway. The nasal septum, which separates the nostrils, should be in the midline, although it can be deviated to one side (usually the left) as a result of normal growth or from acute trauma. The external portion of the nose is formed mostly of cartilage.

Several bones associated with the nose contain cavities known as the paranasal sinuses FIGURE 7-3 ▾. These hollowed out sections of bone, which are lined with mucous membranes, decrease the weight of the skull and provide resonance for the voice. The contents of the sinuses drain into the nasal cavity.

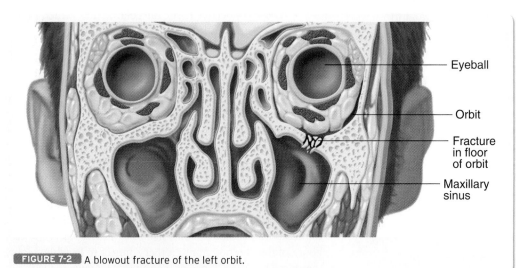

FIGURE 7-2 A blowout fracture of the left orbit.

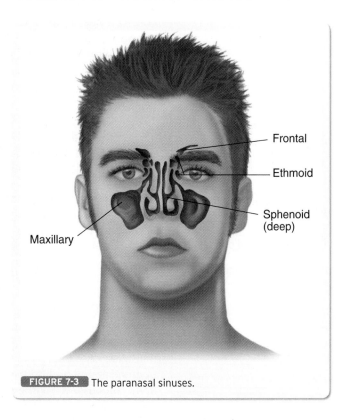

FIGURE 7-3 The paranasal sinuses.

The Brain

The **brain**, which occupies 80% of the cranial vault, contains billions of neurons (nerve cells) that serve a variety of vital functions FIGURE 7-4 ▸. The major regions of the brain are the cerebrum, brain stem, and cerebellum. The cerebrum is the largest part of the brain and controls higher brain functions. The cerebellum controls the primitive functions, coordination, and balance. The brain stem controls the vital body functions such as the cardiorespiratory functions. The remaining intracranial contents include cerebral blood (12%) and cerebrospinal fluid (8%).

The brain accounts for only 2% of total body weight, yet it is the most metabolically active and perfusion-sensitive organ in the body. Because the brain has no storage mechanism for oxygen or glucose, it is totally dependent on a constant source of both fuels via cerebral blood flow provided by the carotid and vertebral arteries. As such, the brain will continually manipulate the physiology as needed to guarantee that a ready supply of oxygen and glucose is available.

As mentioned, the cerebrum is the largest portion of the brain, and is responsible for higher functioning such as reasoning. It is divided into left and right hemispheres. The two hemispheres do not function equally. In a right-handed person, for example, the speech center is usually located in the left hemisphere, which is then said to be dominant. The cerebrum is divided into specialized areas called lobes.

The cerebellum controls more primitive functions, and is sometimes called the "athlete's brain" because it is responsible for the maintenance of posture and equilibrium and the coordination of skilled movements.

The brain stem is located at the base of the brain and connects the spinal cord to the rest of the brain. Many structures critical to the maintenance of vital functions are located here. Two primary components of the brain stem are the medulla and the pons. The medulla (or medulla oblongata) coordinates heart rate, blood vessel diameter, swallowing, vomiting, coughing, and sneezing. The pons acts as a relay between the cerebrum and the cerebellum, and also contains the sleep center of the brain. The medulla directly controls respirations, while the pons has some indirect control, so injury to either can have a negative impact on the casualty's ability to breathe properly.

Surrounding and enfolding the brain and spinal cord is a protective covering called the meninges FIGURE 7-5 ▸. The meninges consist of three layers: the dura mater, the arachnoid membrane, and the pia mater. The meningeal arteries are located between the dura mater and the skull, and there is a potential space between the dura mater and the skull where blood can collect following a head injury.

The arachnoid membrane is so named because the blood vessels it contains resemble a spider web. This membrane is thin and delicate. The innermost layer, the pia mater, is a thin,

translucent, highly vascular membrane that firmly adheres directly to the surface of the brain.

In the space between the arachnoid membrane and the pia mater (the subarachnoid space) is a nutrient-filled fluid called **cerebrospinal fluid (CSF)**. CSF is manufactured in the ventricles (hollow storage areas in the brain), and normally flows freely between the ventricles and through the subarachnoid space. A blockage in this system can cause an increase in the pressure within the brain (intracerebral pressure or ICP), as can bleeds within the cranial cavity. CSF is normally reabsorbed by the arachnoid membrane.

The Eyes

The eyes are delicate organs adapted to provide vision. They are protected by the skull, eyelids, eyelashes, and tears. Their shape is maintained by fluid contained within the eye. The structures of the eye FIGURE 7-6 ▶ include the following:

- The **sclera** (white of the eye) is a tough, fibrous coat that helps maintain the shape of the eye and protect the contents of the eye. It is connected to six muscles that allow the eye to look up, down, and side to side. In some illnesses, such as hepatitis, the sclera becomes yellow.
- The **cornea** is the tough, transparent, colorless portion of the eye that overlies the iris and

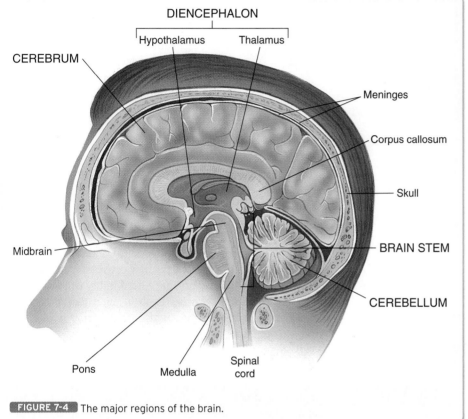

FIGURE 7-4 The major regions of the brain.

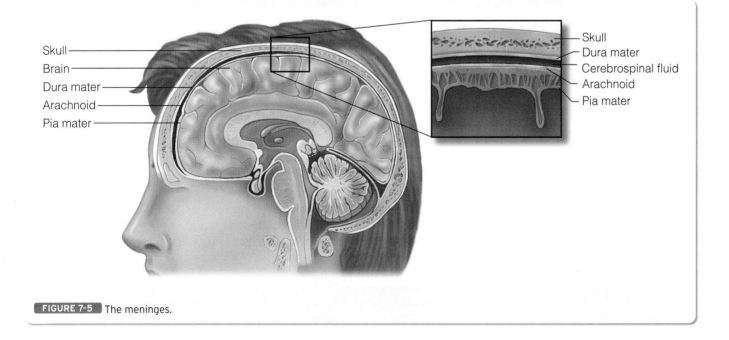

FIGURE 7-5 The meninges.

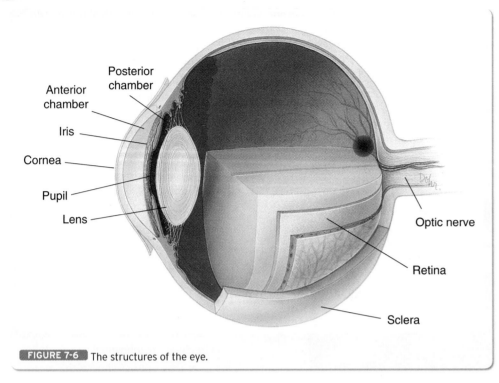

Anterior chamber
Posterior chamber
Iris
Cornea
Pupil
Lens
Optic nerve
Retina
Sclera

FIGURE 7-6 The structures of the eye.

pupil. Injuries may cause opacity and stop light rays from entering the eye.

- The **conjunctiva** is a delicate mucous membrane that lines the eyelid and extends from the eyelid to the front of the eyeball. It covers the anterior portion of the sclera. Cyanosis can be detected in the conjunctiva when it is not easily assessed by the skin of dark-skinned casualties.

- The **iris** is the colored part of the eye located between the cornea and lens. It controls the amount of light entering the eye.

- The **pupil** is the adjustable circular opening within the iris through which light passes to the lens. A normal pupil dilates in dim light to permit more light to enter the eye and constricts in bright light to decrease the amount of light entering the eye.

- Behind the pupil and iris is the **lens**, a transparent circular structure filled with a jelly-like substance that can adjust to focus both near and far objects.

- The **retina** is the inner layer of the eye and contains rods and cones, the specialized receptors that allow us to see. It is a delicate, 10-layered structure of nervous tissue that extends from the optic nerve. It receives light impulses and converts them to nerve signals that are conducted to the brain by the optic nerve and interpreted as vision.

- The **lacrimal glands** (tear glands) are located in the upper, outer aspect of each upper eyelid. Tears prevent infection and keep the eyes moist, and drain through ducts located in the eyelids.

- The **canthus** is the corner of the eye, where the upper and lower eyelids meet. Each eye has a medial canthus and a lateral canthus.

Assess Head Injury

Initial Assessment

The initial assessment of the casualty with a possible head injury includes forming a general impression and determining the level of consciousness. A change in the level of consciousness is the single most important observation you can make when determining the severity of a head injury. Initially, determining the casualty's AVPU score (Alert, responsive to Verbal stimuli, responsive to Pain, and Unresponsive) is adequate because the rapid trauma survey includes a more thorough neurologic exam.

As part of your general impression, ask the casualty what happened and where it hurts. Confused or slurred speech, repetitive questions, and/or amnesia are indicators of a head injury. Although other problems may cause similar symptoms, in the setting of trauma, assume a head injury exists until your assessment proves otherwise. Keep in mind that any casualty with a suspected head injury is also presumed to have a spinal injury, so cervical spine precautions should be observed.

Continue your assessment with the casualty's airway; head injury casualties are more prone to airway obstruction. Open the airway with the jaw-thrust maneuver. An oral airway may be inserted if needed. Nasal airways should not be used in the setting of a likely head injury or severe facial trauma because of the possibility that the casualty has a basal skull fracture, which could result in the nasal airway being inserted directly into the brain instead of the airway as intended. Vomiting is common within the first hour following head trauma, so be alert for the need to log roll the casualty and/or clear the casualty's airway.

Assess the casualty's circulation. As previously discussed, casualties with head injuries are at high risk for spinal injuries, and spinal injuries can cause a loss of blood pressure control, resulting in hypotension and hypoperfusion. Additionally, the injury itself may have caused another bleed elsewhere in the body that results in hypoperfusion. Check the casualty's pulse to see if it is slow, fast, weak, or bounding. One key point to remember is that when a head injury itself causes hypotension, it is often a terminal event. When presented with a head-injured casualty who is hypotensive, you should always look for another cause for the drop in pressure, which generally means looking for a bleed somewhere—something to note in the initial assessment and then keep in mind for the rapid trauma survey.

Rapid Trauma Survey

Alterations in the casualty's level of consciousness are the hallmark of a brain injury.

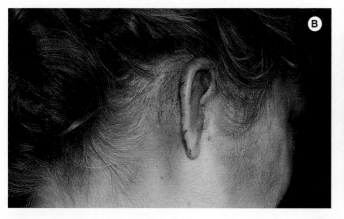
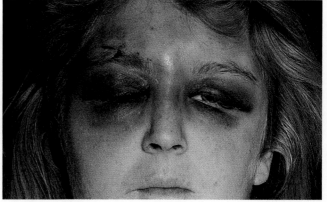

FIGURE 7-7 Signs of a basilar skull fracture include **A.** Battle's sign and **B.** Raccoon eyes.

Look for obvious deformities such as depressed or open skull fractures and lacerations. Do not probe any open lacerations or depressions you find, because this may push bone fragments into the brain. Never remove any impaled objects from an open head injury. As stated before, all casualties with head injuries must be suspected of having a cervical spine injury as well and managed accordingly.

Bleeding from the ear or nose is a sign of head trauma. One technique for detecting CSF that is mixed with blood is the halo or target sign. When a drop of fluid is allowed to fall onto a bed sheet or gauze, the CSF will diffuse from blood and form a halo ring around the blood. Other signs of head trauma are swelling and/or discoloration behind the ear (**Battle's sign**) and swelling and/or discoloration around both eyes (**raccoon eyes**). These signs may indicate a basilar skull fracture   FIGURE 7-7 ▲ .

Frequently monitor the size, equality, and reactivity of the casualty's pupils. The nerves that control dilation and constriction of the pupils are very sensitive to changes in ICP. Pupils that are slow to constrict (sluggish) are a relatively early sign of increased ICP; sluggish pupils could also indicate hypoxia. Brain stem injury is probable if both pupils are dilated and do not react to light. This is an ominous sign of increased ICP   FIGURE 7-8 ▶ . If the pupils are dilated but react to light, injury is often reversible. Other causes of dilated pupils that may or may not react to light include the following:

- Hypothermia
- Anoxia
- Lightning strike (ocular autonomic disturbance may occur after lightning strike, so dilated unresponsive pupils should not be used as a sign of brain death)
- Optic nerve injury
- Direct trauma to the eye
- Drug effects
- A glass eye
- Anisocoria (normal condition where one pupil is larger than the other at baseline)

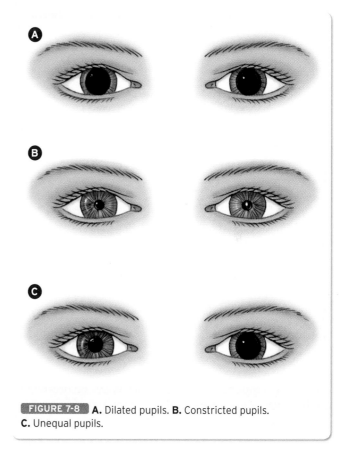

FIGURE 7-8 **A.** Dilated pupils. **B.** Constricted pupils. **C.** Unequal pupils.

If the casualty has a normal level of consciousness (LOC), then the dilated pupils are not due to head injury—you must look for other causes. Reassess the casualty immediately.

Check for DCAP-BTLS from head to toe. See if the casualty has intact sensation and motor functions by pinching the fingers and toes and looking for withdrawal or localization of the pain   FIGURE 7-9 ▶ . This usually indicates there is normal or minimally impaired brain function.

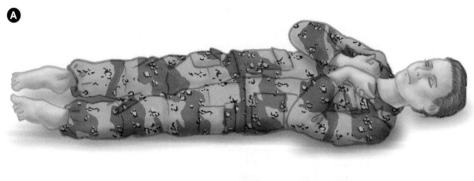

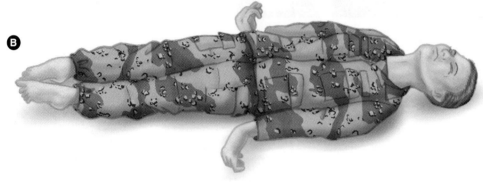

FIGURE 7-9 Posturing in response to painful stimuli can give you information about the casualty's condition. **A.** Decorticate posturing. **B.** Decerebrate posturing.

You may also see posturing in severe cases. There are two types of posturing: **decorticate** and **decerebrate**. The casualty exhibiting decorticate posturing will exhibit hyperextension in the legs and flexion at the arms and elbows with the hands coming in toward the center (core) of the body. This may occur if the injury is at the level of the upper midbrain. Although any posturing is a very bad sign, it is not nearly as bad as decerebrate posturing. In decerebrate posturing, the casualty will present with teeth clenched, arms and legs extended, and wrists flexed. This is usually caused by a severe injury involving the central midbrain. Casualties may have decorticate posturing on one side of the body and decerebrate on the other, or may go back and forth between the two.

Additional Assessment

Baseline vital signs may indicate changes in the status of intracranial pressure.

Observe and record the baseline vital signs during the additional assessment and each time you perform a reassessment. Increasing intracranial pressure causes increased blood pressure (hypertension). The reasons for this are:

- In a closed head injury, intracranial pressure increases as a result of swelling of the brain due to trauma.

- As the pressure increases on the brain, cerebrovascular perfusion may be compromised. The result of this is an autonomic response by the brain to increase perfusion, resulting in a marked hypertension.

When low blood pressure (hypotension) is caused by a head injury, it is usually a terminal event. Hypovolemic shock does not result from an isolated head injury; look for another cause of the hypovolemia. A decrease in pulse rate (bradycardia) may be caused by an increase in intracranial pressure.

Increasing intracranial pressure causes the respiratory rate to increase or decrease, and/or become irregular. Unusual respiratory patterns may reflect the level of brain/brain stem injury. Keep in mind that respirations are not as useful an indicator as other vital signs in monitoring the course of a head injury. Respirations could also be affected by fear, hysteria, chronic illnesses, chest injuries, and spinal cord injuries.

Assess the neurologic status using the Glasgow Coma Scale (GCS):

- **Severe head injury:** GCS is < 9.
- **Moderate head injury:** GCS is 9 to 13.
- **Minor head injury:** GCS is 14 to 15.

Next, reassess the casualty and record the casualty's level of consciousness. Record the casualty's pupil size and reactivity to light, baseline vital signs, and baseline neurologic status because decisions on casualty management are made based on changes in all parameters of the physical and neurologic examination. Future decisions on treatment depend on baseline evaluations and observed changes.

Field Medical Care TIPS

Prior to death, the casualty may develop a rapid, noisy respiratory pattern called central neurogenic hyperventilation.

MACE Assessment Tool

The MACE assessment is a tool developed by the Defense and Veterans Brain Injury Center (DVBIC). The purpose of the MACE is to evaluate a casualty in whom a concussion is suspected. The four cognitive domains tested are: orientation, immediate memory, concentration, and delayed recall. The MACE is used to confirm a diagnosis and assess the current clinical status of the casualty.

The MACE is the recommended tool for use in theatre at Level I, II, and III. This tool can be easily used by combat medics to confirm a suspected diagnosis of concussion and can be administered in 5 minutes. Evaluate any casualty who was dazed, confused, "saw stars," or lost consciousness (even momentarily) as a result of an explosion, blast, fall, motor vehicle crash, or other event involving abrupt head movement or a direct blow to the head.

The MACE assessment tool has 13 sections FIGURE 7-10 ▶:

- **History (I–VIII)**
    - **I** Description of the incident
    - **II** Cause of the injury
    - **III** Was a helmet on?
    - **IV** Amnesia before?
    - **V** Amnesia after?
    - **VI** Loss of consciousness (LOC) or "blacking out"
    - **VII** Observation of LOC or unresponsiveness
    - **VIII** Symptoms
- **Examination (IX–XIII):** Give one point for each correct response for a total of five possible points. It should be noted that a correct response on time of day must be within 1 hour of the actual time.
    - **Orientation (IX):** Assess the casualty's awareness of the accurate time:

      What month is this?

      What is the date or day of the month?

      What day of the week is it?

      What year is it?

      What time do you think it is?
    - **Immediate Memory (X):** Assess the casualty using a brief repeated list learning test. Read the casualty the list of five words once and then ask the casualty to repeat it back to you, as many as the casualty can recall, in any order. Repeat this procedure two more times for a total of three trials, even if the casualty scores perfectly on the first trial. One point is given for each correct answer for a total of 15 possible points.
    - **Neurological Screening (XI):** No points are given for this section:

      Eyes: check pupil size and reactivity.

      Verbal: notice speech fluency and word finding.

      Motor: (pronator drift) ask the casualty to lift arms with palms up, ask the casualty to then close his or her eyes, assess for either arm to "drift" down. Assess the casualty's gait and coordination if possible. Document any abnormalities.
    - **Concentration (XII):** The casualty receives one point for each string length for a total of four points and one point if able to recite *all* months in reverse order. The total possible score for concentration portion is five.

      Inform the casualty that you are going to read a string of numbers and when you are finished, casualty needs to repeat them backwards. That is, in reverse order of how you read them. For example if you say 7-1-9, the casualty will say 9-1-7. Repeat this. If the casualty is correct on the first trial of each string length, proceed to the next string length. Proceed to the next string length if the casualty is correct on the second trial. Discontinue after casualty failure on both trials of the same string. There are a total of four different string lengths.

      Have the casualty tell you the months of the year in reverse order. That is, start with December and end with January.
    - **Delayed Recall (XIII):** Assess the casualty's ability to retain previously learned information by asking him or her to recall as many words as possible from the initial word list, without reading the word list. Give one point for each word remembered for a total of five possible points.

The total possible score for the MACE assessment tool is 30. The mean total score is 28. Scores below 25 may represent clinically relevant neurocognitive impairment and require further evaluation for the possibility of a more serious brain injury. The scoring system also takes on particular clinical significance during serial assessments.

Level 1 Algorithm

The Level 1 Algorithm is an algorithm that can be used at Level I sites by all health care providers to determine if a soldier should be suspected of a traumatic brain injury (TBI) and needs to be further evaluated FIGURE 7-11 ▶. Evaluate any casualty who was dazed, confused, "saw stars," or lost consciousness (even momentarily) as a result of an explosion, blast, fall, motor vehicle crash, or other event involving abrupt head movement or a direct blow to the head.

■ Assess and Provide Care for a Traumatic Head Injury

Your mission in managing head injuries is to prevent secondary injury. It is extremely important to perform a rapid trauma survey and then transport the casualty to a facility capable of managing head trauma.

Impaled Object in the Cheek

The signs and symptoms of an impaled object in the cheek include:

- An obvious object that has passed through an external cheek
- Bleeding into the mouth and throat (blood in the mouth and throat may induce nausea and vomiting)

Ensure an open airway in the casualty that is free of obstructions (eg, broken teeth/dentures or oral cavity bleeding). If necessary, examine the external cheek and the inside of the mouth to determine whether the object passed through the cheek wall. If you see an impaled object in the cheek but cannot see both ends, stabilize the object in place. Do not try to remove the object as long as the airway is not compromised.

Treatment and transport considerations include:

- Checking neurologic status using the GCS
- Immobilizing the head and neck

If the casualty's airway is open, leave the object in place and stabilize it. Pack the inside of the cheek with rolled gauze. Use of standard face masks may be dangerous unless you leave 3″ to 4″ of the dressing outside of the casualty's mouth. Dress the external wound and suction as needed. Provide full spinal immobilization on a long board. Transport the casualty in the lateral recumbent position, with the head of the spine board elevated to allow for drainage and vomitus if

Patient Name: _____

SS#: _____-_____-_____ Unit: _____

Date of Injury: _____/_____/_____ Time of Injury: _____

Examiner: _____

Date of Evaluation: _____/_____/_____ Time of Evaluation: _____

History: (I—VIII)

I. Description of Incident
Ask:
a) What happened?
b) Tell me what you remember.
c) Were you dazed, confused, "saw stars"? ☐ Yes ☐ No
d) Did you hit your head? ☐ Yes ☐ No

II. Cause of Injury: (circle all that apply)
1) Explosion/blast 4) Fragment
2) Blunt object 5) Fall
3) MVC 6) Gunshot wound
7) Other _____

III. Was a helmet worn?
☐ Yes ☐ No Type _____

IV. Amnesia Before: Are there any events just BEFORE the injury that are not remembered? (Assess for continuous memory prior to injury)
☐ Yes ☐ No If yes, how long? _____

V. Amnesia After: Are there any events just AFTER the injuries that are not remembered? (Assess time until continuous memory after the injury)
☐ Yes ☐ No If yes, how long? _____

VI. Does the individual report loss of consciousness or "blacking out"?
☐ Yes ☐ No If yes, how long? _____

VII. Did anyone observe a period of loss of consciousness or unresponsiveness?
☐ Yes ☐ No If yes, how long? _____

VIII. Symptoms: (circle all that apply)
1) Headache 2) Dizziness
3) Memory problems 4) Balance problems
5) Nausea/vomiting 6) Difficulty
7) Irritability concentrating
8) Visual disturbances
9) Ringing in the ears
10) Other _____

Examination: (IX—XIII)

Evaluate each domain. Total possible score is 30.

IX. Orientation: (1 point each)

Month:	0	1
Date:	0	1
Day of week:	0	1
Year:	0	1
Time:	0	1

Orientation Total Score _____/5

X. Immediate Memory: Read all five words and ask the patient to recall them in any order. Repeat steps two more times for a total of three trials. (1 point for each correct word, total over three trials)

List	Trial 1	Trial 2	Trial 3
Elbow	0 1	0 1	0 1
Apple	0 1	0 1	0 1
Carpet	0 1	0 1	0 1
Saddle	0 1	0 1	0 1
Bubble	0 1	0 1	0 1
Trial score	____	____	____

Immediate Memory Total Score _____/15

XI. Neurological Screening As the clinical condition permits, check:
Eyes: pupillary response and tracking
Verbal: speech fluency and word finding
Motor: pronator drift, gait/coordination
Record any abnormalities. **No points are given for this.**

XII. Concentration
Reverse digits: (Go to next string length if correct on first trial. Stop if incorrect on both trials.) One point for each string length.

4-9-3	6-2-9	0	1
3-8-1-4	3-2-7-9	0	1
6-2-9-7-1	1-5-2-8-5	0	1
7-1-8-4-6-2	5-3-9-1-4-8	0	1

Months in reverse order (1 point for entire sequence correct)
Dec-Nov-Oct-Sep-Aug-Jul-Jun-May-Apr-Mar-Feb-Jan
0 1

Concentration Total Score _____/5

XIII. Delayed Recall (1 point each). Ask the patient to recall the 5 words from the earlier memory test. (Do NOT reread the word list.)

Elbow	0	1
Apple	0	1
Carpet	0	1
Saddle	0	1
Bubble	0	1

Delayed Recall Total Score _____/5

TOTAL SCORE _____/30

Notes: _____
_____
_____

Diagnosis: (circle one or write in diagnoses)
No concussion
850.0 Concussion without loss of consciousness (LOC)
850.1 Concussion with loss of consciousness (LOC)
Other diagnoses: _____
_____

FIGURE 7-10 MACE Assessment Tool.

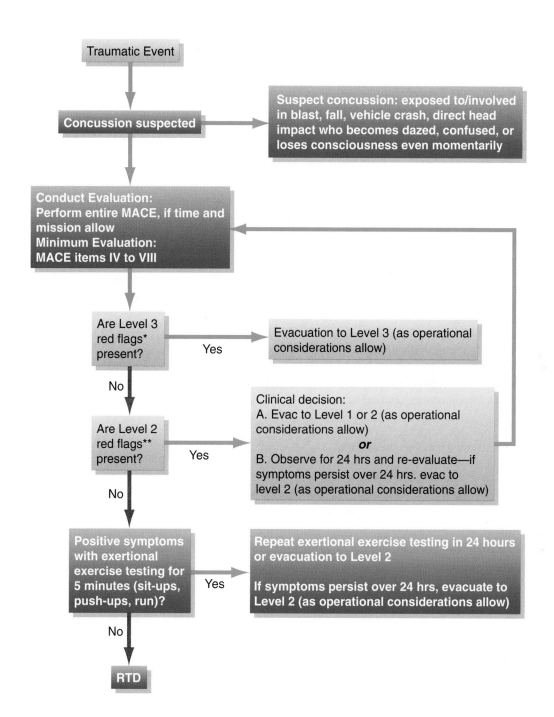

Traumatic Event

Concussion suspected → Suspect concussion: exposed to/involved in blast, fall, vehicle crash, direct head impact who becomes dazed, confused, or loses consciousness even momentarily

Conduct Evaluation:
Perform entire MACE, if time and mission allow
Minimum Evaluation:
MACE items IV to VIII

Are Level 3 red flags* present? — Yes → Evacuation to Level 3 (as operational considerations allow)

No ↓

Are Level 2 red flags** present? — Yes → Clinical decision:
A. Evac to Level 1 or 2 (as operational considerations allow)
or
B. Observe for 24 hrs and re-evaluate—if symptoms persist over 24 hrs. evac to level 2 (as operational considerations allow)

No ↓

Positive symptoms with exertional exercise testing for 5 minutes (sit-ups, push-ups, run)? — Yes → Repeat exertional exercise testing in 24 hours or evacuation to Level 2

If symptoms persist over 24 hrs, evacuate to Level 2 (as operational considerations allow)

No ↓

RTD

* Level 3 Evacuation Decisions Red Flags:
1. Progressively declining levels of consciousness/Neurological exam
2. Pupillary asymmetry
3. Seizures
4. Repeated vomiting

** Level 2 Evacuation Decisions Red Flags:
1. MACE (items IV-VIII)
2. RED FLAGs
   a. Double vision
   b. Worsening headache
   c. Can't recognize people or place disorientation
   d. Behaves unusually or seems confused and irritable
   e. Slurred speech
   f. Unsteady on feet
   g. Weakness or numbness in arms/legs

Treatment:
1. Headache management: Tylenol
2. Avoid tramadol, narcotics, NSAIDs, ASA or other platelet inhibitors until CT confirmed negative
3. Give an educational sheet to all positive mild TBI patients
4. Rest, limited duty activities

FIGURE 7-11 Level 1 Algorithm.

there is no spinal involvement. Give oxygen via a nasal cannula if constant suctioning is required. Monitor the baseline vital signs and airway every 3 to 5 minutes for any changes and document these findings.

Nasal Injuries

The signs and symptoms of nasal injuries include:

- Abrasions, lacerations, and punctures
- Avulsions
- Difficulty breathing through the nares
- Nosebleeds (epistaxis)
- Other traumatic injuries, indicating that the casualty has suffered a traumatic mechanism of injury

Ensure that the airway is patent. Even though the mouth may be clear, blood and mucus released from nasal injuries can flow into the throat causing an airway obstruction. Expect vomiting and be prepared to suction the casualty.

Treatment and transport considerations include:

- **Abrasions, lacerations, and punctures:** Control the bleeding, apply a sterile dressing, and bandage in place.
- **Avulsion:** Return the attached flaps to the normal position. Apply a pressure dressing and bandage. Fully avulsed flaps of skin and avulsed portions of external nose should be kept cool and transported with the casualty.
- **Foreign objects:** Do not pull free or probe. Transport the casualty without disturbing the object unless the object is obstructing the airway.

Fully immobilize the spine if signs of a cervical spine or head injury are present. Monitor the baseline vital signs, airway, and LOC every 3 to 5 minutes. Transport the casualty in a sitting position if no signs or symptoms of a head or spinal injury are present.

Nosebleeds

For a casualty with no signs or symptoms of skull fracture or spinal injury, place the casualty in a slightly forward, seated position to allow for drainage. For an unconscious casualty or if signs and symptoms of spinal injury are present, fully immobilize the casualty on a long spine board. Elevate the board 6″ and turn it to the side to facilitate drainage.

You or the casualty may pinch the nostrils to control bleeding. Apply pressure for at least 5 minutes and *do not* pack the nostrils. However, if there is clear fluid or a mix of blood and clear fluid draining from the nose or the ears, the casualty may have a skull fracture. Do not pinch the nostrils or attempt to stop the drainage flow.

Oral Cavity Injuries

The signs and symptoms of oral cavity injuries include:

- Lacerated lip or gum
- Lacerated or avulsed tongue
- Dislodged teeth

Airway obstruction is a common problem with this type of injury. Look for foreign objects (eg, blood, teeth, vomit, mucus) in the airway. Remove any dislodged teeth and dental appliances. With a gloved hand, remove loose dentures and any parts of broken dentures. Transport any dental appliance and broken teeth with the casualty. Place any teeth in a container of normal saline or milk. Ensure an open airway.

For a lacerated lip or gum, control the bleeding by placing a rolled or folded dressing between the lip and the gum, leaving a dressing "tail" exposed. For profuse bleeding, position the casualty to allow for drainage. Monitor the casualty and dressing closely.

For a lacerated or avulsed tongue, do not pack the mouth with dressings. Position the casualty for drainage. For a fully avulsed tongue, save and wrap the part, keep it cool, and transport it with the casualty.

For an avulsed lip, control the bleeding with a pressure dressing and position for drainage. Do not bandage across the mouth. Save, wrap, label, and transport any fully avulsed tissues, keeping the part cool. Transport the casualty in a sitting position unless signs of spinal or head injury are present.

■ Assess Eye Injuries

Assessment of Ocular Trauma

Ocular trauma is classified as penetrating or nonpenetrating; either type can lead to serious damage and loss of vision. Eye injuries on the battlefield are common in spite of the eyes being protected by the bony orbit.

Take the casualty's history. As with other medical areas, an accurate history often assists you in establishing severity of injury. Determine the mechanism of injury:

- Was it a blunt trauma or penetrating injury?
- Was there a projectile or missile?
- Was it caused by glass from a motor vehicle accident?
- Did the casualty suffer thermal, chemical, or laser burns?
- Does the casualty wear glasses or contact lenses?
- Does the casualty have a history of eye disease or previous eye trauma or surgery?
- Is there eye pain or loss of vision?
- If there is vision loss, is it in one eye or both?

During the rapid trauma survey, determine visual acuity, the most important step in evaluating extent of injury. Screen visual acuity with any available printed material if you are in the field. If the casualty is unable to read print, have the casualty count your raised fingers or distinguish between light and dark. If you are in a garrison clinic, screen the casualty utilizing a standard Snellen chart. Determine DCAP-BTLS, discoloration, foreign bodies, blood in the anterior chamber (hyphema), pupillary response, drainage, or bleeding from the eye.

Specific Ocular Injuries

Eyelid Injuries

The signs and symptoms of eyelid injuries include:

- Ecchymosis
- Swelling
- Pain

Perform an Upper Eyelid Eversion

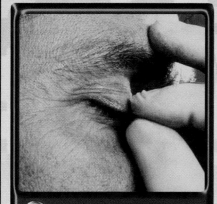

1. Evert the upper eyelid by having the casualty look down. Gently grasp the casualty's upper eyelashes and pull them out and down.

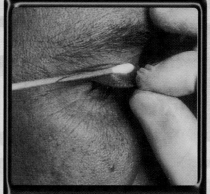

2. Place the shaft of an applicator or tongue blade about 1 cm from the eyelid margin. Pull the eyelid upward using the applicator as a fulcrum to turn the eyelid inside out. Do not press down on the eye itself.

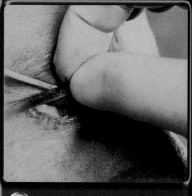

3. Pin the eyelid in this position by pressing the lashes against the eyebrow while you examine the upper eyelid. Ask the casualty to blink several times to return the eyelid to a normal position.

Perform a visual acuity test. Assess DCAP-BTLS, discoloration, and pupillary response, and assess for eyelid foreign bodies. Look at the underlying eye structures for a more serious injury.

Treating Foreign Bodies in the Eyelid

The first step is to locate the foreign body. An upper eyelid eversion is commonly performed to examine the inside of the upper eyelid. To perform this procedure, follow the steps in SKILL DRILL 7-1 ▲ :

1. Evert the upper eyelid by having the casualty look down.
2. Gently grasp the casualty's upper eyelashes and pull them out and down (**Step ①**).
3. Place the shaft of an applicator or tongue blade about 1 cm from the eyelid margin.
4. Pull the eyelid upward using the applicator as a fulcrum to turn the eyelid inside out. Do not press down on the eye itself (**Step ②**).
5. Pin the eyelid in this position by pressing the lashes against the eyebrow while you examine the upper eyelid.
6. Ask the casualty to blink several times to return the eyelid to a normal position (**Step ③**).

If you find a foreign body, perform an eye irrigation; however, do not irrigate an eye that has an impaled object

in it. Eye irrigation is used to flush superficial foreign bodies or toxic chemicals from one or both eyes. Irrigations are occasionally utilized for removing dried mucus or drainage that may accumulate in inflamed or infected eye structures. There are no contraindications to this procedure, but irrigation must be performed gently and carefully. To perform this procedure, follow the steps in SKILL DRILL 7-2 ▶ :

1. Identify the casualty and explain the procedure.
2. Ask the casualty to remove any contact lenses or eyeglasses, if necessary. If the casualty is unable to remove them him- or herself, remove the lenses yourself.
3. Position the casualty. If the casualty is lying on his or her back, tilt his or her head slightly to the side that is being irrigated. If the casualty is seated, tilt his or her head slightly backward and to the side that is being irrigated (**Step ①**).
4. Position the equipment. Drape the areas of the casualty that may be splashed by the solution. Place a catch basin next to the face on the affected side. Position the light source so that it does not shine directly into the casualty's eyes.
5. Put on gloves (**Step ②**).

6. Clean the eyelids gently with cotton balls, and clean debris from the outer eye (**Step ③**).

7. Separate the eyelids using your thumb and forefinger, and hold the lids open.

8. Irrigate the eye by holding the irrigating tip 1″ to 1½″ away from the casualty's eye. Direct the irrigating solution gently from the inner canthus to the outer canthus. Use only enough pressure to maintain a steady flow of solution and to dislodge the secretions or foreign bodies. The irrigator should never touch the casualty's eye (**Step ④**).

9. Instruct the casualty to look up to expose the conjunctival sac and lower surface of the eye.

10. Instruct the casualty to look down to expose the upper surface of the eye.

11. Dry the area around the eye by gently patting with gauze sponges. Do not touch the casualty's eye.

12. Remove your gloves and wash your hands (**Step ⑤**).

13. Record the treatment given on the appropriate form (**Step ⑥**).

Treating Eyelid Lacerations

Cover the affected eye with a loose dressing to stop the bleeding. Cover both eyes and evacuate the casualty as soon as possible. Evacuate the casualty with glasses, if indicated.

Corneal Injuries

Corneal abrasions may occur from trauma or from contact lens wearing. Assessment begins with a visual acuity test. Assess DCAP-BTLS, discoloration, pupillary response, and corneal foreign bodies. The signs and symptoms of corneal injuries include:

- Pain
- Foreign body sensation
- Decreased vision in the affected eye

With corneal foreign bodies, the first step is to locate the foreign body. Examine the inside of the lower lid by pulling the lid down with the thumb while the casualty looks up. Then perform an upper eyelid eversion as described in Skill Drill 7-1.

If the foreign body is superficial, irrigate the eye and eyelid as described in Skill Drill 7-2. If the foreign body is imbedded or if there is a corneal abrasion, cover both eyes and evacuate the casualty as soon as possible. Evacuate the casualty with glasses, if indicated.

Chemical Burns

Chemical spills often cause these burns. This is the only ocular trauma for which you do not perform the visual acuity test and DCAP-BTLS first. The signs and symptoms of chemical burns include:

- Pain
- Decreased vision in the affected eye

Immediately irrigate the eyes gently with large amounts of water or IV solution per Skill Drill 7-2. Evacuate the casualty immediately. Continue irrigation for a minimum of 60 minutes or until arrival at the MTF. Evacuate the casualty with glasses, if indicated.

Penetrating Ocular Trauma

Penetrating ocular trauma can occur from numerous sources (eg, knife and gunshot wounds). Any projectile injury has the potential to penetrate the eye. The signs and symptoms include:

- Pain
- Decreased vision
- Swelling
- Irregular pupils
- Hyphema

The assessment begins with the visual acuity test. Assess DCAP-BTLS, discoloration, and pupillary response. If there is no impalement, cover the affected eye with a loose dressing. Assess the casualty's tetanus status. Patch both of the casualty's eyes and evacuate immediately. Evacuate the casualty with glasses, if indicated.

If an impalement is present, stabilize the object with folded gauze rolls or pads and protect the eye with a cup, as described later in Skill Drill 7-4. Do not remove the impaled object. Assess the casualty's tetanus status. Patch both of the casualty's eyes and evacuate immediately. Evacuate casualty with glasses, if indicated.

Ocular Extrusion

With an ocular extrusion, the eye is protruding from the socket. Assessment begins with the visual acuity test. Assess DCAP-BTLS, discoloration, and pupillary response.

Shield and gently cup the avulsed eye with a loose, moist dressing. Do not attempt to force the eye back into its socket. Patch both eyes and evacuate the casualty immediately. Evacuate the casualty with glasses, if indicated.

With any eye injury, cover both eyes, even if only one eye is injured. The eyes use sympathetic movement. When one eye moves, the other eye duplicates the movement. With both eyes covered, the casualty needs assistance for all activities, so you will have to serve as his or her eyes, keeping the casualty reassured and oriented. In a combat scenario, you may have to keep the casualty's eyes uncovered, so the casualty will be able to escape from any danger presented on the battlefield.

■ Identify Specific Head Injuries

Scalp Wounds

Do not underestimate the potential blood loss from a scalp wound. Control the bleeding with direct pressure.

Skull Injuries

Skull injuries include linear nondisplaced fractures, compound fractures, and depressed fractures. In adults with a large contusion or darkened swelling of the scalp, suspect an underlying skull fracture. Avoid placing direct pressure on an obvious depressed or compound skull fracture. Leave any

Perform an Eye Irrigation

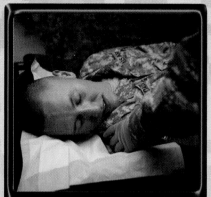

1 Identify the casualty and explain the procedure. Ask the casualty to remove any contact lenses or eyeglasses, if necessary. If the casualty is unable to remove them him- or herself, remove the lenses yourself. Position the casualty. If the casualty is lying on his or her back, tilt his or her head slightly to the side that is being irrigated. If the casualty is seated, tilt his or her head slightly backward and to the side that is being irrigated.

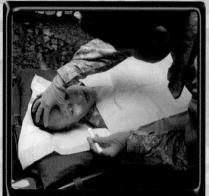

2 Position the equipment. Drape the areas of the casualty that may be splashed by the solution. Place a catch basin next to the face on the affected side. Position the light source so that it does not shine directly into the casualty's eyes. Put on gloves.

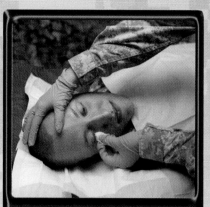

3 Clean the eyelids gently with cotton balls, and clean debris from the outer eye.

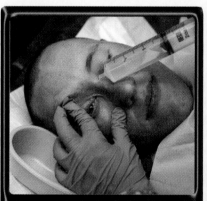

4 Separate the eyelids using the thumb and forefinger, and hold the lids open. Irrigate the eye by holding the irrigating tip 1″ to 1½″ away from the casualty's eye. Direct the irrigating solution gently from the inner canthus to the outer canthus. Use only enough pressure to maintain a steady flow of solution and to dislodge the secretions or foreign bodies. The irrigator should never touch the casualty's eye.

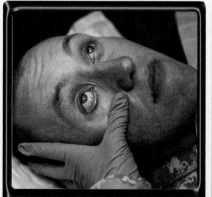

5 Instruct the casualty to look up to expose the conjunctival sac and lower surface of the eye, and then to look down to expose the upper surface of the eye. Dry the area around the eye by gently patting with gauze sponges. Do not touch the casualty's eye. Remove your gloves and wash your hands.

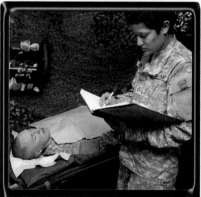

6 Record the treatment given on the appropriate form.

penetrating object of the skull in place and immediately transport to the medical treatment facility (MTF). For a gunshot wound (GSW) to the head, unless there are clear entrance and exit wounds, assume the bullet may have ricocheted and may be lodged near the spinal cord.

Brain Injuries

Traumatic Brain Injury

A **traumatic brain injury (TBI)** is an injury to the brain resulting from an event such as a blast, fall, direct impact, or motor vehicle accident which causes an alteration in the casualty's mental status. This typically results in the temporarily related onset of symptoms such as:

- Headache
- Nausea
- Vomiting
- Dizziness or balance problems
- Fatigue
- Insomnia or sleep disturbances
- Drowsiness
- Sensitivity to light
- Noise
- Blurred vision
- Difficulty remembering
- Difficulty concentrating

TBI can cause a broad range of physical, cognitive, emotional, and social problems for casualties. Casualties complain of:

- Decreased memory
- Decreased attention
- Decreased concentration
- Slower thinking
- Irritability
- Depression
- Impaired vision
- Mood swings
- Equilibrium imbalance
- Headaches
- Nausea

The levels of TBI are:

- **Mild:** Presentations range from asymptomatic to confusion or amnesia for the event. GCS is usually 14 or 15. This level accounts for 80% of head injuries and casualties usually return to full recovery within weeks after the injury.
- **Moderate:** GCS is between 9 to 13. This level accounts for 10% of head injuries. Most casualties should be admitted or observed because of the potential for deterioration.
- **Severe:** GCS is less than 9. This type accounts for 10% of head injuries. The mortality approaches 40%, with deaths usually occurring within 48 hours. Long-term disability is common in casualties with this level of injury.

The causes of TBI include:

- **Transportation accidents:** automobiles, motorcycles, bicycles
- **Falls** (most common in elderly)
- **Violence:** alcohol-related, child abuse, firearms
- **Military-related:** high-velocity blasts, military vehicle rollovers, and traumatic accidents

Concussion

The term *concussion* implies that there is no significant injury to the brain. A concussion is trauma to the head with a variable period of unconsciousness or confusion and then a return to normal consciousness. Amnesia from the injury may occur.

Short-term memory may be affected and there may be associated:

- Dizziness
- Headache
- Ringing in the ears (tinnitus)
- Nausea
- Temporary alterations in personality/behavior

Cerebral Contusion

A cerebral contusion is bruised brain tissue. A history of prolonged unconsciousness or serious alteration in state of consciousness are signs of a cerebral contusion. Other signs include:

- Profound confusion
- Persistent amnesia
- Vomiting
- Abnormal behavior

Brain swelling may be severe and rapid. The casualty may appear to have suffered a cerebrovascular accident (stroke) or have focal neurologic signs. The casualty may have personality changes depending on the location of the cerebral contusion. Injured casualties with an altered level of consciousness should be hyperventilated and transported rapidly to an MTF.

Intracranial Hemorrhage

The four major types of intracranial hemorrhage are epidural hematoma, subdural hematoma, intracranial hematoma, and subarachnoid hemorrhage. The signs and symptoms include:

- Headache
- Visual changes
- Personality/behavioral changes
- Slurring of speech
- Confusion
- Changes in LOC and possible coma
- Decreased pulse rate (bradycardia)
- Increased blood pressure (hypertension)

Suspect brain or cervical spine injuries for all head, face, and neck wounds. Check the casualty's mouth carefully for broken teeth or blood. Do not attempt to clean the surface of a scalp wound; to do so may cause additional bleeding. Do not remove impaled objects; stabilize them in place. Gently palpate for depressions. Do not apply a pressure dressing.

■ Care of Head Injuries

Ensure an open and clear airway. Protect for possible neck or spinal injuries.

Do not lift or attempt to wrap the head of a casualty who is lying down if there are signs of a spinal injury. Neck movement worsens the injury of a casualty with a spinal injury.

Control bleeding by gentle pressure. If brain tissue is exposed or if cranial/facial fracture is suspected, do not apply pressure. Instead, use only sufficient pressure to stop the flow of blood. Underlying fractures may be present.

Initiate a saline lock and/or manage with intravenous fluids as follows:

- Administer Ringer's lactate.
- Restrict to minimal fluid infusion (TKO/KVO) to avoid overload.

Assess for shock and administer fluids as needed to support circulation if hypovolemia is the cause. Apply a dressing or bandage, being careful not to compromise the airway. If brain tissue is exposed, apply a sterile dressing; local protocol will dictate whether the dressing should be moist or dry. Administer a high flow of oxygen. Reassess neurologic status and baseline vital signs frequently. Signs of a worsening condition include:

- Increase in severity of headache
- Change in pupil size
- Progressive weakness on one side

Stabilize any impaled objects. Support the airway with suction of secretions as needed, if available. Administer wound care according to the care described in detail in Chapter 4, *Controlling Bleeding and Hypovolemic Shock*. Evaluate the casualty's last tetanus immunization and give an update, if appropriate. Administer pain control as required.

Provide full spinal immobilization before transport. Transport the casualty with his or her head elevated 30° by elevating the top of the litter or spine board 6″ (reverse Trendelenburg). If a facial wound is present, tilt the spine board toward the side of the injury to allow for drainage.

> **Field Medical Care TIPS**
>
> Due to morphine's effect on ICP and pupillary response, it is not recommended in casualties with intracranial injury.

■ Prevention and Medical Management of Laser Injuries

Lasers are devices that produce an intense, narrow beam of light. Lasers are commonly used in the US Army as rangefinders and target designators. They are also used to simulate live fire during force-on-force exercises. The use of laser devices may result in accidental injury to the eye.

The rapid growth of laser science has resulted in the increased use of laser instruments in all the military branches. If we have devices that can accidentally permanently blind us, it is likely that threat forces have similar equipment. This may increase the potential for laser eye injuries in the field.

Lasers interfere with vision either temporarily or permanently in one or both eyes. At low energy levels, lasers may produce temporary reduction in visual performance in critical tasks, such as aiming weapons or flying aircraft. At higher energy levels, they may produce serious long-term vision loss, even permanent blindness.

Prevention and Protection

Laser-protective eyewear has been developed to protect soldiers against specific laser hazards; however, it does not protect the eye from injury by other laser threat wavelengths. Passive protection consists of taking cover and using any protective gear that is available. Ordinary eyeglasses or sunglasses afford a very limited amount of protection. Active protection consists of applying evasive action, scanning battlefields with one eye, minimizing the use of binoculars in areas known to have lasers in use, using built-in or clip-on filters, and using battlefield smoke screens.

Injuries produced by lasers include:

- **Retina injuries:** Burns or hemorrhage producing loss of vision
- **Cornea injuries:** Burns, vision loss, corneal scarring, and corneal perforation

Burns of the cornea are treated similarly to other types of thermal burns.

All laser injuries need to be evaluated by a medical officer.

■ Visual Acuity Test

The visual acuity test measures distance vision by determining the smallest letters that you can read on a standardized chart at a distance of 20′. It is most often performed in the garrison. This test is performed initially on all casualties presenting with an eye complaint (except for ocular burns). In children and the elderly, this test may be performed routinely to screen for any visual problems. To perform the visual acuity test, follow the steps in **SKILL DRILL 7-3 ▶**:

1. Position the casualty 20′ away from the Snellen chart, making sure the area is well lit (**Step ①**).
2. Test each eye individually by covering one eye with an opaque card or gauze, being careful to avoid applying pressure to the eye (**Step ②**).
3. Ask the casualty to identify all of the letters beginning at the 20/20 vision level. If the casualty can read this line, no further testing needs to be done on this eye for far vision. If the casualty cannot read the 20/20 line, determine the smallest line on which the casualty can identify all of the letters. Record the visual acuity designated by that line.
4. Repeat the preceding steps with the other eye.
5. If a casualty has corrective lenses, test without glasses first, and then test with glasses on (**Step ③**).

SKILL DRILL 7-3

Perform the Visual Acuity Test

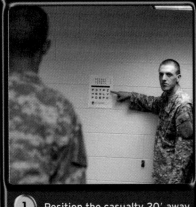

1 Position the casualty 20′ away from the Snellen chart, making sure the area is well lit.

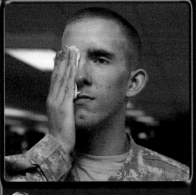

2 Test each eye individually by covering one eye with an opaque card or gauze, being careful to avoid applying pressure to the eye.

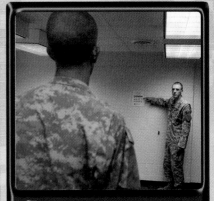

3 Ask the casualty to identify all of the letters beginning at the 20/20 vision level. If the casualty can read this line, no further testing needs to be done on this eye for far vision. If the casualty cannot read the 20/20 line, determine the smallest line on which the casualty can identify all of the letters. Record the visual acuity designated by that line. Repeat with the other eye. If a casualty has corrective lenses, test without glasses first, and then test with glasses on.

Distance vision visual acuity is recorded as a fraction in which the numerator indicates the distance from the chart (20′) and the denominator indicates the distance at which a normal eye can read the line. Thus, 20/200 means that the casualty can read at 20 feet what the average person can read at 200 feet. **TABLE 7-1 ▸** lists the levels of vision.

■ Bandaging an Impaled Object in the Eye

To stabilize an impaled object in the eye, follow the steps in **SKILL DRILL 7-4 ▸** :

1. Stabilize the object by placing a roll of 3″ gauze bandage or folded 4″ × 4″ gauze pads on either side of the object, along the vertical axis of the head in a manner that will stabilize the object. This will help prevent further contamination and minimize movement of the object (**Step 1**).

2. Fit a disposable paper drinking cup or paper cone over the impaled object. In a battlefield setting it is

TABLE 7-1 The Level of Vision

Distance Vision Visual Acuity	Description
20/20	Normal vision. Fighter pilot minimum. This level of vision is required to read numbers in a telephone book.
20/40	Able to pass a driver's license test in all 50 states. Most printed material is at this level.
20/80	Able to read an alarm clock at 10 feet. News headlines are this size.
20/200	Legal blindness. Able to see stop sign letters.

SKILL DRILL 7-4

Stabilizing an Impaled Object in the Eye

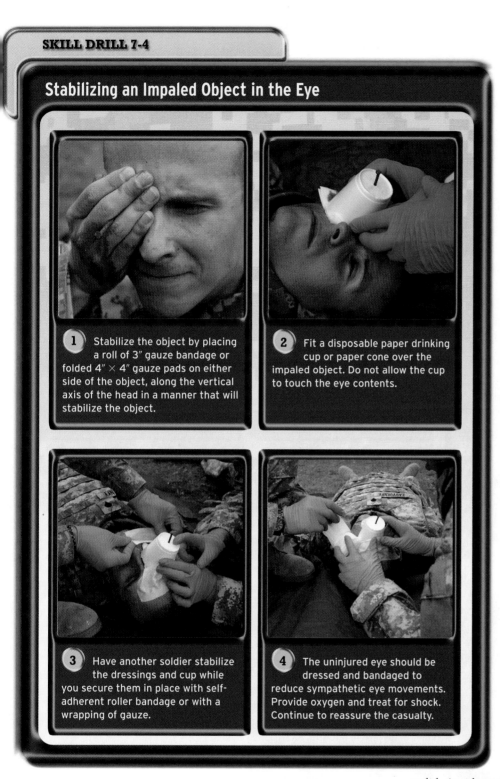

1 Stabilize the object by placing a roll of 3" gauze bandage or folded 4" × 4" gauze pads on either side of the object, along the vertical axis of the head in a manner that will stabilize the object.

2 Fit a disposable paper drinking cup or paper cone over the impaled object. Do not allow the cup to touch the eye contents.

3 Have another soldier stabilize the dressings and cup while you secure them in place with self-adherent roller bandage or with a wrapping of gauze.

4 The uninjured eye should be dressed and bandaged to reduce sympathetic eye movements. Provide oxygen and treat for shock. Continue to reassure the casualty.

roller bandage or with a wrapping of gauze. Do not secure the bandage on top of the cup (Step **3**).

5. The uninjured eye should be dressed and bandaged to reduce sympathetic eye movements.

6. Provide oxygen and treat for shock. Continue to reassure the casualty and provide emotional support (**Step 4**).

■ Instillation of Eye Drops

To instill eye drops, follow the steps in **SKILL DRILL 7-5 ▸**:

1. Identify the casualty and explain the procedure.

2. Position the casualty. If the casualty is lying on his or her back, tilt his or her head slightly to the side. If the casualty is seated, tilt his or her head slightly backward and to the side (**Step 1**).

3. Put on gloves.

4. Identify the medication and check the eyedropper for cracks or chips.

5. Draw the medication into the eyedropper (**Step 2**).

6. Gently pull down on the casualty's lower eyelid using two fingers.

7. Instruct the casualty to look upward (**Step 3**).

8. Instill the prescribed number of drops into the center of the lower eyelid. Avoid touching any part of the container to the eye.

9. Press on the inner canthus of the eye when instilling the eye drops. This prevents the solution from draining into the tear duct and minimizes the risk of systemic effects (**Step 4**).

10. Instruct the casualty to close his or her eyes for 1 minute.

11. Wipe off any excess solution with a gauze pad.

unlikely that a paper cup will be readily available, so you will have to improvise.

3. Do not allow the cup to touch the eye contents. This type of bandaging will offer rigid protection and will call attention to the casualty's problem. Do not use a Styrofoam cup, which will flake (**Step 2**).

4. Have another soldier stabilize the dressings and cup while you secure them in place with self-adherent

Instilling Eye Drops

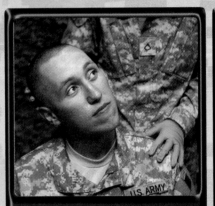

1 Identify the casualty and explain the procedure. Position the casualty. If the casualty is lying on his or her back, tilt his or her head slightly to the side. If the casualty is seated, tilt his or her head slightly backward and to the side.

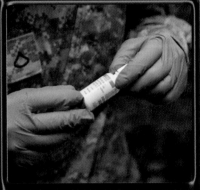

2 Put on gloves. Identify medication.

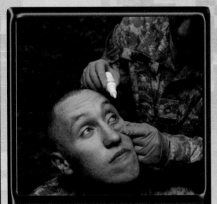

3 Gently pull down on the casualty's lower eyelid using two fingers. Instruct the casualty to look upward.

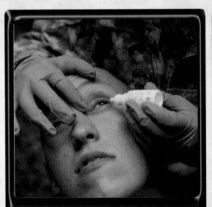

4 Instill the prescribed number of drops into the center of the lower eyelid. Avoid touching any part of the container to the eye. Press on the inner canthus of the eye when instilling eye drops. This prevents the solution from draining into the tear duct and minimizes the risk of systemic effects.

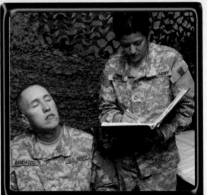

5 Instruct the casualty to close his or her eyes for 1 minute. Wipe off any excess solution with a gauze pad. Repeat the procedure for the other eye, if needed. Remove gloves and wash hands. Record the treatment time, type of medication, strength of medication, and eye into which medication was instilled.

12. Repeat the procedure for the other eye, if needed.

13. Remove gloves and wash hands.

14. Record the treatment time, type of medication, strength of medication, and eye into which medication was instilled (**Step 5**).

■ Instillation of Eye Ointments

To instill eye ointments, follow the steps in **SKILL DRILL 7-6 ▶**:

1. Prepare the casualty.

2. Verify the casualty and the medication requirements.

3. Explain the procedure to the casualty.

4. Position the casualty. If the casualty is lying on his or her back, tilt his or her head slightly to the side. If the casualty is seated, tilt his or her head slightly backward and to the side.

5. Wash your hands and put on gloves (**Step 1**).

6. Expel a small amount of ointment from the tube onto a 4″ × 4″ gauze pad to clear the tube of air bubbles and to clear dried ointment from tube (**Step 2**).

7. Gently pull down the lower lid using two fingers.

8. Instruct the casualty to look upward.

9. Apply the ointment inside the lower lid. Squeeze a thin line of ointment from inner canthus to outer canthus. Avoid touching any part of the eye with the tube (**Step 3**).

10. Ask the casualty to blink a few times. This helps to disperse the ointment.

11. If the medication is to be instilled into the other eye, change your gloves and use another tube of medication to prevent the spread of infection from one eye to the other.

12. Use a gauze pad to wipe away excess medication.

13. Remove gloves and wash your hands.

14. Record the treatment time, type of medication, and eye to which the medication was applied (**Step 4**).

■ Summary

To provide your casualty with the highest chance of recovery, you must know the anatomy of the head and central nervous system. The most important principles for the management of head-injured casualties are rapid assessment, adequate airway management, rapid transport to the appropriate echelon of care, and frequent reassessment. It is important to remember that spinal injuries are often associated with head injuries. You must immobilize the spine to prevent harm and paralysis. Injuries of the eye may be disabling if not treated promptly.

Instilling Eye Ointment

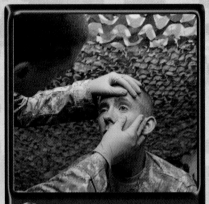

1 Prepare the casualty. Verify the casualty and the medication requirements. Explain the procedure to the casualty. Position the casualty. If the casualty is lying on his or her back, tilt his or her head slightly to the side. If the casualty is seated, tilt his or her head slightly backward and to the side. Wash your hands and put on gloves.

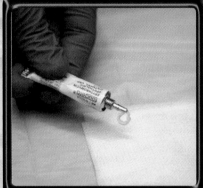

2 Expel a small amount of ointment from the tube onto a 4″ × 4″ gauze pad to clear the tube of air bubbles and to clear dried ointment from the tube.

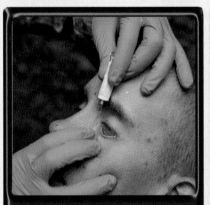

3 Gently pull down the lower lid using two fingers. Instruct the casualty to look upward. Apply the ointment inside the lower lid. Squeeze a thin line of ointment from inner canthus to outer canthus. Avoid touching any part of the eye with the tube.

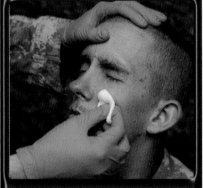

4 Ask the casualty to blink a few times. This helps to disperse the ointment. If the medication is to be instilled into the other eye, change your gloves and use another tube of medication to prevent the spread of infection from one eye to the other. Use a gauze pad to wipe away excess medication. Remove gloves and wash your hands. Record the treatment time, type of medication, and eye to which medication was applied.

YOU ARE THE COMBAT MEDIC

Y ou are assigned to provide medical support to a convoy of both diplomatic and military personnel. Your convoy is hit by an IED embedded in the carcass of an animal. Once within the predetermined safety zone, you quickly assess the personnel in all of the vehicles. One of the diplomats has sustained an eye injury and is in need of immediate treatment.

Assessment

You determine that there is moderate to severe damage to the vehicle with multiple fragmentation penetrations throughout the vehicle. You gain entrance into the SUV with the assistance of two soldiers and observe a female in severe pain holding her right eye, which has visible and active bleeding. You assess her ABCs and note that her airway is patent. You reassure her while assessing her eye. Upon inspection of the right eye, you find multiple metal fragmentation pieces embedded into the both the socket and in the lenses of the pupil in various lengths, from 2″ to 4″. She tells you that she is unable to see and that the pain is burning.

Treatment

You obtain a 4″ x 4″ gauze dressing and instruct her to apply it firmly but gently to the eye to control the bleeding. The Convoy Commander comes alongside and requests a report. You state that you have one casualty, a civilian, and that she has a major injury involving her right eye and request an immediate 9-line MEDEVAC.

You need to secure the casualty's eyes by blinding both of them to protect and prevent further injury. Within your kit, you obtain two thick sterile pads and 2″ tape. You explain in short detail how you are going to blind her to protect both eyes. You take an unopened bottle of water, expel the contents, cut the bottle, puncture the bottom, gently place it over the embedded objects, and secure it to her face. When the helicopter arrives, you give the flight medic a brief but detailed report as you assist her in securing the casualty into the litter.

1. LAST NAME, FIRST NAME		RANK/GRADE		MALE	
Solange, Anne				✓	FEMALE
SSN **000-111-5555**	SPECIALTY CODE			RELIGION	

2. UNIT

FORCE				NATIONALITY	
A/T	AF/A	N/M	MC/M		
	BC/BC		NBI/BNC	DISEASE	PSYCH

3. INJURY

FRONT   BACK

	AIRWAY
X	HEAD
	WOUND
	NECK/BACK INJURY
	BURN
	AMPUTATION
	STRESS
	OTHER (*Specify*)

_____

_____

4. LEVEL OF CONSCIOUSNESS

X	ALERT		PAIN RESPONSE
	VERBAL RESPONSE		UNRESPONSIVE

5. PULSE	TIME	6. TOURNIQUET		TIME
		X NO ☐ YES		

7. MORPHINE		DOSE	TIME	8. IV	TIME
X NO ☐ YES					

9. TREATMENT/OBSERVATIONS/CURRENT MEDICATION/ALLERGIES/NBC (ANTIDOTE)

Multiple metal fragments to the right eye. Unable to see. Possible Blast Injury.

10. DISPOSITION		RETURNED TO DUTY	TIME
	X	EVACUATED	**1536**
		DECEASED	

11. PROVIDER/UNIT **Ray, Raj**	DATE (YYMMDD)

Aid Kit

Ready for Review

- On the battlefield, the structures that regulate the senses are extremely important for a casualty's survival.
- The brain—the most important organ in the body—requires maximum protection from injury.
- A change in the level of consciousness is the single most important observation you can make when determining the severity of a head injury.
- Your mission in managing head injuries is to prevent secondary injury.
- Eye injuries on the battlefield are common in spite of the eye being protected by the bony orbit.
- The use of laser devices may result in accidental injury to the eye.

Vital Vocabulary

Battle's sign Bruising over the mastoid bone behind the ear commonly seen following a basilar skull fracture; also called retroauricular ecchymosis.

brain Part of the central nervous system located within the cranium; contains billions of neurons that serve a variety of vital functions.

canthus The corner of the eye.

cerebrospinal fluid (CSF) Fluid produced in the ventricles of the brain that flows in the subarachnoid space and bathes the meninges.

conjunctiva A thin, transparent membrane that covers the sclera and internal surfaces of the eyelids.

cornea The transparent anterior portion of the eye that overlies the iris and pupil.

decerebrate (extensor) posturing Abnormal posture characterized by extension of the arms and legs; indicates pressure on the brain stem.

decorticate (flexor) posturing Abnormal posture characterized by flexion of the arms and extension of the legs; indicates pressure on the brain stem.

foramen magnum The large opening at the base of the skull through which the spinal cord exits the brain.

iris The colored portion of the eye.

lacrimal glands The structures in which tears are secreted and drained from the eye.

lens A transparent body within the globe of the eye that focuses light rays.

pupil The circular opening in the center of the eye through which light passes to the lens.

raccoon eyes Bruising under or around the orbits that is commonly seen following a basilar skull fracture; also called periorbital ecchymosis.

retina A delicate 10-layered structure of nervous tissue located in the rear of the interior of the globe of the eye that receives light and generates nerve signals that are transmitted to the brain through the optic nerve.

sclera The white part of the eye.

skull The structure at the top of the axial skeleton that houses the brain and consists of 28 bones that comprise the auditory ossicles, the cranium, and the face.

traumatic brain injury (TBI) An injury to the brain from an event such as a blast, fall, direct impact, or motor vehicle accident which causes an alteration in mental status.

COMBAT MEDIC *in Action*

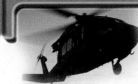

You are on patrol with your unit on a HMMWV. The gunner complains of vision problems. After your initial assessment rules out any vision-threatening injuries, you perform a visual acuity test with the soldier and determine that his field of vision is within 20/20. The soldier complains that he feels like something is in his eye and it is burning. His left eye is tearing and there is redness. You evaluate for a foreign body within the pupil and see what appears to be sand trapped in the upper eyelid.

1. True or false? When performing an eye irrigation, contact lenses must remain in the casualty's eyes.
   A. True
   B. False

2. The first step in assessing an ocular injury is to:
   A. palpate the eye.
   B. perform a visual acuity test.
   C. bandage the eye.
   D. evert the eyelid.

3. When treating a foreign body in the eyelid, you should:
   A. evert the eyelid and irrigate the eye.
   B. wipe the foreign body out with a cotton swab.
   C. have the casualty rub his eyes until the foreign body is removed.
   D. evacuate the casualty immediately.

4. The signs of upper eyelid injury include:
   A. pain.
   B. ecchymosis.
   C. swelling.
   D. all of the above.

5. True or false? Always irrigate an eye with an impaled object before stabilizing the object.
   A. True
   B. False

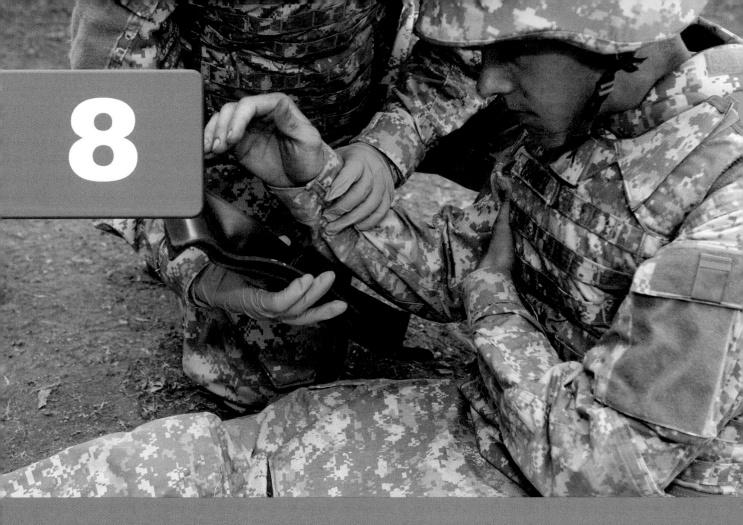

8

Musculoskeletal Injuries

Objectives

Knowledge Objectives

- [ ] Describe the anatomy and physiology of the musculoskeletal system.
- [ ] Describe how to assess a musculoskeletal injury.
- [ ] Identify life-threatening extremity trauma.
- [ ] Describe emergency care for extremity injuries.
- [ ] Discuss the principles of splinting.

Skills Objective

- [ ] Apply a splint.
- [ ] Apply a SAM splint.

Introduction

As a combat medic, you will encounter musculoskeletal injuries on the battlefield more frequently than any other injury category. Your knowledge of the underlying anatomy, assessment principles, and appropriate management techniques can prevent further painful injury and even prevent permanent disability or death. The ability to accurately recognize and treat musculoskeletal injuries is one of the many skills that you will need to perform on the battlefield.

Anatomy and Physiology of the Musculoskeletal System

The musculoskeletal system gives the human body its shape and allows for its movement. It is essential that you understand its basic anatomy and physiology.

Functions of the Musculoskeletal System

The musculoskeletal system performs many important functions within the body. Bones help *support* the soft tissues of the body and form a framework that gives the human body its shape and allows it to maintain an erect posture. *Movement* is generated because muscles are attached to bones by **tendons**. When a muscle contracts, the force generated by the muscle is transferred to a bone on the opposite side of the **joint** from the muscle, leading to motion. Bones also offer *protection* to the more fragile organs and structures beneath them—for example, the skull protects the brain, the rib cage protects the heart and lungs, and the spinal column protects the spinal cord.

The Body's Scaffolding: The Skeleton

The integrated structure formed by the 206 bones of the body is called the skeleton. It may be divided into two distinct portions: the **axial skeleton** and the **appendicular skeleton**. The axial skeleton is composed of the bones of the central part, or axis, of the body; its divisions include the vertebral column, skull, ribs, and sternum. The skull is composed of the cranium, mandible, basilar skull, face, and inner ear **FIGURE 8-1 ▾**.

The spine is composed of 33 spinal vertebrae: 7 cervical, 12 thoracic, 5 lumbar, 5 sacral, and 4 coccygeal. The thorax is formed by the sternum and 12 pairs of ribs, which are connected to the spine posteriorly.

The appendicular skeleton is divided into the **pectoral girdle**, the **pelvic girdle**, and the bones of the upper and lower extremities.

Shoulder and Upper Extremities

The pectoral girdle **FIGURE 8-2 ▸**, also referred to as the shoulder girdle, consists of two scapulae and two clavicles. The **scapula** (shoulder blade) is a flat, triangular bone held to the rib cage posteriorly by powerful muscles that buffer it against injury. The **clavicle** (collarbone) is a slender, S-shaped bone attached by ligaments at the medial end to the sternum and at the lateral end to the raised tip of the scapula, called the **acromion**. The acromion process of the scapula is the highest portion of the shoulder. It forms the acromioclavicular (AC) joint with the clavicle and is a frequent area of shoulder injury (AC separation). The clavicle acts as a strut to keep the shoulder propped up; however, because it is slender and very exposed, this bone is vulnerable to injury.

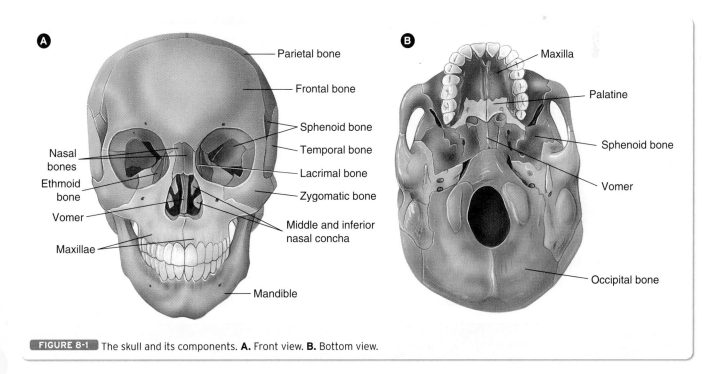

FIGURE 8-1 The skull and its components. **A.** Front view. **B.** Bottom view.

The upper extremity **FIGURE 8-3** joins the shoulder girdle at the glenohumeral joint. The proximal portion contains the **humerus**, a bone that articulates proximally with the scapula and distally with the bones of the forearm—the radius and ulna—to form the hinged elbow joint.

The **radius** and **ulna** make up the forearm. The radius, the larger of the two forearm bones, lies on the thumb side of the forearm. Distally, the ulna is narrow and is on the small-finger side of the forearm. It serves as the pivot around which the radius turns at the wrist to rotate the palm upward or downward. Because the radius and the ulna are arranged in parallel, when one is broken, the other is often broken as well.

The hand **FIGURE 8-4** contains three sets of bones: wrist bones (**carpals**), hand bones (**metacarpals**), and finger bones (**phalanges**). The carpals, especially the scaphoid, are vulnerable to fracture when a casualty falls on an outstretched hand. Phalanges are more apt to be damaged by a crushing injury.

Pelvis and Lower Extremities

The pelvic girdle **FIGURE 8-5** is actually three separate bones—the **ischium**, **ilium**, and **pubis**—fused together. The ilium is the superior bone that contains the iliac crest. It is a wide bony wing that can be felt near the waist. The ischium is the inferior and posterior portion of the pelvis. The pubis

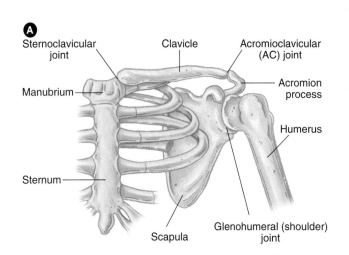

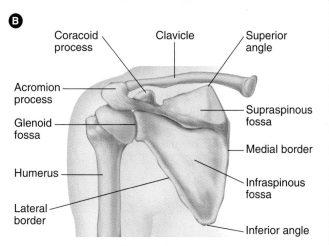

FIGURE 8-2   The pectoral girdle. **A.** Anterior view, including the clavicle. **B.** Posterior view, including the scapula.

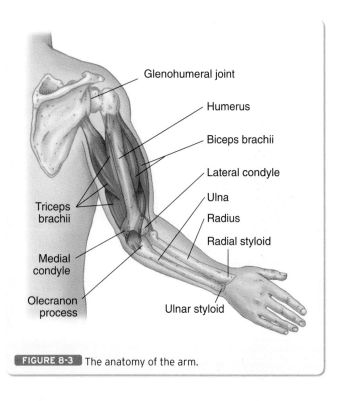

FIGURE 8-3   The anatomy of the arm.

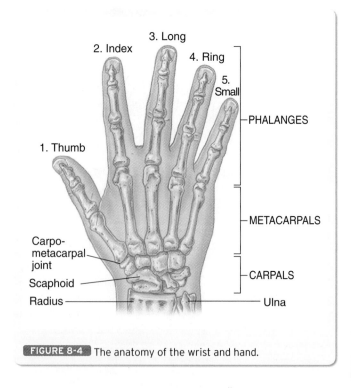

FIGURE 8-4   The anatomy of the wrist and hand.

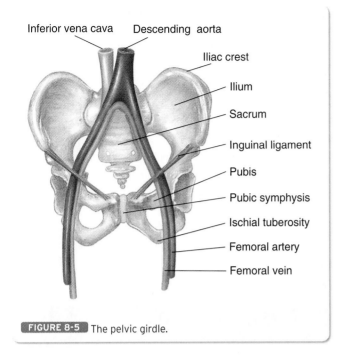

FIGURE 8-5   The pelvic girdle.

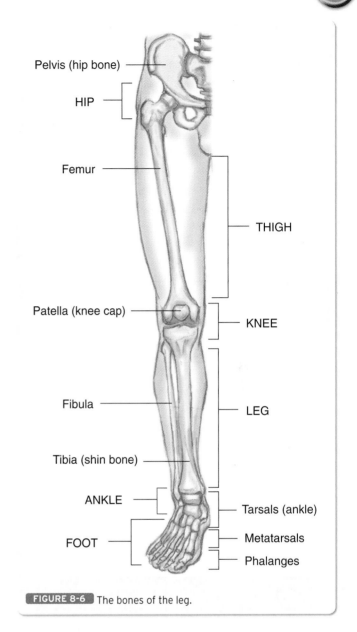

FIGURE 8-6   The bones of the leg.

is formed by the joining of the bones of the anterior pubis. The pelvis is joined posteriorly to the sacral spine (sacroiliac joint). The hip joint, which is the only moveable joint in the pelvis, consists of the **acetabulum** (socket of the hip joint) and the ball at the proximal end of the femur (femoral head).

The lower extremity consists of the bones of the thigh, leg, and foot **FIGURE 8-6 ▸**. The **femur** (thigh bone) is a long, powerful bone that articulates proximally in the ball-and-socket joint of the pelvis and distally in the hinge joint of the knee. The *head* of the femur is the ball-shaped part that fits into the acetabulum. It is connected to the *shaft*, or long tubular portion of the femur, by the femoral *neck*. The femoral neck is a common site for fractures.

The lower leg consists of two bones, the **tibia** and the **fibula**. The tibia (shin bone) forms the inferior component of the knee joint and is the larger bone of the lower leg. The fibula is the smaller bone of the lower leg. Anterior to this joint is the **patella** (knee cap), a bone that is important for knee extension. The tibia runs down the front of the lower leg, where it is vulnerable to direct blows, and can be felt just beneath the skin.

The ankle is the joint of the tibia and fibula of the leg with the talus of the foot. The two distinct landmarks are two protrusions that you can see on the lateral and medial aspects of the ankles. The lateral malleolus is at the lower end of the fibula. The medial malleolus is at the lower end of the tibia.

The foot **FIGURE 8-7 ▸** consists of three classes of bones: seven *foot bones* (**tarsals**), five *forefoot bones* (**metatarsals**), and 14 *toe bones* (phalanges). The largest of the tarsal bones is the heel bone, or **calcaneus**, which is subject to injury when a person jumps from a height and lands on his or her feet.

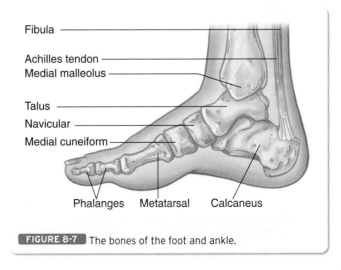

FIGURE 8-7   The bones of the foot and ankle.

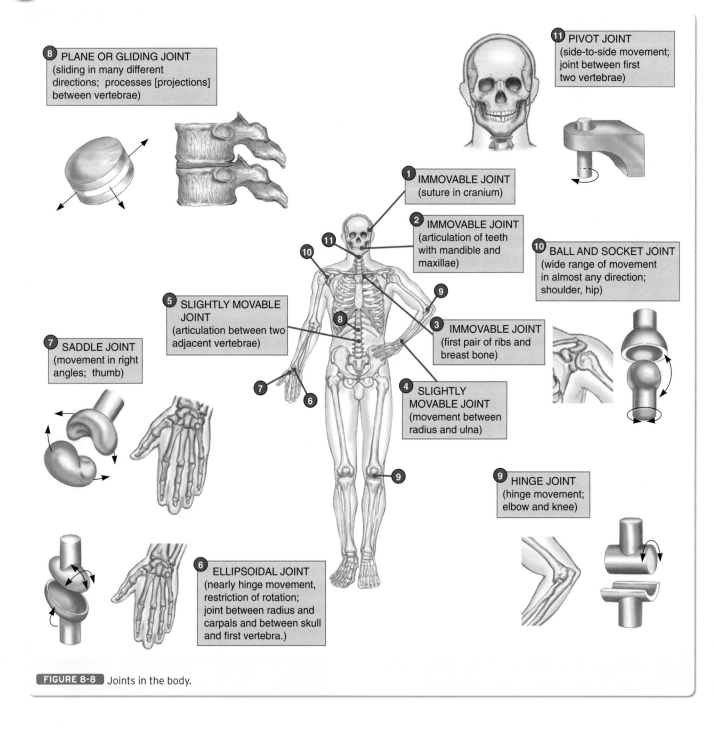

8 PLANE OR GLIDING JOINT
(sliding in many different
directions; processes [projections]
between vertebrae)

11 PIVOT JOINT
(side-to-side movement;
joint between first
two vertebrae)

1 IMMOVABLE JOINT
(suture in cranium)

2 IMMOVABLE JOINT
(articulation of teeth
with mandible and
maxillae)

10 BALL AND SOCKET JOINT
(wide range of movement
in almost any direction;
shoulder, hip)

5 SLIGHTLY MOVABLE
JOINT
(articulation between two
adjacent vertebrae)

3 IMMOVABLE JOINT
(first pair of ribs and
breast bone)

7 SADDLE JOINT
(movement in right
angles; thumb)

4 SLIGHTLY
MOVABLE JOINT
(movement between
radius and ulna)

9 HINGE JOINT
(hinge movement;
elbow and knee)

6 ELLIPSOIDAL JOINT
(nearly hinge movement,
restriction of rotation;
joint between radius and
carpals and between skull
and first vertebra.)

FIGURE 8-8 Joints in the body.

Joints

Joints are where ligaments connect bones to other bones. The
types of joints include **FIGURE 8-8** :

- **Ball-and-socket joint:** The ball rotates in a round socket
  (shoulder/hip joint).
- **Hinge joint:** Bends and straightens (elbow/knee joint).
- **Pivot joint:** Rotation (atlantoaxial and proximal radio-
  ulnar joint radius rotates around ulna).
- **Condyloid joint:** Motion in two planes at right angles
  (radius and carpal bone joint).

- **Saddle joint:** Motion in two planes at right angles, but
  no axial rotation.
- **Gliding joint:** Limited motion for gliding (vertebrae,
  carpal, and tarsal bones).

Possible Joint and Muscle Injuries
Dislocations

With a **dislocation**, the bone is forcibly displaced from its joint.
Shoulder dislocation is the most common type. A dislocation is
likely to bruise or tear the muscles, ligaments, blood vessels,
tendons, and nerves near a joint. Signs include rapid swelling

(edema), discoloration (ecchymosis), loss of ability to use the joint, severe pain, muscle spasms, possible numbness and loss of pulses below the joint, or a stiff and immobile joint.

Sprains

Sprains are a stretching or tearing injury to ligaments and soft tissues that support a joint. Signs include pain or pressure at joint, pain upon movement, swelling, tenderness, possible loss of movement, and discoloration. Strains can be caused by a forcible overstretching or tearing of a muscle or tendon. Additional signs are pain, lameness or stiffness (sometimes involving knotting of muscles), moderate swelling at place of injury, discoloration, and a possible loss of strength in the affected area. If significant muscle tearing is present, a distinct gap will be felt at the site.

Contusions

Contusions are caused by blunt trauma and may involve damage to bones, muscles, tendons, blood vessels, nerves, and other tissues. Signs of contusions include immediate pain and swelling. Swelling occurs because the blood from broken vessels oozes into soft tissues underneath the skin. There may be initial skin reddening due to irritation. Later, the characteristic black and blue marks (ecchymosis) appear. The skin eventually turns yellowish or greenish. Contusions may cause a limited range of motion (ROM).

■ Assess the Musculoskeletal Injury

Initial Assessment

After performing the situational assessment, begin the initial assessment. Consider the casualty's mechanism of injury (MOI). With musculoskeletal injuries, common mechanisms of injury include bullet or shrapnel wounds, falls, motor vehicle accidents, and sports injuries. Assess the casualty's level of consciousness (LOC) and airway, breathing, and circulation.

Rapid Trauma Survey

After the initial assessment, perform a rapid trauma survey. When assessing musculoskeletal injuries, be sure to check the joints above and below the injury. Assess whether the casualty has evidence of a fracture. Signs of fractures in different bones are covered in TABLE 8-1 ▸ . Fractures can cause more than pain in a casualty. A femur fracture, for example, can cause a loss of 1 to 2 liters of blood. Pelvic fractures can cause severe hemorrhage and can be fatal. With a **closed fracture**, the bone injury is entirely internal and there is no break in the skin. The signs of a closed fracture include deformity, discoloration, and crepitus FIGURE 8-9 ▸ .

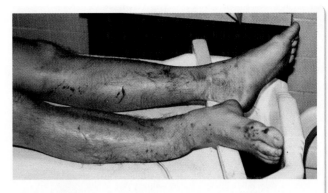
FIGURE 8-9 Obvious deformity is a sign of bone fracture.

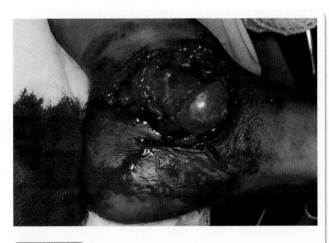
FIGURE 8-10 An open fracture.

An **open fracture** occurs when the sharp ends of broken bones protrude (push out) through the skin FIGURE 8-10 ▲ . An open fracture may be caused by an object such as a bullet that penetrates from the outside. Open fractures usually involve extensive damage to tissues and may become infected. Antibiotics may be indicated. Fractured bone ends are extremely sharp and pose a serious threat to surrounding tissue. Nerves, arteries, and veins located near the bone or near the skin are often injured.

Neurologic injuries may be due to lacerations from bone fragments or from pressure caused by hematomas or swelling called **compartment syndrome**. The neurovascular bundle and the muscles run through different compartments in the arms and legs, and increased pressure from swelling within these compartments can injure these structures. Be certain to check the pulse, motor, and sensation (PMS) of extremities.

Assess Amputations

Amputations are potentially life-threatening injuries due to the severe tissue damage with subsequent hemorrhage and shock FIGURE 8-11 ▸ . Massive hemorrhage can occur, but most often the bleeding will control itself with a spontaneous retraction of major vessels and ordinary pressure applied to the stump. If major bleeding continues, rapidly apply a

TABLE 8-1 Specific Fractures

Fracture Site	Signs	Concerns
Clavicle	• Injured shoulder lower than the uninjured shoulder • Usually unable to raise arm above level of shoulder • May attempt to support injured shoulder by holding elbow with other hand • Deformity • Localized pain • Swelling	• Look for signs of lung or neck injury.
Humerus	• Pain • Swelling • Crepitus at the point of fracture	
Radius and/or ulna	• Pain • Swelling • Inability to use forearm and wrist	• Often occurs during a fall on an outstretched arm. • When both the radius and ulna are fractured, the arm usually appears deformed. • When only one bone is broken, the other acts as a splint and the arm retains a more natural appearance. • Watch for compartment syndrome.
Simple rib fracture	• Pain localized at the site of the fracture • Possible rib deformity • Coughing or movement is usually painful. • The casualty will remain still and will often lean toward the injured side.	• Be alert to pulmonary contusion.
Pelvis	• Severe pain during a gentle pelvic rock	• Bone fragments from a fractured pelvis may perforate or lacerate the bladder (blood in the urine). • Can cause extensive bleeding in the retroperitoneal space or the abdomen, which is difficult to control. • Usually fractures in more than one place. • Casualty may be unable to sit or stand. • Use a pneumatic antishock garment (PASG), if available. This is most effective in splinting pelvic fractures. If a PASG is not available, then anatomic splinting will be necessary. This can be accomplished with a pelvic sling such as a SAM sling or with improvised materials such as a poncho and a windlass device.
Femur	• Muscle spasms • Excruciating pain • Swelling at the site of the fracture	• The fractured leg is typically shorter than the uninjured leg because of the contraction of the thigh muscle. • Damage to the blood vessels and nerves may result. • A loss of 1 to 2 L of blood is possible. • Isolated knee pain may be referred pain from hip injuries.
Patella	• Pain • Swelling • Deformity of patella • Inability to straighten the knee	
Tibia and fibula	• Pain • Swelling • Deformity • Crepitus at point of fracture	• Assess the casualty's joints. • Watch for signs of compartment syndrome.

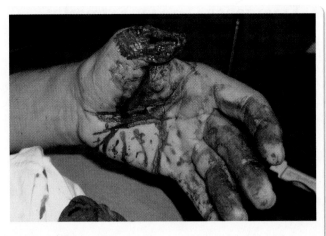

FIGURE 8-11 An amputation involving the thumb.

tourniquet. If possible, locate the amputated part and transport with the casualty. Don't let the obvious amputation distract you from other life-threatening conditions like airway or breathing problems.

Continuing the Rapid Trauma Survey

One of the simplest ways to assess an extremity is to compare one side with the other, noting any discrepancy in length, position, or skin color. Next, note the DCAP-BTLS (Deformity, Contusions, Abrasions, Penetrating injury, Burns, Tenderness, Lacerations, Swelling) as you observe and palpate the soft tissue from head to toe and assess the casualty for limitations, such as the inability to move a joint. While performing the DCAP-BTLS exam, be sure to consider the **six Ps of musculoskeletal assessment**: Pain, Paralysis, **Paresthesias** (numbness or tingling), Pulselessness, Pallor, and Pressure.

Pain

A casualty experiences acute pain when peripheral pain receptors (nocioceptors) convert painful stimuli into electrical impulses that are transmitted via the peripheral nerve fibers to the spinal cord. The signal ascends along the spinal cord to the pain-sensing region of the brain. When a tissue is injured, various chemical mediators are released that facilitate the conduction of the painful stimulus to the brain.

When assessing a casualty's pain, remember the OPQRST acronym: Onset of the pain; Provoking or palliating factors; Quality of the pain (such as sharp, pressure, crampy); Region of the pain, including its primary location and areas where pain radiates or refers; Severity of the pain; and the Time (duration) that the casualty has been experiencing pain. It is also useful to have the casualty quantify the severity of the pain by using a scale of 0 to10 or visual images such as faces that appear to be happy or in pain.

Inspection

When inspecting an injured extremity, always evaluate the joint above and the joint below the site of injury because the injuring force may have affected these sites as well. In particular, compare the injured side with the uninjured side. While inspecting a casualty's injuries, look for the following signs:

- Deformity, including asymmetry, angulation, shortening, and rotation
- Skin changes, including contusions, abrasions, avulsions, punctures, burns, lacerations, and bone ends
- Swelling
- Muscle spasms
- Abnormal limb positioning
- Increased or decreased range of motion
- Color changes, including pallor and cyanosis
- Bleeding, including estimating the amount of blood loss

Palpation

Palpation of an injured extremity should include the injury site and the regions above and below it. Regions of **point tenderness** should be identified. Reassess any tender areas frequently to determine whether there are changes in the location or severity of the pain or tenderness. Note that although point tenderness is one of the best indicators of an injury, it may be absent in patients who are intoxicated or who have an injury to the spinal cord.

When palpating an injured site, attempt to identify instability, deformity, abnormal joint or bone continuity, and displaced bones. Feel for crepitus, which is commonly found at the site of a fracture. Palpate distal pulses on all extremities, with special attention to comparing the strength of the pulses in the injured extremity with those in a normal one.

On occasion, an arterial injury may be identified while palpating an extremity. Signs of an arterial injury include a pulsatile expanding hematoma, diminished distal pulses, a palpable thrill (vibration) over the site of injury that correlates with the casualty's heartbeat, and difficult-to-control bleeding.

The purpose of palpating the pelvis is to identify instability and point tenderness. Apply pressure over the pubic symphysis to evaluate for tenderness and crepitus. Next, press the iliac wings toward the midline and then posteriorly. Any gross instability found during this examination should be reported because it may indicate a severe pelvic injury. Do not repeatedly examine the pelvis if instability is found because the manipulation may disrupt blood clots and cause further bleeding.

The upper and lower extremity exam should include palpation of the entire length of each arm and leg to identify any sites of injury. The most efficient way to accomplish this is to place your hands around the extremity and squeeze. Repeat this procedure every few centimeters until you reach the end of the extremity. When evaluating the upper extremities, always examine the cervical spine and shoulder because complaints within the arm may be caused by a more proximal disorder. Likewise, with the lower extremities, always conduct an exam of the pelvis and hip if the patient complains of pain in the leg.

Motor Function and Sensory Exam

It is essential to assess a casualty's distal pulse, as well as motor and sensory function, in the case of a musculoskeletal injury. A motor function exam should be performed whenever a casualty has an injury to an extremity, provided the casualty does not also have a life-threatening injury. While performing a motor exam, carry out each test with and without resistance because some casualties may be too weak to overcome any outside resistance. Also, perform the test on both sides of the body simultaneously so that each extremity can be compared.

A sensory exam should be performed on all casualties who have an injury or complaint related to an extremity, assuming that it does not take attention away from a potentially fatal condition. It is important to assess not only for the presence or absence of sensation, but also for the quality and symmetry of sensation.

To perform a sensory exam, first ask the casualty if he or she feels any abnormal sensations, such as numbness, tingling, or burning. Next, conduct a gross sensory exam by lightly touching the injured extremity and the unaffected side simultaneously; have the casualty report whether the two sides feel the same or different. In some cases, a casualty may complain of an abnormally severe sensation of pain when just lightly touched. Such hyperesthesia may be a sign of an injury to the spinal cord.

■ Emergency Care for Extremity Injuries

The overall goal in the treatment of a musculoskeletal injury is to identify the type and extent of the injury. First, expose the injury area. Control bleeding per the procedures presented in Chapter 4, *Controlling Bleeding and Hypovolemic Shock*. These techniques include:

- Direct pressure
- Pressure dressing
- Pressure points
- Elevation
- Tourniquet
- Hemostatic agents (Chitosan dressing or QuikClot powder)
- Splinting

To treat specific fractures, see **TABLE 8-2 ▾** .

Splinting

The objective of splinting is to prevent motion in the broken bone ends. The nerves that cause the most pain in a fractured

TABLE 8-2 Treat Specific Fractures

Fracture Site	Treatment
General principles of treatment for all fractures	• If fracture is open, control bleeding and immobilize. • If extremity is grossly angulated, gently realign. If the extremity is grossly angulated it will be difficult to effectively splint the fracture, which is why it is necessary to gently realign the fracture site. In addition, if the blood flow has been restricted by a grossly deformed injury, gentle realignment may improve the blood flow to the distal parts of the extremity. • Carefully straighten the extremity; apply splints.
Clavicle	• If fracture is open, control bleeding. • Apply sling and swathe, if possible. • Bend the casualty's elbow on the injured side and place the forearm across the chest. • Raise the hand about 4″ above the level of the elbow. • Support the forearm in position by means of a wide sling. A wide roller bandage or cravat may be used to secure the casualty's arm to the chest. • Use pain medication as needed. • The type of pain medications available may depend on the tactical situation. You may only have oral meds (acetaminophen or ibuprofen), or you may have injectable meds such as morphine. • Evacuate casualty to the nearest medical treatment facility (MTF).

Humerus	• Control bleeding and immobilize.
	• If fracture is in upper part of arm near shoulder:
	  – Place a pad or folded towel in armpit.
	  – Bandage arm securely to body.
	  – Support forearm in narrow sling.
	  – Provide pain medication as needed.
	  – Evacuate to nearest MTF.
	• If fracture is in middle of humerus:
	  – Fasten two wide splints or four narrow splints around the arm (sugar tong splint).
	  – Support the forearm in a narrow sling.
	  – Be certain the splint does not extend too far up the armpit (this may cause compression of blood vessels and nerves).
	  – Provide pain medication as needed.
	  – Evacuate to nearest MTF.

(continues)

TABLE 8-2 **Treat Specific Fractures** *(continued)*

Fracture Site	Treatment

Humerus *(continued)*	• If fracture is at or near elbow:
	  – You may need to splint in the extended position or may place in sling if possible.
	  – Soft splints may allow you to mold the splint around the elbow.
	  – In all cases, assess for signs and symptoms of shock.
	  – Provide pain medication as needed.
	  – Transport to nearest MTF.

Radius and/or ulna	• If fracture is open, control bleeding and immobilize. • If extremity is grossly angulated, gently realign the arm. If a fractured extremity is grossly angulated it will be difficult to effectively splint the fracture, which is why it is necessary to gently realign the fracture site. In addition, if the blood flow has been restricted by a grossly deformed injury, gentle realignment may improve the blood flow to the distal parts of the extremity. • Apply splint to area (SAM splint, air splint, basswood splint, wire ladder). • Splints should be long enough to extend from elbow to wrist. • Use bandages to hold splints in place. • Place forearm across the chest. • Support forearm in position by means of a wide sling and cravat bandage. • Raise hand about 4″ above level of elbow. • Provide pain medication as needed. • Transport to nearest MTF.
Simple rib fractures	• Ordinarily, rib fractures are not bound, strapped, or taped. • Provide pain medication as needed. • Place casualty in position of comfort. • Transport to nearest MTF.
Pelvis	• Initiate large-bore IV. • Provide pain medication as needed. • Minimize movement. • Assess for signs and symptoms of shock. • Keep casualty supine. • Legs may be straight or bent, depending on patient's comfort. • Immobilize. • Fractures of the pelvis and hip are best treated with PASG or anatomic splints. • Adequate immobilization can also be obtained by placing folded ponchos, poncho liners, or blankets between legs. • Use cravats, roller bandages, or straps to hold the legs together. • Fasten casualty securely to stretcher or improvised support. • Provide pain medication as needed. • Transport to nearest MTF.
Femur	• If fracture is open, control bleeding and immobilize. • Carefully straighten the leg; apply splints. • Use a traction splint. • PASG can be used to splint a femur fracture. • The legs can be tied together to support the injured leg (anatomic splint). • Assess for signs and symptoms of shock. • Initiate large-bore IV. • Provide pain medication as needed. • Transport to nearest MTF.
Patella	• Straighten the injured limb if possible. (Slow, gentle, passive extension of the lower extremity will be possible if the patient does not have to contract their quadriceps.) • Because the patella does not articulate with other bones, immobilizing the knee is the preferred method to splint this fracture (air splint, rigid splint, or knee immobilizer works well). • Provide pain medication as needed. • Transport to nearest MTF.
Tibia and fibula	• If fracture is open, control bleeding. • Carefully straighten the leg. • Splint the fracture (air splint, rigid splint, or a pillow works well). • Provide pain medication as needed. • Transport to nearest MTF. • Treat specific joint injury.

extremity lie in the membrane surrounding the bone. The broken bone ends irritate these nerves, causing a very deep and distressing type of pain. Splinting not only decreases pain, but also eliminates further damage to muscles, nerves, and blood vessels and helps to control hemorrhage.

Rules of Splinting

You must adequately visualize the injured part. Clothes should be cut off, not pulled off, unless there is only an isolated injury that presents no problems with maintaining immobilization. Check and record distal movement, sensation, and circulation before and after splinting. Pulses may be marked with a pen to identify where they were last checked. If the extremity is grossly angulated or pulses are absent, you should apply gentle traction in an attempt to realign it. If resistance is encountered, splint the extremity in the angulated position. Remember: it takes very little force to lacerate the wall of a blood vessel or to interrupt the blood supply to a large nerve.

If an open fracture is present, do not pull the exposed bone ends back into the wound. Open wounds should be covered with a sterile dressing before splinting. Try to splint on the side of an extremity away from open wounds. Use a splint that will immobilize the joints above and below the injury. Pad the splint well, especially when splinting over bony prominences. If applying traction to an open fracture, the bone may retract back into the wound. This is acceptable. In a life-threatening situation, injuries may be splinted while the patient is being transported. If in doubt, splint a possible injury.

Treating Joint Injuries

Dislocations

To treat a dislocation, loosen the clothing around the injured part. Place the casualty in a position of comfort. Support the injured part by means of a sling, pillows, bandages, or splints. Treat all dislocations as fractures. Administer pain medication as needed, and evacuate the casualty to the nearest MTF.

Sprains

Follow the acronym RICE: Rest, Ice, Compression, and Elevation. RICE is an easy way to remember how to manage soft-tissue injuries. Treat all sprains as fractures on the battlefield. Apply cold packs for the first 24 to 48 hours to reduce swelling and to control internal bleeding. Elevate and rest the affected area. Apply a compressive dressing (elastic wrap) to control swelling, and immobilize the area. Administer pain medication as needed, and transport the casualty to the nearest MTF.

Strains

Follow the acronym RICE. Keep the affected area elevated and at rest. Apply cold packs for the first 24 to 48 hours to control bleeding and swelling. Apply a compressive dressing (elastic wrap) to the injured area, and administer pain medications as needed. If the strain is severe and the casualty is unable to function, transport the casualty to the nearest MTF.

Contusions

Slight contusions (bruises) do not require treatment. Apply a compressive dressing (elastic wrap) to the contused area as needed for comfort. Elevate the injured part and apply ice to the injured area for the first 24 to 48 hours. Administer pain medication as needed.

Treating Amputations

A tourniquet should be applied rapidly. Apply pressure to the stump to control bleeding, and cover the stump with damp sterile dressing and elastic wrap. Wrap the dressing tight enough to apply uniform, reasonable pressure across the entire stump. A damp sterile dressing is needed to prevent the internal tissues from being exposed to the air and drying out. This can be accomplished by using sterile $4'' \times 4''$ gauze covered by a battle dressing and wrapped with an elastic wrap.

Initiate a large-bore IV and treat for shock. Administer pain medication as needed. Care for the amputated part by placing it in a plastic bag, if available. Place the bag in a larger bag or container containing ice and water. Cooling slows the chemical processes and will increase the part's viability in excess of 4 hours. Do not place the amputated part directly on ice and never use dry ice.

■ Principles of Splinting

Splints are used to immobilize fractures to prevent further damage and to control bleeding. On the battlefield, some splints may need to be improvised. Splints may be improvised from such items as:

- Boards
- Poles
- Sticks
- Tree limbs
- Rolled magazines
- Newspapers
- Cardboard
- Pillows

Narrow materials such as wire or cord should not be used to secure a splint in place. If raw materials are not available, anatomic splints may be utilized. For example, the chest wall can be used to immobilize a fractured arm and the uninjured leg can be used to immobilize (to some extent) a fractured leg. Splints should be padded in order to prevent pressure points on bony prominences. If standard padding materials are unavailable, padding may be improvised from such items as:

- Clothing
- Blankets
- Poncho liners
- Ponchos
- Shelter halves
- Leafy vegetation

Slings are bandages suspended from the neck to support an upper extremity. Slings may be improvised by using the tail of a coat, a belt, a battle dress uniform (BDU) shirt, or pieces torn from such items as clothing and blankets. The triangular bandage is ideal for this purpose. Remember when applying a sling that the casualty's hand should be higher than his or her elbow, and the sling should be applied so that the supporting pressure is on the uninjured side.

Swathes are bands (pieces of cloth, pistol belts) that are used to further immobilize a splinted fracture. Triangular and cravat bandages are often used as swathe bandages. The purpose of the swathe is to immobilize. The swathe bandage is placed above and/or below the fracture, not over it.

To splint a fracture, follow the steps in **SKILL DRILL 8-1 ▸** :

1. Prepare the casualty for splinting the suspected fracture. Reassure the casualty. Loosen any tight or binding clothing. Remove all jewelry from the casualty distal to the fracture site. If the jewelry is not removed at this time and swelling continues, further injury can occur.

2. Gather splints or material for an improvised splint.

3. Ensure that the splints are long enough to immobilize the joint above and below the suspected fracture.

4. If possible, use at least four ties (two above and two below the fracture) to secure the splints. The ties should be nonslip knots and should be tied away from the body on the splint. If splinting material is not available, then swathes or a combination of swathes and slings can be used to immobilize an extremity with an anatomic splint.

5. Pad the splints where they touch any bony prominences. Padding prevents excessive pressure to the area.

6. Check the circulation distal to the injury. Note any pale, white, or bluish-gray color of the skin, which may indicate impaired circulation. Assess capillary refill.

7. Check the temperature of the injured extremity. Use your hand (ungloved portion) to compare the temperature of the injured side with the uninjured side of the body. The body area below the injury may be cooler to the touch, indicating poor circulation.

8. Question the casualty about the presence of numbness, tightness, cold, or tingling sensations. Casualties with fractures to the extremities may show impaired circulation, such as numbness, tingling, cold, and/or pale to blue skin distal to the injured site. These casualties should be treated and evacuated as soon as possible. Prompt medical treatment may prevent loss of the limb (**Step ①**).

9. Apply the splint in place.

10. Align the long bones to anatomic position under gentle traction if severe deformity exists or distal circulation is compromised.

Field Medical Care TIPS

Do not delay lifesaving treatment to apply splints to casualties.

11. If it is an open fracture, stop the bleeding and protect the wound. Cover the wound before applying a splint. If bones are protruding (sticking out), do not attempt to push them back under the skin.

12. Apply padding to protect the area.

13. Place one splint on each side of the arm or leg. Make sure that the splints reach, if possible, beyond the joints above and below the fracture (**Step ②**).

14. Tie the splints. Secure each splint in place above and below the fracture site with improvised or actual cravats. Improvised cravats, such as strips of cloth, belts, or whatever else you have, may be used. With minimal motion to the injured areas, tie the splints with the bandages. Push the cravats through and under the natural body curvatures (spaces), and then gently position the improvised cravats and tie in place. Use nonslip knots. Tie all knots on the splint on the outside of the casualty. Do not tie cravats directly over a suspected fracture/dislocation site (**Step ③**).

15. Check the splint for tightness. Check to be sure that bandages are tight enough to securely hold splinting materials in place, but not so tight that circulation is impaired (**Step ④**).

16. Recheck the circulation after application of the splint. Check the skin color and temperature to ensure that the bandages holding the splint in place have not been tied too tightly. A fingertip check can be made by inserting the tip of the finger between the wrapped tails and the skin. Make any adjustment without allowing the splint to become ineffective. (**Step ⑤**)

17. Apply a sling, if applicable. An improvised sling may be made. A sling should place the supporting pressure on the casualty's uninjured side. The supported arm should have the hand positioned slightly higher than the elbow.

18. Insert the splinted arm in the center of the sling.

19. Bring the ends of the sling up and tie them at the side (or hollow) of the neck on the uninjured side.

20. Twist and tuck the corner of the sling at the elbow (**Step ⑥**).

21. Apply a swathe, if applicable. You may use any large piece of cloth to improvise a swathe. The swathe should not be placed directly on top of the injury, but positioned either above or below the fracture site. Apply swathes to the injured arm by wrapping the

SKILL DRILL 8-1

Apply a Splint

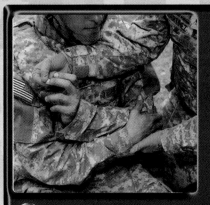

1. Prepare the casualty for splinting the suspected fracture. Gather splints or material for an improvised splint. Ensure that the splints are long enough to immobilize the joint above and below the suspected fracture. If possible, use at least four ties (two above and two below the fracture) to secure the splints. Pad the splints where they touch any bony prominences. Padding prevents excessive pressure to the area. Check the circulation distal to the injury. Assess capillary refill. Check the temperature of the injured extremity. Question the casualty about the presence of numbness, tightness, cold, or tingling sensations. Prompt medical treatment may prevent loss of the limb.

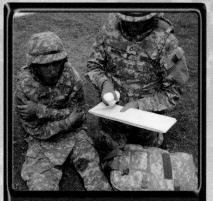

2. Apply the splint in place. Align the long bones to anatomic position under gentle traction if severe deformity exists or distal circulation is compromised. If it is an open fracture, stop the bleeding and protect the wound. Apply padding to protect the area.

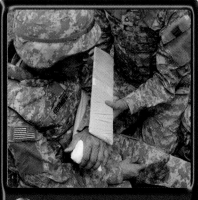

3. Place one splint on each side of the arm or leg. Make sure that the splints reach, if possible, beyond the joints above and below the fracture.

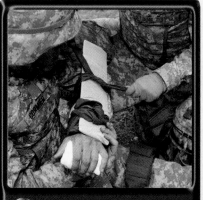

4. Tie the splints.

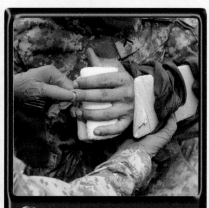

5. Check the splints for tightness. Check to be sure that bandages are tight enough to securely hold splinting materials in place, but not so tight that circulation is impaired. Recheck the circulation after application of the splint.

Apply a Splint (continued)

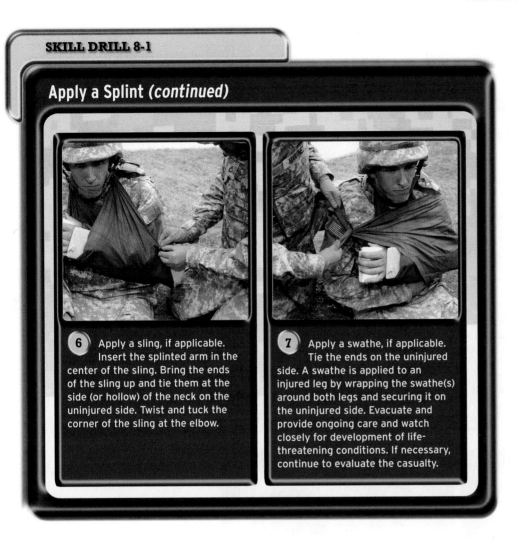

6 Apply a sling, if applicable. Insert the splinted arm in the center of the sling. Bring the ends of the sling up and tie them at the side (or hollow) of the neck on the uninjured side. Twist and tuck the corner of the sling at the elbow.

7 Apply a swathe, if applicable. Tie the ends on the uninjured side. A swathe is applied to an injured leg by wrapping the swathe(s) around both legs and securing it on the uninjured side. Evacuate and provide ongoing care and watch closely for development of life-threatening conditions. If necessary, continue to evaluate the casualty.

swathe over the injured arm, around the casualty's back, and under the arm on the uninjured side.

22. Tie the ends on the uninjured side.

23. A swathe is applied to an injured leg by wrapping the swathe(s) around both legs and securing it on the uninjured side.

24. Evacuate and provide ongoing care and watch closely for development of life-threatening conditions. If necessary, continue to evaluate the casualty (**Step 7**).

SAM Splint

A SAM splint can be molded to fit the extremity and can be very useful in the battlefield. To apply a SAM splint, follow the steps in **SKILL DRILL 8-2 ▶**:

1. Applying self-stabilization techniques, the casualty immobilizes the injured extremity, if possible.

2. Take the SAM splint and mold it around the casualty's uninjured extremity (**Step 1**).

3. Splint the injured extremity with the molded SAM splint and then secure the injured extremity to the SAM splint. If the casualty is able, he or she can help to stabilize the injured extremity (**Step 2**).

4. Apply a sling to immobilize the extremity (**Step 3**).

5. Apply a swathe to secure the injured extremity to the casualty's body (**Step 4**).

■ Summary

The ability to accurately recognize a musculoskeletal injury and apply the appropriate management can prevent further painful injury and even prevent permanent disability and/or death. Injuries to bones and joints should be splinted prior to moving the casualty; however, if life-threatening injuries exist, address them first and, if the casualty is a high priority for evacuation, immobilize the whole casualty on a long spine board. Always save a life over a limb.

SKILL DRILL 8-2

Apply a SAM Splint

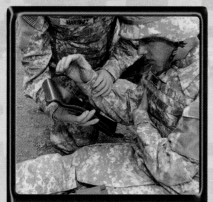

1 Applying self-stabilization techniques, the casualty immobilizes the injured extremity, if possible. Take the SAM splint and mold it around the casualty's uninjured extremity.

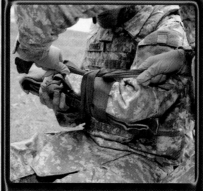

2 Splint the injured extremity with the molded SAM splint and then secure the injured extremity to the SAM splint. If the casualty is able, he or she can help to stabilize the injured extremity.

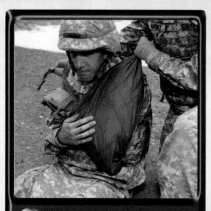

3 Apply a sling to immobilize the extremity.

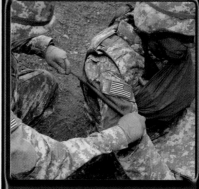

4 Apply a swathe to secure the injured extremity to the casualty's body.

YOU ARE THE COMBAT MEDIC

You are the combat medic supporting an infantry patrol. During a routine patrol, the platoon commander encounters a casualty in an overturned HMMWV. The convoy commander shouts out, "Medic, medic, come quick!" The convoy commander leads you to the overturned vehicle where you locate the casualty. You perform your situational assessment. The possibility of enemy contact is unknown at this time. Perimeter defense is established by the rest of the infantry patrol. The situation is safe and you are attending to only one casualty. You inspect the inside of the vehicle, where you notice a bent steering wheel and that the vehicle is stable. Your general impression reveals that your casualty is suffering from a bleeding laceration to the left forearm. The closest medical transport facility (MTF) is 40 minutes away and the MEDEVAC is available upon request.

Assessment

Upon further evaluation of the casualty, you notice that he responds to verbal stimuli, is tachypneic, skin is cool and moist, with bright red bleeding noted to the left forearm. Respirations are 28 breaths/min with good chest rise. The rapid trauma survey reveals an abrasion to the left side of the face. No cerebrospinal fluid (CSF) or active bleeding is noted. The casualty's neck appears to have no obvious injuries, trachea is midline, and jugular veins are flat. Chest wall is stable, no crepitus noted, breath sounds are present and equal bilaterally, with normal heart tones. Abdomen is soft and nontender, without rigidity, distension, or bruising. Pelvis is stable and without crepitus. A laceration and weak radial pulse is noted in the casualty's left arm.

Treatment

Treatment of this casualty follows the ABCs of care. The casualty has a patent airway, and is suffering from arterial bleeding to the left forearm. You make the determination that this casualty warrants immediate evacuation and the platoon commander calls for immediate MEDEVAC evacuation. While awaiting arrival of the MEDEVAC, you apply immediate direct pressure to the left forearm. It seems as though you are having trouble controlling the bleeding with direct pressure alone, so you apply a tourniquet to the bleeding extremity which seems to stop the hemorrhage. You also administer oxygen through a bag-valve-mask device.

While waiting to evacuate the casualty, you obtain vascular access in the right antecubital fossa space, and give enough normal saline to maintain a blood pressure high enough for adequate peripheral perfusion. Reassessment reveals a conscious, well-oriented casualty with a respiratory rate of 22 breaths/min, nonlabored; radial pulse of 108 beats/min and strong; and blood pressure of 120/66 mm Hg. The MEDEVAC chopper arrives and assumes care for the casualty.

1. LAST NAME, FIRST NAME		RANK/GRADE	X	MALE
Dwight, Theo		PFC		FEMALE
SSN 000-111-0000	SPECIALTY CODE ØZ		RELIGION Methodist	

2. UNIT

FORCE				NATIONALITY	
A/T	AF/A	N/M	MC/M		
	BC/BC		NBI/BNC	DISEASE	PSYCH

3. INJURY

	AIRWAY
	HEAD
X	WOUND
	NECK/BACK INJURY
	BURN
	AMPUTATION
	STRESS
	OTHER (Specify)

FRONT   BACK

4. LEVEL OF CONSCIOUSNESS

	ALERT		PAIN RESPONSE
X	VERBAL RESPONSE		UNRESPONSIVE

5. PULSE 108 bpm	TIME 1640	6. TOURNIQUET ☐ NO X YES	TIME 1635
7. MORPHINE X NO ☐ YES	DOSE	TIME	8. IV NS	TIME 1638

9. TREATMENT/OBSERVATIONS/CURRENT MEDICATION/ALLERGIES/NBC (ANTIDOTE)

Casualty in a motor vehicle rollover. Laceration to the left forearm.

10. DISPOSITION	RETURNED TO DUTY		TIME
	X	EVACUATED	
		DECEASED	

11. PROVIDER/UNIT Martin, Joe	DATE (YYMMDD)

Aid Kit

Ready for Review

- As a combat medic, you will encounter musculoskeletal injuries frequently on the battlefield.
- With musculoskeletal injuries, common mechanisms of injury include bullet or shrapnel wounds, falls, motor vehicle accidents, and sports injuries.
- The overall goal in the treatment of a musculoskeletal injury is to identify the type and extent of the injury.
- Splints are used to immobilize fractures to prevent further damage and to control bleeding. On the battlefield, some splints may need to be improvised.

Vital Vocabulary

acetabulum The cup-shaped cavity in which the rounded head of the femur rotates.

acromion Lateral extension of the scapula that forms the highest point of the shoulder.

amputation Severing of a part of the body.

appendicular skeleton The part of the skeleton comprising the upper and lower extremities.

axial skeleton The part of the skeleton comprising the skull, spinal column, and rib cage.

calcaneus The heel bone; the largest of the tarsal bones.

carpals The eight small bones of the wrist.

clavicle The collar bone.

closed fracture A fracture in which the skin is not broken.

compartment syndrome An increase in tissue pressure in a closed fascial space or compartment that compromises the circulation to the nerves and muscles within the involved compartment.

contusion Bruise.

dislocation The displacement of a bone from its normal position within a joint.

femur The proximal bone of the leg that extends from the pelvis to the knee.

fibula The smaller of the two bones of the lower leg.

humerus The bone of the upper arm.

ilium The broad, uppermost bone of the pelvis.

ischium The lowermost dorsal bone of the pelvis.

joint The point at which two or more bones articulate, or come together.

metacarpals The five bones that form the palm and back of the hand.

metatarsals The five long bones extending from the tarsus to the phalanges of the foot.

open fracture Any break in a bone in which the overlying skin has been damaged.

paresthesia Abnormal sensation such as burning, numbness, or tingling.

patella The kneecap.

pectoral girdle The shoulder girdle.

pelvic girdle The large bone that arises in the area of the last nine vertebrae and sweeps around to form a complete ring.

phalanges The bones of the fingers or toes.

point tenderness Tenderness that is sharply localized at the site of an injury; found by gently palpating along the bone with the tip of one finger.

pubis One of two bones that form the anterior portion of the pelvic ring.

radius The bone on the thumb side of the forearm.

scapula The shoulder blade.

six Ps of musculoskeletal assessment Pain, Paralysis, Paresthesias, Pulselessness, Pallor, and Pressure.

sprain An injury, such as a stretch or a tear, to the ligaments of a joint that commonly leads to pain and swelling.

tarsals The ankle bones.

tendon The fibrous portion of muscle that attaches to bone.

tibia The shin bone.

ulna The larger bone of the forearm, on the side opposite the thumb.

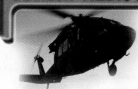

While attempting to take down a door with his shoulder, a soldier in your unit injures himself. He is conscious, well-oriented, answers all questions appropriately, and obeys all commands. Your perimeter is safe and this is your only casualty. You make the determination that this casualty is stable for ground transport which is 15 minutes away from the closest MTF.

After taking body substance isolation precautions, you decide to splint the injured shoulder. You instruct the casualty to apply stabilization with his uninjured hand. You assess motor, sensory, and distal circulation prior to immobilization and note no abnormalities. You use a sling and swathe for immobilization. You reassess motor, sensory, and distal circulation in the immobilized arm and note no abnormalities.

1. A partial dislocation of a joint is called a:
   A. subluxation.
   B. dislocation.
   C. stress fracture.
   D. sprain.

2. A complete disruption of the integrity of a joint is called a:
   A. sprain.
   B. dislocation.
   C. fracture.
   D. subluxation.

3. A fracture is considered complicated if it involves any one or more of the following conditions, EXCEPT:
   A. a crushing injury.
   B. painful, swollen deformity.
   C. decreased distal pulse.
   D. diminished distal sensory or motor function.

4. Prior to splinting a casualty who had dislocated his shoulder, you assessed positive distal pulses, motor, and sensation in the extremity. After the application of a sling and swathe, the casualty complains of paresthesia and numbness in the arm and fingers. What action should you now take?
   A. Apply ice and administer morphine IM or IV.
   B. Loosen the sling, then swathe and reassess.
   C. Remove the splint and pull traction on the arm, and resplint.
   D. Resplint the injury.

5. Which of the following is NOT a typical finding at the site of a musculosketal injury?
   A. Pain or tenderness
   B. Crepitation
   C. Diaphoresis
   D. Capillary refilling

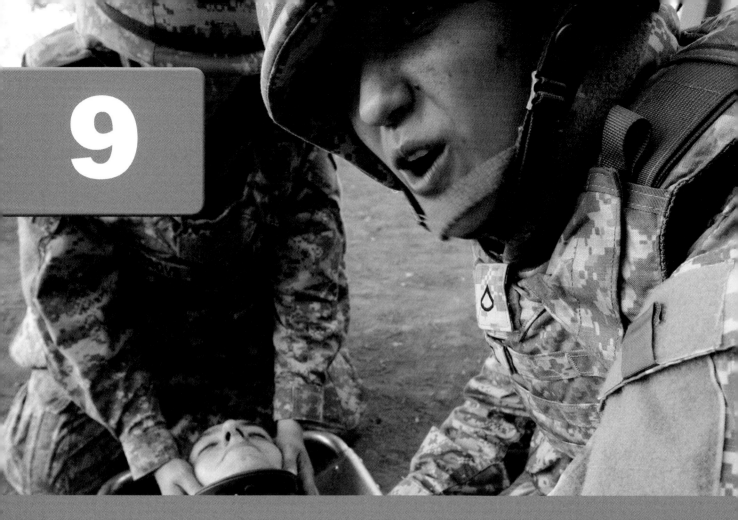

9

Spinal Injuries

Objectives

Knowledge Objectives

- [ ] Describe the anatomy and physiology of the spine.
- [ ] Identify the mechanisms of spinal injury.
- [ ] Identify and treat spinal injuries.
- [ ] Identify immobilization devices.

Skills Objective

- [ ] Transport a casualty with a suspected spinal injury.

■ Introduction

The nervous system is well protected by the bony structures of the skeletal system. The brain lies within the skull. The spinal cord lies inside the spinal column with the major nerves lying deep within the body. Despite being well protected, the nervous system can be injured from trauma. These injuries are extremely serious and can lead to paralysis and death.

■ Anatomy and Physiology Review

An understanding of the form and function of spinal anatomy coupled with a high level of suspicion for spinal cord injury (SCI) is required to decipher the often subtle findings associated with SCI.

The Spine

The spine consists of 33 irregular bones (vertebrae) articulating to form the vertebral column, which is the major structural component of the axial skeleton **FIGURE 9-1 ▾**. These skeletal components are stabilized by both ligaments and muscle. Together these components support and pro-

tect neural elements while allowing for fluid movement and erect stature.

Vertebrae are identified according to their location as cervical, thoracic, lumbar, sacral, or coccyx. The **vertebral body**, the anterior weight-bearing structure, is made of bone that provides support and stability. Components of each vertebra include the **lamina**, **pedicles**, and spinous processes **FIGURE 9-2 ▾**. Each vertebra is unique in appearance, with the exception of the atlas and axis (C1 and C2) **FIGURE 9-3 ▾**, shares basic structural characteristics but with adjacent vertebrae. Each vertebra (except the C1 and C2) has a drum-shaped body located toward the front serving as the weight-bearing part. Disks of cartilage between the vertebral bodies act as shock absorbers and provide flexibility. At the center of each vertebra is a large hole (foramen) for the spinal cord.

The cervical spine includes the first seven bones of the vertebral column and its supporting structures. In addition to protecting the vital cervical spinal cord, the cervical spine

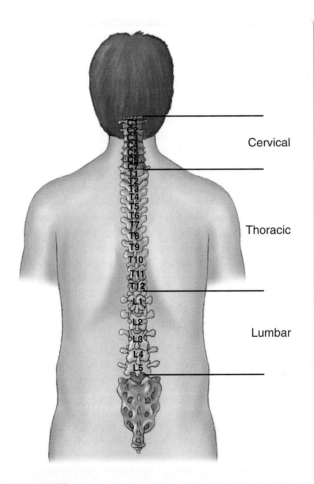

FIGURE 9-1 The spinal column consists of 33 bones divided into five sections. Each vertebra is numbered and referred to by a letter corresponding to the section of the spine where it is located plus its number. For example, the fifth thoracic vertebra is referred to as T5.

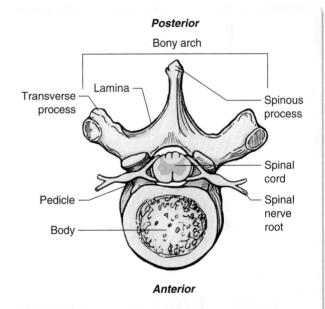

FIGURE 9-2 The human vertebra. Vertebrae in different sections of the spinal column vary in shape; this is a general representation. The space through which the spinal cord passes is called the foramen.

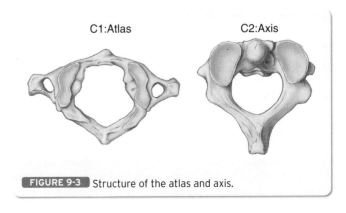

FIGURE 9-3 Structure of the atlas and axis.

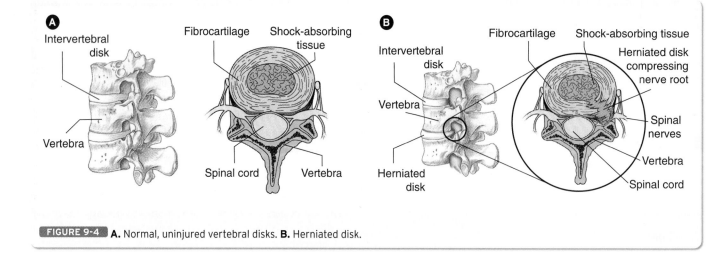

FIGURE 9-4   **A.** Normal, uninjured vertebral disks. **B.** Herniated disk.

Field Medical Care TIPS

C7 is the most prominent point of reference.

supports the weight of the head and permits a high degree of mobility in multiple planes. The atlas (C1) and axis (C2) are uniquely suited to allow for rotational movement of the skull. In Greek mythology, Atlas was a Titan who held up the earth. The atlas supports the head and the axis serves as a pivot for turning the head side to side.

The thoracic spine consists of 12 vertebrae in addition to the supporting muscles and ligaments found in the vertebral column; the thoracic spine is further stabilized by the rib attachments. The spinous processes on the thoracic vertebrae are slightly larger than those on the cervical, reflecting their role as attachment points for muscles that hold the upper body erect and assist with the movement of the thoracic cavity during respiration.

The lumbar spine includes the five largest bones in the vertebral column, and is integral in carrying a large portion of the upper body weight. The lumbar spine is especially susceptible to injury because of this weight-bearing capacity. It is located at the small of the back and is heavier and larger than the rest of the spine to support more weight.

The sacrum is composed of five fused vertebrae that form the posterior plate of the pelvis. As a child, the five bones are separate but they fuse to form one bone in adults. The coccyx (tailbone) is made up of four small fused vertebrae. Coccyx injuries, although often extremely painful, are typically clinically insignificant.

Each vertebra is separated and cushioned by intervertebral disks that limit bone wear and act as shock absorbers. As the body ages, these disks lose water content and become thinner, causing the height loss associated with aging. Stress on the vertebral column may cause a disk to herniate into the spinal canal, resulting in a spinal cord or nerve root injury FIGURE 9-4 ▲ .

The muscles, tendons, and ligaments that connect the vertebrae allow the spinal column a degree of flexion and extension, limited to an extent by the stabilization they must provide to the spinal column.

The Brain and Meninges

The **central nervous system (CNS)** consists of the brain and the spinal cord, both of which are encased in and protected by bone. The brain, located within the cranial cavity, is the largest component of the CNS. It contains billions of neurons that serve a variety of vital functions, voluntary and involuntary.

The **brain stem**, which consists of the medulla, pons, and midbrain, connects the spinal cord to the remainder of the brain. The brain stem is vital for numerous basic body functions. Damage to this critical structure can easily result in death. All but two of the 12 cranial nerves exit from the brain stem.

The entire CNS is enclosed by a set of three membranes collectively known as the meninges FIGURE 9-5 ▶ . The outer membrane, called the **dura mater**, is tough and fibrous. The middle layer, called the **arachnoid**, contains blood vessels that give it the appearance of a spider web. The innermost layer, resting directly on the brain or spinal cord, is the **pia mater**. The meninges float in **cerebrospinal fluid (CSF)**. The meninges and CSF form a fluid-filled cushion that protects the brain and spinal cord.

The Spinal Cord

The **spinal cord** transmits nerve impulses between the brain and the rest of the body. Located at the base of the brain, it represents the continuation of the CNS. This bundle of nerve fibers leaves the skull through a large opening at its base called the **foramen magnum**. The spinal cord extends from the base of the skull to L2; here it separates into the **cauda equina**, a collection of individual nerve roots. Thirty-one pairs of spinal nerves arise from the different segments of the

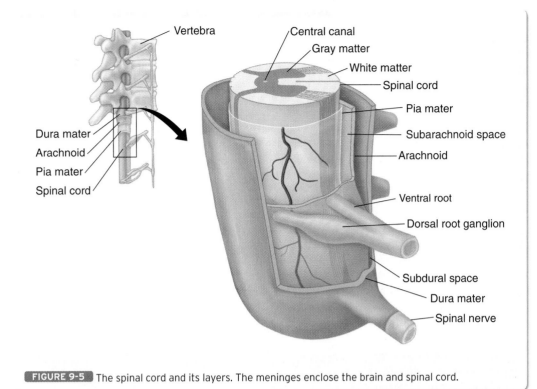

Vertebra

Central canal
Gray matter
White matter
Spinal cord
Pia mater
Subarachnoid space
Arachnoid
Ventral root
Dorsal root ganglion
Subdural space
Dura mater
Spinal nerve

Dura mater
Arachnoid
Pia mater
Spinal cord

FIGURE 9-5 The spinal cord and its layers. The meninges enclose the brain and spinal cord.

spinal cord; each pair is named according to its corresponding segment.

The spinal cord conducts sensory impulses to the brain and conducts motor impulses from the brain to the muscles. These signals travel back and forth rapidly. Some are purely within the spinal cord and never involve the brain, called reflexes. A strong tap just below the knee causing the lower leg to jerk can demonstrate this. It is also manifested by placing your hand on a stove and your reflex system moving it away before your brain receives the warning signal.

The **peripheral nervous system** includes all of the nerves outside the central nervous system. The **cranial nerves** carry impulses to and from specialized organs to the brain. The **spinal nerves** carry messages to and from the spinal cord. The **autonomic nervous system** consists of nerves, ganglia, and plexuses that carry impulses to all smooth muscles, secretory glands, and the heart. It regulates the activity of these visceral organs. These activities are usually automatic and are not subject to conscious control.

■ Mechanism of Injury

Acute injuries of the spine are classified according to the associated mechanism, location, and stability of the injury. Vertebral fractures can occur with or without associated SCI. Because stable fractures do not involve the posterior column, they pose less risk to the spinal cord. Unstable injuries involve the posterior column of the spinal cord and typically include damage to portions of the vertebrae and ligaments that directly protect the spinal cord and nerve roots. Unstable injuries carry a higher risk of complicating SCI and

progression of injury without appropriate treatment. Mechanisms of spinal injury are listed in **TABLE 9-1 ▼**.

Flexion Injuries

Flexion injuries result from forward movement of the head, typically as the result of rapid deceleration (eg, in a car crash) or from a direct blow to the occiput. At the level of C1–C2, these forces can produce an unstable dislocation with or without an associated fracture. Farther down the spinal column, flexion forces are transmitted anteriorly through the vertebral bodies and can result in an anterior wedge fracture. Depending on their severity, anterior wedge fractures can be stable or unstable. Loss of more than half the original size of the vertebral body or multiple levels of injury suggest involvement of the posterior column.

Hyperflexion injuries of greater force can result in teardrop fractures—avulsion fractures of the anterior-inferior border of the vertebral body. The injuries to ligaments associated with teardrop fractures raise concern for possible SCI and are often unstable fractures. Severe flexion can also result in a potentially unstable dislocation of vertebral joints. This situation does not involve fracture but can severely injure the ligaments. Strong forces can result in the anterior displacement of **facet joints**. A bilateral facet dislocation is an extremely unstable injury.

TABLE 9-1	Mechanisms of Spinal Injury
Hyperextension	Excessive posterior movement of the head or neck
Hyperflexion	Excessive anterior movement of the head or neck
Compression	The weight of the head or pelvis driven into a stationary neck or torso
Rotation	Excessive rotation of the torso, or the head and neck moving in different directions from each other
Lateral stress	Direct lateral force on the spinal column, typically shearing one level of the cord from another.
Distraction	Excessive stretching of the column or the cord

Rotation with Flexion

The only area of the spine that allows for significant rotation is C1–C2. Injuries to this area are considered unstable due to its high cervical location and scant bony and soft-tissue support. **Rotation-flexion injuries** often result from high acceleration forces. Rotation with abrupt flexion can produce an unstable dislocation in the cervical spine. In the thoracolumbar spine, rotation-flexion forces typically cause fracture rather than dislocation.

Vertical Compression

Vertical compression forces are transmitted through vertebral bodies and directed either inferiorly through the skull or superiorly through the pelvis or feet. They typically result from a direct blow to the crown of the skull or rapid deceleration from a fall through the feet, legs, and pelvis. Forces transmitted through the vertebral body cause fractures, ultimately shattering and producing a "burst" or compression fracture without associated SCI **FIGURE 9-6 ◀**. Compression forces can cause the herniation of disks, subsequent compression on the spinal cord and nerve roots, and fragmentation into the canal.

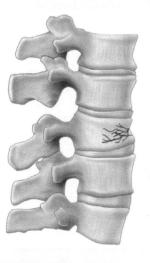

FIGURE 9-6 A compression fracture.

Although most fractures resulting from these injuries are stable, primary SCI can occur when the vertebral body is shattered and fragments of bone become embedded in the cord. Some compression injuries may be associated with significant retropharyngeal edema, and serious airway compromise is a consideration.

Hyperextension

Hyperextension of the head and neck can result in fractures and ligamentous injury of variable stability. The hangman's fracture (C2), or distraction, results from hyperextension due to rapid deceleration of the skull, atlas, and axis as a unit. The resulting bilateral pedicle fracture of C2 is an unstable fracture but is rarely associated with SCI. A teardrop fracture of the anterior-inferior edge of the vertebral body results from hyperextension, resulting in rupture or tear of the anterior longitudinal ligament. The injury is stable with the head and neck in flexion, but unstable in extension due to loss of structural support.

■ Spinal Column Injury

The head is a relatively large ball perched on top of the neck; a sudden movement of the head or trunk will produce flexion, extension, or lateral stresses that may damage the bony

Field Medical Care TIPS

Fortunately, spinal column injury can occur without injuring the spinal cord. Statistically, only 14% of all column injuries have evidence of spinal cord damage. In the cervical spine region, it is much more common to have cord injuries with almost 40% of column injuries having spinal cord damage. Conversely, only 63% of injuries have evidence of spinal column damage. This means that almost half of the patients with some degree of paralysis have no obvious bone or ligament injury to the spinal column, even on x-ray. The unconscious trauma patient carries a high risk (15% to 20%) of spinal column injuries. These injuries are frequently in more than one place, and therefore the unconscious casualty should be immediately and consistently immobilized.

or connective tissue component of the spinal column. Injury to the spinal column is like an injury to any other bone in the body—it may involve fractures, sprains, strains, or dislocations. Spinal column injury requires a significant amount of force unless there is a preexisting weakness or defect in the bone. For that reason, the elderly and those with severe arthritis are at a high risk for spinal injuries.

Like other bone injuries, pain is the most common symptom. Other symptoms include:

- Localized pain and/or muscle spasm
- Loss of sensation
- Paresthesias
- Paralysis
- Priapism
- Incontinence (loss of bladder or bowel control)

■ Spinal Cord Injury

Spinal cord injury results in a defective connection of signals, presenting as a loss of motor function and reflexes, loss of change in sensation, and/or neurogenic shock.

The delicate structure of the spinal cord's tracts makes it very sensitive to any form of trauma. Primary damage occurs at the time of injury and may result in the cord being cut, torn, or crushed, or its blood supply being cut off. Secondary damage occurs from hypotension, generalized hypoxia, injury to blood vessels, swelling, or compression of the cord from surrounding hemorrhage. Emergency efforts are directed at preventing secondary damage through attention to the ABCs and careful packaging of the casualty.

Clues to spinal cord injury include:

- The mechanism of injury:
  - Blunt trauma above the clavicles
  - Diving accident
  - Motor vehicle or bicycle accident
  - Fall
  - Stabbing or impalement anywhere near the spinal column

- Shooting or blast injury to the torso
- Any violent injury with forces that could act on the spinal column
- When the casualty complains of:
  - Neck or back pain
  - Numbness or tingling
  - Loss of movement or weakness
- When you find the following signs and symptoms:
  - Pain on movement or palpation of the spinal column
  - Obvious deformity of the back or spinal column
  - Guarding against movement of the back
  - Loss of sensation (may be unilateral)
  - Erection of the penis (priapism)

■ Neurogenic Shock

Injury to the thoracic or cervical spinal cord can produce **neurogenic shock**, which results from the malfunction of the automatic nervous system in regulating blood vessel tone and cardiac output. This results in a casualty who is hypotensive, with normal skin color and temperature and an inappropriately slow heart rate, versus a hypovolemic casualty with cool, clammy skin and a rapid heart rate.

In hypovolemic shock, catecholamines (epinephrine and norepinephrine) are released from the adrenal glands, which causes the blood vessels to constrict and the heart rate to increase. In neurogenic shock, there is no signal to the adrenal glands to release these hormones. Consequently the blood vessels dilate, blood pools due to the larger diameter of the blood vessels, and blood pressure falls. The brain cannot correct this because it has no way to get the signal to the adrenal glands. The casualty with neurogenic shock cannot show signs of pale skin, fast heartbeat, and sweating because the spinal cord injury prevents the release of catecholamines.

■ Identify and Treat Injuries to the Spine

Situational Assessment

Provide emergency care to the casualty. Determine if a rapid extrication is necessary. See Chapter 16, *Evacuation*, for detailed evacuation and casualty packaging procedures. During the situational assessment, identify any condition that may immediately endanger the casualty or you:

- Fire or immediate danger of fire
- Danger of explosion
- Danger of drowning
- Structure in danger of collapse
- Continuing toxic exposure

Initial exam of the casualty identifies a condition that requires immediate intervention that cannot be done in the entrapped area:

- Airway obstruction that cannot be relieved by modified jaw thrust or finger sweep
- Cardiac or respiratory arrest
- Chest or airway injuries requiring ventilation or assisted ventilation
- Deep shock or bleeding that cannot be controlled

Initial Assessment

Perform an initial assessment of the casualty. Ensure an open airway. If necessary, open the airway using the jaw thrust. Assess the casualty's breathing. Diaphragmatic breathing may be present due to damage to the nerves that innervate the intercostal muscles. Assess the casualty's circulation and look for major hemorrhage. Treat any life-threatening conditions at this time.

Rapid Trauma Survey

Assessment of the Responsive Casualty

Consider the mechanism of injury:

- Falls
- Blunt trauma
- Penetrating trauma to the head, neck, or torso
- Vehicle accidents

The casualty's ability to walk should not rule out spinal injury because 20% of all casualties with spinal injuries are seen walking around the accident scene.

- Does your neck or back hurt? Where?
- Can you move your hands and feet?
- Can you feel me touching your fingers/toes? Paralysis or loss of sensation of the upper and/or lower extremities are the most reliable signs of a spinal cord injury if the casualty is conscious.

Inspect the casualty for:

- Deformities
- Contusions
- Abrasions
- Punctures
- Burns
- Tenderness
- Swelling
- Lacerations

Palpate the casualty for areas of tenderness, instability, crepitus, or deformity. Assess the casualty for the equality of the strength of the extremities. Assess the casualty's handgrip and gently push feet against your hands. Assess the casualty's level of consciousness (LOC).

Assessment of the Unresponsive Casualty

Determine the mechanism of injury from witnesses. Inspect the casualty for:

- Deformities
- Contusions
- Abrasions
- Punctures
- Burns
- Tenderness
- Lacerations
- Swelling

Palpate the casualty for areas of tenderness, instability, crepitus, or deformity.

Assess for tenderness with gentle palpation in the area of injury. Assess the casualty for deformity. Obvious deformities (eg, "step offs") are rare. Check the casualty's response to painful stimuli by pinching between the thumb and index finger or pinching the skin on top of each foot.

Check the casualty for impaired breathing. This may indicate damaged spinal nerves, which send information to the respiratory center of the brain. Signs of impaired breathing include diaphragmatic breathing and panting.

Check for life-threatening spinal cord injuries. These occur with spinal column injuries from C1 to T8 due to damage to the spinal nerves and/or brain stem, which interrupt nerve transmission to the respiratory center.

Other signs to look for include:

- Priapism (persistent erection of the penis often associated with a spinal cord injury)
- Incontinence (bowel and/or bladder loss of control)
- Soft-tissue injury with trauma

Protect the Spine

Establish and maintain manual in-line stabilization of the casualty's head and neck during the initial assessment. Continue to maintain stabilization until the casualty is properly secured to a long spine board. Proper manual stabilization of the cervical spine is accomplished by grasping the casualty's shoulder with each hand and gently positioning the casualty's head between your forearms FIGURE 9-7 ▶. This technique allows the head, neck, and torso to move as one unit. Apply the proper size rigid cervical collar.

If the casualty is found in a lying position, immobilize the casualty to a long spine board using the log roll method FIGURE 9-8 ▶. If the casualty is found in a sitting position, immobilize the casualty to a short spine board or Kendrick extrication device (KED) FIGURE 9-9 ▶. If the casualty is found in a standing position, immobilize the casualty to a long spine board FIGURE 9-10 ▶.

Use the scoop litter if you are unable to log roll the casualty. Adjust the scoop litter to the correct length, and ensure that it is separated, inserted, and fastened according to its design. The casualty is immobilized to the scoop litter in the same manner as to a long spine board FIGURE 9-11 ▶.

Lift the scoop litter from the side, about 4″ to 6″ off the ground while a long spine board is slid lengthwise under it. The scoop litter should not be lifted from the head and foot ends or used to carry the casualty before it has been placed on a long spine board because it can sag without center support. Secure the scoop litter to the long spine board. Because the casualty is already immobilized on the scoop litter, no additional immobilization should be necessary. The long spine board, scoop litter, and casualty are then secured to a cot.

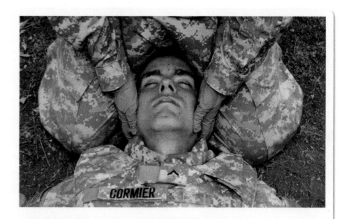

FIGURE 9-7   Proper manual stabilization of the cervical spine is accomplished by grasping the casualty's shoulder with each hand and gently positioning the casualty's head between your forearms.

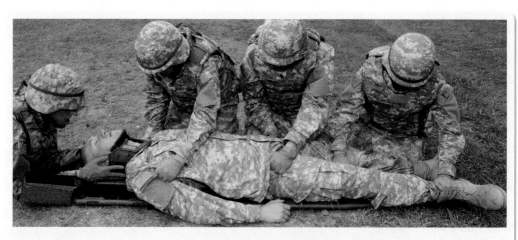

FIGURE 9-8   If the casualty is found in a lying position, immobilize the casualty to a long spine board using the log roll method.

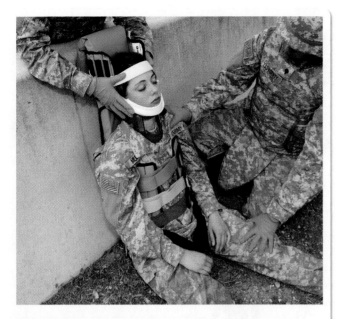

FIGURE 9-9 If the casualty is found in a sitting position, immobilize the casualty to a short spine board or KED.

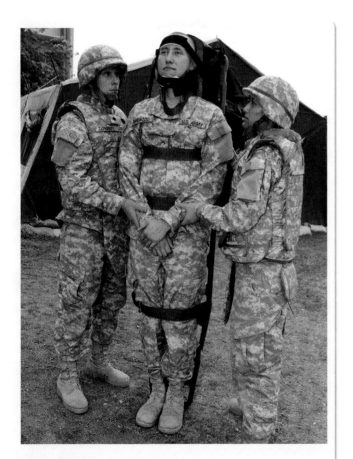

FIGURE 9-10 If the casualty is found in a standing position, immobilize the casualty to a long spine board.

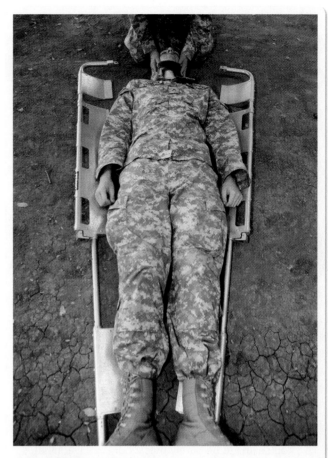

FIGURE 9-11 The casualty is immobilized to the scoop litter in the same manner as to a long spine board.

Transport Considerations

After immobilizing the casualty, continually assess the casualty's pulse, motor, and sensory (PMS) functions in all extremities. Care for other injuries. The best treatment you can provide to a casualty with a spinal injury is swift evacuation. Transport the casualty immediately. Monitor the casualty for signs and symptoms of neurogenic shock. Continue the neurologic assessment and monitor vital signs every 3 to 5 minutes.

■ Summary

To provide your casualty with the best chance of recovery, you must know the anatomy of the spine and central nervous system. The most important point in management of spine trauma is rapid assessment, treatment of decreased level of consciousness, adequate airway management, rapid transport to the appropriate echelon of care, and frequent reassessment. You must immobilize the spine to prevent harm and paralysis. Neck movement can worsen the condition of a casualty with a spinal injury.

YOU ARE THE
COMBAT MEDIC

During a house-to-house search of an insurgent camp, a member of your team starts up the staircase to begin a search of the second floor. As he approaches the top stair, the staircase collapses, sending the soldier to the ground. You make your way to the casualty and find him conscious, breathing, and lying on his left side.

The situational assessment reveals that the casualty is alert, oriented to time, place, and person; with no airway or breathing issues; and no life-threatening bleeding found. The captain, fearing the position of the team is vulnerable, orders you to prep the casualty for immediate evacuation. A combat lifesaver (CLS) brings you the emergency backboard from the HMMWV. Once the casualty is secure on the backboard, he is moved to the HMMWV for transport to the Medical Treatment Facility (MTF) 10 miles away.

Assessment

Now you have an opportunity to perform an initial assessment. The soldier is stable and the immobilization seems to be purely precautionary. Five minutes into transport, the casualty complains of a sharp pain traveling down his right arm. Also, the last two digits on his hand are numb. You checked his pulses, neurologic function, and sensory on his upper extremities after placing him on the backboard and did not find any deficits. The casualty is becoming anxious and his breathing rate is now 32 breaths/min and shallow. His pulse rate is 103 beats/min and regular and his blood pressure is 130 mm Hg. The road is very bumpy and you do not dare to try and adjust the casualty on the board.

Upon arrival at the MTF, you transfer the casualty over to the medical officer and inform him of the change in the casualty's condition during transport.

1. LAST NAME, FIRST NAME		RANK/GRADE	✓	MALE
Wilson, Troy		PFC/E3		FEMALE
SSN	SPECIALTY CODE			RELIGION
000-555-1234	00A			Baptist

2. UNIT

FORCE				NATIONALITY		
A/T	AF/A	N/M	MC/M			
	BC/BC		NBI/BNC		DISEASE	PSYCH

3. INJURY

	AIRWAY
	HEAD
FRONT BACK	WOUND
X	NECK/BACK INJURY
	BURN
	AMPUTATION
	STRESS
	OTHER (Specify)

Possible neck/back

injury after fall

4. LEVEL OF CONSCIOUSNESS

✓	ALERT		PAIN RESPONSE
	VERBAL RESPONSE		UNRESPONSIVE

5. PULSE	TIME	6. TOURNIQUET		TIME
103 bpm	1805	X NO ☐ YES		

7. MORPHINE	DOSE	TIME	8. IV	TIME
X NO ☐ YES				

9. TREATMENT/OBSERVATIONS/CURRENT MEDICATION/ALLERGIES/NBC (ANTIDOTE)

Evacuated on backboard. Complains of pain in right arm. Last two fingers are numb in right hand. Breathing rate is 32 breaths/min & shallow. Blood pressure is 130 mm Hg.

10. DISPOSITION		RETURNED TO DUTY		TIME
	X	EVACUATED		1820
		DECEASED		

11. PROVIDER/UNIT	DATE (YYMMDD)
Smith, Reed	

Ready for Review

- Despite being well protected, the nervous system can be injured from trauma. These injuries are extremely serious and can lead to paralysis and death.
- Acute injuries of the spine are classified according to the associated mechanism, location, and stability of the injury.
- Establish and maintain manual in-line stabilization of the casualty's head and neck during the initial assessment.
- After immobilizing the casualty, continually assess the casualty's pulse, motor, and sensory (PMS) functions in all extremities.
- Care for other injuries.
- The best treatment you can provide to a casualty with a spinal injury is swift evacuation.

Vital Vocabulary

arachnoid The middle membrane of the three meninges that enclose the brain and spinal cord.

autonomic nervous system Consists of nerves, ganglia, and plexus that carry impulses to all smooth muscles, secretory glands, and the heart.

brain stem The portion of the brain that connects the spinal cord to the rest of the brain, and contains the medulla, pons, and midbrain.

cauda equina The location where the spinal cord separates; composed of nerve roots.

central nervous system (CNS) The system containing the brain and spinal cord.

cerebrospinal fluid (CSF) Fluid produced in the ventricles of the brain that flows in the subarachnoid space and bathes the meninges.

cranial nerves Carry impulses to and from specialized organs and the brain.

dura mater The outermost of the three meninges that enclose the brain and spinal cord; it is the toughest membrane.

facet joint The joint on which each vertebra articulates with adjacent vertebrae.

flexion injury A type of injury that results from forward movement of the head, typically as the result of rapid deceleration, such as in a car crash, or with a direct blow to the occiput.

foramen magnum A large opening at the base of the skull through which the spinal cord exits the brain.

hyperextension Extension of a limb or other body part beyond its usual range of motion.

lamina Components of the spine that rise from the posterior pedicles and fuse to form the posterior spinous processes.

neurogenic shock The malfunction of the automatic nervous system in regulating blood vessel tone and cardiac output.

pedicles Thick lateral bony struts that connect the vertebral body with spinous and transverse processes and make up the lateral and posterior portions of the spinal foramen.

peripheral nervous system All the nerves outside of the central nervous system.

pia mater The innermost of the three meninges that enclose the brain and spinal cord; it rests directly on the brain and spinal cord.

rotation-flexion injury A type of injury typically resulting from high acceleration forces; can result in a stable unilateral facet dislocation in the cervical spine.

spinal cord The part of the central nervous system that extends downward from the brain through the foramen magnum and is protected by the spine.

spinal nerves Carry messages to and from the spinal cord.

vertebral body Anterior weight-bearing structure in the spine made of cancellous bone and surrounded by a layer of hard, compact bone that provides support and stability.

vertical compression A type of injury typically resulting from a direct blow to the crown of the skull or rapid deceleration from a fall through the feet, legs, and pelvis, possibly causing a burst fracture or disk herniation; forces are transmitted through vertebral bodies and directed either inferiorly through the skull or superiorly through the pelvis or feet.

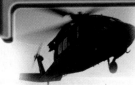

COMBAT MEDIC *in Action*

During some off-duty time, you and a few soldiers go swimming down by the river. There is a small cliff that many are jumping off and into the water. One soldier dives head first off the cliff and fails to reappear from below the water. You and your other friends realize what has happened and begin to search the water for the soldier. Suddenly the victim floats to the top of the water. You swim over and notice he is unconscious and not breathing. He is also bleeding from a 4" gash to the left side of his head.

1. What is the priority for this casualty?

   A. Circulation
   B. Immobilization
   C. Airway
   D. Bleeding

2. There is not a backboard around. How will you move the casualty out of the water?

   A. Do not move him and try to work on him in the water.
   B. Use available personnel to float the casualty to the shore, stabilizing the neck and body.
   C. Use the two-man arm and leg carry once you are close enough to put your feet down.
   D. Use the fireman's carry once you are close enough to put your feet down.

3. You have been able to get the casualty to the shore. You administer the two rescue breaths and they go in. Your pulse check reveals there is a pulse. What is your next step in the care of this casualty?

   A. Leave the casualty alone, he will be fine.
   B. Maintaining stabilization, reassess the breathing. If the casualty is not breathing administer rescue breaths at the rate of 1 every 5 seconds.
   C. Reassess the breathing and make sure it is adequate. If not, start to administer rescue breaths at the rate of 1 every 5 seconds.
   D. None of the above.

4. While administering the rescue breathing, the casualty vomits. What would be the proper way to clear the airway when there is no suction unit available?

   A. Quickly move the casualty's head to the side and dump the contents out. Return the head to the inline position. Do this while keeping the body supine.
   B. Finger sweep the mouth while someone maintains stabilization of the head.
   C. Using the soldiers at the scene, instruct them to help you log roll the casualty on his side, keeping the head and body inline. Clear the contents of the airway then roll the casualty back on his back, again keeping the head and body inline.
   D. Attempt to suck out the obstruction using your mouth.

5. It has been a couple of minutes and you recheck the casualty's pulse and cannot find one. What is your next course of action?

   A. Begin chest compressions.
   B. Continue with just rescue breathing.
   C. Give up and state the casualty is dead.
   D. Give abdominal thrusts.

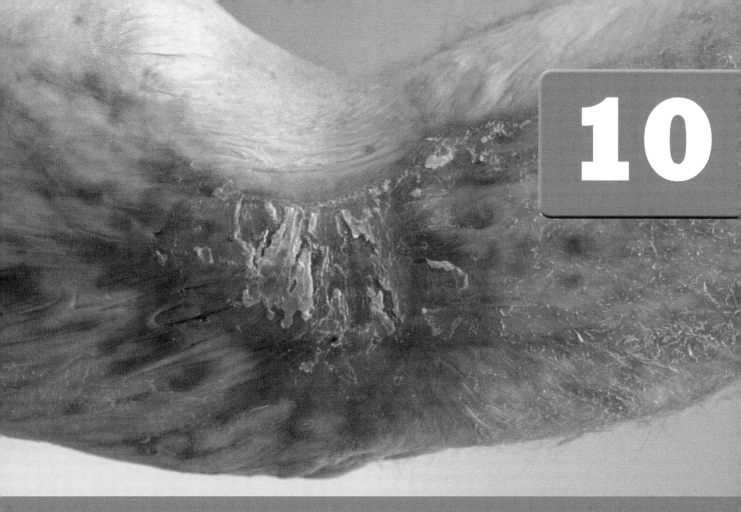

10

Burns

Objectives

Knowledge Objectives
- ☐ Describe the anatomy and physiology of the skin.
- ☐ Identify and eliminate the source of a burn.
- ☐ Describe the assessment of a burn in a casualty.
- ☐ Describe the management of a casualty with thermal burns.
- ☐ Describe the management of a casualty with chemical burns.
- ☐ Describe the management of a casualty with electrical burns.
- ☐ Describe the management of a casualty with lightning injury.
- ☐ Describe the management of a casualty with inhalation burns.

Skills Objectives
- ☐ Insert a Foley catheter.
- ☐ Insert a nasogastric tube.

■ Introduction

More than 1 million burn injuries occur each year in the United States, resulting in more than 5,000 deaths. Many who survive their burns are severely disabled and/or disfigured. Applying the basic principles taught here will decrease death, disability, and disfigurement from burns.

Burns are among the most serious and painful of all injuries. The sources of these injuries are heat, toxic chemicals, electricity, and ultraviolet and nuclear radiation. Caring for a burn casualty may present other problems: the scene may be hazardous, the fire or substance that caused the burn may have to be extinguished or removed, the casualty may be experiencing shock or respiratory arrest caused by the burn, and he or she may have sustained fractures from falling. You must also be aware of and avoid energized wires, toxic fumes and smoke, or the exposure to radioactivity that may have caused the burn.

■ Anatomy and Physiology Review

The human skin is much more than a wrapping that keeps the inside of the body from falling out. The skin, also known as the **integument**, is the largest and one of the most complex organs in the body. It has a crucial role in maintaining **homeostasis** (balance) within the body. The skin is durable, flexible, and usually able to repair itself. It varies in thickness from almost 1 cm on the heel to 1 mm on the eye's surface. The skin has four functions:

- It acts as an all-purpose fortress to protect the underlying tissue from injury and exposure from extremes of temperature, ultraviolet radiation, mechanical forces, toxic chemicals, and invading microorganisms.
- The skin aids in temperature regulation (**thermoregulation**), preventing heat loss when the core body temperature starts to fall and facilitating heat loss when the core temperature rises.
- As a watertight seal, the skin prevents excessive loss of water from the body and drying of tissues, thereby helping maintain the chemical stability of the internal environment. Without skin, a person would become water-logged after the first rain and would resemble a prune after the first hot day of summer.
- The skin serves as a sense organ, keeping the brain informed about the external environment. Changes in temperature and sensations of pain are mediated through skin sense receptors.

Significant damage to the skin may make the body vulnerable to bacterial invasion, temperature instability, and major disturbances of fluid balance. People who survive serious burns must live with the ramifications of the damage to large portions of the integument:

- Difficulty with thermoregulation
- Inability to sweat from the scarred portions of the skin
- Impaired vasoconstriction and vasodilation in the areas of severe damage

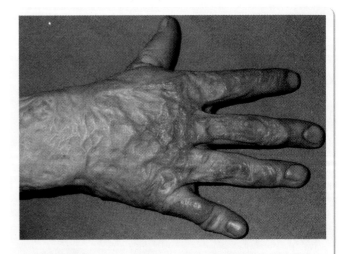

FIGURE 10-1 People who survive serious burns must live with the ramifications of the loss.

- Little or no melanin (pigment) in the scar tissue, which makes the skin susceptible to sunburn
- Inability to grow hair on the injured site and little or no sensation in the scarred areas

All of these factors may restrict a person's ability to function even many years after the burn trauma has healed **FIGURE 10-1 ▲**. People who survive serious burns also have a high rate of depression.

Layers of the Skin

To carry out its functions, the skin needs a specialized structure **FIGURE 10-2 ▶**. The skin is composed of two principal layers: the epidermis and the dermis. The **epidermis**, or outermost layer, is the body's first line of defense, constituting the major barrier against water, dust, microorganisms, and mechanical stress. The epidermis is itself composed of several layers: an outermost layer of hardened, nonliving cells, which are continuously shed through a process called **desquamation**, and three inner layers of living cells that constantly divide to give rise to new "dead layer" skin cells. The deeper layers of the epidermis also contain variable numbers of cells bearing **melanin** granules. The darkness of a person's skin is directly proportional to the amount of melanin present.

Underlying the epidermis is a tough, highly elastic layer of connective tissues called the **dermis**. The dermis is a complex material composed chiefly of collagen fibers, elastin fibers, and a mucopolysaccharide gel. **Collagen** is a fibrous protein with a very high tensile strength, so it gives the skin high resistance to breakage under mechanical stress. **Elastin** imparts elasticity to the skin, allowing it to spring back to its usual contours. The **mucopolysaccharide gel** gives the skin resistance to compression.

Enclosed within the dermis are several specialized skin structures. Nerve endings mediate the senses of touch, temperature, pressure, and pain, for example. Blood vessels carry oxygen and nutrients to the skin and remove the carbon dioxide and metabolic waste products. **Cutaneous** blood vessels also

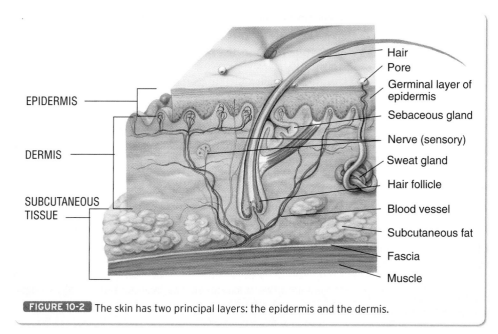

EPIDERMIS

DERMIS

SUBCUTANEOUS
TISSUE

Hair
Pore
Germinal layer of
epidermis
Sebaceous gland
Nerve (sensory)
Sweat gland
Hair follicle
Blood vessel
Subcutaneous fat
Fascia
Muscle

FIGURE 10-2 The skin has two principal layers: the epidermis and the dermis.

The tissue beneath the dermis, called the **subcutaneous layer**, consists mainly of **adipose tissue** (fat). Subcutaneous fat insulates the underlying tissues from extremes of heat and cold. It also provides a substantial cushion for underlying structures, while serving as an energy reserve for the body.

Finally, beneath the subcutaneous layer are the muscles, tendons, bones, and vital organs. Muscles have thick, fibrous capsules that are prone to hypoxia and **anaerobic metabolism** in a burn state. Bones are living tissue that can be severely affected by burn injury. Vital organs may also be damaged by thermal, chemical, or electrical energy.

serve a crucial role in regulating body temperature by regulating the volume of blood that flows from the body's warm core to its cooler surface.

Also in the dermis, sweat glands produce sweat and discharge it through ducts passing to the surface of the skin in a process regulated by the sympathetic nervous system. Sweat consists of water and salts. The average volume of sweat lost during 24 hours under normal conditions ranges from 500 to 1,000 mL. During strenuous exercise, sweat glands may secrete as much as 1,000 mL in an hour. Evaporation of water from the skin surface is one of the body's major mechanisms for shedding excess heat.

Hair follicles are structures that produce hair and enclose the hair roots. Each follicle contains a single hair. Attached to the hair follicle is a small muscle that, on contraction, causes the follicle to assume a more vertical position. Sensations such as cold and fright stimulate the autonomic nervous system, which in turn brings about contraction of those muscles and results in "gooseflesh." Hairs in each part of the body have definite periods of growth, after which they are shed and replaced; scalp hair, for example, has a life span of 2 to 5 years and grows at an average rate of 1.5 to 3.9 mm per week. Hair melts when it burns, yet sometimes appears to remain on the casualty. When you brush your hand over it, you may find that what you thought was a mustache is now simply a streak of ash. Closely observe nasal hair, eyebrows, and eyelashes in burn casualties because damage to them may indicate airway injury. When hair on the arms or legs "falls out" or can be removed without pain, deeper skin structures have been damaged.

At the neck of each hair follicle is a **sebaceous gland** that produces an oily substance called **sebum**. The secretions of the sebaceous glands empty into the hair follicles and ultimately reach the surface of the skin. Sebum is believed to keep the skin supple so it doesn't dry out and crack.

The Eye

The specific anatomy and physiology of the eye are covered in Chapter 7, *Head Injuries*. Clearly, the eyes are sensitive to burn injuries—from a flame, superheated gases, a light source, or chemicals. The tear ducts and eyelids combine to constantly lubricate the surface of the eyes **FIGURE 10-3 ▾**. Unfortunately, intense heat, light, or chemical reactions on the surface of the eye can quickly burn the thin membrane or skin covering the surface of the eye. Ocular damage is a common result of alkali (base) injury. The higher the pH of the substance, the more severe the damage to the eye. When a casualty gets a substance like lime in the eyes, the damage is worsened by repeatedly rubbing the eyes as opposed to initiating copious irrigation and essential treatment.

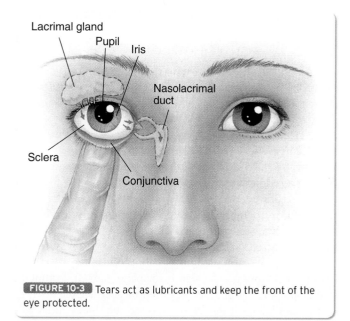

Lacrimal gland
Pupil
Iris
Nasolacrimal
duct
Sclera
Conjunctiva

FIGURE 10-3 Tears act as lubricants and keep the front of the eye protected.

■ Pathophysiology

As a combat medic, you are likely to provide care to casualties who have been burned. A **burn** occurs when the body, or a body part, receives more energy than it can absorb without injury. Potential sources of this energy include thermal, inhalation, toxic chemicals, radiation exposure, and electricity (including lightning). Mechanisms of burn injury include scalding, steam, flame, flash, retained heat, and other trauma. The proper care of a burn may increase a casualty's chances of survival and decrease the risk or duration of long-term disability. Although a burn may be the casualty's most obvious injury, you should always perform a complete assessment to determine whether there are other, more serious injuries.

Any time large surface areas are burned, the risk of shock increases. These risks come from local and systemic responses. Initially, during the emergent phase, there is a release of **catecholamines** (that is, epinephrine and norepinephrine) in response to the pain and stress of the situation. Because of the overall vasoconstriction, there is a decrease in blood flow to the injured area. During the next several hours there follows a fluid shift phase. Damaged cells in the area release vasoactive substances, creating an inflammatory response and increasing capillary permeability. Massive edema is the result of fluid shifting from the intravascular space into the extravascular space. Sodium moves into the injured cells, creating even more fluid loss as osmotic pressure increases. This also causes a loss of electrolytes and may lead to **hypovolemia**.

Tissue damage reduces the ability of the body to regulate its core temperature. Fluid seeps into the damaged area where it is exposed to surface air, causing evaporation and loss of heat. In severe burns, this can rapidly lead to hypothermia. As fluid volume decreases, there is less oxygen transported to the tissues and organs, leading to hypoxia, acidosis, and possibly anoxia. Hypovolemia causes a decrease in cardiac output, resulting in hypotension. In an attempt to maintain homeostasis, the body responds with vasoconstriction in an effort to elevate blood pressure and increase perfusion to vital organs and with tachypnea to offset the metabolic acidosis and hypoxia.

The burn process also releases **myoglobin** from dead or dying cells into the bloodstream that may plug tubules in the kidneys, leading to renal failure. Myoglobin, along with the hypovolemia, can lead to liver failure, and excessive potassium released from the cells can create dysrhythmias and heart failure.

As the burn destroys skin, a tough leathery substance known as eschar is produced. Eschar is not pliable like normal skin. As edema increases, pressure is exerted on the underlying structures. Circulatory compromise secondary to circumferential eschar around an extremity may require an escharotomy, or surgical incision to relieve the pressure and restore circulation. A circumferential burn may result in compartment syndrome. The skin is unable to stretch, leading to eventual compression and decreased or absent circulation in the tissues below. If the burn is around the thorax, tidal volume and chest excursion may be drastically reduced by the eschar formation, thus resulting in ventilatory insufficiency.

Inhalation injury is present in the majority of burn deaths. This is generally the result of carbon monoxide or cyanide toxicity. If the casualty survives the initial injury, death is usually the result of secondary infection. The barrier of protection offered by intact skin is breeched, which results in an invasion of various types of infectious agents. Pathogens invade the wound shortly after the burn and may do so until the area is healed. The best protection for the casualty is the use of sterile dressings and avoidance of any preventable contamination of the site.

Mechanism of Burn Injury

Removing the burn source is the first step in treating any burn casualty. The most important concept of removing the burn source is the maintenance of safety. This involves both maintaining your safety and maintaining the casualty's safety. There are significant dangers in removing the burn source in all types of burn injuries.

Thermal Burns

A **thermal burn** is sometimes called trauma by fire. However, heat energy can be transmitted in a variety of ways in addition to fire. Although these burns are all caused by heat (as opposed to electricity, chemicals, or radiation), many different situations can cause thermal burns and pose a safety hazard.

The removal of casualties from burning buildings or cars always takes priority over all other treatments. If the casualty's clothing is on fire, cover the casualty with a field jacket or any large piece of nonsynthetic material and roll the casualty on the ground to put out the flames. Nonadherent clothing, jewelry, and watches should be removed. Clothing adhering to the burn should be left undisturbed.

Chemical Burns

Chemicals are not always easy to detect, either on casualties or on the objects in the environment. Severe chemical burns to rescuers have occurred because of the inability of the rescuer to identify a chemical source. Remove liquid chemicals from the burned casualty by flushing with as much water as possible. Remove dry chemicals by carefully brushing them off with a clean, dry cloth. If large amounts of water are available, flush the area. Otherwise, apply no water. Small amounts of water applied to a dry chemical burn may cause a chemical reaction, transforming the dry chemical into an active burning substance.

White phosphorus is a chemical substance that burns when exposed to oxygen. Phosphorus contained in grenades, shells, or bombs can cause severe thermal and chemical burns. Phosphorus contained in munitions (certain grenades) are designed to fragment and may penetrate deep tissues with both metal and phosphorus fragments. Because of this, white phosphorus burns should be covered with water, saline, a wet cloth, or wet mud. Keep the area covered with the wet material to exclude air and to prevent the particles from further burning or possibly igniting.

Six mechanisms of injury may damage the body's tissues in cases of chemical burns:

- **Reduction:** Protein denaturation caused by the reduction of the amide linkages following exposure to a reducing agent (such as alkyl mercuric compounds, diborane, lithium aluminum hydride, and other metallic hydrides).
- **Oxidation:** Caused when a chemical inserts oxygen, sulfur, or halogen (such as chlorine) atoms (such as from sodium hypochlorite, potassium permanganate, peroxides, or chromic acid) into the body's proteins.
- **Corrosion:** Caused by chemicals that corrode the skin and cause massive protein denaturing (such as phenols, hydroxides, sodium, potassium, ammonium, and calcium).
- **Protoplasmic poisons:** Chemicals that form esters with proteins (such as formic acid and acetic acid) or that bind or inhibit the inorganic ions needed for the body's normal functions (such as oxalic acid and hydrofluoric acid).
- **Desecration:** Caused by desiccants that damage the body by extracting water from tissues (such as concentrated or fuming sulfuric acid); the reaction often causes heat (exothermic), which adds insult to the injury.
- **Vesication:** Vesicants rapidly produce cutaneous blisters and typically are referred to as chemical warfare agents or weapons of mass destruction (such as mustard gas).

With a chemical burn injury, it is difficult to estimate the extent of the burn—it may have penetrated deep into the body's tissues. By using the rule of nines (discussed later in this chapter), estimate the body surface area affected, but be aware that the extent of the injury may be much more severe. Do not underestimate the power of a small quantity of chemical. Chemicals such as phenols and highly corrosive acids can cause considerable damage to the skin and its underlying tissues very quickly. Flush, flush, and then flush some more!

Typically, chemical burns react with the skin and tissues quickly. In some cases, however, the injury may take time to develop, as in a person who is exposed to cement (calcium oxide). Cement tends to penetrate through clothing and can react with sweat on the surface of the skin. Hours later, the casualty may notice that a burn injury has occurred.

Considerations that influence the management and affect the prognosis of a casualty with a chemical burn injury

---

Field Medical Care TIPS

Prolonged contact with petroleum products such as gasoline or diesel fuel may produce a chemical injury to the skin that is actually a full-thickness burn but initially appears to be only a partial-thickness injury. Sufficient absorption of the hydrocarbon may cause organ failure and even death.

Field Medical Care TIPS

Chemicals known to cause burning injuries to the eyes include acids (such as concentrated liquid chlorine), alkalis (such as cement powder or a strong cleaning agent), dry chemicals (such as lye or lime), and phenols.

---

include the specific chemical involved, the duration and amount of exposure, and the delay in neutralizing the chemical or decontaminating the casualty. This is especially important when considering an injury that may have occurred to the casualty's eyes.

Electrical Burns

Electrical burns pose a particular hazard to the combat medic. Electrical wire is hazardous and dangerous. Unless you are trained to do so, do not attempt to remove wires. Objects commonly felt to be safe (wooden sticks, manila rope, and fire fighters' gloves) may not be protective and may result in electrocution. If at all possible, turn off the source of electricity before any rescue attempt is made.

There are two types of electrical current:

- Alternating current (AC) is a range that includes house current in most locales and tends to cause ventricular fibrillation if the pathway includes the heart.
- Direct current (DC) is much less dangerous than AC; however, electrothermal skin burns have been reported from DC current.

Electrical injury may cause disruption of the body's normal electrical activities. The neurologic system is affected most commonly. Neurologic dysfunction is present in some form, even if only temporarily, in virtually all casualties. Transient nerve injuries resulting in temporary numbness and tingling are most common. Mass depolarization of the brain may lead to a loss of consciousness, amnesia, and coma. Spinal cord involvement may result in transverse myelitis (inflammation of the spinal cord), which may have a delayed onset and is associated with a poor prognosis for recovery.

Electrical injuries may also affect the heart, resulting in cardiac dysrhythmias. Some may be transient, but others may result in cardiac arrest. Sudden death from an AC electrical injury is usually the result of ventricular fibrillation, although asystole and other dysrhythmias are common. Ventricular fibrillation is three times more likely to occur if the flow of current is arm to arm, because the electrical current flows directly across the heart.

Heat is also generated by the flow of electrical current through body tissues, resulting in direct thermal injury. At higher voltages, higher temperatures are achieved, resulting in greater injury. High-tension voltages cause devastating injuries from huge amounts of internal thermal damage.

Vascular injury occurs as the result of vascular spasm. Heat generated by the injury can also cause coagulation and vascular occlusion. Damage to the vascular wall may produce

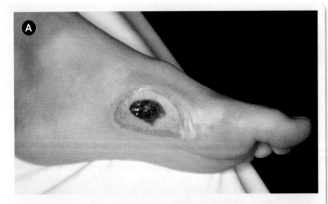

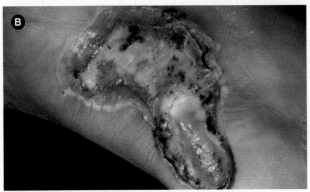

FIGURE 10-4 Electrical burns have entrance and exit wounds. **A.** The entrance wound is often quite small. **B.** The exit wound can be extensive and deep.

delayed thrombosis and bleeding. Compartment syndrome may develop as a result of injury to the musculature.

Renal injuries may occur as a result of rhabdomyolysis, which causes myoglobinuria from massive release of myoglobin. Myoglobin crystallization in the kidney tubules may cause acute renal failure.

Not all electrical or lightning injuries are the same. A detailed history, including all of the specific information associated with the event, is essential. Determine the voltage and type of current, if possible. Identify whether the injury was brief or sustained and an approximate time of contact. Determine conditions associated with the injury that may have influenced the amount of energy transferred. These may include conditions such as wet skin or a puddle of water.

If possible, determine the mechanism of injury. Was this a direct contact, an arc, or a flash burn? Also ask about any loss of consciousness and any pre-existing medical conditions that may exacerbate the problem and hinder effective resuscitation.

Other electrical burn injuries may include:

- Skin burns at entrance and exit sites **FIGURE 10-4 ▲** . Direct contact and passage through tissue may produce extensive areas of necrosis. The entrance site is often a characteristic bulls-eye wound that appears dry, leathery, charred, or depressed. The exit wound

may be ulcerated and have an "exploded" appearance with areas of tissue missing.
- Surface flame burns (casualty's clothing being ignited).
- Dislocations and/or fractures (due to violent muscle contractions).
- Numerous internal structures may be injured secondary to electrical injury including the abdominal organs and urinary bladder.

Inhalation Injuries

Inhalation injuries are often classified as carbon monoxide poisoning, heat, or smoke inhalation injuries. Most frequently, inhalation injuries occur when a casualty is injured in a confined space; however, even victims of fires in open spaces may have inhalation injuries. Inhalation injuries account for more than half of the 5,000 burn-related deaths per year in the United States.

Supraglottic Inhalation Injury

Because of the location of supraglottic structures, they are very susceptible to inhalation injuries. The upper airway is very vascular and has a large surface area. Inhaling superheated steam or air can damage tissues, resulting in irritation and edema. This can quickly lead to partial or complete airway obstruction. Upper airway edema is the earliest consequence of inhalation injury. The tissue damage from inhaling hot air is not immediately reversible by introducing fresh, cool air.

Infraglottic Inhalation Injury

Because of the location, thermal injury to the lower airway is rare. However, inhalation of toxins and smoke is just as hazardous. Systemic toxins affect the ability of the blood to absorb oxygen. Because carbon monoxide is colorless, odorless, and tasteless, your only clue may be the environment in which the casualty is found. Burning materials also give off toxins that damage the lung parenchyma. This is especially true of petroleum-based products, such as wool, rubber, and polyurethane foam.

Smoke intoxication is frequently hidden by more visible injuries such as burns. The condition of a casualty who appears unharmed may later deteriorate as a result of smoke inhalation. Most of the smoke at a fire is a suspension of small particles of carbon and tar, but there is also some ordinary dust floating in a combination of heated gases. Some of the suspended particles in smoke are merely irritating, but others may be lethal. The size of the particle determines how deeply into the lungs it will be inhaled.

■ Assessment

The evaluation of the burn casualty is often complicated by the vivid nature of the burn injuries. You must remember that even casualties with major burns rarely die in the initial postburn period from the burn injury. They die as a consequence of related trauma or the associated conditions such as airway compromise or smoke inhalation. Perform an initial assessment and rapid trauma survey immediately upon arrival in a safe staging area. The care of the burn itself has a lower priority.

Critical problems in the burn casualty that require immediate intervention are airway compromise, altered level of consciousness (LOC), or the presence of major injuries in addition to the burn. Clues to the mechanism of injury (MOI) that point to critical problems include a history of being confined in a closed space with fire or smoke, electrical burns, falls from a height, or other major blunt force trauma.

Signs and Symptoms

The first complaint in a burn casualty is usually pain at the site. The skin condition changes in relation to the affected burn site. As cells and tissues are destroyed, they slough off. Other soft-tissue injuries may occur depending on the extent of the burn. If the burn is the result of a fall, blast, or other trauma, the casualty might also present with musculoskeletal injuries. In severe burns, the musculoskeletal system sustains significant damage in the absence of actual musculoskeletal trauma. Any burns near the face expose the airway to potential damage. Expect to hear adventitious (abnormal) sounds as the airway swells and narrows. Hoarseness, **dyspnea**, **dysphagia**, and **dysphasia** all are common. Other signs and symptoms associated with burns include burned hair, nausea and vomiting, altered levels of consciousness, edema, **paresthesia**, possible hemorrhage, and chest pain.

Carbon monoxide poisoning and asphyxiation are by far the most common causes of early death associated with a burn injury. Most inhalation injuries are caused by smoke particles, carbon monoxide, and toxic fume inhalation, and these injuries are not immediately apparent. Always assume an inhalation injury has occurred when the casualty was in an enclosed space fire. Explosions and lightning may throw casualties some distance from the original injury, thus causing musculoskeletal injuries.

Electrical burns are usually more serious than they appear on the skin surface. Extremities usually have significant tissue damage because their small size results in higher electrical current accumulation. Chemicals not only may injure the skin, but also may be absorbed into the body and cause internal organ failure.

The initial assessment of a burn wound and the possibilities for complications include:

- Burn depth
- Burn size
- Age of the casualty
- Pulmonary injury
- Associated trauma
- Special considerations (electrical, chemical)
- Pre-existing illnesses

Burn Depth

The depth of the burn is important for evaluating the severity of the burn and planning for wound care. Burns are first classified according to their depth FIGURE 10-5 ▶ :

- **First-degree burns** involve minor tissue damage to the epidermal layer only, causing an intense and painful inflammatory response. The cause is a minor flash or sunburn and the skin color is red. The skin surface does not have any blisters and is dry. The sensation is mild discomfort to very painful. Healing takes 3 to 6 days.
- **Second-degree burns** involve damage through the epidermis and into a variable depth of the dermis but no underlying tissue. It is characterized by a red or mottled appearance with associated swelling and blister formation. The burn will heal with or without scarring, which will be related to the size and depth of the injury. Surgical repair or grafting may be necessary. It is also described as a partial-thickness burn because there are layers of skin cells left that can multiply with resultant healing. The causes include flashes, flame, or hot liquids. The skin color is mottled red. The skin surface will have weeping blisters. The sensation is extremely painful. Significant fluid loss and subsequent shock may occur. Depending on the depth of the burn, healing takes 2 to 4 weeks.
- **Third-degree burns** involve damage to all layers of the epidermis and dermis. Subcutaneous tissue, muscle, bone, and/or organs may be involved. Healing is impossible except in small third-degree burns that usually scar in from the sides. All third-degree burns leave scars. Deeper third-degree burns usually result in the skin protein becoming denatured and hard, leaving a firm leather-like covering that is referred to as eschar. All layers of skin are destroyed with this type of burn. No skin cells remain to allow healing. It is also referred to as a full-thickness burn. The causes include electricity, chemicals, hot metals, and flame. The casualty's skin color is charred, translucent, and/or pearly white, and parchment like. The skin surface is dry with thrombosed blood vessels. The sensation is anesthetic. Skin grafting is required for healing.

A pure third-degree burn is unusual. Severe burns are typically a combination of first-degree, second-degree, and third-degree burns. First-degree burns heal well without scarring. Small second-degree burns also heal without scarring. However, deep second-degree burns and all third-degree burns are best managed surgically and frequently require skin grafting.

Suspect significant airway burns if there is singed hair within the nostrils, soot around the nose and mouth, hoarseness, or hypoxia. It may be impossible to accurately estimate the depth of a particular burn. Even experienced burn specialists sometimes underestimate or overestimate the extent of a particular burn.

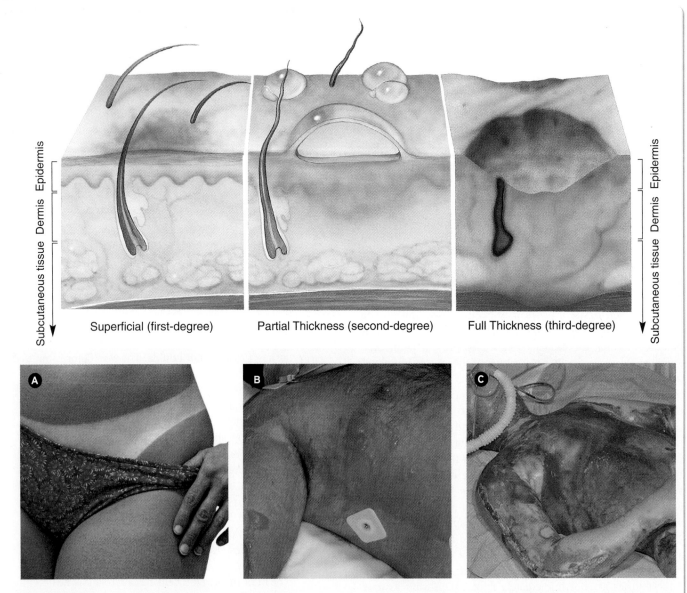

FIGURE 10-5 Classification of burns. **A.** First-degree burns involve only the epidermis. The skin turns red but does not blister, and the burn doesn't go through to the dermis. **B.** Second-degree burns involve some of the dermis, but they do not destroy the entire thickness of the skin. The skin is mottled, white to red, and often blistered. **C.** Third-degree burns extend through all layers of the skin and may involve subcutaneous tissue and muscle. The skin is dry, leathery, and often white or charred.

Superficial (first-degree)

Partial Thickness (second-degree)

Full Thickness (third-degree)

Epidermis Dermis Subcutaneous tissue

Burn Size

One quick way to estimate the surface area that has been burned is to compare it with the size of the casualty's palm, which is roughly equal to 1% of the casualty's total body surface area. This is known as the **rule of palms**, sometimes called the palmar method. This method is especially useful with irregularly shaped burns. Another useful measurement system is the **rule of nines**, which divides the body into sections, each of which is approximately 9% of the total surface area **FIGURE 10-6 ▸**. Remember that the head of an infant or child is relatively larger than the head of an adult, and the

Field Medical Care **TIPS**

When estimating scattered burns, remember that the casualty's palm surface represents approximately 1% of his or her total body surface area (BSA). Therefore, by using the palmar surface as a guideline, even the extent of irregularly disposed burns can be estimated.

legs are relatively smaller. **TABLE 10-1 ▸** covers the rule of nines in adults and **TABLE 10-2 ▸** covers the rule of nines in children.

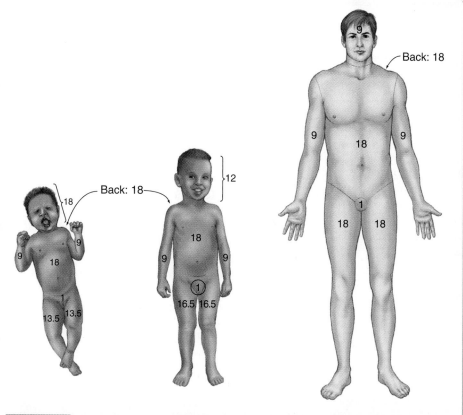

FIGURE 10-6 The rule of nines is a quick way to estimate the amount of surface area that has been burned. It divides the body into sections, each approximately 9% of the total body surface area.

Manage the Casualty With Thermal Burns

Initial Assessment

Begin by securing the airway, while simultaneously checking the initial level of consciousness (LOC) and protecting the c-spine. Assessment of breathing, circulation, and control of major hemorrhage are then carried out. High-flow oxygen should be initiated, if available. Check pulses distal to the burn sites and fully expose the casualty, removing all nonadherent clothing, watches, and jewelry as the combat situation dictates. Initiate IV hydration with two large-bore needles and Ringer's lactate solution. IV administration is covered in depth in Chapter 13, *Intravenous Access.* IV lines should be placed through noninjured and nonburned skin, if possible. Initiate cardiac monitoring, if available.

Rapid Trauma Survey

Be watchful for airway and circulatory compromise. Warning signs are the presence of facial and scalp burns, sooty sputum, and singed nasal hair and eyebrows. Examine the oral cavity, looking for soot, swelling, or erythema. Ask the casualty to speak. A raspy, hoarse voice suggests a lower airway injury. On auscultation of the chest, crackles, wheezing, or abnormal breath sounds suggest an inhalation injury. Cover the casualty in a space blanket, poncho liner, sheets, or blanket. The casualty should not be allowed to become chilled or hypothermic. The casualty should never be transported on wet sheets or clothing.

Obtain a SAMPLE history and also record the mechanism of injury, depth of burn, extent of burn, age of the casualty, any associated pulmonary injury, pre-existing illnesses, and chemical/electrical details. Obtain the casualty's baseline vital signs. Perform a burn wound assessment by estimating the depth based on appearance. Roughly calculate the burn size by using the rule of nines.

TABLE 10-1 **Rule of Nines in an Adult**
Head and neck equals 9%
Anterior trunk equals 18%
Posterior trunk equals 18%
Anterior upper extremities equal 9%
Posterior upper extremities equal 9%
Anterior lower extremities equal 18%
Posterior lower extremities equal 18%
Perineum (groin) equals 1%

TABLE 10-2 **Rule of Nines in Children**
Head and neck equals 18%
Anterior trunk equals 18%
Posterior trunk equals 18%
Anterior upper extremities equal 9%
Posterior upper extremities equal 9%
Anterior lower extremities equal 14%
Posterior lower extremities equal 14%
Perineum (groin) equals 1%

Field Medical Care TIPS

The heads of infants and young children are larger in relationship to the rest of the body than adults and require a modification to the rule of nines in estimating the extent of burns.

IV Hydration

IV administration is covered in detail in Chapter 13, *Intravenous Access*. IV fluids should be administered to the burned casualty based on the **Parkland formula**, which recommends giving 4 mL of Ringer's lactate solution for each kilogram of body weight and for each percent of total body surface area burned in the first 24 hours to maintain blood volume and urinary output. Multiply 4 mL by the casualty's weight by the percentage of body surface area (BSA) burned:

4 mL × casualty's weight (kg) × BSA burned = Total fluid in 24 hours

Thus, for a 75-kg casualty with 45% BSA burned, the calculation is as follows:

4 (mL) × 75 (kg) × 45 (BSA) = 13,500 mL during the first 24 hours

The Parkland formula further states that the casualty should receive half of this amount of fluid in the first 8 hours following the burn; therefore, using the above example, the casualty would receive 6,750 mL during the first 8 hours (approximately 850 mL per hour). The remainder of the fluid is infused over the next 16 hours. Calculate fluid requirements based on the time of injury, not the time fluid resuscitation started. For example, if the injury occurred 4 hours before IV fluids were able to be started, the rate would double to 1,700 mL per hour for 4 hours. Urinary output in an adult should be 30 to 50 cc/hour.

Wound Care

Wrap the casualty's burns in a dry sterile dressing. If the casualty's hands or toes are burned, separate the casualty's digits with sterile gauze pads applied loosely. The hands should be placed in the position of function. Do not apply ointments or solutions if evacuation time is less than 24 hours. If evacuation time is greater than 24 hours, dress the wound in burn cream (Silvadene) and wrap in Kerlix. Do not open blisters.

Do not open eyelids if they are burned. Be certain that the burn is thermal and not chemical. Apply moist sterile gauze pads to both eyes.

Morphine sulfate may be given for pain. Morphine may be administered in small, frequent amounts, 2 to 5 mg by the intravenous route. Do not exceed 20 mg every 4 hours unless cleared by a medical officer. Side effects of morphine include respiratory depression, nausea, and vomiting. Monitor the casualty closely for respiratory depression.

Regardless of immunization status, all burn casualties should receive a 0.5 mL tetanus toxoid booster intramuscularly (IM) because burns are at high risk for tetanus infection. If the casualty is able to swallow liquids and medications, administer gatifloxin orally as a single daily dose. If the casualty has greater than a 20% BSA burn, is unconscious, or is unable to swallow, administer cefotetan at 2 g via an IV push over 3 to 5 minutes every 12 hours until evacuation. Burns commonly acquire secondary bacterial infections.

Frequent monitoring of extremity pulses is required in circumferential burns to legs and arms. This is due to the increased chance of compromise to distal circulation due to swelling and edema. A procedure called an **escharatomy** may be required to release the pressure due to swelling. This procedure is performed by a medical officer at a Battalion Aid Station or Forward Support Medical Company (FSMC).

Monitor urinary output by inserting a Foley catheter, if available. Adjust IV hydration to achieve a urinary output of 30 to 50 cc/hour for an adult. To insert a catheter in a male casualty, follow the steps in **SKILL DRILL 10-1 ▶** :

1. Help position the casualty supine with legs slightly spread apart. Maintain privacy as much as possible.

2. Wash your hands and apply a mask, goggles, and clean nonlatex gloves.

3. Open supplies including the urinary catheter and placement kit. Place necessary supplies onto a clean area within reach. Connect a syringe filled with saline to the balloon port. Also connect the indwelling catheter to the drainage system.

4. Wash the penis with soap and water (or have the casualty do so if he is able), making sure that the foreskin has been retracted.

5. Coat the end of the catheter with a water-soluble gel. An anesthetic gel is preferred for casualties with sensation in the penile area.

6. Hold the penis at a 90° angle to the body and insert the catheter (**Step ①**).

7. When urine is evident in the tubing, insert the catheter until the Y between the drainage port and the balloon port is at the tip of the penis (**Step ②**).

8. Inflate the balloon and gently pull back on the catheter until you feel resistance, which indicates that the balloon is snug against the neck of the bladder.

9. Allow urine to drain. Note the amount and color (**Step ③**).

10. To remove a catheter, remove the saline in the balloon port and pull back gently until the catheter is free of the tip of the penis. Never remove an indwelling

SKILL DRILL 10-1

Insert a Foley Catheter

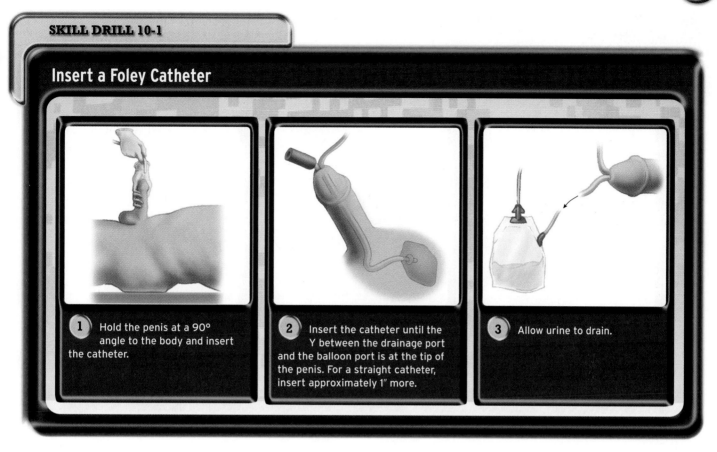

1 Hold the penis at a 90° angle to the body and insert the catheter.

2 Insert the catheter until the Y between the drainage port and the balloon port is at the tip of the penis. For a straight catheter, insert approximately 1″ more.

3 Allow urine to drain.

catheter without using a syringe to remove the saline from the balloon, because it may damage the urinary sphincter.

11. Remove your gloves and wash your hands, following BSI precautions.

12. If the catheter is to remain in place, secure it to the casualty's leg.

To catheterize a female casualty, follow the steps in **SKILL DRILL 10-2 ▶** :

1. Help position the female casualty supine with legs spread apart or side lying with the top knee flexed. Maintain privacy as much as possible.

2. Wash your hands and apply clean nonlatex gloves.

3. Open supplies including the urinary catheter and placement kit. Place necessary supplies onto a clean area within reach. If you are inserting an indwelling catheter, connect a syringe filled with saline to the balloon port. Also connect the indwelling catheter to the drainage system. There are no connecting ports for either a balloon or a drainage bag on a straight catheter.

4. Wash the perineal area with soap and water (or have the female casualty do so if she is able). First cleanse

the outer area of the perineum, and then spread the labia minora and thoroughly wash the mucosa surrounding the vagina and the urinary meatus. Dry with a clean towel.

5. Coat the end of the catheter with a water-soluble gel. An anesthetic gel is preferred for female casualty with sensation in the perineal area.

6. Locate the urinary meatus anterior to the vagina and insert the catheter (**Step 1**).

7. When urine is evident in the tubing, insert the catheter another 1″ to 3″ (**Step 2**).

8. Inflate the balloon and gently pull back on the catheter until you feel resistance, which indicates that the balloon is snug against the neck of the bladder. This step is unnecessary when using a straight catheter.

9. Allow urine to drain. Note the amount and color (**Step 3**).

10. To remove a catheter, remove the saline in the balloon port and pull back gently until the catheter is free of the tip of the meatus. Never remove an indwelling catheter without using a syringe to remove the saline from the balloon, as it may damage the urinary sphincter. For a straight catheter, simply pull back

Catheterizing a Female Casualty

1 Locate the urinary meatus anterior to the vagina and insert the catheter.

2 When urine is evident in the tubing, insert the catheter another 1" to 3".

3 Allow urine to drain.

gently to remove the catheter. If the catheter is to be reused, it should be cleaned.

11. Remove your gloves and wash your hands.

12. If the catheter is to remain in place, secure it to the female casualty's leg or abdomen according to the female casualty's needs.

In thermal burns over less than 20% of BSA, insert a nasogastric tube, and do not give the casualty anything by mouth (NPO) until evacuation. To insert a nasogastric tube, follow the steps in **SKILL DRILL 10-3 ▶** :

1. Explain the procedure to the casualty, and oxygenate him or her, if necessary and possible. Ensure that the casualty's head is in a neutral position. Suppress the gag reflex with a topical anesthetic spray.

2. Constrict the blood vessels in the nares with a topical alpha agonist.

3. Measure the tube for the correct depth of insertion (nose to ear to xiphoid process) (**Step ①**).

4. Lubricate the tube with a water-soluble gel (**Step ②**).

5. Advance the tube gently along the nasal floor (**Step ③**).

6. Encourage the casualty to swallow or drink to facilitate passage of the tube into the esophagus (**Step ④**).

7. Advance the tube into the stomach.

8. Confirm proper placement: auscultate over the epigastrium while injecting 30 to 50 mL of air into the tube and/or observe for gastric contents in the tube (**Step ⑤**).

9. Apply suction to the tube to aspirate the stomach contents, and secure the tube in place (**Step ⑥**).

■ Manage the Casualty With Chemical Burns

The body sites most often burned by chemicals are the face, eyes, and extremities. In general, a chemical burn size is small and the mortality rate is lower than for thermal burns. However, wound healing and recovery time may be longer. The severity of the chemical burn is related to the chemical agent, concentration and volume of the chemical, and the duration of contact.

First, stop the burning process. Wear protective gloves, eyewear, and the like. Remove all clothing covered with chemicals, especially shoes, which can trap concentrated chemicals.

Irrigate copiously with any source of available water to flush chemicals off the body. Wipe or scrape any retained agent that sticks to the skin. Continue flushing a minimum of 60 minutes (unless a critical or unstable situation warrants transport sooner). Brush off dry chemicals on the skin before performing irrigation. Perform an initial assessment and rapid trauma survey as discussed with thermal burns.

SKILL DRILL 10-3

Nasogastric Tube Insertion

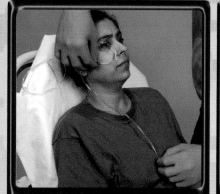

1 Explain the procedure to the casualty, and oxygenate the casualty if necessary. Ensure that the casualty's head is in a neutral position and suppress the gag reflex with a topical anesthetic spray. Constrict the blood vessels in the nares with a topical alpha agonist. Measure the tube for correct depth of insertion (nose to ear to xiphoid process).

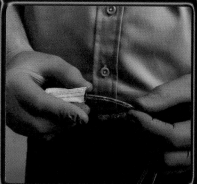

2 Lubricate the tube with a water-soluble gel.

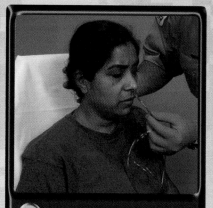

3 Advance the tube gently across the nasal floor.

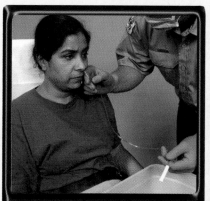

4 Encourage the casualty to swallow or drink to facilitate passage of the tube. Advance the tube into the stomach.

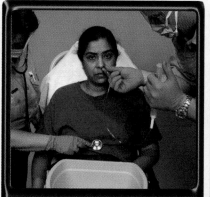

5 Confirm proper placement: Auscultate over the epigastrium while injecting 30 to 50 mL of air and/or observe for gastric contents in the tube. There should be no reflux around the tube.

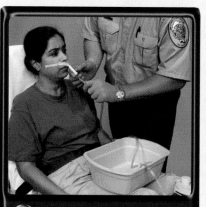

6 Apply suction to the tube to aspirate the gastric contents and secure the tube in place.

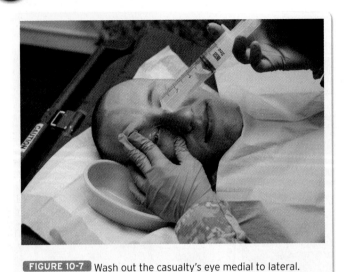

FIGURE 10-7 Wash out the casualty's eye medial to lateral.

Chemical Burns to the Eye

Protect yourself during the washing process. Immediately flush the casualty's eyes with water. Irreversible damage will occur in the eye quickly because of caustic chemicals so irrigate to prevent severe and permanent damage to the cornea. Use a mild water flow from a hose, IV tubing, or water from a container. Hold the casualty's eyelids open; wash medial (nasal) to lateral **FIGURE 10-7 ▲**. Irrigate the eyes for at least 60 minutes and transport the casualty while irrigating. Do not use neutralizers such as vinegar or baking soda. During irrigation, remove contact lenses. Although soldiers will not generally be wearing contact lenses, be aware of this precaution when treating aircrew members.

■ Manage the Casualty With Electrical Burns

Electricity entering the body and traveling through the tissues causes tissue damage. Because of their small size, the extremities usually have more significant tissue damage with electrical burns. The damage is due to the higher local current density. The severity of electrical injury is determined by the type and amount of current, the path of the current, and the duration of contact with the current.

Immediate cardiac dysrhythmias are the most serious injury that occurs due to electrical contact. A careful, immediate evaluation of a casualty's cardiac status and continuous monitoring of cardiac activity is necessary because the casualty may initially appear to be stable. Common life-threatening dysrhythmias are premature ventricular contractions and ventricular fibrillation. Initiate aggressive advanced life support management of these dysrhythmias according to your local protocols. These casualties usually have normal healthy hearts and the chances for resuscitation are excellent. To manage a casualty in ventricular fibrillation with only basic life support available, start cardiopulmonary resuscitation (CPR) and transport immediately.

Perform a rapid trauma survey, as discussed with thermal burns, once the efforts at managing cardiac status are complete. Fluid requirements for casualties with electrical burns are higher than fluid requirements for casualties with thermal burns due to the high risk of kidney failure in casualties with electrical burns.

Other electrical burn injuries may include skin burns at entrance and exit sites. Direct contact and passage through tissue may produce extensive areas of necrosis. The entrance site is often a characteristic bulls-eye wound that appears dry, leathery, charred, or depressed. The exit wound may be ulcerated and have an "exploded" appearance with areas of tissue missing.

Other electrical burn injuries may include:

- Surface flame burns (casualty's clothing being ignited)
- Dislocations and/or fractures (due to violent muscle contractions)
- Numerous internal structure injuries secondary to electrical injury, including injury to the abdominal organs and urinary bladder

■ Manage the Casualty With a Lightning Injury

Lightning kills more Americans each year than any other weather-related phenomenon. Injuries from lightning are different from other electrical burns in that they involve very high voltage and currents, but very short duration. The casualty does not need to be hit directly to sustain an injury. Lightning may strike an adjacent object or nearby ground and still produce injury. The most serious effect of a lightning strike is cardiac arrest, with the massive current acting like a defibrillator to briefly stop the heart. Lightning strikes often become multiple casualty events.

The signs and symptoms of lightning injury include:

- The pathway of tissue damage is often over rather than through the skin. Third-degree burns are rare.
- First-degree burns occur where electrical energy enters and exits the body. Exit wound burns are usually larger.
- Disrupted nerve pathways are displayed as paralysis.
- Muscle tenderness, with or without twitching.
- Respiratory difficulties or arrest.
- Cardiac arrhythmia or arrest.
- Loss of consciousness.
- Visual difficulties.
- Fractured bones and dislocations from severe muscle contractions or from falling (can include spinal column).
- Seizures.

Perform an initial assessment. Immediate cardiac dysrhythmias are the most serious injury that occurs due to electrical contact. A careful, immediate evaluation of a casualty's cardiac status and continuous monitoring of cardiac activity is necessary because the casualty may initially appear to be stable. Common life-threatening dysrhythmias are premature ventricular contractions and ventricular fibrillation. Initiate aggressive advanced life support management of these dysrhythmias based on your local protocols. These casualties usually have normal healthy hearts and the chances for resuscitation are excellent. To manage a casualty in ventricular fibrillation with only basic life support available, start cardiopulmonary resuscitation (CPR) and transport immediately.

Perform a rapid trauma survey, as discussed with thermal burns, once the efforts at managing cardiac status are complete. Initiate large-bore IV access with IV running open to aid in preventing renal failure from muscle damage. The major problems caused by lightning injury are usually not from the burn. Respiratory and cardiac arrest are real possibilities. Be prepared to provide basic cardiac life support measures at any time.

Manage the Casualty With Inhalation Burns

Inhalation injuries are classified as carbon monoxide poisoning and heat or smoke inhalation injuries. These injuries account for more than half of the 5,000 burn-related deaths per year in the United States. Asphyxiation and carbon monoxide poisoning are the most common cause of early death associated with burn injury.

Inhalation injuries most often occur when a casualty is injured in a confined space or is trapped. Inhalation injury can also occur in an open space; therefore, all burn victims should be evaluated for this injury. Carbon monoxide is a byproduct of combustion and is one of numerous chemicals in common smoke. Its presence is impossible to detect because it is odorless, colorless, and tasteless.

Casualties quickly become hypoxic. (Alteration in the level of consciousness is the most predominant sign of hypoxia.) A cherry-red color or cyanosis is rarely present as a result of carbon monoxide poisoning. Death usually occurs from a myocardial infarction secondary to cardiac hypoxia.

By having the casualty breathe fresh air only, it will take up to 7 hours to reduce the carbon monoxide buildup to a safe level. Having the casualty breathe 100% oxygen decreases this time to about 90 to 120 minutes. Carbon monoxide poisoning can be caused from fumes, steam, or smoke in the air. Assume that the casualty has carbon monoxide poisoning in all closed space fires.

Signs and symptoms include:
- Difficulty breathing (dyspnea)
- Coughing, stridor
- Breath has "smoky" or "chemical" smell
- Black residue in casualty's nose and mouth
- Singed nasal or facial hairs
- Burns to the head, the face, or the front of the trunk

Treatment begins by moving the casualty to a safe area. Do an additional assessment and supply life support measures as needed. Give high-flow oxygen by mask, if available. Begin basic life support ventilation using 100% oxygen if the casualty has lost consciousness. Institute cardiac monitoring, if available. Care for possible spinal injuries and any other injury or illness requiring care at the scene. Provide care for shock. Stay alert for behavioral changes. If difficulty breathing increases, be prepared to intubate with a Combitube (see Chapter 3, *Airway Management*). Transport the casualty in a position of comfort if other injuries allow it. Most conscious casualties are able to breathe more easily when placed in an upright (seated) position.

Summary

Burn injury is the fourth leading cause of trauma death. Prompt recognition and management of burns, based on this knowledge, will reduce the potential for shock development, burn contamination, and chance of other complications.

YOU ARE THE
COMBAT MEDIC

An intense rebel mortar attack hits your base. One of the rounds impacts the dining facility and explodes with a deafening roar. The chow hall erupts into a huge ball of flames and there are many soldiers trapped under the rubble. You and two of your partners grab your medic bags and run to the scene. The mortar attack is now suppressed by an AC-130 gunship and ground forces. At the scene, you see a group of soldiers pulling three soldiers from the remains of the structure.

After checking the first two and finding superficial injuries, you focus on the third. She is unconscious and burned on the arms, legs, and head. You notice black soot near her nose and mouth. She has labored breathing at a rate of 10 breaths/min. Knowing that this could mean she inhaled superheated gases from the fire, you elect to immediately intubate her. You do so successfully and assist the casualty's breathing with a bag-valve-mask (BVM) device. Cutting away what is left of her uniform, you effectively stop the burning process. Finally, you place an emergency blanket on her.

Four soldiers quickly arrive at your side with a litter to help carry the casualty to the Battalion Aid Station (BAS) for further evaluation. Arriving in the BAS, you see it overrun with other casualties from the attack. Your team leader states that you are to stay with your casualty and treat accordingly. One of the litter bearers stays to help you. You hook the BVM up to an oxygen source and pass off to the litter bearer.

Assessment

Uncovering the casualty, you quickly get an idea of the extent of the burns. Her left arm has second degree (partial thickness) burn that goes from the palm to the shoulder. Her right arm is only burned on the forearm but it is a third degree (full thickness) burn. Both anterior thigh regions have first degree (superficial) burns. There is also still the suspected inhalation risk because of the soot around the nares and mouth.

Treatment

After completing your assessment, you cover her with dry, sterile burn sheets and then blankets. You initiate an IV in the right arm and try to find a location for a second line. Due to both arms having injury, an external jugular vein is selected and entered successfully. You quickly obtain a set of vital signs and get pulse of 120 beats/min, respirations are assisted at 24 breaths/min, and blood pressure is 90/60 mm Hg. The casualty is now showing signs of hypovolemia and is decompensating. This casualty needs fluid.

1. LAST NAME, FIRST NAME		RANK/GRADE	MALE	
May, Helen		PFC/E3	FEMALE ✓	
SSN 000-555-1234	SPECIALTY CODE OOA		RELIGION Christian	

2. UNIT

FORCE				NATIONALITY		
A/T	AF/A	N/M	MC/M			
	BC/BC		NBI/BNC		DISEASE	PSYCH

3. INJURY		
	X	AIRWAY
		HEAD
FRONT BACK		WOUND
		NECK/BACK INJURY
	X	BURN
		AMPUTATION
		STRESS
		OTHER (Specify)

4. LEVEL OF CONSCIOUSNESS			
ALERT		PAIN RESPONSE	
VERBAL RESPONSE		UNRESPONSIVE	✓

5. PULSE 120	TIME 1220	6. TOURNIQUET [X] NO ☐ YES	TIME

7. MORPHINE [X] NO ☐ YES	DOSE	TIME	8. IV NS	TIME 1215

9. TREATMENT/OBSERVATIONS/CURRENT MEDICATION/ALLERGIES/NBC (ANTIDOTE)

Evacuated out of a structure that sustained a mortar attack. Black soot near nose & mouth. Breathing labored at 10 breaths/min. Intubated and provide O_2 by BVM.

10. DISPOSITION		RETURNED TO DUTY		TIME
	X	EVACUATED		1230
		DECEASED		

11. PROVIDER/UNIT Smith, John	DATE (YYMMDD)

Ready for Review

- Burns are among the most serious and painful of all injuries.
- A burn occurs when the body, or a body part, receives more energy than it can absorb without injury.
- The evaluation of the burn casualty is often complicated by the vivid nature of the burn injuries.
- Managing burn injuries begins by securing the airway, while simultaneously checking the initial level of consciousness (LOC) and protecting the c-spine.
- The body sites most often burned by chemicals are the face, eyes, and extremities.
- Electricity entering the body and traveling through the tissues causes tissue damage. Because of their small size, the extremities usually have more significant tissue damage with electrical burns.
- Lightning kills more Americans each year than any other weather-related phenomenon. Injuries from lightning are different from other electrical burns in that they involve very high voltage and currents, but very short duration.
- Inhalation injuries are classified as carbon monoxide poisoning and heat or smoke inhalation injuries. Asphyxiation and carbon monoxide poisoning are the most common causes of early death associated with burn injury.

Vital Vocabulary

adipose tissue Fat tissue.

anaerobic metabolism The metabolism that takes place in the absence of oxygen; the principal product is lactic acid.

burn An injury to the body that occurs when the body or a body part receives more energy than it can absorb without injury.

cathecholamines Epinephrine and norepinephrine.

collagen A protein that gives tensile strength to the connective tissues of the body.

cutaneous Pertaining to the skin.

dermis The inner layer of skin containing hair follicle roots, glands, blood vessels, and nerves.

desquamation The continuous shedding of the dead cells on the surface of the skin.

dysphagia Difficulty swallowing.

dysphasia Impairment of speech.

dyspnea Any difficulty in respiratory rate, regularity, or effort.

elastin A protein that gives the skin its elasticity.

epidermis The outermost layer of the skin.

escharotomy A surgical cut through the eschar or leathery covering of a burn injury to allow for swelling and minimize the potential for development of compartment syndrome in a circumferentially burned limb or the thorax.

first-degree burn A burn involving only the epidermis, producing very red, painful skin.

homeostasis A tendency to constancy or stability in the body's internal environment.

hypovolemia A large drop in body fluids.

integument The skin.

melanin The pigment that gives skin its color.

mucopolysaccharide gel One of the complex materials found, along with the collagen fibers and elastin fibers, in the dermis of the skin.

myoglobin A protein found in muscle that is released into the circulation after crush injury or other muscle damage and whose presence in the circulation may produce kidney damage.

paresthesia Sensation of tingling, numbness, or "pins and needles" in a body part.

Parkland formula A formula that recommends giving 4 mL of normal saline for each kilogram of body weight, multiplied by the percentage of body surface area burned; sometimes used to calculate fluid needs during lengthy transport times.

rule of nines A system that assigns percentages to sections of the body, allowing calculation of the amount of skin surface involved in a burn area.

rule of palms A system that estimates total body surface area burned by comparing the affected area with the size of the patient's palm, which is roughly equal to 1% of the patient's total body surface area.

sebaceous gland A gland located in the dermis that secretes sebum.

sebum An oily substance secreted by sebaceous glands.

second-degree burn A burn that involves the epidermis and part of the dermis, characterized by pain and blistering; previously called a partial-thickness burn.

subcutaneous layer Beneath the skin.

thermal burn An injury caused by radiation or direct contact with a heat source on the skin.

thermoregulation The ability of the body to maintain temperature through a combination of heat gain by metabolic processes and muscular movement, and heat loss through respiration, evaporation, conduction, convection, and perspiration.

third-degree burn A burn that extends through the epidermis and dermis into the subcutaneous tissues beneath; previously called a full-thickness burn.

COMBAT MEDIC in Action

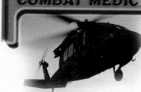

A five-man team of explosive ordinance disposal (EOD) personnel enters a bunker to disarm some shells that were discovered during a raid. The shells are suspected to carry a blister agent. As they are taking the shell casing apart, it explodes, covering three soldiers with the agent. You hear the radio call for help and are just a few hundred yards from the entrance of the bunker. When you arrive you see the three wounded being assisted from the bunker by the two soldiers who did not get hit with the agent.

1. What is the first step in treating these casualties?
   A. Circulation
   B. Decontamination
   C. Airway
   D. Breathing

2. The first and second casualties have reddening to the arms and face. The other casualty, who was turned around at the time of explosion, just has reddening to the back of his neck. What is the priority of the casualties for this scene?
   A. The third casualty is the priority because the agent will get to the spinal cord through his neck.
   B. The first casualty should be treated first because he is the team leader.
   C. The first and second casualties are the priority due to the agent splashing on the face.
   D. All of the casualties should be treated together as the same priority. All of the casualties will develop symptoms at the same time and require the same treatment.

3. What would you use to decontaminate the casualties?
   A. Soap and water
   B. M-100
   C. M-291
   D. Reactive skin decontamination lotion (RSDL)
   E. All the above

4. You start to transport the victims to the MTF, when you notice blisters starting to appear on the arms of the first two casualties. What should you do?
   A. Pop the blisters. They are full of agent and need to be cleaned off.
   B. Cover the blisters with dry sterile gauze, taking care not to pop them.
   C. Continue to wipe the casualties with an M-291 kit.
   D. Administer the casualties NAAK to prevent more blisters.

5. All the casualties describe feeling immediate pain when exposed to the agent against the skin. Is this significant?
   A. Not really, all blister agents cause pain on contact.
   B. Yes, anything the casualties tell you can help treat them.
   C. No, you suspect they were hit by the shrapnel of the shell casing.
   D. No, they are delirious and you cannot trust the their history of events.

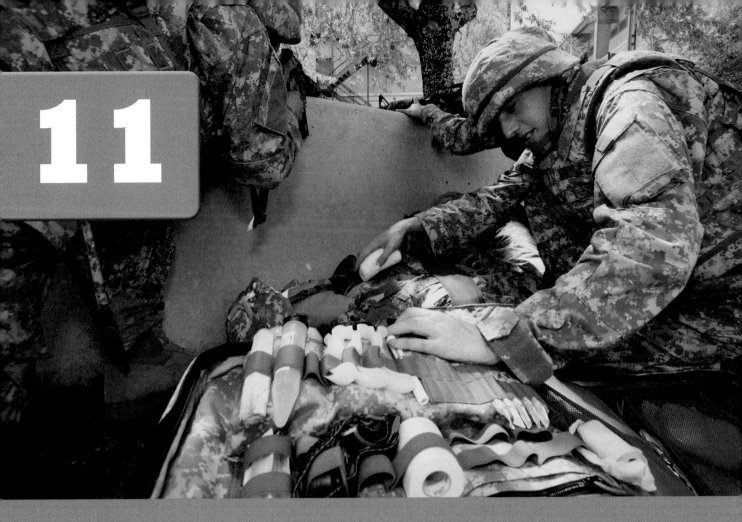

11

Ballistic and Blast Injuries

Objectives

Knowledge Objectives

- [ ] Identify small arms, their wounding agents, and their effects.
- [ ] Identify explosive munitions, their wounding agents, and their effects.
- [ ] Define a ballistic injury.
- [ ] Define a blast injury.
- [ ] Identify flame and incendiary munitions, their agents, and their effects.
- [ ] Identify the medical implications of conventional weapons.

Introduction

As a combat medic, you need to understand the potential injuries that casualties may have based on the type of projectile that caused the injury. This chapter is a fundamental guide for preparing you to make educated decisions that will save the lives of casualties. You are a highly trained medical operative who is skilled in the treatment of a wide range of injuries and illnesses. In many cases, you can treat a casualty without the threat of hostile engagement. However, when faced with the threat of personal injury, you will be forced to make critical decisions concerning the immediate medical care and evaluation of the casualty while attempting to avoid danger. You must also manage to stabilize the casualty for a safe evacuation from the battlefield.

While managing to care for the wounded and make efforts to evacuate them, you are also responsible for the situational assessment and determining the mechanism of injury. This information is important to relay to the other members of the medical team. You must provide this information so that any potential injuries can be evaluated and treated more effectively in the medical treatment facility (MTF). You are the eyes and ears of the medical team. The information you gather will result in a more thorough exam and treatment of the casualty.

It is important that you understand the mechanisms of all types of weapons and projectiles that can cause injury. This provides you the ability to quickly evaluate and treat the casualty. In some cases, this may mean that the casualty can be evaluated, treated, and released back to duty. In other cases, the casualty's injuries can be repaired in the field. You also need to be able to accurately estimate the resources needed to treat multiple casualties based on the types of weapons used.

With more serious trauma, you must stabilize the casualty effectively to minimize blood loss and prevent further tissue damage. Often the only definitive treatment for traumatic injury is surgery. These surgical repairs can be as simple as suturing a bleeding wound or as extensive as a complete bowel resection. The goal is to keep the casualty alive to be transported to an MTF to receive surgical repair or to return to duty.

You are responsible for treating the entire casualty. Your knowledge of traumatic injuries and organ systems allows for the proper care of the casualty. Treat the obvious injuries and be wise enough to suspect the not-so-obvious internal injuries. Treat shock before it becomes irreversible and keep the casualty stable until he or she can receive higher level care. You are the vital link in getting the casualty from the battlefield to the operating room alive.

Introduction to Ballistic and Blast Injuries

Ballistics is the study of projectiles and/or firearms. During combat operations, these projectiles and firearms are the most common causes of injuries that you will encounter. There are a wide range of ballistic injuries, which are seen both in the combat zone and in more and more domestic areas. You will treat

---

Field Medical Care TIPS

Here are some reasons why you should know how weapons are used as well as their effects on the human body:

- You are required to protect and defend the lives of casualties.
- You will be better able to treat the casualties you encounter if you have a solid understanding of the effects of ballistic and blast injuries.
- You will be able to more accurately predict the number and type of casualties that may result from specific types of weapons used in a combat action so that adequate medical support can be arranged.
- Your knowledge can lead to development of countermeasures and protective equipment. For example, Israeli medical officers helped to develop fireproof clothing to reduce the incidence of burns in tank crews.

---

wounds from small arms to heavy artillery, including blasts and explosions from incendiary devices, mines, and bombs.

The study of ballistics refers to the study of the **velocity** and trajectory of a projectile from the weapon to the target. This is termed **external ballistics**. External ballistics is very complex and is highly studied. This chapter focuses on the effects of **internal ballistics** or the effects of projectiles on human tissue.

The **kinetic energy** of a projectile is the energy of motion. This energy is transferred to anything that comes in contact with the projectile. For our purposes, the effects discussed will be on solid and hollow organs, bones, and soft tissue. The mass of the projectiles can vary greatly. The differences in mass and velocity have a profound effect on the penetration of the projectile in the human body. As a bullet enters and passes through the body, the kinetic energy that it possesses is transferred to the surrounding tissue. This creates a temporary cavity at the point in which the most kinetic energy is released and transferred. As the bullet slows, there is less of a cavity surrounding the path of the bullet. If the bullet begins to tumble, it slows down dramatically and transfers a larger amount of kinetic energy into the surrounding tissue.

It has been highly emphasized that the velocity of a projectile is the most important factor in determining the extent of injury. This is not entirely true. Although this is a very important component, a number of other factors have an effect on the damage that a projectile can inflict.

Types of Weapons

Small Arms

Small arms are individually carried weapons commonly used by military personnel FIGURE 11-1 ▶ . These include pistols, rifles, and machine guns. These types of firearms shoot solid

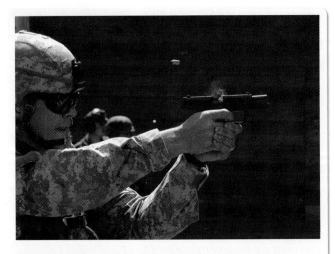

FIGURE 11-1   Small arms are commonly used by military personnel.

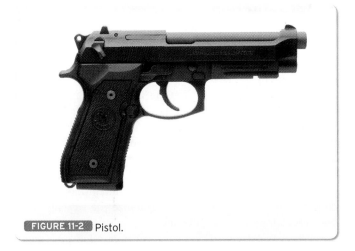

FIGURE 11-2   Pistol.

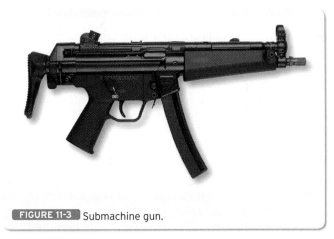

FIGURE 11-3   Submachine gun.

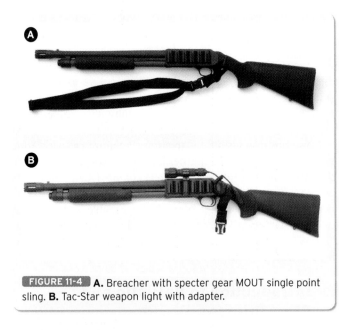

FIGURE 11-4   **A.** Breacher with specter gear MOUT single point sling. **B.** Tac-Star weapon light with adapter.

or hollow-point projectiles generally less than 20 mm in diameter. The magazine capacity for some of these weapons can be 99 or more rounds. Small arms are designed to be used in close combat situations where offensive, defensive, and cover fire are needed.

Small arms are capable of firing many rounds and can generate multiple casualties. Multiple wounds require more resources and personnel to treat and evacuate casualties. With small arms, a casualty can be hit with many rounds in a very short amount of time. The likelihood of hitting a vital organ becomes exponentially greater with the increased number of rounds that are fired. This can result in multiple wounds in a soldier and creates a greater risk of injuring so many organs that the soldier has little chance of survival.

Some examples of small arms are:

- **Pistol (9.0 mm, 0.40 or 0.45 cal):** A small-caliber hand weapon capable of discharging multiple rounds. A pistol uses relatively low-velocity ammunition and is modestly lethal. The accuracy varies depending on the user, but the pistol is generally not an accurate weapon. This weapon may be employed using one or both hands FIGURE 11-2 ▸.
- **Submachine gun (Uzi or MAC-10):** This weapon is either shoulder- or hip-fired and is used in tactical situations. It is equipped to fire in semi-automatic or fully automatic modes. The ammunition is small handgun ammunition (9 mm) that is relatively low velocity. This weapon is capable of firing a large number of rounds without reloading. It is usually issued to specialized personnel and is commonly used by terrorist organizations and gangs because of its small size and ability to be concealed FIGURE 11-3 ▸.
- **Shotgun (12-gauge or 20-gauge):** The shotgun is rarely used in combat; traditionally it is used as a hunting weapon. It is capable of holding multiple rounds and can fire as quickly as the user can pull the

trigger or pump the action. The shotgun can eject a multitude of different projectiles. It is shoulder-fired FIGURE 11-4 ▲.

- **Assault rifle (M-16, AK-47):** This may be the most commonly utilized military weapon, and is the weapon of most infantry and snipers. The average assault rifle uses a 7.62-mm NATO round, an extremely high-velocity bullet. Muzzle velocities are greater than 3,000 feet per second (fps) and they can fire up to 800 to 900 rounds per minute. This is a shoulder-fired weapon FIGURE 11-5 ▾.

- **Sniper rifle (M24 SWS):** The sniper rifle is built for greater accuracy than any other small firearm. It possesses a high muzzle velocity. It is also fitted with a telescopic sight for targets at extremely long ranges FIGURE 11-6 ▾.

Machine Guns

Machine guns are fully automatic, individual, or crew-served weapons used to suppress enemy fire rather than hit specific targets. There are three categories of machine gun:

- **Light machine gun (squad automatic weapon [SAW]):** Capable of semi-automatic or fully automatic firing. Considered to be a medium-range weapon. Can deliver about 725 rounds per minute FIGURE 11-7 ▸.
- **General purpose (M-60, general purpose machine gun [GPMG]):** Fires semi-automatic or fully automatic modes at about 550 rounds per minute FIGURE 11-8 ▸.
- **Heavy machine gun (M-2 heavy barrel 0.50-caliber machine gun [HMG]):** A fully automatic weapon that can deliver a larger projectile at approximately 500 rounds per minute FIGURE 11-9 ▾.

Muzzle Velocities

The wound-causing agent from small arms fire is the projectile or bullet, which is discharged when the weapon is fired. The severity of wounds depends on several factors:

- Caliber (size)
- Shape
- Design and construction
- Weight
- Velocity
- Type of tissue struck or impacted
- Fragmentation of the bullet

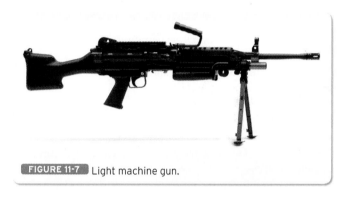
FIGURE 11-7 Light machine gun.

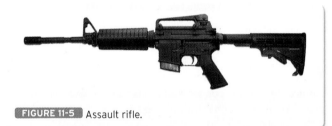
FIGURE 11-5 Assault rifle.

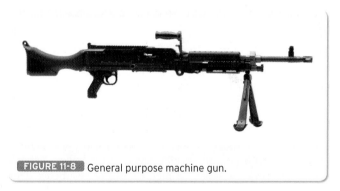
FIGURE 11-8 General purpose machine gun.

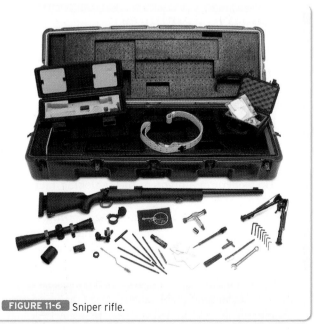
FIGURE 11-6 Sniper rifle.

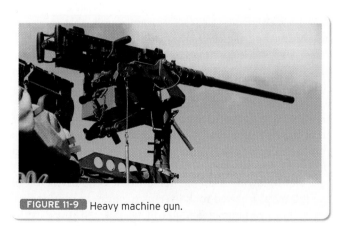
FIGURE 11-9 Heavy machine gun.

The pistol and shotgun have the slowest muzzle velocities of all the small arms. This means that their muzzle velocity measured at the end of the gun barrel is generally below 1,000 fps. Their bullets generally have less energy and penetration than rifled ammunition. Most of the damage caused by these slower rounds is by crushing and lacerating soft tissue. Wounds and complications of wounds resulting from pistols and shotguns may manifest in a variety of ways:

- Simple penetrating wounds
- Through-and-through penetrating wounds with disproportionately large exit wounds
- Fractures, amputations, and substantial soft-tissue injuries when extremities are involved
- Eviscerations of body cavities
- Substantial soft-tissue and internal organ injuries
- Severe blood loss, shock, and death

Medium-velocity cartridges are known to have muzzle velocities between 1,000 and 2,000 fps. They cause most of their damage by **cavitation**, a destructive force that results when a projectile travels over 1,000 fps. It causes a temporary cavity that forms when the pressure wake from the bullet stretches the skin outward. The skin and tissue can quickly return to their normal position but are often damaged. This can cause contusions to solid organs or rupture hollow organs. Large areas of hematomas also can form in the temporary cavity.

Any high-velocity cartridge that travels over 2,000 fps can cause **shock waves** in the soft tissue. These bullets cause the same crushing and lacerations as the slower velocity bullets but with increased cavitation, and they can cause a shock wave and hydrostatic energy that precedes the bullet. A shock wave can cause pressures as high as 200 atmospheres. This is highly effective in stretching tissue but lasts for only a few microseconds.

Most military rifles fire projectiles that reach greater than 2,000 fps. With the NATO 7.62-mm round, this results in a very fast bullet that can yaw and tumble FIGURE 11-10 ▶ . These effects create unpredictable wound patterns and large areas of cavitation. The bullets also can hit bones and can deflect to other unpredictable areas of the body to cause damage. This makes finding an exit wound very important when trying to determine the path of the bullet. You should place importance on determining the path that the bullet took through your casualty in order to help you determine which organs may be affected.

The following example demonstrates the cavitation of the full metal jacketed round versus the heavier hunting-type round from a shotgun. The full metal jacketed round pene-

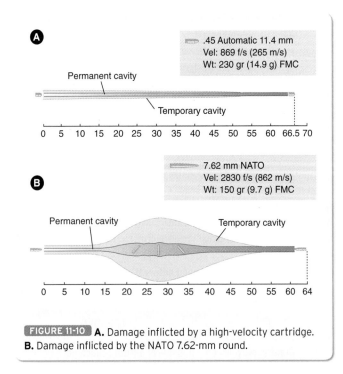

FIGURE 11-10 **A.** Damage inflicted by a high-velocity cartridge. **B.** Damage inflicted by the NATO 7.62-mm round.

trates much deeper before slowing down due to tumbling. At the point where the bullet slows, it releases most of its kinetic energy, putting the greatest area of the wound deep below the surface tissue.

The heavier, hunting round is a slower projectile and still penetrates deeply through the tissue, but the greatest area of cavitation is near the skin or initial contact surface. The shotgun round has most of its destructive effects near the surface due to less concentrated mass and slower velocity. Its penetration is also significantly less than the higher velocity solid bullets.

■ Explosive Munitions

Explosive munitions consist of explosive projectiles and other explosive devices such as bombs, rockets, grenades, and mines that are fired from ordinance (eg, artillery pieces), dropped from aircraft, launched (eg, multiple launch rocket system), thrown, or planted in order to cripple or destroy personnel and equipment. These types of weapons are not as accurate as some other forms of weaponry, but use their explosive force to create destruction on a large scale in order to cause as much damage as possible in concentrated areas. The generic prototype of the exploding munition is the shell.

There are two basic types of exploding antipersonnel munitions, which are most commonly encountered in the form of grenades, rockets, bombs, and mines FIGURE 11-11 ▶ :

- With *random-fragmentation munitions* the shell casing splinters unpredictably, and the resulting fragments vary in size, shape, and velocity (generally larger

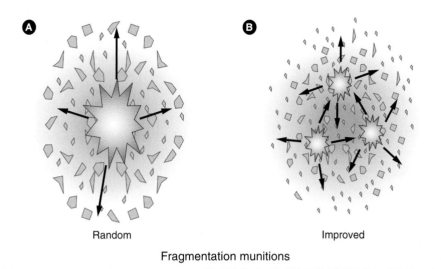

FIGURE 11-11 **A.** Random-fragmentation munitions. **B.** Improved-fragmentation munitions.

fragments). There is less chance of a hit, but the wounds are generally critical.

- With *improved-fragmentation munitions* either the shell casing is made of a fragmented material that breaks up in a more controlled fashion or the shell is filled with preformed fragments, which disperse evenly in the target area (generally smaller, more uniform fragments). More injuries are created, requiring the use of greater resources.

Antimaterial munitions have antipersonnel effects. Kinetic-energy antimaterial warheads (eg, armor piercing, fin stabilized, discarding-sabot round fired by tanks) rely on the speed and the density of the projectile to disable or destroy the target **FIGURE 11-12 ▸**. The principle injuring mechanisms are:

- **The penetrator:** The projectile is made of hardened material, tungsten, steel, or depleted uranium.
- **Fragments:** From the target when struck.
- **Blast overpressure:** The penetrator is traveling at supersonic speeds, so the shock waves produce a blast overpressure that is enhanced when the waves are reflected from a vehicle's inner walls.
- **Secondary fires:** Fires that occur after the explosion.

Explosive antimaterial warheads (eg, light anti-tank weapon [LAW], anti-tank 4 rocket [AT4], or TOW 2) are most commonly found in the form of a shaped-charge or hollow-charge warhead. The principle wounding agents from these weapons are:

- **Fragments from the casing and/or target, called spall:** A high-velocity jet is formed, which takes the shape of a long, thin rod. The front of the jet travels at a velocity of 20,000 fps. This allows the warhead to penetrate thick armor.
- **Blast overpressure:** This is usually sufficient to blow the vehicle's hatch open, and personnel who are sitting in the openings are propelled out of the vehicle.

- **Flame:** Anyone in the path of the high-temperature jet will suffer catastrophic burns, similar to injury from a blowtorch.
- **Secondary fires:** Fires that occur after the explosion.

Enhanced blast weapons (EBWs) rely primarily on the blast and secondarily on heat for their effects, whereas conventional weapons rely on explosively driven projectiles, fragments, or shaped charges to attack targets **FIGURE 11-13 ▸**. Confined spaces intensify the blast effects by reflecting the pressure waves from interior surfaces. In particular, these weapons kill by causing massive damage to the lungs and other internal organs. The primary kill mechanism of enhanced blast munitions is internal crushing injuries.

There are primarily four types of EBWs:

- **Metallized explosives:** Contain a reactive metal, usually aluminum powder
- **Reactive surround explosives:** Contain a reactive metal powder similar to metallized explosives
- **Fuel-air explosives:** Contain a fuel-rich reactive compound that is dispersed via a burster charge, which is subsequently detonated by a second charge
- **Thermobaric explosives:** Contain energetic metal fuel particles and an energetic binder

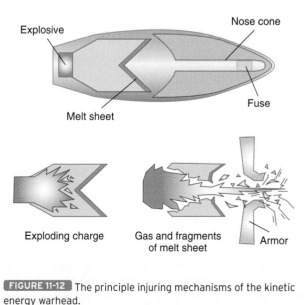

FIGURE 11-12 The principle injuring mechanisms of the kinetic energy warhead.

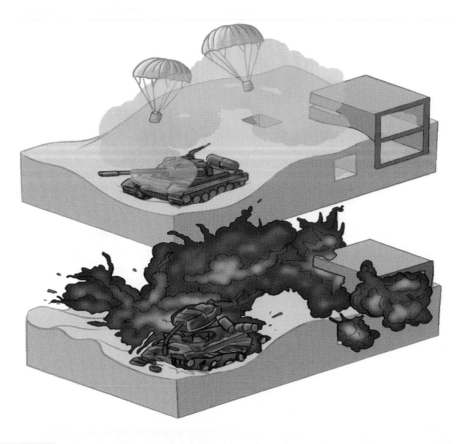

FIGURE 11-13   EBWs rely primarily on blast and secondarily on heat for their effects.

Ballistic injuries sustained from the primary and secondary missiles created by exploding munitions are in principle the same type of ballistic injuries sustained from small arms fire. However, the size of the projectile striking the casualty may be considerably larger and the injuries sustained are proportional. The nature and extent of ballistic injuries generated by explosive munitions will vary considerably. Factors that influence these are:

- Proximity to the explosion
- Size and shape of the missile or fragment
- Velocity of the missile or fragment
- Tissue struck (vital organs)

We will discuss blast injuries in great detail because ballistic and burn injuries sustained from these weapons are essentially the same as any other form of blunt or penetrating trauma and/or burn injury that a casualty might experience under other circumstances. Blast injuries occur in a number of ways.

- **Primary blast injury:** Due solely to the direct effects of the pressure wave on the body. The injury from the primary blast is seen almost exclusively in the gas-containing organs of the body—the lungs, intestines, and inner ears. An injury to the lungs causes the greatest morbidity and mortality.
- **Secondary blast injury:** Penetrating or nonpenetrating injury caused by ordinance projectiles or secondary missiles, which are energized by the explosion and strike the casualty.
- **Tertiary blast injury:** Results from whole body displacement and subsequent traumatic impact with environmental objects (eg, trees, buildings, vehicles). Other indirect effects include crush injury from the collapse of structures (buildings, bunkers, or tunnels) and toxic effects from the inhalation of combustion gases FIGURE 11-14 ▶.

The Physics of an Explosion

When a substance is detonated, a solid or liquid is chemically converted into large volumes of gas under pressure with resultant energy release. Propellants, like gunpowder, are explosives designed to release energy relatively slowly compared with

These weapons are usually known as two-stage explosive systems. The initial explosion disperses the fuel, which mixes with the surrounding atmosphere, and then the second explosion ignites the fuel–air mixture, which results in significant blast overpressure over relatively large areas. Consequently, these explosive mixtures are most effective in confined spaces such as caves, tunnels, buildings, and bunker interiors where surfaces enable the shock wave reflection and reinforcement process. The duration of the shock/combustion process is generally greater by a factor of one and one half or more compared to a conventional high explosive in the same structure.

Mechanisms of Injury

The principle injuring mechanisms are caused by a complicated mix of ballistic, blast, and burn injuries. The type and severity of wounds sustained primarily depend on the casualty's distance from the epicenter of the explosion. Casualties close to the epicenter of the explosion are likely to suffer from all wound-causing agents of the munitions (ballistic, blast, and thermal). Casualties who sustain wounds from all three of the wound-causing agents usually suffer from mutilating blast injury and are not likely to survive. Casualties who are farther away from the epicenter are likely to experience a combination of blast from the explosion and penetrating trauma from primary and secondary missiles created by the explosion.

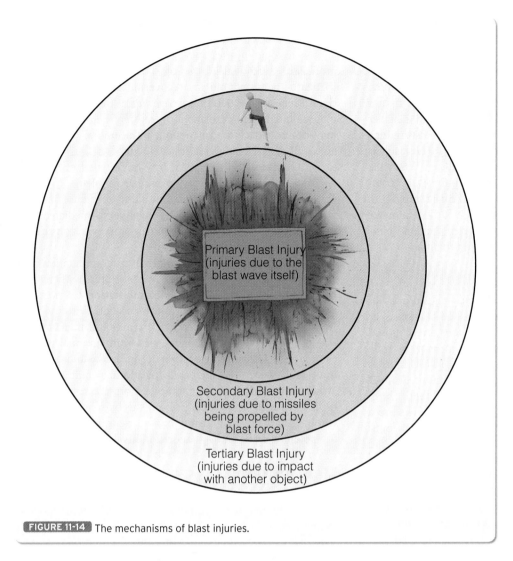

Primary Blast Injury
(injuries due to the
blast wave itself)

Secondary Blast Injury
(injuries due to missiles
being propelled by
blast force)

Tertiary Blast Injury
(injuries due to impact
with another object)

FIGURE 11-14 The mechanisms of blast injuries.

spheric; it may last 10 times as long as the positive wave pulse. It occurs as air displaced by the positive wave pulse returns to fill the space of the explosion. It can lead to massive movements of air resulting in high-velocity winds.

The speed, duration, and pressure of the shock wave are affected by the following:

- The *size* of the explosive charge. The larger the explosion, the faster the shock waves and the longer they will last.
- The nature of the *surrounding medium*. Pressure waves travel much more rapidly in water, for example, and are effective at greater distances in water.
- The *distance* from the explosion. The farther one is from the explosion, the slower the shock wave velocity and the longer its duration.
- The presence or absence of *reflecting surfaces*. If the pressure wave is reflected off a solid object, its pressure may be multiplied several times. For example, a shock wave that might cause minimal injury in the open can cause devastating trauma if the casualty is standing beside a wall or similar solid object.

The changes in pressure produced by the shock wave are accompanied by transient *winds*, sometimes of very high velocity, that can accelerate small objects to speeds of hundreds of feet per second. A missile traveling at 50 fps can easily penetrate human skin; at 400 fps, a missile can enter any of the major body cavities and cause serious internal injury. Blast winds can also send the human body flying against larger, more stationary objects, or amputate limbs.

In an *underwater explosion*, a shock wave travels at greater velocity than in open air, thereby making it possible to receive injuries at three times the distance that would normally be required to receive such injuries. This is because positive pressures are higher and there is no negative pressure or high-velocity wind. Blast fragments and gases move shorter distances in water, however.

An explosion is significantly more damaging in *closed spaces* because of a limited dissipation environment for the forces involved and for the generation of toxic gases and

high explosives (eg, trinitrotoluene), which are designed to detonate very quickly. Composition C4 can create initial pressures of more than 4 million lb/in^2. This generates a pressure pulse in the shape of a spherical blast wave that expands in all directions from the point of explosion. Flying debris and high winds commonly cause conventional blunt and penetrating trauma.

Components of a Blast Shock Wave

The leading edge of the shock wave is called the **blast front**. A **positive wave pulse** refers to the phase of the explosion in which there is a pressure front higher than atmospheric pressure. The peak magnitude of the wave experienced by a casualty becomes lessened the farther the casualty is from the center of the explosion. The increase in pressure from a blast can be so abrupt that high-explosive blast waves are also referred to as shock waves. Shock waves possess a characteristic, **brisance**, that describes the shattering effect of the wave and its ability to cause disruption of tissues as well as structures. Tissue damage depends on the magnitude of the pressure spike and the duration of force application. The **negative wave pulse** refers to the phase in which pressure is less than atmo-

smoke. The blast wave is magnified when it comes into contact with a solid surface such as a wall, causing casualties near a wall to be hit with significantly higher pressure, resulting in increased risk of injury and death.

Blast pressures cause destruction at the interface between tissues of different densities or the interface between tissues and trapped air. When the shock wave passes from a higher to a lower density medium, a severe pressure disturbance develops at the interface of the denser medium. The result is fragmentation of the heavier medium, or **spalling**. When the shock wave contacts small gas bubbles, the bubbles are compressed and high local pressures are created, called implosion. The bubbles can then re-expand and cause further damage. Acceleration and deceleration of organs at their fixation points will occur in a manner similar to that in blunt trauma.

Tissues at Risk

Air-containing organs such as the middle ear, lung, and gastrointestinal tract are most susceptible to pressure changes. The junction between tissues of different densities and exposed tissues such as the head and neck are prone to injury as well. The ear is the organ system most sensitive to blast injuries. The **tympanic membrane** evolved to detect minor changes in pressure and will rupture at pressures of 5 to 7 lb/in^2 above atmospheric pressure. Thus, the tympanic membranes are a sensitive indicator of the possible presence of other blast injuries. The casualty may complain of ringing in the ears, pain in the ears, or some loss of hearing, and blood may be visible in the ear canal. Dislocation of structural components of the ear may occur. Permanent hearing loss is possible.

Primary **pulmonary blast injuries** occur as contusions and hemorrhages. When the explosion occurs in an open space, the side toward the explosion is usually injured, but the injury can be bilateral when the casualty is located in a confined space. The casualty may complain of tightness or pain in the chest and may cough up blood and have tachypnea or other signs of respiratory distress. Subcutaneous emphysema (crackling under the skin) over the chest can be palpated, indicating air in the thorax. Pneumothorax is common and may require emergency decompression (see Chapter 3, *Airway Management*). Pulmonary edema may ensue rapidly.

One of the most concerning pulmonary blast injuries is **arterial air embolism**, which occurs on alveolar disruption with subsequent air embolization into the pulmonary vasculature. Even small air bubbles can enter a coronary artery and cause myocardial injury. Air embolisms to the cerebrovascular system can produce disturbances in vision, changes in behavior, changes in state of consciousness, and a variety of other neurologic signs.

Solid organs are relatively protected from shock wave injury but may be injured by secondary missiles or a hurled body. Hollow organs, however, may be injured by similar mechanisms as for lung tissue. Petechiae, or pinpoint hemorrhages that show up on the skin, to large hematomas are the dominant form of pathology. Perforation or rupture of the bowel and colon is a risk. Underwater explosions can result in very severe abdominal injuries.

Neurologic injuries and head trauma are the most common causes of death from blast injuries. Subarachnoid (beneath the arachnoid layer covering the brain) and subdural (beneath the outermost covering of the brain) hematomas are often seen. Permanent or transient neurologic deficits may be secondary to concussion, intracerebral bleeding, or air embolism. Instant but transient unconsciousness, with or without retrograde amnesia, may be initiated not only by head trauma, but also by cardiovascular problems. Bradycardia and hypotension are common after an intense pressure wave from an explosion. This is a vagal nerve–mediated form of cardiogenic shock without compensatory vasoconstriction (for example, vasovagal syncope).

Extremity injuries, including traumatic amputations, are common. Other injuries are often associated with tertiary blasts. Casualties with traumatic amputation by postblast wind are likely to sustain fatal injuries secondary to the blast. In present combat, improved body armor has increased the number of survivors of blast injuries from shrapnel wounds to the torso. The number of severe orthopaedic and extremity injuries, however, has increased. In addition, although body armor may limit or prevent shrapnel from entering the body, it also "catches" more energy from the blast wave, possibly resulting in the casualty being thrown backward, thus increasing potential spine and spinal cord injury.

■ Munitions

Flame, incendiary, and phosphorus-containing munitions are weapons that use a combustible material source to expel people from strongholds or hidden positions and destroy material. Although flame and incendiary munitions theoretically constitute separate classes of weapons, they both use fire as the means to achieve the objectives of the user. The fear of being burned is the crucial incapacitating factor in the effectiveness of these weapons. The types of flame and incendiary munitions are listed in **TABLE 11-1 ▼**.

The wounding agent for all flame, incendiary, and phosphorus-containing munitions is the intense heat and fires that they generate and the fumes produced by the fires.

TABLE 11-1 Flame and Incendiary Munitions	
Type	**Means of Delivery**
Flame munitions	• Aerial-delivered bombs (such as Napalm) • Flame throwers • Rocket-launched warheads
Incendiary weapons	• Aerial-delivered bombs • Grenades
Phosphorus-containing munitions	• Aerial-delivered bombs • Artillery shells • Grenades

The injuries and complications of injuries produced by flame, incendiary, or phosphorus-containing munitions include burns and smoke inhalation. The specific treatment for burns is discussed in Chapter 10, *Burns*.

■ Medical Implications of Conventional Weapons

The weapons of conventional land warfare are designed to inflict physical harm on personnel by wounding with bullets or fragments, or damaging internal organs with blast effects or burns. You must be adequately prepared to treat all of these types of injury.

Ballistic Injuries

Most casualties in modern conventional hostilities are caused by weapons that cause ballistic wounds [FIGURE 11-15 ▼]. The severity of the wound depends to some extent on the nature of the projectile or fragment. The most important factor in a ballistic injury is the anatomical site hit.

The care for small arms wounds is essentially the same as for any other form of trauma and revolves around:

- Airway.
- Breathing.
- Circulation (bleeding is controlled).
- Shock is prevented or treated appropriately. (IV therapy is initiated if appropriate.)
- Evacuation is accomplished in a timely manner with care being constantly provided.

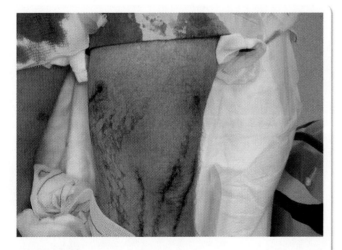

FIGURE 11-15   Most casualties in modern conventional hostilities are by weapons that cause ballistic wounds.

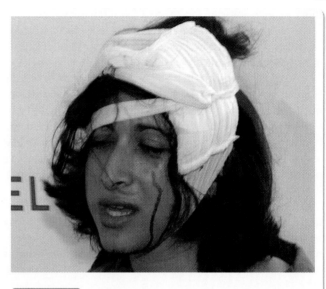

FIGURE 11-16   Air-filled organs such as lungs, intestines, and inner ears are susceptible to blast injuries.

Blast Injuries

Blast injuries may not be obvious at first. As weapons increasingly take advantage of the physical properties of blast waves, be aware that a blast injury may be present in a casualty whose only overt injuries are blunt, penetrating, or thermal trauma. Bleeding from the ears may be a subtle sign of a blast injury, and you should continue to search for further injuries. Remember, air-filled organs such as lungs, intestines, and inner ears are susceptible to blast injuries [FIGURE 11-16 ▲].

The care for blast injuries is essentially the same as for any other form of trauma and revolves around:

- Airway.
- Breathing (be on guard for pneumothorax, hemothorax, flail chest, and pulmonary contusion).
- Circulation (be on guard for hemorrhage, hypovolemia, cardiac tamponade, and embolus).
- Shock is prevented or treated appropriately. (IV therapy is initiated if appropriate.)
- Evacuation is accomplished in a timely manner with care being constantly provided.

■ The Casualty Mortality Curve

The casualty mortality curve is an important concept to understand and accept. About 20% of casualties are expected to die within 6 minutes of injury no matter what care they receive. These casualties include those who have sustained major trauma to the heart or brain. It is best in situations such as this to not waste resources or risk the lives of lifesavers to treat the dead or dying. You must be able to quickly determine the signs incompatible with life.

The second stage of this curve is when you will have the most profound effect on the casualty. During the hour following a major trauma, approximately 10% will die from hemorrhage or from obstruction of the airway. It is the casualties in this category you can treat with IV fluids, airway interventions, and wound care. You must provide aggressive care of casualties with such life-threatening injuries. This will result in better outcomes and survival.

After 6 hours, another 10% have died from breathing problems. These injuries may be airway burns or hemopneumothoraces. Once again, this progression can either be treated or at least recognized in order to secure a rapid extrication to a MTF. By this time there will also be some casualties who will start to show the first signs of shock that may have been caused by more subtle bleeding or unrecognized injuries, if they have not received adequate resuscitation with IV fluids.

Between 6 and 24 hours there may be deaths from untreated shock, but after this the casualties' conditions may remain relatively stable. By 72 hours, deaths are more likely to result from infections than trauma. This means that wounds that have been stabilized in the battlefield must continue to receive attention at an MTF.

■ Summary

As a combat medic, you need to understand the potential injuries that casualties may have based on the type of projectile that caused the injury. You are a highly trained medical operative who is skilled in the treatment of a wide range of injuries and illnesses. In many cases, you can treat a casualty without the threat of hostile engagement. However, when faced with the threat of personal injury, you will be forced to make critical decisions concerning the immediate medical care and evaluation of the casualty while attempting to avoid danger. You must also manage to stabilize the casualty for a safe evacuation from the battlefield.

You are the combat medic in a five-vehicle convoy. You are riding in the second vehicle. The convoy is travelling quickly down a main road, taking every precaution against an attack. While making a tight right turn, you hear an earsplitting roar and feel your vehicle lurch forward. The fifth vehicle in the convoy has been hit by an IED that was embedded in the curbing. After the commander states that the scene is secure, you head toward the disabled vehicle with your medical aid bag and a combat lifesaver (CLS). The engine block is completely gone from the front of the vehicle and the windshield is shattered. From the mechanism of injury, you are expecting to find blast injuries.

Assessment

The priority casualty is the driver. The soldiers riding in the vehicle with him have exited the vehicle on their own and are loudly complaining of ringing in their ears. Since they are talking and able to state their chief complaint, you know that they are alert and that their airways are patent. The driver is still in the vehicle and isn't speaking. His eyes are closed and you can see blood coming out of his ears.

Treatment

While the CLS stabilizes the casualty's c-spine, you open the airway with a jaw thrust. There are no visible obstructions, so you insert an OPA and ventilate the casualty with a bag-valve-mask device. The casualty's pulse rate is 58 beats/min, so he may be suffering from a head injury. This casualty needs to be evacuated to a medical treatment facility quickly. A KED is brought and the casualty is immobilized and extricated from the vehicle onto a longboard. As you await the MEDEVAC, you continue to provide ventilations with the BVM device and monitor the casualty's vital signs.

| 1. LAST NAME, FIRST NAME | RANK/GRADE | X | MALE |
| Wolf, Nathan | SGT | | FEMALE |

| SSN | SPECIALTY CODE | RELIGION |
| 000-111-0000 | 00A | Jewish |

2. UNIT

FORCE				NATIONALITY	
A/T	AF/A	N/M	MC/M		
	BC/BC		NBI/BNC		DISEASE	PSYCH

3. INJURY	AIRWAY
	HEAD
FRONT BACK	X	WOUND
	NECK/BACK INJURY
	BURN
	AMPUTATION
	STRESS
	X	OTHER (Specify)

Blast Injury

4. LEVEL OF CONSCIOUSNESS		
ALERT		PAIN RESPONSE
VERBAL RESPONSE	X	UNRESPONSIVE

| 5. PULSE | TIME | 6. TOURNIQUET | | TIME |
| 38 bpm | 0630 | X NO | ☐ YES | |

| 7. MORPHINE | | DOSE | TIME | 8. IV | TIME |
| X NO | ☐ YES | | | | |

9. TREATMENT/OBSERVATIONS/CURRENT MEDICATION/ALLERGIES/NBC (ANTIDOTE)

Driver in vehicle hit by an IED. Vehicle suffered massive frontal damage. Unresponsive, able to establish airway & ventilate. Secured to KED & longboard.

10. DISPOSITION	RETURNED TO DUTY	TIME
	X	EVACUATED	0646
	DECEASED	

| 11. PROVIDER/UNIT | DATE (YYMMDD) |
| Han, Tim | |

Aid Kit

Ready for Review

- As a combat medic, you need to understand the potential injuries that casualties may have based on the type of projectile that caused the injury.
- You will treat wounds from small arms to heavy artillery, including blasts and explosions from incendiary devices, mines, and bombs.
- Small arms are capable of firing many rounds and can generate multiple casualties.
- Multiple wounds require more resources and personnel to treat and evacuate casualties.
- Explosive munitions consist of explosive projectiles and other explosive devices such as bombs, rockets, grenades, and mines that are fired from ordinance (eg artillery pieces), dropped from aircraft, launched (eg multiple launch rocket system), thrown, or planted in order to cripple or destroy personnel and equipment.
- Flame, incendiary, and phosphorus-containing munitions are weapons that use a combustible material source to expel people from strongholds or hidden positions and destroy material.
- The weapons of conventional land warfare are designed to inflict physical harm on personnel by wounding with bullets or fragments, or damaging internal organs with blast effects or burns.
- The casualty mortality curve is an important concept to understand and accept. About 20% of casualties are expected to die within 6 minutes of injury no matter what care they receive. These casualties include those who have sustained major trauma to the heart or brain.

Vital Vocabulary

arterial air embolism Air bubbles in the arterial blood vessels.

ballistics The study of the dynamic properties and characteristics of bullets or projectiles.

blast front The leading edge of the shock wave.

brisance The shattering effect of a shock wave and its ability to cause disruption of tissues and structures.

cavitation A temporary cavity that forms from the pressure wake from a bullet that stretches the skin outward.

external ballistics The study of projectiles in the phase between the weapon and the intended target. This includes velocity, trajectory, and many other factors.

internal ballistics The study of projectiles and their effect on human tissue.

kinetic energy The energy of motion; this energy is transferred to anything that the projectile comes in contact with.

negative wave pulse The phase of an explosion in which pressure from the blast is less than atmospheric pressure.

positive wave pulse The phase of an explosion in which there is a pressure front with a pressure higher than atmospheric pressure.

primary blast injury Injuries caused by an explosive pressure wave on the gas-containing organs of the body.

pulmonary blast injuries Pulmonary trauma resulting from short-range exposure to the detonation of explosives.

secondary blast injury Penetrating or nonpenetrating injuries caused by ordinance projectiles or secondary missiles.

shock wave Waves of pressure from muzzle velocities above 2,000 fps that precede the bullet and compress the tissue ahead of and around the bullet. Shock waves can reach pressures above 200 atmospheres.

small arms Individually carried weapons commonly carried by military personnel, including pistols, rifles, and machine guns; they shoot solid or hollow-point projectiles generally less than 20 mm in diameter.

spall Fragments from the shell casing and/or target.

spalling Delaminating or breaking off into chips and pieces.

tertiary blast injury Injury from whole body displacement and subsequent traumatic impact with environmental objects.

tympanic membrane The eardrum; a thin, semitransparent membrane in the middle ear that transmits sound vibrations to the internal ear by means of the auditory ossicles.

velocity The rate of change of position or speed. Commonly measured in meters per second (m/s).

COMBAT MEDIC *in Action*

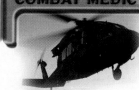

Your unit is travelling on a main road. Before travelling underneath an overpass, soldiers inspect the area for possible explosive devices on the overpass or near the overpass. While searching the area, a soldier is hit by sniper fire from the overpass. The sniper is quickly taken out and you rush to attend to the casualty. He is lying on the ground, holding his bleeding leg.

1. The damage caused by small arms fire is from:
   A. crushing and lacerating soft tissue.
   B. temporary cavities.
   C. shock waves.
   D. blast pressure.

2. Small arms fire can cause:
   A. fractures and amputations.
   B. severe blood loss, shock, and death.
   C. simple penetrating wounds.
   D. all of the above.

3. The muzzle velocity of small arms is generally below:
   A. 2,000 fps.
   B. 3,500 fps.
   C. 1,000 fps.
   D. 100 fps.

4. Your first concern with this type of trauma is:
   A. airway.
   B. circulation.
   C. contamination.
   D. evacuation.

5. The severity of a small arms fire wound depends upon:
   A. shape.
   B. weight.
   C. velocity.
   D. all of the above.

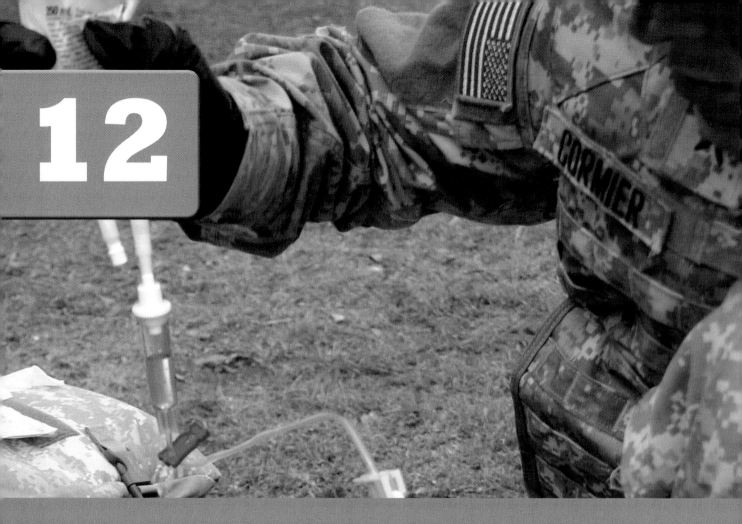

12

Battlefield Medications

Objectives

Knowledge Objectives

- ☐ List the indications for administration of battlefield medications.
- ☐ Describe the administration of morphine.
- ☐ Discuss the administration of acetaminophen.
- ☐ Explain the administration of promethazine.
- ☐ Discuss the administration of naloxone.
- ☐ Describe the administration of antibiotics.

Skills Objectives

- ☐ Draw medication from an ampule.
- ☐ Draw medication from a vial.
- ☐ Administer medication via the subcutaneous route.
- ☐ Administer medication via the intramuscular route.
- ☐ Administer medication via the intravenous bolus route.
- ☐ Administer medication via the intraosseous route.
- ☐ Perform the FAST1 procedure.
- ☐ Remove the FAST1 device.

Introduction

As a combat medic, in combat or in remote peacekeeping operations, you may be responsible for administering medications. You must become an expert in administering medication safely while understanding the medications' indications, contraindications, and side effects.

How Medications Work

Pharmacology is the study of the properties (characteristics) and effects of drugs and medications on the body. **Drugs** are chemical agents used in the diagnosis, treatment, and prevention of disease. Although the terms *drugs* and *medications* are often used interchangeably, drugs may make some people think of narcotics or illegal substances. For this reason, you should use the word *medications*. In general terms, a medication is a chemical substance that is used to treat or prevent disease or relieve pain.

The **dose** is the amount of medication that is given. The dose depends on the casualty's size and age, as well as the desired action of the medication. The **action** is the therapeutic effect that a medication is expected to have on the body. **Indications** are the therapeutic uses for a particular medication.

There are times when you should not give a casualty medication, even if it usually is indicated for that casualty's condition. Such situations are called **contraindications**. A medication is contraindicated when it would harm the casualty or have no positive effect on the casualty's condition.

Field Medical Care TIPS

An *indication* is a reason for giving a drug. A *contraindication* is a reason not to give a drug. The number one contraindication for any medication is hypersensitivity (allergy) to that drug.

Side effects are any actions of a medication other than the desired ones. Side effects may occur even when a medication is administered properly and under the appropriate circumstances. For example, giving **epinephrine** to a casualty who is having an allergic reaction should dilate the bronchioles and decrease wheezing. However, two side effects of epinephrine are cardiac stimulation and constriction of the arteries, which may elevate the casualty's heart rate and blood pressure. These side effects are predictable; others are not.

Medication Names

Medications have been identified or derived from four major sources: plants (alkaloids, glycosides, gums, oils), animals and humans, minerals and mineral products, and chemical and synthetic substances made in the laboratory. For instance, morphine is derived from plants.

Medications have different types of names. A **trade name** is the brand name that a manufacturer gives to a medication, such as Tylenol. As a proper noun, a trade name begins with a capital letter. Trade names are used in every aspect of our daily lives, not just in medications. Well-known examples include Jell-O gelatin, Band-Aid adhesive bandages, and Hershey's chocolate candy. A medication may have many different trade names, depending on how many companies manufacture it. Advil, Nuprin, and Motrin all are trade names for the same generic medication, ibuprofen.

The **generic name** of a medication (such as ibuprofen) is usually its original chemical name, which is not capitalized, and is usually suggested by the first manufacturer and approved by the US Food and Drug Administration (FDA). Sometimes a medication is called by its generic name more often than by any of its trade names.

Indications for Administration of Battlefield Medications

Normally a licensed medical provider such as a nurse practitioner, physician's assistant, or physician administers medication. However, federal and state law allow a licensed medical provider to authorize administration of medications from a distance (eg, via radio) or to delegate that authority under strict protocols in certain situations, including combat. This means that your medical officer can authorize you to administer certain medications under strict guidelines on the battlefield. Indications for battlefield administration of medications include analgesics to combat pain, antiemetics to combat nausea or vomiting, narcotic antagonists to combat narcotic side effects, and antibiotics for infection prophylaxis.

Morphine is an effective pain-relieving medication (analgesic) and should be used in casualties suffering from severe pain. You may be required to administer morphine to severely injured casualties under the following circumstances:

- Operational and combat injuries
- Traumatic amputation
- Ballistic injuries
- Severe burns
- Crush injuries
- Long evacuation delays
- Expectant causalities to minimize terminal suffering

For mild to moderate pain in a casualty who is still able to fight, acetaminophen (Tylenol) should be given orally. These medications do not cause sedation or confusion and allow the casualty to continue on the battlefield.

Although morphine is the most potent painkiller, it commonly causes severe nausea and vomiting. Morphine acts on the central nervous system and also can cause hypotension, bradycardia, and respiratory depression if given in excess amounts. Promethazine (Phenergan) is used to combat the side effects of morphine, including nausea and vomiting. If the casualty experiences adverse effects following administration of morphine, naloxone (Narcan) is given. Naloxone is also given to casualties with a suspected morphine overdose. Morphine overdose may result in a casualty with respiratory depression.

To prevent infection, oral antibiotics (eg, gatifloxacin) are given to all casualties who have minor to moderate open wounds and are able to swallow medications. Oral antibiotics are usually not given to casualties with penetrating cavity injuries (chest or abdomen). These injuries must be judged on a case-by-case basis.

Intravenous antibiotics are given to severely injured casualties who cannot take oral medications, such as casualties with head injuries with altered mental status or unconscious casualties. Care of casualties in the tactical combat environment should include the use of prophylactic antibiotics for all open wounds. Infections are a common cause of late morbidity and mortality in combat trauma. For antibiotics to be practical and effective, the antibiotic should be administered as soon as possible after the injury occurs. Antibiotics must be continued until the casualty reaches a medical treatment facility (MTF). A **Combat Pill Pack** may be issued to every soldier prior to deployment. Soldiers are instructed to take the pill pack if they sustain any penetrating injury.

Medication Administration

Before administering any medication to a casualty, you must have a thorough understanding of how the medication will affect the human body—both negatively and positively. This includes familiarity with the medication's mechanism of action, indications, contraindications, route(s) of administration, dose, and antidotes for adverse reactions.

In addition to knowledge of the medications you may administer, you must also have an understanding of basic math for pharmacology to calculate the appropriate medication dose. Medication doses and flow rate calculations are common areas of confusion for many, yet they are skills you will need to perform. You must learn to quickly and accurately calculate doses to maximize the chance for a positive outcome. Disastrous results, including death, may be the outcome if you administer an inappropriate medication or dose, give it by the wrong route, or give the medication too rapidly or too slowly.

The Five Rights of Medication Administration

Prior to giving any medications, verify the following five rights of medication administration:

- **Right casualty:** Verify that the casualty does not have any contraindications to the medication.
- **Right medication:** Check to ensure that the medication you are about to administer is correct.
- **Right dosage:** Check the concentration for the medication to be administered.
- **Right time:** Check the casualty's field medical card (FMC) to see whether any medication has been given previously. Consider how long it will take to evacuate the casualty to an MTF where a licensed provider can treat him or her.
- **Right route:** Confirm whether the medication should be given by the oral, intramuscular (IM), or intravenous (IV) route.

TABLE 12-1 Symbols Used in the Metric System	
Symbols of Weight (smallest to largest)	**Abbreviations**
microgram	μg (or mcg)
milligram	mg
gram	g (or gm)
kilogram	kg
Symbols of Volume (smallest to largest)	
milliliter	mL
deciliter	dL
liter	L

The Metric System

The **metric system** is a decimal system based on multiples of 10. It is used to measure length, volume, and weight, which are represented as follows:

- **Meter (m):** The basic unit of length
- **Liter (L):** The basic unit of volume
- **Gram (g):** The basic unit of weight

In the metric system, prefixes demonstrate the fraction of the base being used. Commonly used prefixes, from smallest to largest, include the following:

- micro- = 0.000001
- milli- = 0.001
- centi- = 0.01
- kilo- = 1,000

TABLE 12-1 ▲ illustrates the symbols of weight and volume used in the metric system. It is important to be able to recognize these symbols, because medications will be supplied in a variety of weights and volumes, and you will be required to convert these weights to volume to administer the appropriate dose of a medication to your casualty.

TABLE 12-2 ▶ illustrates the metric units of weight and volume and their equivalents. Again, you must be able to understand these metric unit equivalents for proper medication conversion and subsequent administration.

Weight and Volume Conversion

To administer the appropriate dose of a medication to a casualty, you must be able to convert larger units of weight to smaller ones (for example, g to mg) and larger units of volume to smaller ones (for example, L to mL). Conversely, you must also be able to convert smaller units of weight to larger ones (for example, mg to g) and smaller units of volume to larger ones (for example, mL to L).

Medications are packaged in different units of weight and volume; however, the weight (for example, μg, mg, g) and volume (for example, mL) of the medication to be

TABLE 12-2 **Metric Units and Their Equivalents**	
Units of Weight (smallest to largest)	**Equivalents**
1 μg	0.001 mg
1 mg	1,000 μg
1 g	1,000 mg
1 kg	1,000 g
Units of Volume (smallest to largest)	
1 mL	1 cc*
100 mL	1 dL
1,000 mL	1 L

*Cubic centimeter (cc) is a unit also used to represent milliliters (mL); therefore, 1 cc is the same as 1 mL (1 cc = 1 mL).

administered is usually only a fraction of the total amount of its packaged form.

Weight Conversion

Converting weight is generally simply a matter of multiplying or dividing by 1,000 *or* moving the decimal point three places to the right or left. To convert a gram to milligrams (or a milligram to micrograms), multiply the larger unit of weight by 1,000 *or* simply move the decimal point three places to the right, as demonstrated in the following examples:

EXAMPLE 1

Converting 2 g to mg (2 g = X mg)

2 g × 1,000 = 2,000 mg *or* 2.000 g = 2,000 mg
→

EXAMPLE 2

Converting 5 mg to μg (5 mg = X μg)

5 mg × 1,000 = 5,000 μg *or* 5.000 mg = 5,000 μg
→

Conversely, to convert a smaller unit of weight to a larger one, divide the smaller unit of weight by 1,000 or simply move the decimal point three places to the left, as demonstrated in the following examples:

EXAMPLE 1

Converting 200 μg to mg (200 μg = X mg)

200 μg ÷ 1,000 = 0.2 mg *or* 200.0 μg = 0.2 mg
←

EXAMPLE 2

Converting 250 mg to g (250 mg = X g)

250 mg ÷ 1,000 = 0.25 g *or* 250.0 mg = 0.25 g
←

Volume Conversion

You will usually be dealing with only two measurements of volume: milliliters and liters. The formula is the same as with converting units of weight—simply dividing or multiplying by 1,000 *or* moving the decimal point three places to the left or right.

When converting a smaller unit of volume to a larger one (for example, mL to L), divide the smaller unit of volume by 1,000 *or* simply move the decimal point three places to the left, as demonstrated in the following examples:

EXAMPLE 1

Converting 100 mL to L (100 mL = X L)

100 mL ÷ 1,000 = 0.1 L *or* 100 mL = 0.1 L
←

EXAMPLE 2

Converting 250 mL to L (250 mL = X L)

250 mL ÷ 1,000 = 0.25 L *or* 250 mL = 0.25 L
←

Conversely, when converting a larger unit of volume to a smaller one (for example, L to mL), multiply the larger unit of volume by 1,000 *or* simply move the decimal point three places to the right, as demonstrated in the following examples:

EXAMPLE 1

Converting 1.5 L to mL (1.5 L = X mL)

1.5 L × 1,000 = 1,500 mL *or* 1.500 L = 1,500 mL
→

EXAMPLE 2

Converting 25 L to mL (25 L = X mL)

25 L × 1,000 = 25,000 mL *or* 25.000 L = 25,000 mL
→

■ Calculating Medication Doses

There are multiple formulas for calculating medication doses, but it is beyond the scope of this chapter to demonstrate *every one* of them. Our discussions are limited to formulas that most combat medics find easy to understand. For other calculation formulas, you are encouraged to consult with the instructor. The method of drug dose calculation demonstrated is based on the following three factors:

1. **Desired dose:** Amount of the medication you give the casualty. It is expressed as a standard dose (for example, 5 mg of morphine).

2. **Concentration of the medication available (dose on hand):** You must know the medication's <u>concentration</u>—the total weight (µg, mg, or g) of the medication contained in a specific volume (mL or L). *To administer a medication, you must know the weight of the medication that is present in each milliliter.* This will tell you the concentration of the medication that you have on hand. The formula for calculating this is as follows:

> Total Weight of the Medication ÷ Total Volume in Milliliters = Weight per Milliliter

3. **Volume to be administered:** After determining the concentration of the medication present in each milliliter (dose on hand), you must calculate how much volume is needed to give the amount of the desired dose. Use the following formula to calculate the volume to be administered:

> Desired Dose (µg, mg, g) ÷ Dose on Hand (mg/mL) = Volume to Be Administered (mL)

Calculating the Dose and Rate for a Medication Infusion

Following the administration of certain medications, you may need to begin a continuous infusion to maintain a therapeutic blood level of the medication to prevent a recurrence of the condition. Medication infusions are usually ordered to be administered in a specified period of time, usually per minute.

When administering a continuous medication infusion, remember these rules:

1. When adding a certain number of grams of a medication to a bag of IV fluid, *you must convert the medication into milligrams.* For example, if you place 2 g of morphine into the IV fluid, you must use 2,000 mg (2 g) to determine the concentration/dose on hand.

2. Always divide the amount of the medication by the *total number of minutes* over which the medication will be infused. For example, do not divide by 1 hour, divide by 60 minutes.

Oral Administration of Medications

Forms of solid and liquid oral medications include capsules, timed-release capsules, lozenges, pills, tablets, elixirs, emulsions, suspensions, and syrups FIGURE 12-1 ▸. To give oral medications, you may use a small medicine cup. Gather the appropriate equipment for the form of medication you are administering. Check for indications, contraindications, precautions, and the five rights before administering any medication.

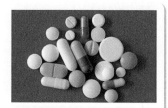

FIGURE 12-1 Tablets and capsules, oral medications typically taken by mouth, enter the bloodstream through the digestive system.

Follow these steps when administering an oral medication FIGURE 12-2 ▾:

1. Take BSI precautions.
2. Determine the need for the medication.
3. Check the medication to be sure it is the right medication, it is not cloudy or discolored, and that its expiration date has not passed. Check the five rights.
4. Determine the appropriate dose. If using a liquid medication, pour the desired amount into a calibrated cup.
5. Instruct the casualty to swallow the medication with water, if administering a pill or tablet.
6. Monitor the casualty's condition, and document the medication given, route, time of administration, and response of the casualty.

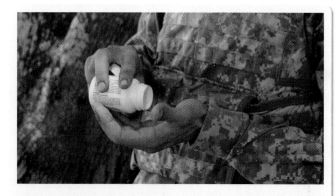

FIGURE 12-2 Administering an oral medication. Administer with a cup of water, if necessary.

Parenteral Administration of Medications

<u>Parenteral</u> medications are those given through any route other than the gastrointestinal tract. Parenteral routes used by the combat medic include subcutaneous, intramuscular,

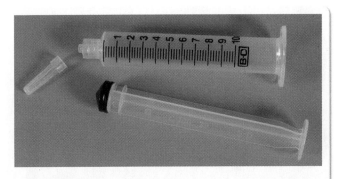

FIGURE 12-3 A syringe consists of a plunger, body or barrel, flange, and tip.

Field Medical Care **TIPS**

Any medication administered directly through the skin, such as through the subcutaneous or intramuscular route, is referred to as percutaneous administration.

IV bolus, and intraosseous (IO). Of the parenteral drug routes, IV administration is the most commonly used and generally is the quickest route for getting medication into the central circulation. IV administration is further covered in Chapter 13, *Intravenous Access*.

Equipment

A variety of needles and syringes are used for administering parenteral medications. Most syringes come prepackaged in color-coded packs with a needle already attached. The needles and syringes may also be packaged separately. You must choose the appropriate size of syringe and appropriate needle length for the desired route. Syringes consist of a plunger, body or barrel, flange, and tip FIGURE 12-3 ▲ . All hypodermic syringes are marked with 10 calibrations per milliliter on one side of the barrel. Each small line represents 0.1 mL. The 3-mL syringe is the most common used for injections, but others are available as needed. Needle lengths vary from 3/8″ to 1″ for standard injections. The gauge of the needle refers to the diameter; the smaller the number, the larger the diameter.

Packaging of Parenteral Medications

Parenteral medications are most commonly packaged in ampules, vials, and prefilled syringes. **Ampules** are breakable sterile glass containers that are designed to carry a single dose of medication FIGURE 12-4 ◀ . **Vials** may contain single or multiple doses FIGURE 12-5 ▶ . Vials have a rubber-stopper

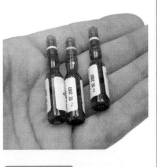

FIGURE 12-4 Ampules.

top and are made of glass or plastic. Prefilled syringes are designed for ease of use. There are also single-dose disposable cartridges that use a reusable syringe such as a Tubex or Aboject FIGURE 12-6 ▼ . Some medications, such as ertapenem (Invanz), may need to be reconstituted. These come with two vials, one with a powdered form of the drug and one with sterile water.

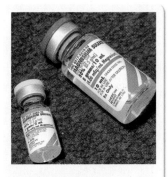

FIGURE 12-5 Vials (single-dose and multidose).

Drug reconstitution involves injecting the sterile water from one vial into another vial that contains the powder, making a solution for injection.

Ampules

When drawing a medication from an ampule, follow the steps in SKILL DRILL 12-1 ▶ :

1. Check the medication to be sure that the expiration date has not passed and that it is the correct medication and concentration.

2. Shake the medication down into the base of the ampule. If some of the medication appears to be stuck in the neck, gently thump or tap the stem (**Step ①**).

Field Medical Care **TIPS**

Any time you are using a needle to draw up medication or to inject blood into blood tubes, always hold the syringe against your palm with the needle pointing up and draw the vial or blood tube down onto the needle using the thumb and forefinger of the palm the syringe is braced against to avoid sticking yourself.

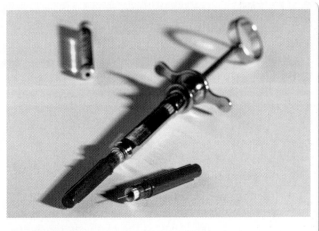

FIGURE 12-6 A Tubex syringe.

SKILL DRILL 12-1

Drawing Medication From an Ampule

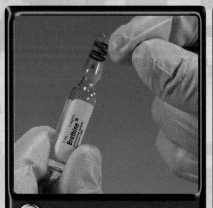

1 Gently thump or tap the stem of the ampule to shake medication down into the base.

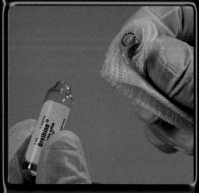

2 Grip the neck of the ampule using a 4″ × 4″ gauze pad and snap the neck off.

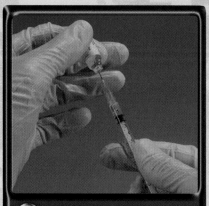

3 Without touching the outer sides of the ampule, insert the needle into the medication in the ampule, and draw the solution in the syringe.

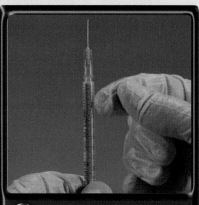

4 Holding the syringe with the needle pointing up, gently tap the barrel to loosen air trapped inside.

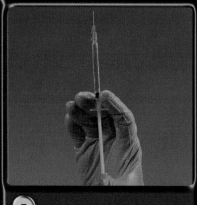

5 Gently press on the plunger to dispel any air bubbles, and recap the needle using the one-handed method.

3. Using a 4″ × 4″ gauze pad or an alcohol prep, grip the neck of the ampule and snap it off. Drop the stem in the sharps container (**Step ②**).

4. Insert the needle into the ampule without touching the outer sides of the ampule. Draw the solution into the syringe, and dispose of the ampule in the sharps container (**Step ③**).

5. Hold the syringe with the needle pointing up, and gently tap the barrel to loosen air trapped inside and cause it to rise (**Step ④**).

6. Press gently on the plunger to dispel any air bubbles (**Step ⑤**).

7. Recap the needle using the one-handed method and avoiding contamination.

Vials

When using a vial of medication, you must first determine how much of the medication you will need and how many doses are in the vial. For a single-dose vial, you will draw up the entire amount in the vial. For multiple-dose vials, you should draw out only the amount needed. Remember that once you remove the cover from a vial, it is no longer sterile. If you need a second dose, the top of the vial should be cleaned with alcohol before withdrawing the medication.

When drawing medication from a vial, follow the steps in **SKILL DRILL 12-2 ▶**:

1. Check the medication to be sure that the expiration date has not passed and that it is the correct medication and concentration (**Step ①**).

2. Remove the sterile cover, or clean the top with alcohol if it was previously opened.

3. Determine the amount of medication you will need, and draw that amount of air into the syringe (**Step ②**). Allow a little extra room to expel some while removing air bubbles.

4. Invert the vial, and insert the needle through the rubber stopper into the medication. Expel the air in the syringe into the vial and then release the plunger, keeping the tip of the needle within the medication (**Step ③**).

5. Once you have the correct amount of medication in the syringe, withdraw the needle and expel any air in the syringe (**Step ④**).

6. Recap the needle using the one-handed method and avoiding contamination (**Step ⑤**).

Prefilled Syringe

Prefilled syringes come in tamper-proof boxes and are separated into the glass medication cartridge and a syringe **FIGURE 12-7 ▼**. Pop the tops off of the syringe and the medication cartridge, and screw them together. Remove the needle cover, and expel air in the manner previously described. Follow the steps for the route the medication is to be given.

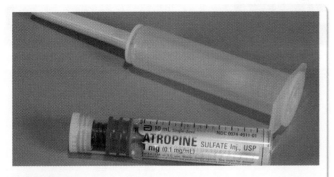

FIGURE 12-7 Prefilled syringes come in two parts, the glass medication cartridge and a syringe.

■ Administration of Medication by the Subcutaneous Route

<u>Subcutaneous</u> injections are given into the loose connective tissue between the dermis and the muscle layer **FIGURE 12-8 ▼**. Volumes of a medication administered subcutaneously are usually 1 mL or less. The injection is performed using a 24- to 26-gauge ½″ to 1″ needle. Common sites include the upper arms, anterior thighs, and abdomen **FIGURE 12-9 ▼**.

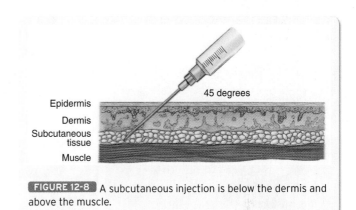

FIGURE 12-8 A subcutaneous injection is below the dermis and above the muscle.

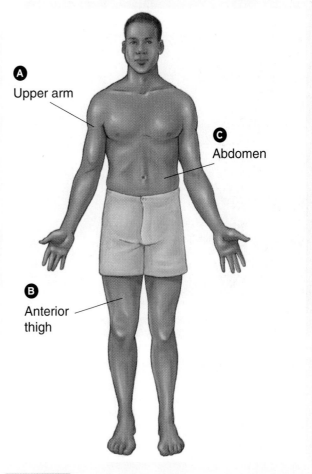

FIGURE 12-9 Common sites for subcutaneous injections. **A.** Upper arm. **B.** Anterior thigh. **C.** Abdomen.

SKILL DRILL 12-2

Drawing Medication From a Vial

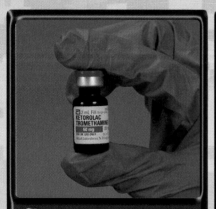

1 Check the medication and its expiration date.

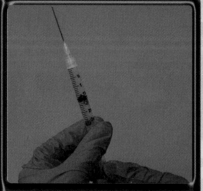

2 Determine the amount of medication needed, and draw that amount of air into the syringe.

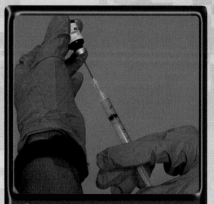

3 Invert the vial, and insert the needle through the rubber stopper. Expel the air in the syringe and release the plunger, keeping the tip of the needle within the medication.

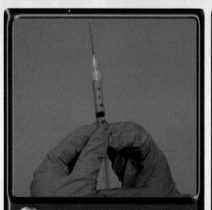

4 Once you have the correct amount of medication in the syringe, withdraw the needle, and expel any air in the syringe.

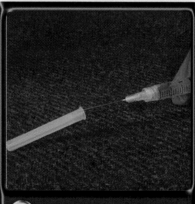

5 Recap the needle using the one-handed method.

Follow the steps in **SKILL DRILL 12-3 ▸** to administer a medication via the subcutaneous route:

1. Take BSI precautions.

2. Determine the need for the medication.

3. Check the medication to be sure that it is not cloudy, that the expiration date has not passed, and that it is the correct drug and concentration, and determine the appropriate dose (**Step ①**).

4. Assemble and check equipment needed: alcohol preps and a 3-mL syringe with a 24- to 26-gauge needle. Draw up the correct dose of medication (**Step ②**).

5. Cleanse the area for the administration (usually the upper arm or thigh) using **aseptic technique** (**Step ③**).

6. Pinch the skin surrounding the area, advise the casualty of a stick, and insert the needle at a 45° angle (**Step ④**).

7. Pull back on the plunger to aspirate for blood. The presence of blood in the syringe indicates you may have entered a vein. Remove the needle, and hold pressure over the site. Discard the syringe and needle in the sharps container. Prepare a new syringe and needle and select another site.

8. If there is no blood in the syringe, inject the medication and remove the needle. Immediately place it in the sharps container.

9. To disperse the medication through the tissue, rub the area in a circular motion with your gloved hand (**Step ⑤**).

10. Properly store any unused medication.

11. Monitor the casualty's condition, and document the medication given, route, administration time, and response of the casualty.

■ Administration of Medication by the Intramuscular Route

By penetrating a needle through the dermis and subcutaneous tissue into the muscle layer, a casualty is given medication via the **intramuscular (IM) route**. This allows administration of a larger volume of medication (up to 5 mL) than the subcutaneous route. There is also the potential for damage to nerves because of the depth of the injection, so it is important to choose the appropriate site. Common anatomic sites for IM injections include the following:

- **Vastus lateralis muscle:** The large muscle on the lateral side of the thigh
- **Rectus femoris muscle:** The large muscle on the anterior side of the thigh
- **Gluteal area:** The buttocks, specifically the upper lateral aspect of either side
- **Deltoid muscle:** The muscle of the upper arm that covers the prominence of the shoulder. The site for injection is approximately 1½″ to 2″ below the acromion process on the lateral side **FIGURE 12-10 ▾**.

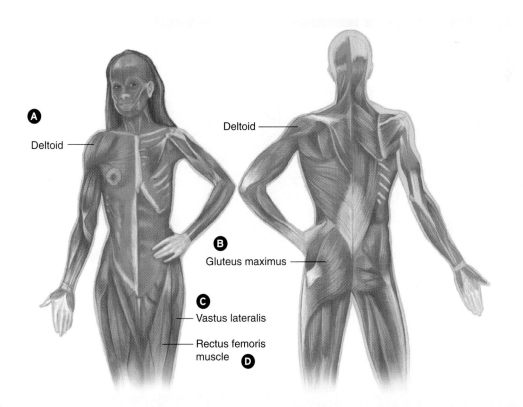

FIGURE 12-10 Common sites for intramuscular injections. **A.** Deltoid muscle. **B.** Gluteal area. **C.** Vastus lateralis muscle. **D.** Rectus femoris muscle.

SKILL DRILL 12-3

Administering Medication Via the Subcutaneous Route

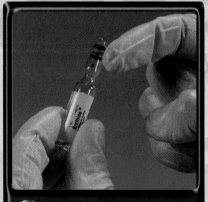

1 Check the medication to be sure that it is the correct one, that it is not discolored, and that the expiration date has not passed.

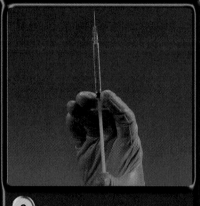

2 Assemble and check the equipment. Draw up the correct dose of medication.

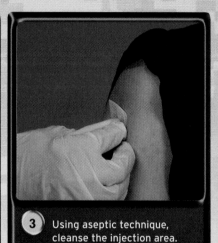

3 Using aseptic technique, cleanse the injection area.

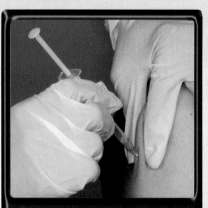

4 Pinch the skin surrounding the area, and insert the needle at a 45° angle. Pull back on the plunger to aspirate for blood. If there is no blood, inject the medication, remove the needle, and hold pressure over the area.

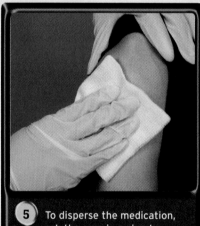

5 To disperse the medication, rub the area in a circular motion. Monitor the casualty's condition.

Follow the steps in **SKILL DRILL 12-4 ▶** to administer an IM injection:

1. Take BSI precautions.

2. Determine the need for the medication.

3. Check the medication to be sure it is the correct one, that it is not discolored, and that the expiration date has not passed, and determine the appropriate dose.

4. Assemble and check equipment needed: alcohol preps and a 3- to 5-mL syringe with a 21-gauge, 10 or 20 needle. Draw up the correct dose of medication.

5. Cleanse the area for the administration (usually the upper arm or the hip) using aseptic technique (Step ①).

6. Stretch the skin over the cleansed area, advise the casualty of a stick, and insert the needle at a 90° angle.

Administering Medication Via the Intramuscular Route

1 Check the medication to be sure it is the correct one, that it is not discolored, and that its expiration date has not passed. Assemble and check the equipment. Draw up the correct dose of medication. Using aseptic technique, cleanse the injection area.

2 Stretch the skin over the area, and insert the needle at a 90° angle. Pull back on the plunger to aspirate for blood. If there is no blood, inject the medication and remove the needle.

3 To disperse the medication, rub the area in a circular motion. Monitor the casualty's condition.

7. Pull back on the plunger to aspirate for blood. The presence of blood in the syringe indicates you may have entered a blood vessel. Remove the needle, and hold pressure over the site. Discard the syringe and needle in the sharps container. Prepare a new syringe and needle, and select another site.

8. If there is no blood in the syringe, inject the medication and remove the needle. Immediately place it in the sharps container (**Step 2**).

9. To disperse the medication through the tissue, rub the area in a circular motion with your gloved hand.

10. Store any unused medication properly.

11. Monitor the casualty's condition, and document the medication given, route, administration time, and response of the casualty (**Step 3**).

■ Administration of Medication by Intravenous Bolus

The **intravenous (IV) route** places the medication directly into the circulatory system. Chapter 13, *Intravenous Access*, covers intravenous access in detail. This is the fastest route of medication administration to administer because it bypasses most barriers to medication absorption. This also means that there is no room for error. Medications are administered by direct injection with a needle and syringe into an established peripheral IV line. When using a needleless system, the syringe simply screws into the injection port.

In terms of medication administration, a **bolus** is a single dose given by the IV route. A bolus (in one mass) can be a small or large quantity of a medication. Some medications require an initial bolus and then a continuous IV infusion to maintain a therapeutic level of the medication.

Complications may arise from using the IV route. These include phlebitis (inflammation of a vein) or infection, extravasation of fluid or medication into the surrounding tissues, air in tubing that may lead to an air embolus, allergic reaction to a fluid or medication, pulmonary embolism, or a failure to infuse properly for any reason.

Follow the steps in **SKILL DRILL 12-5 ▶** when administering a medication via the IV bolus route. Chapter 13, *Intravenous Access*, discusses IV boluses in detail.

1. Take BSI precautions.

2. Determine the need for the medication.

3. Check the medication to be sure that it is the correct one, that it is not cloudy or discolored, and that its

SKILL DRILL 12-5

Administering Medication Via the Intravenous Bolus Route

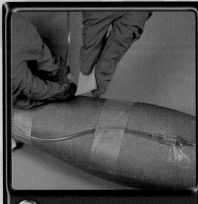 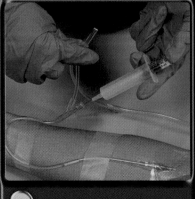 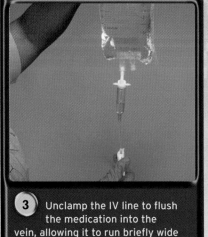

1 Assemble and check the equipment. Cleanse the injection port, or remove the protective cap if using the needleless system.

2 Insert the needle into the port, and pinch off the IV tubing proximal to the administration port. Administer the correct dose at the appropriate rate.

3 Unclamp the IV line to flush the medication into the vein, allowing it to run briefly wide open, or flush with a 20-mL bolus of normal saline. Readjust the IV flow rate to the original setting, and monitor the casualty's condition.

expiration date has not passed, and determine the appropriate dose.

4. Assemble needed equipment, and draw up medication. Expel any air in the syringe. Draw up 20 mL of normal saline to use as a flush for the medication.

5. Cleanse the injection port with alcohol, or remove the protective cap if using the needleless system (**Step ①**).

6. Insert the needle into the port, and pinch off the IV tubing proximal to the administration port. Failure to shut off the line will result in the medication taking the pathway of least resistance and flowing into the bag instead of into the casualty.

7. Administer the correct dose of the medication at the appropriate rate. Some medications must be administered very quickly, while others must be pushed slowly to prevent adverse effects (**Step ②**).

8. Place the needle and syringe into the sharps container.

9. Unclamp the IV line to flush the medication into the vein. Allow it to run briefly wide open, or flush with a 20-mL bolus of normal saline.

10. Readjust the IV flow rate to the original setting (**Step ③**).

11. Properly store any unused medication.

12. Monitor the casualty's condition, and document the medication given, route, time of administration, and response of the casualty.

■ Administration of Medication by the IO Route

Any fluid or medication that may be given through an IV line can also be given by the **intraosseous (IO)** route. Shock and status epilepticus are only two of the reasons for establishing IO access. Unlike an IV line, fluid does not flow well into the bone because of resistance; therefore, it is necessary to use a large syringe to infuse the fluid.

Complications of using the IO route are similar to those of the IV route. Along with the complications discussed in the previous section, there is also the potential for compartment syndrome if fluid leaks outside of the bone and into the osteofascial compartment, fracture of the tibia from improper technique, and pulmonary embolism due to the bone and fat particles.

Follow the steps in **SKILL DRILL 12-6 ▸** to administer a medication via the IO route:

1. Take BSI precautions.

2. Determine the need for the medication.

SKILL DRILL 12-6

Administering Medication Via the IO Route

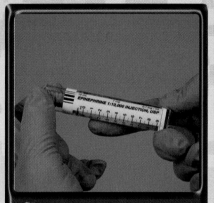

1. Check the medication to make sure it is the correct one, that it is not discolored, and that the expiration date has not passed. Assemble the equipment, and draw up the medication. Draw enough fluid from the IV line for a flush.

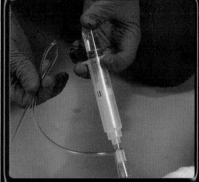

2. Cleanse the injection port, or remove the protective cap if using the needleless system. Insert the needle into the port, and pinch off the IV tubing proximal to the administration port. Administer the correct dose at the proper push rate.

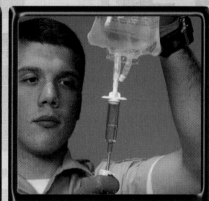

3. Unclamp the IV line to flush the medication into the body, allowing it to run briefly wide open, or flush with a 20-mL bolus of normal saline (or the fluid being given). Readjust the IV flow rate to the original setting, and monitor the casualty's condition.

3. Check the medication to be certain that it is the correct one, that it is not cloudy or discolored, and that the expiration date has not passed, and determine the appropriate dose.

4. Assemble needed equipment, and draw up the medication. Also draw enough fluid from the IV line for a flush (**Step 1**).

5. Cleanse the injection port of the extension tubing with alcohol, or remove the protective cap if using the needleless system.

6. Insert the needle into the port, and clamp off the IV tubing proximal to the administration port. This is usually managed with a three-way stopcock. Failure to shut off the line will result in the medication taking the pathway of least resistance and flowing into the bag instead of into the casualty.

7. Administer the correct dose of the medication at the proper push rate. Some medications must be administered very quickly, while others must be pushed slowly to prevent adverse effects (**Step 2**).

8. Place the needle and syringe into the sharps container.

9. Unclamp the IV line to flush the medication into the body. Flush with at least a 20-mL bolus of normal saline (or the fluid being administered).

10. Readjust the IV flow rate to the original setting.

11. Store any unused medication properly.

12. Monitor the casualty's condition, and document the medication given, route, time of administration, and response of the casualty (**Step 3**).

The FAST1 Procedure

The **FAST1 device** (First Access for Shock and Trauma) was the first IO device approved for use in adults. Four design elements allow for this device's IO placement in the sternum: an infusion tube and subcutaneous portal, an introducer, a target/strain relief patch, and a protective dome **FIGURE 12-11 ▶**. The company that developed the FAST1 chose sternum placement based on the ease of locating the manubrium and the easier penetration than with other bones.

To perform the FAST1 procedure, follow the steps in **SKILL DRILL 12-7 ▶**:

1. Prepare the site.

2. Undo or cut the casualty's shirt to expose the sternum.

3. Identify the sternal notch.

4. Use aseptic technique to prepare the site (**Step 1**).

5. Place the target patch.

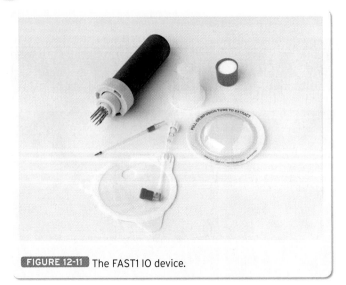

FIGURE 12-11 The FAST1 IO device.

6. Remove the top half of the backing (labeled *remove 1*) from the patch (**Step** ②).

7. Locate the sternal notch using your index finger.

8. Holding your index finger perpendicular to the skin, align the locating notch in the target patch with the sternal notch, keeping your index finger perpendicular (**Step** ③).

9. Verify that the target zone (circular hole) on the patch is directly over the casualty's midline.

10. Secure the top half of the patch to the body by pressing firmly downward on the patch, engaging the adhesive.

11. Remove the remaining backing (labeled *remove 2*) and secure the patch to the casualty (**Step** ④).

12. Verify the correct patch placement by checking the alignment of the patch locating the notch with the casualty's sternal notch and making sure the target zone is over the midline of the casualty's body. The correct patch placement is critical for safe and effective placement of the device (**Step** ⑤).

13. Insert the introducer.

14. Remove the sharps cap from the introducer (**Step** ⑥).

15. Place the bone probe cluster needles in the target zone of the target patch, and ensure that all the bone probe needles are within the target zone (**Step** ⑦).

16. Hold the introducer perpendicular to the skin of the casualty to ensure proper functioning of the depth-control mechanism (**Step** ⑧).

17. Pressing straight along the introducer axis, with hand and elbow in line, push with firm constant force until a distinct release is heard and felt. Apply the force perpendicular to the skin and along the long axis of the introducer. Avoid extreme force, twisting, or jabbing motions (**Step** ⑨).

18. After the release, expose the infusion tube by gently withdrawing the introducer along the same path used to insert it (perpendicular to the skin). The stylet supports will fall away (**Step** ⑩).

19. Locate the orange sharps plug, and place it on a flat surface with the foam facing up. Keep both hands behind the needles, and push the bone probe cluster straight into the foam. After the sharps plug has been engaged and the sharps are safely covered, reattach the clear sharps cap to the introducer. This completes the dual sharps protection (**Step** ⑪).

20. Connect the infusion tube to the right-angle female connector on the target patch. This connection is a slip luer (**Step** ⑫).

21. Use saline to flush bone marrow out of the infusion site (**Step** ⑬).

22. *Optional step*: Verify correct placement of the infusion tube by attaching the enclosed syringe to the straight female connector and withdraw marrow into the infusion tube. Attach the straight female connector to the source of fluids or drugs. Fluid can now flow to the site.

23. Secure the protector dome. Place the protector dome directly over the target patch and press down firmly to engage the Velcro fastening. Ensure that the infusion tubing and the right-angle female connector are contained under the dome. The dome can be removed by holding the patch against the skin and peeling back the dome Velcro (**Step** ⑭).

24. Attach the remover package to the casualty for transport. The remover package must be transported with the casualty. It will be used later to remove the FAST1 system. Do not breach the packaging because the remover is sterile (**Step** ⑮).

25. *Optional step*: Increase the flow rate. Attach the syringe to the straight female connector on the patch. Increase fluid flow rate by flushing the system with 10 cc of saline. Reattach IV fluid line when flush is complete.

To remove the FAST1, follow the steps in **SKILL DRILL 12-8 ▶**:

1. Remove the protector dome from the patch by peeling the Velcro ring away from the patch. Make sure one hand is holding the patch against the casualty's skin while the other hand peels the dome Velcro up so the patch does not come away from the skin during the process (**Step** ①).

2. Ensure that the clamp controlling the IV fluid flow is turned off (**Step** ②).

3. Disconnect the IV line from the straight female connector tube on the patch (**Step** ③).

4. Disconnect the infusion tube from the right-angle female connector on the patch (**Step** ④).

5. Remove the infusion tube. *Do NOT pull on the infusion tube to remove it. Open the remover package while maintaining sterile technique* (**Step** ⑤).

SKILL DRILL 12-7

Insert a FAST1 Device

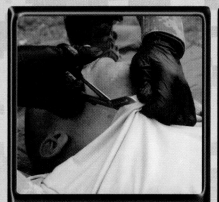

1 Prepare the site. Undo or cut the casualty's shirt to expose the sternum. Identify the sternal notch. Use aseptic technique to prepare the site.

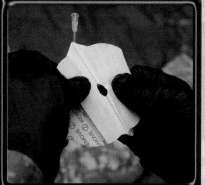

2 Place the target patch. Remove the top half of the backing (labeled remove 1) from the patch.

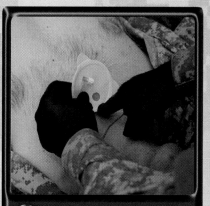

3 Locate the sternal notch using your index finger. Holding your index finger perpendicular to the skin, align the locating notch in the target patch with the sternal notch, keeping your index finger perpendicular.

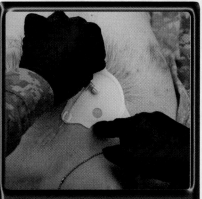

4 Verify that the target zone (circular hole) on the patch is directly over the casualty's midline. Secure the top half of the patch to the body by pressing firmly downward on the patch, engaging the adhesive. Remove the remaining backing (labeled remove 2) and secure the patch to the casualty.

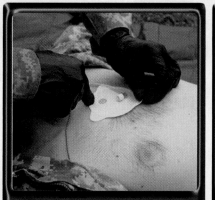

5 Verify the correct patch placement by checking the alignment of the patch locating notch with the casualty's sternal notch and making sure the target zone is over the midline of the casualty's body.

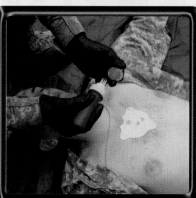

6 Insert the introducer. Remove the sharps cap from the introducer.

Insert a FAST1 Device (*continued*)

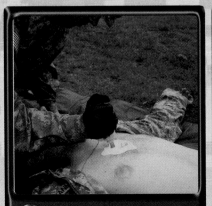

7 Place the bone probe cluster needles in the target zone of the target patch, and ensure that all the bone probe needles are within the target zone.

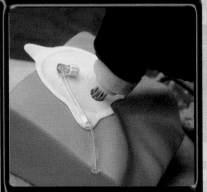

8 Hold the introducer perpendicular to the skin of the casualty to ensure proper functioning of the depth-control mechanism.

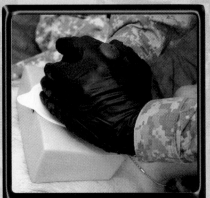

9 Pressing straight along the introducer axis, with hand and elbow in line, push with firm constant force until a distinct release is heard and felt. Apply the force perpendicular to the skin and along the long axis of the introducer.

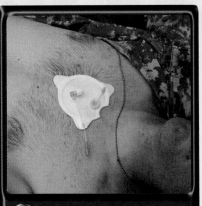

10 After the release, expose the infusion tube by gently withdrawing the introducer along the same path used to insert it (perpendicular to the skin). The stylet supports will fall away.

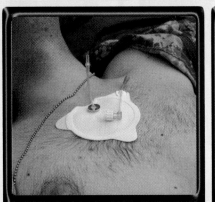

11 Locate the orange sharps plug, and place it on a flat surface with the foam facing up. Keep both hands behind the needles, and push the bone probe cluster straight into the foam. After the sharps plug has been engaged and the sharps are safely covered, reattach the clear sharps cap to the introducer.

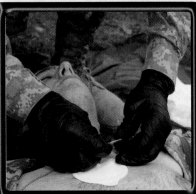

12 Connect the infusion tube to the right-angle female connector on the target patch. This connection is a slip luer.

SKILL DRILL 12-7

Insert a FAST1 Device (*continued*)

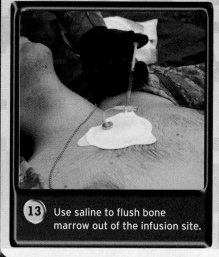
13 Use saline to flush bone marrow out of the infusion site.

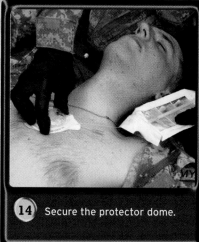
14 Secure the protector dome.

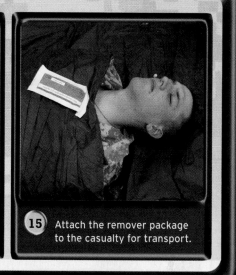
15 Attach the remover package to the casualty for transport.

6. Remove the tubing protecting the remover tip. Insert the remover into the infusion tube while holding the infusion tube straight out (90°) from the casualty (**Step 6**).

7. Advance the remover and turn it clockwise until it stops. This will engage the threads in the proximal tip of the infusion tube (**Step 7**).

8. Use one hand to press down lightly on the target patch and the other to pull the remover straight out to dislodge the infusion tube.

9. Hold the remover by the T-shaped knob. *Do NOT hold the luer or tubing.* If the remover disengages from the infusion tube without removing it, reattempt. Make sure that you pull the remover in the direction perpendicular to the infusion site to avoid bending the remover tip (**Step 8**).

10. Gently peel the target patch away from the casualty and discard the patch (**Step 9**).

11. Apply pressure to the infusion site. Reassess to check for bleeding from the site. Dress the infusion site using aseptic technique.

12. Dispose of the remover and infusion tube using contaminated sharps protocols (**Step 10**).

■ Analgesics

Morphine

Indications

You may need to administer morphine to severely injured casualties who **FIGURE 12-12 ▾**:

- Have serious injuries
- Are in severe pain
- Expect a long delay in evacuation times

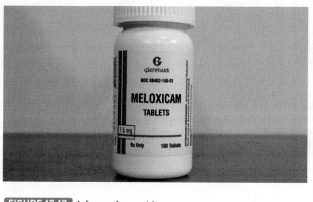

FIGURE 12-12 A form of morphine.

SKILL DRILL 12-8

Remove the FAST1 Device

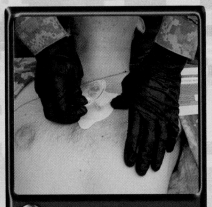

1 Remove the protector dome from the patch by peeling the Velcro ring away from the patch. Make sure that one hand is holding the patch against the casualty's skin while the other hand peels the dome Velcro up so the patch does not come away from the skin during the removal process.

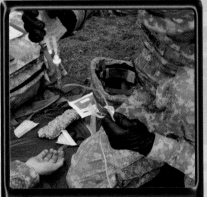

2 Ensure that the clamp controlling the IV fluid flow is turned off.

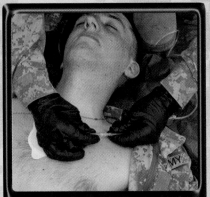

3 Disconnect the IV line from the straight female connector tube on the patch.

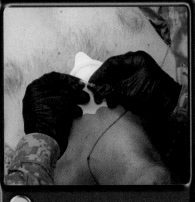

4 Disconnect the infusion tube from the right-angle female connector on the patch.

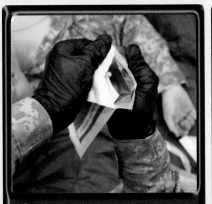

5 Remove the infusion tube. Do NOT pull on the infusion tube to remove it. Open the remover package while maintaining sterile technique.

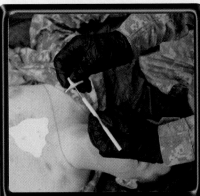

6 Remove the tubing protecting the remover tip. Insert the remover into the infusion tube while holding the infusion tube straight out (90°) from the casualty.

SKILL DRILL 12-8

Remove the FAST1 Device (*continued*)

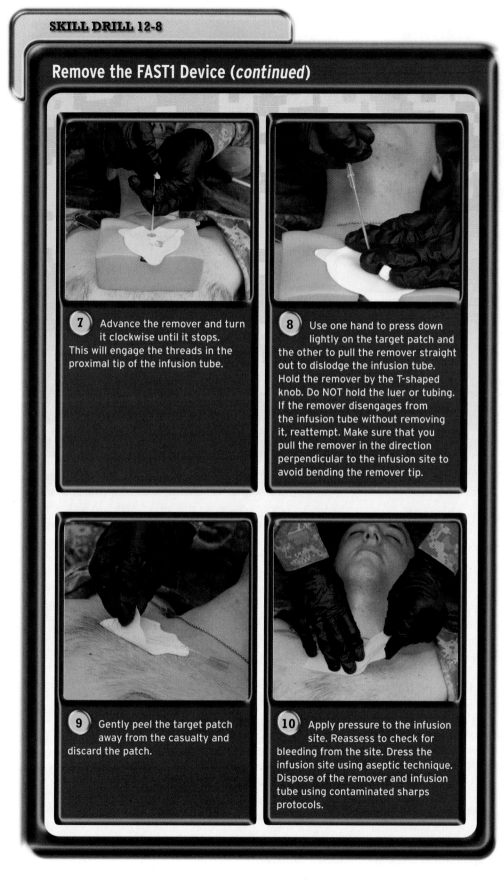

7 Advance the remover and turn it clockwise until it stops. This will engage the threads in the proximal tip of the infusion tube.

8 Use one hand to press down lightly on the target patch and the other to pull the remover straight out to dislodge the infusion tube. Hold the remover by the T-shaped knob. Do NOT hold the luer or tubing. If the remover disengages from the infusion tube without removing it, reattempt. Make sure that you pull the remover in the direction perpendicular to the infusion site to avoid bending the remover tip.

9 Gently peel the target patch away from the casualty and discard the patch.

10 Apply pressure to the infusion site. Reassess to check for bleeding from the site. Dress the infusion site using aseptic technique. Dispose of the remover and infusion tube using contaminated sharps protocols.

Contraindications and Adverse Effects

Morphine has serious adverse effects and therefore should be administered cautiously to casualties with head injuries. Administration of morphine may cause increased intracranial pressure (ICP) and may induce vomiting. Administration of morphine causes constriction of the pupils and inhibits pupillary reactions. Using pupillary response for casualty assessment is therefore an unreliable parameter for the assessment of head injuries.

Although morphine is a powerful pain reliever, it can depress respirations. This rarely is a problem for those in severe pain, because the pain itself usually blocks the respiratory effect of the morphine. For casualties in less pain, the respiratory rate must be constantly monitored. Relative and absolute contraindications to the use of morphine include:

- Upper airway obstruction
- Burns to the respiratory tract
- Wounds to the throat, nasal passages, oral cavity, or jaw
- Bronchial asthma
- Significant chest injuries
- Altered mental status (morphine may cause mental confusion and may interfere with making a proper assessment)
- Shock (morphine is a peripheral vasodilator and therefore lowers the blood pressure, increasing the effects of shock)
- Known allergies to morphine (absolute contraindication)

Most soldiers who claim to have an allergy to morphine will either develop a rash or experience nausea, vomiting, and/or pruritis (itching) when morphine is administered. In combat, these soldiers can still take morphine. Early in the predeployment

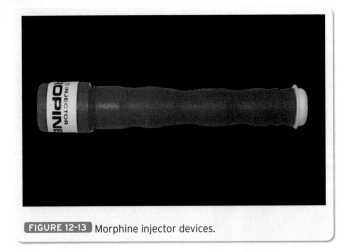

FIGURE 12-13   Morphine injector devices.

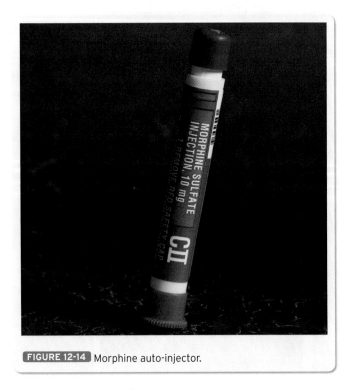

FIGURE 12-14   Morphine auto-injector.

process you need to identify soldiers who have had a previous **anaphylactic** reaction to morphine and have other injectable pain medications supplied for their use. The specific type of alternate medication to carry and administer will depend on the area of deployment and the decision of the battalion medical officer.

The side effects of morphine include:

- Sedation (morphine may cause considerable mental confusion and therefore should not be given to ambulatory casualties)
- Nausea, vomiting, and constipation
- Pruritis and skin flushing

Routes of Administration

Morphine comes in multiple strengths and may be administered in a variety of ways. In combat situations, the IV route is the preferred method of administration due to a more rapid pain relief response over the more traditional IM methods.

IV Morphine Dosage

Administer an initial dose of 5 mg IV via a slow IV push over 4 to 5 minutes. Morphine given by IV should be diluted in 5 mL of sterile water for injection or in normal saline (NaCl) prior to administration. When morphine is given intravenously, repeat doses may be given every 10 minutes. Most adults will experience pain relief at a total dose of 10 to 20 mg, although higher doses may be required. Document every dose given and the time given on the field medical card (FMC). Monitor the casualty closely for any adverse effects.

IM Morphine Dosage

Load the prefilled cartridge into the injector device (usually at a dose of 5 or 10 mg) FIGURE 12-13 ▲. If you are not giving the full 10-mg dose to the casualty, place the unused portion in another syringe (if possible) to utilize the full amount of morphine at a later time. In other words, never waste medical supplies if you don't have to. Select the appropriate site: deltoid muscle, buttocks, or outer thigh. Administer the injection to the casualty. Document the injection amount and the time given on the casualty's FMC. Monitor the casualty for adverse

reactions. Write the letter "M" and the time of the injection on the casualty's forehead.

Auto-Injectors

The US military also utilizes auto-injectors to administer morphine FIGURE 12-14 ▲. The dosage is usually 10 mg. Be aware that auto-injectors come in multiple strengths, so make certain that you always double-check the dosage on the auto-injector.

To administer the auto-injector, remove the safety cap. Press the colored end into the outer aspect of the casualty's thigh and press firmly. This will depress the black firing plunger, which causes a release of gas within the injector that drives the hypodermic needle through the protective cap and about an inch into the muscle. It also pushes 1 mL of the fluid, containing 10 mg of morphine, through the needle and into the muscle tissue. Document the injection and the time given on the casualty's FMC. Monitor the casualty for adverse reactions. Write the letter "M" and the time of the injection on the casualty's forehead.

Fentanyl (Actiq) Narcotic Lozenge

Indications

You may administer fentanyl:

- To casualties who are severely injured but alert/conscious
- For severe pain control
- For casualties with morphine allergies

Contraindications

Contraindications to administering fentanyl include allergy to the medication or any components. Exercise caution in giving to a casualty who has already been given morphine. Fenta-

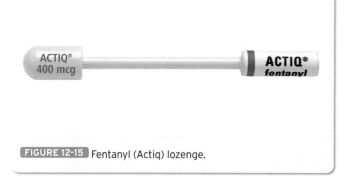

FIGURE 12-15 Fentanyl (Actiq) lozenge.

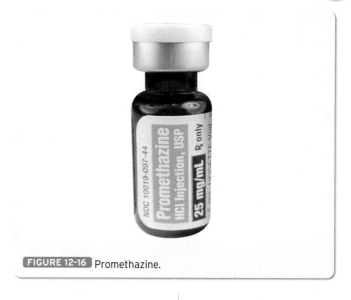

FIGURE 12-16 Promethazine.

nyl increases the chance of respiratory depression and other adverse side effects.

Route of Administration

The route of administration is the fentanyl (Actiq) lozenge on a handle **FIGURE 12-1 5 ▲**. Give 800 µg transbucally (via the mouth). It is recommended to tape the lozenge or handle to the casualty's finger to prevent choking. Reassess the casualty every 15 minutes. Monitor for respiratory depression.

Acetaminophen and Meloxicam

Indications

The analgesics meloxicam (Mobic) and acetaminophen (Tylenol) are used for mild to moderate pain in casualties still able to fight. These medications do not cause sedation.

Adverse Effects

Meloxicam can cause serious gastrointestinal issues if given in high doses. Acetaminophen can cause liver damage if given at high doses for an extended period of time.

Route of Administration

Give the casualty 15 mg of meloxicam by mouth daily. Give 650 mg of acetaminophen (two 325 mg caplets) by mouth every 8 hours. Document every dose given and the time given on the casualty's FMC.

■ Antiemetics

Promethazine (Phenergan)

Indications

Promethazine is used to combat nausea and vomiting associated with the administration of narcotic medications like morphine **FIGURE 12-16 ▶**.

Contraindications and Adverse Effects

The adverse effects of promethazine include:

- Sedation
- Disorientation
- Dizziness

Do not use in ambulatory casualties.

Route of Administration

When administering via IM or IV push, administer 25 or 50 mg. If the dose is given via IM, inject the medication deep into a large muscle mass. If the medication is given via IV, it should be given by a slow IV push (IVP) over 1 to 2 minutes. When administering the medication via IVP, dilute the medication with several mL of normal saline. Document every dose given and the time given on the casualty's FMC.

■ Narcotic Antagonist

Naloxone (Narcan)

Indications

Naloxone is given as a narcotic antagonist to morphine or fentanyl. Narcotics act on the central nervous system and may cause hypotension, bradycardia, and respiratory depression in excess amounts.

Contraindications and Adverse Effects

Naloxone has no absolute contraindications for administration and has minimal side effects. The adverse effects include:

- Nausea
- Vomiting
- Tachycardia

Route of Administration

Give 0.4 to 2 mg of naloxone via slow IVP over 1 to 2 minutes. It may need to be repeated three to four times. Some authorities recommend up to 10 to 20 mg to treat a suspected morphine overdose. An immediate positive response is usually seen when giving naloxone for morphine poisoning, and the duration of action is 1 to 2 hours. Naloxone's effect may wear off earlier than the morphine, permitting the casualty to lapse back into a respiratory depression. Continuous monitoring of a casualty being given naloxone to counteract morphine toxicity is crucial. After every dose of naloxone is given, thoroughly reassess the casualty. Naloxone should be adjusted according to the casualty's respiratory status, not his or her level of consciousness. Document every dose given and the time given on the casualty's FMC.

■ Antibiotics

Infection is a common cause of wound complications and death on the battlefield. It has been proven that early antibiotic prophylaxis in combat saves lives. It is your responsibility to understand the side effects and contraindications for all antibiotic medications that you administer. Both oral and IM/IV antibiotics will be used depending on the deployment and the casualty's injuries TABLE 12-3 ▸ . TABLE 12-4 ▾ lists the antibiotics commonly used on the battlefield. Keep in mind that this list changes often and will be updated by your medical officer.

Most soldiers who claim to have an allergy to antibiotics, especially penicillins, will either develop a rash or experience nausea and vomiting when given penicillin or a cephalosporin. In combat, these soldiers can still take antibiotics. The soldiers who have had a previous anaphylactic reaction to antibiotics are the soldiers to identify early in the deployment. The specific type of alternate antibiotic to give will depend on the area of deployment and the decision of the battalion medical officer.

■ Immunizations

Immunizations are administered to protect and maintain the health of the individual soldier and the population in which they live and work. Control or elimination of disease through an effective immunization program is essential to the accomplishment of a successful mission. As a combat medic, you will have a major impact on protecting soldiers and maintaining their readiness by maintaining immunization records and ensuring that all soldiers receive their immunizations.

TABLE 12-3 Advantages and Disadvantages of Antibiotic Administration Methods

	Oral Antibiotics	IM/IV Antibiotics
Advantages	• Easy to administer. • Allergic reactions are usually less severe.	• Faster absorption of medication.
Disadvantages	• Gastrointestinal upset. • Slow absorption through the GI tract.	• More difficult and time-consuming to administer. • Higher incidence of anaphylaxis. Have epinephrine available for treatment of anaphylaxis. • Once administered, it is impossible to recover the medication.

TABLE 12-4 Common Antibiotics

Antibiotic	Advantage	Disadvantage (concerns)	Route of Administration
Moxifloxacin (Avelox)	• For casualties who can take medications by mouth. • Recommended for casualties with open combat wounds.	• Do not use on casualties younger than 18. • Do not give to pregnant women.	• Give 400 mg (1 tablet) by mouth daily.
Cefotetan (Cefotan)		• Have epinephrine available. • Carefully document.	• PO: 400 mg once a day. • IV: 2 g slow IVP over 4 to 5 minutes. May be repeated at 12-hour intervals until evacuation. • IM: 2 g deep IM.
Ertapenem (Invanz)	• Provides greater broad-spectrum antibiotic coverage.	• Ensure you have medications available in case of an anaphylactic reaction. • Must be reconstituted with at least 50 cc of IV fluid prior to administration.	• IM: 1 g deep every 24 hours. • IV: 1 g daily.

Field Medical Care **TIPS**

Immunizations and chemoprophylaxis are key elements in protecting and maintaining the health of soldiers.

Principles and Classification of Vaccines

<u>Active immunity</u> is the protection produced by the person's own immune system that is usually permanent. The active immunity produced by vaccination is similar to that produced by acquiring the natural infection without the actual risk of disease. <u>Passive immunity</u> is the protection transferred from another person or animal via an antibody. An <u>antigen</u> is a live or inactivated substance (eg, protein, polysaccharide) capable of producing an immune response. An <u>antibody</u> is a protein molecule (immunoglobulin) produced to help eliminate an antigen. A general rule is: the closer a vaccine is to the natural disease, the more effective the immune response will be to the vaccine.

<u>Inactivated vaccines</u> use a form of the virus or bacteria that cannot replicate. They are generally not as effective as live vaccines and often require three to five doses. In addition, the antibody titer falls over time, thus requiring booster shot(s). Examples of inactivated vaccines include:

- **Viral:** polio (IPV), hepatitis A, rabies
- **Bacterial:** typhoid, cholera, plague

<u>Live (attenuated) vaccines</u> use the weakened form of the virus or bacteria. These vaccines must replicate to be effective. The immune response is similar to a natural infection. Live vaccines are usually effective with one dose. However, severe reactions are possible and the vaccine is unstable. Examples of live vaccine include:

- **Viral:** measles, mumps, rubella, vaccinia (smallpox), varicella (chicken pox), yellow fever, polio (OPV), influenza
- **Bacterial:** tuberculosis (Bacillus Calmette-Guerin [BCG]), typhoid (oral)

Personnel Subject to Immunizations and Required Shots

All active duty personnel are required to have current immunizations in order to be considered deployable. Medical exemptions can only be granted by a medical officer (MO). Immunizations include:

- Adenovirus
- Anthrax
- Cholera
- Hepatitis A
- Hepatitis B
- Influenza
- Japanese B encephalitis (JE)
- Measles, mumps, and rubella (MMR)
- Meningococcus
- Plague
- Polio
- Rabies
- Smallpox
- Tetanus-diphtheria
- Typhoid
- Yellow fever

Adenovirus

The vaccine for adenovirus is based on the likelihood of transmission. Adenovirus types 4 and 7 vaccines are administered orally on a one-time basis to recruits.

Anthrax

This vaccine is administered to persons 18 to 65 years of age with the potential for exposure to large amounts of *B anthracis* bacteria on the job, such as laboratory workers. The anthrax vaccine is also administered to deploying military personnel who may be at risk of anthrax exposure. If a dose is not given at the scheduled time, the series does not have to be started over. Simply resume the series as soon as practical. Full immunity requires six doses. The first three doses are given at 2 week intervals. Three additional doses are given, each one 6 months after the previous dose. Annual boosters are required for the vaccine to remain effective. Doses of the vaccine should not be administered on a compressed or accelerated schedule, for example, shorter intervals between doses or more doses than required.

Adverse events include localized injection site reactions: redness, pain, itching, or a lump at the injection site. Additional adverse events include muscle or joint aches, headaches, fatigue, chills, or nausea. Serious adverse reactions are rare. Contraindications include a previous allergic reaction or anyone who has a history of cutaneous (skin) anthrax. As a precaution, pregnant women should not be routinely vaccinated with anthrax. This is not an absolute contraindication in pregnant woman—refer to the medical officer for determination.

Cholera

The cholera vaccine is not administered routinely; it is only administered to military personnel upon travel or deployment to countries requiring cholera vaccination as a condition for entry. Adverse events include:

- Pain at injection site, mild systemic complaints, and temperature > 100.4°F
- Local reaction may be accompanied by fever, malaise, and headache
- Serious reactions, including neurologic reactions, after cholera vaccination are extremely rare

Hepatitis A

Hepatitis A vaccine is required for all deployments. Adverse events are rare. The dosage schedule is:

- First dose at least 4 weeks prior to deployment
- Second dose 6 to 12 months after the initial dose

Hepatitis B

The Hepatitis B is given to health care workers and soldiers. The dosage is a series of three injections. The second injection is given 30 days after the first. The third injection is given 6 months after the first shot. Adverse events include pain at the injection site, mild systemic complaints, and a temperature > 100.4°F.

Influenza

All active duty and reserve military personnel entering active duty for periods in excess of 30 days are immunized against influenza soon after entry on active duty. The vaccine is provided to all military personnel and all others considered being at high risk for influenza infection. The vaccine is provided annually beginning in October. Adverse events include local reactions, fever or malaise, severe allergic reactions (egg allergies), and neurologic reactions (rare).

Japanese B Encephalitis

The Japanese B encephalitis (JE) is required for the military during deployments and travel to endemic areas in Eastern Asia and the Western Pacific Islands. Common adverse events include fever, headache, myalgia, and malaise. Rare adverse events include general urticaria, angioedema, respiratory distress, and anaphylaxis.

Measles, Mumps, and Rubella (MMR)

Measles and rubella are administered to all recruits regardless of prior medical history. Mumps vaccine or MMR vaccine is administered to persons considered to be mumps susceptible. Written documentation of physician-diagnosed mumps or a documented history of prior receipt of the live virus mumps vaccine or MMR vaccine is adequate evidence of immunity. All military and civilian personnel engaged in the delivery of health care and having patient contact are appropriately immunized against measles, mumps, and rubella. Adverse events include low grade fever, parotitis (inflammation of the parotid gland located near the ear), rash, pruritis (mild), and deafness (rare).

Meningococcus

The meningococcal vaccine is administered on a one-time basis to recruits. This vaccine is given as soon as practical after in-processing. Adverse events are rare.

Plague

There are no requirements for routine immunization. The plague vaccine is administered to soldiers who are likely to be assigned to areas where the risk of endemic transmission or other exposure is high. The addition of antibiotic prophylaxis is recommended for such situations. The primary series consists of three doses of the plague vaccine. The first dose is followed by the second dose 4 weeks later. The third dose is administered 6 months after the first dose. Adverse events include general malaise; headache; fever; mild lymphadenopathy and/or erythema; and induration at the injection site.

Polio

A single dose of oral polio vaccine (OPV) is administered to all enlisted recruits. Officer candidates, ROTC cadets, and other reserve components on initial active duty for training receive a single dose of OPV unless prior booster immunization as an adult is documented. Booster doses of OPV are not routinely administered. Adverse events include paralytic poliomyelitis, which is more likely in immunodeficient persons. There is no procedure available for identifying persons at risk of paralytic disease and this disease is rarely vaccine induced. The live OPV is currently being phased out and being replaced with an injectable inactivated polio vaccine (IPV).

Rabies

The rabies vaccine is available preexposure and postexposure. In the preexposure series, the rabies vaccine is administered to personnel with a high risk of exposure (animal handlers; certain laboratory, field, and security personnel; and personnel frequently exposed to potentially rabid animals in a nonoccupational or recreational setting). In the postexposure series, the rabies vaccine and rabies immune globulin (RIG) administration are coordinated with appropriate medical authorities following current Advisory Committee on Immunization Practices (ACIP) recommendations. Adverse events include anaphylaxis, which is rare.

Smallpox

The smallpox vaccine is currently administered only under the authority of the Immunization Program for Biological Warfare Defense. Adverse events include becoming infected with the vaccinia virus. Patients may experience soreness, fatigue, fever, and body aches.

Tetanus-Diphtheria

A primary series of tetanus-diphtheria (Td) toxoid is initiated for all recruits lacking a reliable history of prior immunization. Individuals with previous history of Td immunization receive a booster dose upon entry to active duty and every 5 to 10 years thereafter. Adverse events include local reactions (erythema, induration) and a nodule at injection site. Fever and systemic symptoms are uncommon. There is a current hold on boosters for adults due to a shortage; however, in the event of an injury, the tetanus booster will be given if indicated.

Typhoid

The typhoid vaccine is administered to alert forces and personnel deploying to endemic areas. Either an oral or intramuscular (IM) vaccine is used. For the IM vaccine, one shot is administered with a booster every 2 years. With the oral vaccine, 4 tablets per day are given on days 0, 3, 5, and 7. With the oral vaccine, a booster is required every 5 years. Adverse events include local reactions which may be accompanied by fever, malaise, and headache; nausea and vomiting; abdominal cramps; skin rash; and urticaria (hives).

Yellow Fever

The yellow fever immunization is required for all alert forces, active duty personnel, or reserve components traveling to yellow fever endemic areas. The yellow fever vaccine is administered subcutaneously with a booster in 10 years. Adverse events include mild headache, myalgia, low grade fever, and other minor symptoms. Immediate hypersensitivity reactions include rash, urticaria, and asthma. These reactions are uncommon and occur periodically among people with a history of egg allergies.

Chemoprophylactic Requirements

Chemoprophylaxis is the use of a drug or a chemical to prevent a disease. The following diseases have historically been shown to be of military significance:

- Influenza
- Meningococcal diseases
- Leptospirosis
- Plague
- Scrub typhus
- Traveler's diarrhea
- Malaria
- Group A streptococcal disease

Comprehensive malaria prevention counseling includes mosquito avoidance and personal protective measures including clothing, repellents, bed netting, etc. Chemoprophylaxis is provided to military and civilian personnel considered to be at risk of contracting malaria. Specific chemoprophylactic regimens are determined by each of the services based on degree and length of exposure and the prevalence of drug resistance strains of *Plasmodia* in the area of travel.

Preadministration Screening

Preadminstration screening begins with a medical record screening. What immunizations are required for this individual? Routine immunizations are identified in AR 40-562 and in local policies. Additional requirements are specific for deployment and based on disease prevalence in specific geographic regions. These requirements are determined by the Preventive Medicine Unit using Federal, Department of Defense, and other relevant sources of information.

The current immunization status of the soldier needs to be determined. Ask:

- What has been given?
- When?
- Was the initial series completed?

If an immunization series has been started, and the time since the last dose is greater than the recommended interval for administration of the next dose, do not restart the series. Instead, give the next dose and inform the patient when he or she must return for the remainder of the series, if additional doses are required.

Determine if the soldier's boosters are current. What immunizations are needed, if any, to meet current deployment requirements? Does the patient's medical record reflect any contraindications for immunization?

It is your responsibility to ask the patient about any allergies, possible pregnancy, or current illness before administering the vaccine. Refer all patients with any risk factors to the MO for disposition.

Vaccine Handling, Administrative, and Patient Care Procedures

Vaccine Handling

Before administering any vaccinations, check expiration date and time. The yellow fever vaccine must be used within 1 hour after reconstitution. Any yellow fever vaccine not used within this time must be discarded. Evaluate the vaccine for potential mishandling or contamination.

Ensure that the vaccine is stored at the proper storage temperature. Refrigerated vaccines must be kept at 35.6°F to 46.4°F. Frozen vaccines must be kept at 0°F to 5°F or as directed by the manufacturer. Inspect the vaccine for evidence of bacterial growth. Inspect the vaccines for color change or clarity of the solution. Vaccines that are expired or show signs of contamination or mishandling will be discarded in accordance with (IAW) local standard operating procedure (SOP).

Some facilities authorize predrawing of vaccines to prepare for mass immunization. It is advisable not to predraw immunizations more than 4 hours before administration due to risk of bacterial growth and settling out of particles in the vaccine while in the syringe. If predrawing is allowed, make sure that filled syringes are stored within the proper temperature requirements for the specific vaccine.

After administering immunizations, store partially used vials at the proper temperature. Vaccines must be maintained at required temperature, even in a field environment. All live virus vaccine containers should be handled as infectious waste and disposed in biohazard containers to be burned, boiled, or autoclaved, following local SOP.

Administrative Procedures

Before administering vaccines, screen the medical records of the patients. Select the correct equipment (needles and syringes) for the immunizations to be administered.

Document the vaccine lot number and other identifying information as required by your local SOP.

After administering immunizations, document all vaccines given in the patient medical records (SF 601) IAW local SOP. In addition, record immunizations in the individual shot record (PHS 731). Record any patient adverse reactions or side effects.

Patient Care Procedures

Before administering vaccines, ask the patient about contraindications for immunization (allergies, pregnancy, illness, etc.). Implement appropriate infection control procedures. Explain the vaccine procedure to the patient. Position the patient and administer the required immunizations.

After administering immunizations, inform the patient when he or she is to return for the next injection in the series or for a booster. Instruct the patient to wait in facility for observation for 20 minutes or IAW local SOP. Ensure that the patient is evaluated during and at the end of the designated waiting period for signs of an adverse reaction.

Reactions and Possible Side Effects

Vaccine components can cause allergic reactions in some recipients. Prior to the administration of any immunizing agents, determine if the patient has previously shown any adverse reactions to a specific agent or vaccine component. The most common animal protein allergen is egg protein. Additional vaccine components that can cause reactions include:

- Vaccine antigen (a substance that causes the formation of an antibody)
- Animal proteins
- Antibiotics (eg, penicillin or penicillin derivatives)
- Preservatives (eg, thimerosal, a mercury compound)
- Stabilizers

Contraindications

A known pregnancy is a contraindication for all live virus vaccines. If a live virus vaccine is administered, counsel the woman to avoid becoming pregnant for 3 months and document this in the patient's health record. Ideally, all immunizations should precede pregnancy. Refer all pregnant soldiers to the MO for disposition. Refer all breastfeeding patients to the MO for disposition.

Patients should not be vaccinated if they have moderate or severe febrile illness (usually 101°F or higher, per local SOP). Patients should be vaccinated as soon as they recover from the acute phase of the illness. Minor illnesses, such as diarrhea, mild upper-respiratory infection with or without low grade fever, or other low grade febrile illness are not contraindicated to vaccination.

Due to the compromised immune system of patients with HIV-positive status, vaccines should not be administered, unless specifically ordered by the attending physician with knowledge of the patients' diagnosis.

Do not administer cholera, plague, and/or typhoid vaccines together unless the soldier is deploying immediately. Multiple live virus vaccines (OPV, yellow fever, measles, mumps, rubella, and adenovirus) may be given the same day. If they are not given the same day, then they must be separated by 30 days.

Gamma globulin (immune serum globulin) and MMR must be given at least 14 days apart. If these vaccines are administered closer together, then the MMR may be partially or completely ineffective in protecting against disease. If closer administration is unavoidable, then the MMR must be repeated after 3 months. Gamma globulin administration does not reduce the effectiveness of inactivated vaccines.

Field Medical Care TIPS

No more than one vaccine should be administered in any one anatomic site.

A tuberculosis (TB) test and live vaccines may be given the same day. If they are not given the same day, then the TB test must be deferred for 6 weeks after the live vaccine is given, to prevent a false negative result from the TB test.

If the soldier is receiving immediate predeployment immunizations, then local policy may authorize administration of a greater number of vaccines than routinely permitted, or combinations of vaccines that create increased risk of undesirable side effects. This should be the *exception* and not simply done for convenience.

Documentation

DHHS Form PHS 731 is prepared for each member of the Armed Forces and for nonmilitary personnel. It is a valid certificate of immunization for international travel and quarantine purposes. This form remains in the custody of the individual, who is responsible for its safekeeping and for keeping it in his or her possession when performing international travel. Entries based on prior official records have the following statement added: "Transcribed from official US Department of Defense records." This form is obtained through normal publication supply channels. The DOD immunization stamp is available through medical supply channels.

Issuance of DHHS Form PHS 731 to Military Personnel

At the time of initial immunization of a person entering military services, DHHS Form PH 731 and SF 601, *Health Records-Immunization Records*, are initiated. Written statements from civilian physicians attesting to patient immunization with approved vaccines, providing dates and dosages, are accepted as evidence of immunization. Such information is transcribed to the soldier's official records.

Army SF 601 is prepared in accordance with AR 40-66, *Medical Records and Quality Assurance Administration*. When prepared, SF 601 and DHHS Form 731 contain the soldier's social security number (SSN) as identifying data.

At the time of initial immunization of nonmilitary personnel, entries are made on DHHS Form PHS 731, which is retained by the individual. All subsequent immunizations are recorded on this form which can be presented as an official record of immunizations received. In addition to DHHS Form PHS 731, SF 601 is prepared and permanently maintained for each individual. Individuals preparing the DHHS Form PHS 731 and SF 601(600) ensure that appropriate entries are recorded on both forms and both forms are current and agree with one another.

■ Summary

The administration of medications requires strict attention to detail and an acute awareness of the effects certain medications can have. Administering medications by routes such as IM or IV in many ways is like firing a round downrange; once fired, you cannot recall it. Always review the five rights of medication administration before dispensing or administering any medication.

YOU ARE THE
COMBAT MEDIC

A landmine has exploded. The casualty was thrown clear and impacted the ground 50' away. The scene is as safe as possible. The casualty on the ground appears to be unconscious and unresponsive. The closest MTF is 25 minutes away from your location and the MEDEVAC is grounded due to incoming bad weather.

Assessment

Upon initial assessment of the casualty, you notice that he is unconscious and responsive to painful stimuli. His airway is patent, his breathing rate is 40 breaths/min, and his pulse is 130 beats/min. Exposing his wounds reveals an obvious abdominal evisceration. You cover the exposed organs with moist, sterile gauze to prevent further contamination and drying. Using normal saline IV fluid, you remoisten the gauze periodically to prevent them from drying out.

Treatment

You elect to establish an IV of normal saline (NS) and run it at a KVO (keep vein open) rate. You also have a standing order for administration of cefotetan. There are several dosing regimens for this medication. For IV administration, administer 2 g slow IV push over 3 to 5 minutes. While administering the medication, look for an allergic reaction and have epinephrine ready in case of a reaction. Once the casualty is stabilized, you transport him via ground vehicle to the MTF.

1. LAST NAME, FIRST NAME: Khan, Amir	RANK/GRADE: PFC	X MALE / FEMALE
SSN: 000-111-000	SPECIALTY CODE: 00A	RELIGION: Muslim

Injury: X WOUND. Level of consciousness: X PAIN RESPONSE. Pulse 130 bpm, Time 0400. Tourniquet: X NO. Morphine: X NO. IV: X, Time 0405.

9. TREATMENT/OBSERVATIONS: Abdominal evisceration. Thrown 50 feet by a landmine. Administered 2 g cefotetan via IV.

10. DISPOSITION: X EVACUATED, TIME 0415.
11. PROVIDER/UNIT: Michaels, Andrew

Aid Kit

Ready for Review

- As a combat medic, in combat or in remote peacekeeping operations, you may be responsible for administering medications.
- Pharmacology is the study of the properties (characteristics) and effects of drugs and medications on the body.
- Medications have been identified or derived from four major sources: plants (alkaloids, glycosides, gums, oils), animals and humans, minerals and mineral products, and chemical and synthetic substances made in the laboratory.
- Your medical officer can authorize you to administer certain medications under strict guidelines on the battlefield.
- Before administering any medication to a casualty, you must have a thorough understanding of how the medication will affect the human body—both negatively and positively. This includes familiarity with the medication's mechanism of action, indications, contraindications, route(s) of administration, dose, and antidotes for adverse reactions.
- Forms of solid and liquid oral medications include capsules, timed-release capsules, lozenges, pills, tablets, elixirs, emulsions, suspensions, and syrups.
- Parenteral routes used by the combat medic include subcutaneous, intramuscular, IV bolus, and IO. Of the parenteral drug routes, IV administration is the most common route used and generally is the quickest route for getting medication into the central circulation.
- Subcutaneous injections are given into the loose connective tissue between the dermis and the muscle layer.
- Intramuscular injections are made by penetrating a needle through the dermis and subcutaneous tissue into the muscle layer.
- Any fluid or medication that may be given through an IV line can also be given by the intraosseous route.

Vital Vocabulary

action The expected therapeutic effect of a medication on the body.

active immunity Protection produced by the person's own immune system that is usually permanent.

ampules Small glass containers that are sealed and the contents sterilized.

anaphylactic A severe hypersensitivity reaction that involves bronchoconstriction and cardiovascular collapse.

antibody Protein molecules (immunoglobulin) produced to help eliminate an antigen.

antigen A live or inactivated substance (eg, protein, polysaccharide) capable of producing an immune response.

aseptic technique A method of cleansing used to prevent contamination of a site when performing an invasive procedure, such as inserting an IV line.

bolus A term used to describe ìin one massî; in medication administration, a single dose given by the IV route; may be a small or large quantity of the medication.

chemoprophylaxis The use of a drug or a chemical to prevent a disease.

Combat Pill Pack Medications that soldiers bring into battle.

concentration The total weight of a medication contained in a specific volume of liquid.

contraindications Situations in which a medication should not be given because it would not help or may actually harm a casualty.

dose The amount of medication given on the basis of the casualty's size and age.

drug reconstitution Injecting sterile water (or saline) from one vial into another vial containing a powdered form of the drug.

drugs Chemical agents used in the diagnosis, treatment, and prevention of disease.

epinephrine Medication that increases heart rate and blood pressure but also eases breathing problems by decreasing the muscle tone of the bronchiole tree.

FAST1 device A sternal IO device used in adults; stands for First Access for Shock and Trauma.

generic name The original chemical name of a medication (in contrast with one of its trade names); not capitalized.

immunization Taking substances related to a biologic agent to develop resistance or antibodies in the body.

inactivated vaccines Produced from a form of the virus or bacteria that cannot replicate, they are generally not as effective as live vaccines and often require three to five doses and/or require booster shot(s).

indications Therapeutic uses for a specific medication.

intramuscular (IM) route Injection into a muscle; a medication delivery route.

intraosseous (IO) route Injection into the bone; a medication delivery route.

intravenous (IV) route Injection directly into a vein; a medication delivery route.

live (attenuated) vaccines Produced from a weakened form of the virus or bacteria that must replicate to be effective, they have an immune response similar to natural infection, are usually effective with one dose, can produce severe reactions, and are unstable.

metric system A decimal system based on tens for the measurement of length, weight, and volume.

parenteral Drug administration through any route other than the gastrointestinal tract; parenteral routes include intravenous, intramuscular, intraosseous, subcutaneous, transdermal, intrathecal, inhalation, intralingual, intradermal, and umbilical.

passive immunity Protection transferred from another person or animal via an antibody.

pharmacology The study of the properties and effects of medications.

side effects Any effects of a medication other than the desired ones.

subcutaneous (SC) injection Injection into the tissue between the skin and muscle; a medication delivery route.

trade name The brand name that a manufacturer gives a medication; capitalized.

vials Small glass bottles for medications; may contain single or multiple doses.

COMBAT MEDIC in Action

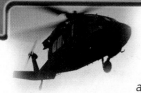

A blast injury leaves one casualty with an amputation injury to the right leg. After applying a tourniquet and stopping the bleeding, you ensure that the casualty's airway and breathing are patent and stable. The MEDEVAC is delayed and this casualty is in considerable pain. Your main focus now is giving the casualty morphine for pain relief. What are the effects of the morphine on the casualty? How much morphine will be given before transport? How will it be administered?

1. The side effects of morphine include all but:
   A. sedation.
   B. increased respirations.
   C. vomiting.
   D. skin flushing.

2. Morphine can be administered via:
   A. IV.
   B. IM.
   C. auto-injectors.
   D. all of the above.

3. The standard dose of morphine in an auto-injector is:
   A. 5 mg.
   B. 10 g.
   C. 5 g.
   D. 10 mg.

4. If the casualty is ambulatory, the best pain medication to administer is:
   A. morphine.
   B. acetaminophen.
   C. phenergan.
   D. naloxone.

5. Fentanyl is another pain medication option. It is administered via:
   A. lozenge.
   B. pill.
   C. auto-injector.
   D. IM.

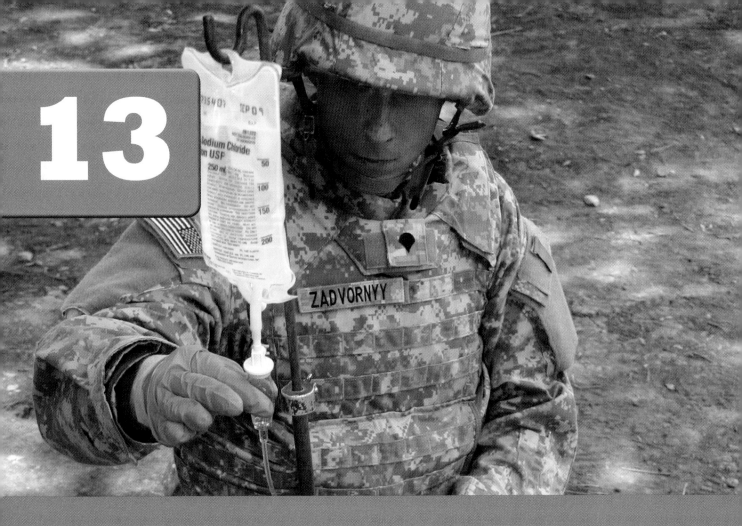

13

Intravenous Access

Objectives

Knowledge Objectives

- [ ] Identify indications for administering an intravenous (IV) infusion.
- [ ] Identify commonly used IV solutions.
- [ ] Calculate an IV drip rate.
- [ ] Identify common complications of IV therapy.

Skills Objectives

- [ ] Initiate an IV.
- [ ] Establish a saline lock.
- [ ] Manage an IV.
- [ ] Change IV tubing.

Introduction

Intravenous (IV) therapy is one of the most invasive procedures you will learn. To accomplish it successfully requires training and practice. Proficiency in IV therapy and technique is required for most procedures associated with advanced life support. A medical problem of any type alters an individual's established balance among the systems of the body.

This balance, called **homeostasis**, produces optimal physical performance. It is the job of the combat medic to fully assess a casualty's condition and to find and treat life-threatening injuries that alter homeostasis. As a combat medic, you will be the first line of defense for soldiers who need to have their homeostatic balance restored.

Basic Cell Physiology

A human cell can exist only in a special balanced environment. Understanding how this environment is created and maintained will give you the foundation you need to perform IV therapy.

Because cells are completely enclosed by cell membranes, compounds must move through the membranes to enter the cells. Small compounds such as water (H_2O), carbon dioxide (CO_2), hydrogen ions (H^+), and oxygen (O_2) can easily pass through cell membranes. Larger charged compounds need assistance to enter cells.

The cell membrane is a selective barrier. It chooses which compounds to allow across, depending on the needs of the particular cell. This **selective permeability** of the cell membrane is due to its composition FIGURE 13-1 ▾. The cell membrane is a **phospholipid bilayer**, that is, it has two parts:

- A **hydrophilic** outer layer made up of phosphate groups
- A **hydrophobic** inner layer made up of lipids or fatty acids

This bilayer is a very important barrier to fluid movement and is very important in maintaining acid-base balance. Everything discussed in this chapter will in some way be related to the cell membrane barrier and movement across it.

Electrolytes

Atoms carry charges—some positive, some negative. Two or more atoms that bond together form a molecule. When atoms bond together, they share and disperse their charges throughout the molecule. Molecules containing carbon atoms—for example, table sugar—are called organic molecules. Molecules created without carbon—for example, table salt—are called inorganic molecules. Inorganic molecules give rise to **electrolytes** when they disassociate in water into their charged components. For example, table salt disassociates into sodium and chloride.

Charged atoms and charged compounds are called electrolytes because of their ability to conduct electricity. Electrolytes, also called **ions**, are reactive and dangerous if left to circulate in the body, but the body uses the energy stored in these charged particles. Electrolytes help to regulate everything from water levels to cardiac function and muscle contractions. Water in the body helps to stabilize electrolyte charges so that the electrolytes can be used to perform the **metabolic** functions that are necessary to life.

Each electrolyte has a unique property or value to the body and is used in a different way. If the electrolyte has an overall positive charge, it is called a **cation**; an electrolyte with an overall negative charge is called an **anion**. The major cations of the body include sodium, potassium, and calcium; bicarbonate, chloride, and phosphorus are the major anions.

Sodium

Sodium is the principal extracellular cation needed to regulate the distribution of water throughout the body in the **intravascular** and **interstitial** fluid compartments, making it a major factor in adequate **cellular perfusion**. This gives rise to the saying, "Where sodium goes, water follows." Sodium is also a major component of the circulating **buffer**, sodium bicarbonate.

Potassium

About 98% of all the body's potassium is found inside the cells of the body, making it the principal intracellular cation. Potassium plays a major role in neuromuscular function as well as in the conversion of glucose into glycogen. Cellular potassium levels are regulated by insulin. The **sodium/potassium pump** is helped by the presence of insulin and **epinephrine**. Low potassium levels—**hypokalemia**—in the serum (blood plasma) can lead to decreased skeletal muscle function, gastrointestinal (GI) disturbances, and

FIGURE 13-1 The phospholipid bilayer.

alterations in cardiac function. High potassium levels in the serum—**hyperkalemia**—can lead to hyperstimulation of neural cell transmission, resulting in cardiac arrest.

Calcium

Calcium is the principal cation needed for bone growth. It plays an important part in the functioning of heart muscle, nerves, and cell membranes and is necessary for proper blood clotting.

Low serum calcium levels—**hypocalcemia**—can lead to overstimulation of nerve cells, resulting in the following signs and symptoms:

- Skeletal muscle cramps
- Abdominal cramps
- Wrist or foot spasms
- Hypotension
- Vasoconstriction

High serum calcium levels—**hypercalcemia**—can lead to decreased stimulation of nerve cells, resulting in the following signs and symptoms:

- Skeletal muscle weakness
- Lethargy
- **Ataxia**
- Vasodilation
- Hot, flushed skin

Bicarbonate

Bicarbonate levels are the determining factor between **acidosis** and **alkalosis** in the body. Sodium bicarbonate is the primary buffer used in all circulating body fluids.

Chloride

Chloride primarily regulates the **pH** of the stomach. It also regulates extracellular fluid levels.

Phosphorus

Phosphorus is an important component in the formation of adenosine triphosphate (ATP), the powerful energy supplier of the body.

Fluid and Electrolyte Movement

Water and electrolytes move among the body's fluid compartments according to some basic chemical and biologic tenets. One of these governing principles is that unequal concentrations on different sides of a cell membrane will move to balance themselves equally on both sides of the membrane. Balance across a cell membrane has two components:

- Balance of compounds (water, electrolytes, etc) on either side of the cell membrane
- Balance of charges (the one or two charges carried on the atoms) on either side of the cell membrane

When concentrations of charges or compounds are greater on one side of the cell membrane than on the other, a gradient is created. The natural tendency for materials is to flow from an area of higher concentration to one of lower concentration. This movement establishes a **concentration gradient**. Gradients are categorized according to the type of material that flows down them—chemical compounds flow down chemical gradients; electrical currents flow down electrical gradients. The process of flowing down a gradient depends on whether the cell membrane will allow the material to pass through it. Certain compounds can travel freely across the cell membrane, a kinetically favorable situation that requires little energy, whereas others require active transport across the membrane, either because of the size of the compound or because of an incompatible charge.

Diffusion

Compounds or charges concentrated on one side of a cell membrane will move across it to an area of lower concentration to balance themselves across the membrane, a process called **diffusion**. To visualize this, imagine that too many people show up for a theater performance. The management decides to open another seating area to accommodate the crowd. Patrons (charges or compounds) are concentrated in the small seating area (the cell) outside the door (the cell membrane) leading to the new seating area. When the theater manager opens the door, patrons can move through (selective cell membrane permeability) from the congested seating area (down a concentration gradient). The patrons spread themselves out evenly (diffuse) throughout the total area, some choosing to stay behind in the original seating area as others move into the new area, so that they all have an equal amount of room.

Filtration

Filtration is another type of diffusion, commonly used by the kidneys to clean blood. Water carries dissolved compounds across the cell membranes of the **tubules** of the kidney. The tubule membrane traps these dissolved compounds but lets the water pass through in much the same way that a coffee filter traps the grounds as water passes through it. This cleans the blood of wastes and removes the trapped compounds from circulation so they can be flushed out of the body. The **antidiuretic hormone (ADH)** prevents the loss of water from the kidneys by causing its reabsorption into the tubules. ADH plays an important role in **diabetes insipidus**.

Active Transport

Often, a cell must maintain an imbalance of compounds across its membrane to achieve some metabolic purpose. An example of such an imbalance is the sodium/potassium pump. Cells use sodium outside and potassium inside the cell for an important cellular function called **depolarization**. To maintain this imbalance, a cell must use energy in the form of ATP and actively transport compounds across its membrane. Even though active transport demands a high energy expenditure, the benefits outweigh the initial utilization of ATP. Pumping sodium out of a cell and potassium into a cell has the added benefit of moving glucose into a cell at the same time.

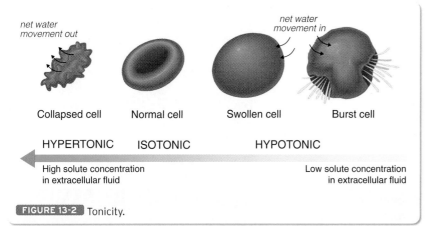

net water movement out

net water movement in

Collapsed cell   Normal cell   Swollen cell   Burst cell

HYPERTONIC   ISOTONIC   HYPOTONIC

High solute concentration in extracellular fluid

Low solute concentration in extracellular fluid

FIGURE 13-2 Tonicity.

Osmosis

Osmosis is the diffusion of water across a cell membrane. When molecules of solute are added to a solution, an equal number of molecules of solvent are displaced from the solution. For example, if 10 sodium ions are added to the fluid surrounding a cell, 10 molecules of water are displaced from that fluid. Therefore, the fluid surrounding the cell contains 10 fewer water molecules relative to the fluid within the cell. Water will diffuse down its concentration gradient to balance itself across the cell membrane. In this example, 5 water molecules will diffuse out of the cell into the surrounding fluid. Increasing the concentration of sodium in the surrounding (extracellular) fluid decreases the concentration of water in that fluid. Water diffuses out of the cell to create a balance of water molecules and to dilute the increased concentrations of sodium. Remember, where sodium goes, water follows.

The diffusion of water adds molecules to the extracellular compartment to create a balanced solution. This increased, yet balanced, volume puts pressure against the cell wall, called **osmotic pressure**. Osmotic pressure drives several important metabolic functions in the body, including cellular perfusion.

The effects of osmotic pressure on a cell are referred to as the **tonicity** of the solution **FIGURE 13-2 ▲** . Tonicity is related to the concentration of sodium in a solution and the movement of water in relation to the sodium levels inside and outside the cell:

- An **isotonic solution** has the same concentration of sodium as does the cell. In this case, water doesn't shift, and no change in cell shape occurs.
- A **hypertonic solution** has a greater concentration of sodium than does the cell. Water is drawn out of the cell, and the cell collapses from the increased extracellular osmotic pressure.
- A **hypotonic solution** has a lower concentration of sodium than does the cell. Water flows into the cell, causing it to swell and possibly burst from the increased intracellular osmotic pressure.

IV fluids introduced into the circulatory system can affect the tonicity of the extracellular fluid, resulting in dire consequences unless care is used.

Fluid Compartments

The body stores water in various locations called fluid compartments. The fluid compartments are defined by their relationship to cells—the water is either inside the cell (intracellular) or outside the cell (extracellular). Although water levels in these compartments constantly shift, homeostatic control mechanisms ensure that balance is restored whenever water is lost.

The body's circulatory (vascular) system functions as a fluid highway, but it also contains cells. Thus, it can be thought of as another fluid compartment. Blood cells contain intracellular water and are surrounded by extracellular water. To differentiate between these two cellular areas, the extracellular compartment is broken down into:

- **Intravascular:** The water portion of the circulatory system surrounding the blood cells (eg, in the heart, arteries, or veins)
- **Interstitial:** Water outside the vascular system and between surrounding cells (eg, between the membranes of two cells in muscle tissue)

In summary, there are three fluid compartments in the human body: intravascular (extracellular), interstitial (extracellular), and intracellular **FIGURE 13-3 ▼** . The fluids within these compartments account for 60% of total body weight.

Intracellular fluid (ICF) accounts for 40% of total body weight, or 75% of all fluid weight. ICF is within all the cells of the body. Large proteins within a cell can draw fluid into the cell because their overall negative charge attracts positively charged atoms like potassium, sodium, and the positive end of the water molecule (H_2O). The cell membrane prevents too many positively charged compounds, including water, from entering the cell and causing it to rupture. The sodium ions

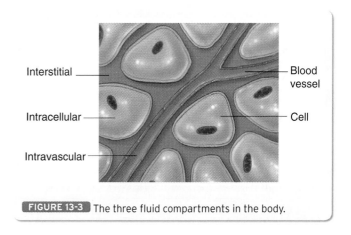

Interstitial

Intracellular

Intravascular

Blood vessel

Cell

FIGURE 13-3 The three fluid compartments in the body.

drawn into the cell are quickly removed via the sodium/potassium pump to prevent cellular **lysis**.

Extracellular fluid (ECF) occupies any area that is not inside the cells and equals 20% of total body weight, or 25% of all fluid weight. ECF compartments act as conduits for transferring gases and nutrients between the vascular and ICF compartments. ECF is found in the interstitial and intravascular compartments. ECF levels in the intravascular and interstitial compartments are regulated by the presence of sodium. Interstitial fluid accounts for 16% of total body weight and occupies the microscopic spaces between the cells. Interstitial fluid consists of a gel-type protein that helps disperse the water evenly throughout the interstitial compartment. This protein gel helps move water freely between the cells and vasculature. Intravascular fluid is also called plasma and accounts for 4% of total body weight.

Perfusion occurs in the capillaries as a result of high hydrostatic pressures and osmosis in the **capillary beds**. The high arterial capillary pressures (hydrostatic pressures) placed on the capillary beds push fluids from the vascular compartment into the interstitial compartment. Dissolved oxygen and nutrients are carried along with the fluids. The resulting shift of fluids from the vascular system creates a high concentration of blood proteins in the venous side of the capillary, which pulls fluid back into the capillary circulation via osmosis.

Fluid Balance

Several factors influence the balance between ICF and ECF. The balance among intracellular, intravascular, and interstitial compartments is dynamic. Changes always occur, and the body adjusts to these changes by retaining or eliminating water. Fluid levels in the body are balanced when intakes equal outputs. Daily intakes of water include fluid from liquid, food, and cellular metabolism; daily outputs occur from respiration and excretion of urine and feces. **TABLE 13-1 ▾** demonstrates how fluid levels are controlled in the body. Amounts shown are estimates for fluid intake versus fluid output.

The interstitial compartment is unique because it acts as a buffer between the other compartments. As fluid levels fluctuate between the intravascular and intracellular compartments, the interstitial compartment first responds by shifting fluid

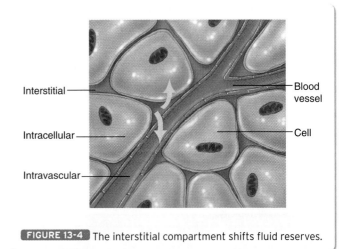

FIGURE 13-4 The interstitial compartment shifts fluid reserves.

reserves between the two compartments **FIGURE 13-4 ▴**. One clinical manifestation of a fluid imbalance is edema, which is defined as increased interstitial fluid levels.

Causes of edema include:

- Increased arterial capillary pressures that push fluid out into the tissues (heart failure and/or unmonitored IV lines are possible causes)
- Decreased production of circulating blood proteins created in the liver, as seen with advanced liver diseases and severe burns
- Increased capillary permeability associated with capillary-dilating compounds, such as histamines released during allergic reactions

■ Principles of Fluid Balance

The role of water in the body is diverse; it plays a part in both cellular metabolism and the maintenance of homeostasis. Without the presence of water in the body, people would quickly succumb to illness and disease, cellular function would cease, and body systems would shut down.

The role water plays in helping to maintain homeostasis is related to the size of the water molecule itself. Composed of only three atoms (two hydrogens and one oxygen), water has some unique properties **FIGURE 13-5 ▸**. Water is a polar molecule; that is, it has two positive poles (hydrogen) and a negative pole (oxygen). This property means that water can surround charged particles and stabilize their charges, allowing the particles to remain in solution. Water can also move across cell membranes easily, because it is a relatively small molecule.

Internal Environment of the Cell

The environment of the cells is one of water; some form of water surrounds all cells. Cells survive as long as this environment remains stable and is compatible with the life of the cell; any alteration in the supply of water, nutrients, oxygen, or food can lead to cellular death. Water exists both inside and outside of cells.

TABLE 13-1 Daily Fluid Balances			
Fluid Gains	Daily Intake (mL)	Fluid Losses	Daily Output (mL)
Actual fluid intake	500–1,700	Water vapor	850–1,200
Fluid from solid food	800–1,000	Urine	600–1,600
Metabolism	200–300	Feces	50–200
Totals	1,500–3,000	Totals	1,500–3,000

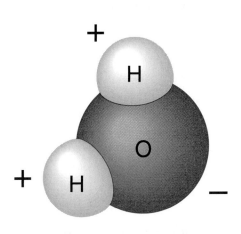

FIGURE 13-5 Water is a polar molecule with two positive poles and one negative pole.

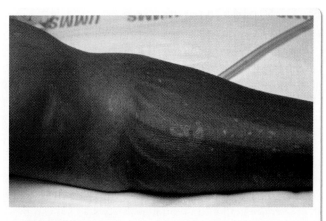

FIGURE 13-6 In an overhydrated casualty, fluid backup occurs and edema develops.

Homeostasis

Maintenance of the internal environment of a cell is regulated by elaborate systems of checks and balances. As systems in the body become imbalanced and begin to shift, feedback systems create an appropriate response to return the internal environment to normal. This normally balanced condition is referred to as homeostasis, or the resistance to change. These checks and balances can be seen in the way the body regulates blood glucose: too little circulating blood glucose and the feedback system responds to create glucose; too much circulating blood glucose and the feedback system responds to store the excess glucose. When disturbances in homeostasis occur as a result of water shifting within the body, certain conditions develop related to the type of shifting that occurs.

Dehydration

Dehydration is defined as depletion of the body's total systemic fluid volume. Dehydration is usually a chronic condition of the elderly or the very young and may take days to manifest. As fluid is lost from the vascular compartment, the body reacts by shifting interstitial fluid into the vascular area. This then forces a shift of fluid from the intracellular to the extracellular compartments. A total systemic fluid deficit results. Signs and symptoms of dehydration include:

- Decreased level of consciousness (LOC)
- **Postural hypotension**
- **Tachypnea**
- Dry mucous membranes
- **Tachycardia**
- Poor skin turgor
- Flushed, dry skin

Causes of dehydration include:

- Diarrhea
- Vomiting
- GI drainage

- Hemorrhage
- Insufficient fluid/food intake

Overhydration

When the body's total systemic fluid volume increases, overhydration occurs. Fluid fills the vascular compartment, filters into the interstitial compartment, and finally is forced from the engorged interstitial compartment into the intracellular compartment. Fluid backup occurs, and the casualty can succumb from these increased fluid levels **FIGURE 13-6**. Signs and symptoms of overhydration include:

- Shortness of breath
- Puffy eyelids
- Edema
- **Polyuria**
- Moist crackles (rales)
- Acute weight gain

Causes of overhydration include:

- Unmonitored IVs
- Kidney failure
- Prolonged hypoventilation

Body Fluid Composition

The fluids found in the body are composed of dissolved elements and water, a combination known as a solution. A solution is a mixture of two things:

- **Solvent:** The fluid that does the dissolving, or the solution that contains the dissolved components (in the body, the solvent is water)
- **Solute:** The dissolved particles contained in the solvent

A good example of making a solution is the process of brewing a cup of coffee. Passing hot water (solvent) over the coffee grounds leaches out the oils (the solute) to create the solution known as coffee. Remember, as the solute concentration increases, the solvent concentration decreases. Is a strong cup of coffee created by using less water (solvent) or by adding more coffee (solute)? Either one could be true, as they both end up creating stronger coffee.

■ IV Fluid Composition

IV solutions are tools designed to facilitate casualty treatment. The use of IV fluids can significantly alter the casualty's condition. It is critical that each bag of IV solution is sterile and safe; therefore, each bag of IV solution is individually sterilized. Compounds and ions dissolved in the solution are identical to the ones found in the body. Each solution is a concentration of solute and solvent.

Because sodium is the primary extracellular cation and regulates water levels in the body, it is used as the benchmark to calculate a solution's tonicity. The concentration of sodium in the cells of the body is approximately 0.9%. Altering the concentration of sodium in the IV solution can move the water into or out of any fluid compartment in the body. Remember, where sodium goes, water follows.

Types of IV Solutions

There are five basic types of IV solutions, each with a different tonicity and dissolved components: isotonic, hypotonic, hypertonic, crystalloid, and colloid. IV fluids use combinations of these five types of solutions to create the desired effects inside the body.

Isotonic Solutions

Isotonic solutions such as **normal saline (NS)** (0.9% sodium chloride) possess close to the same **osmolarity** as serum and other body fluids. Normal saline contains 90 g of sodium chloride per 100 mL of water. Because there is no alteration of serum osmolarity, the fluid stays inside the intravascular compartment. Isotonic solutions expand the contents of the intravascular compartment without shifting fluid to or from other compartments. Awareness of this fact is useful when dealing with hypotensive or hypovolemic casualties. Because this fluid remains in the vascular compartment, you must be careful to avoid fluid overloading. Casualties with hypertension and congestive heart failure are at greatest risk of fluid overload. The extra fluid increases the workload of the heart, creating fluid backup in the lungs.

Normal saline is the solution of choice for blood loss. It is the only solution to be used in conjunction with a blood transfusion. It is indicated for restoring the loss of body fluids.

Lactated Ringer's (LR) solution is generally used for casualties who have lost large amounts of blood. It contains the buffering compound lactate, which is metabolized in the liver to form bicarbonate—the key buffer that combats the intracellular acidosis associated with severe blood loss. This isotonic solution replaces electrolytes in amounts similarly found in plasma. It contains sodium chloride, potassium chloride, calcium chloride, and sodium lactate. The indications for LR include burns, dehydration, and supportive treatment of trauma. LR solution should not be given to casualties with liver problems because they cannot metabolize the lactate.

D$_5$W, 5% dextrose in water, is a special type of isotonic solution. As long as it remains in the bag, it is considered an isotonic solution. Once it is administered, the dextrose is quickly metabolized, and the solution becomes hypo-tonic. With this isotonic solution, the glucose is metabolized quickly, leaving a solution of dilute water. It contains 5 g of dextrose per 100 mL of water. The indications include calorie replacement and when glucose is needed for metabolism during hypoglycemia.

Hypotonic Solutions

A hypotonic fluid has an osmolarity less than that of serum, which means the fluid has less sodium ion concentration than serum. When this fluid is placed in the vascular compartment, it begins diluting the serum. Soon the serum osmolarity is less than the interstitial fluid; water is pulled from the vascular compartment into the interstitial fluid compartment and eventually the same process is repeated, pulling water from the interstitial compartment into the cells.

Hypotonic solutions hydrate the cells while depleting the vascular compartment. They are commonly used for hyperglycemic conditions such as diabetic ketoacidosis, in which high serum glucose levels draw fluid out of the cells and into the vascular and interstitial compartments. Hypotonic solutions can be dangerous to use because they can cause a sudden fluid shift from the intravascular space to the cells, causing cardiovascular collapse and increased intracranial pressure (ICP) from shifting fluid into the brain cells. For example, giving D$_5$W for an extended period can cause increased ICP. This makes hypotonic solutions dangerous to use with casualties experiencing any head trauma. Using hypotonic solutions on casualties with burns or trauma is also hazardous, because these casualties are at risk for developing **third spacing**, an abnormal fluid shift into the extracelluar fluid compartments.

Hypertonic Solutions

A hypertonic solution has an osmolarity higher than serum, which means the solution has more **ionic concentration** than serum and pulls fluid and electrolytes from the intracellular and interstitial compartments into the intravascular compartment. Hypertonic solutions shift body fluids into the vascular spaces and help stabilize blood pressure, increase urine output, and reduce edema. These fluids are rarely, if ever, used on the battlefield. Often, the term *hypertonic* refers to solutions that contain high concentrations of proteins. They have the same effect on fluid as sodium. Careful monitoring is needed to guard against fluid overloading when using hypertonic fluids, especially with casualties who suffer from impaired heart or kidney function. Also, hypertonic solutions should not be given to casualties with diabetic ketoacidosis or others at risk of cellular dehydration. Fluid movement across a cell membrane resulting from hypertonic, isotonic, and hypotonic solutions is shown in **FIGURE 13-7 ▶**.

Crystalloid Solutions

Crystalloid solutions are dissolved crystals (eg, salts or sugars) in water. They contain compounds that quickly disassociate in solution. The ability of these fluids to cross membranes and alter the various fluid levels makes them the best choice for the care of injured casualties who need fluid replacement for body fluid loss. Isotonic solutions will not cause a sig-

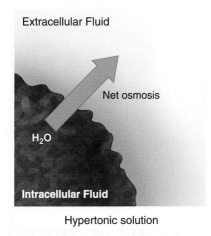 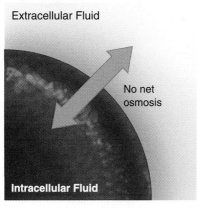 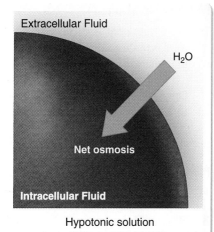

FIGURE 13-7 Fluid movement with hypertonic, isotonic, and hypotonic solutions.

nificant fluid or electrolyte shift, making them an excellent fluid replacement. When using an isotonic crystalloid for fluid replacement to support blood pressure from blood loss, remember the 3 to 1 replacement rule: 3 mL of isotonic crystalloid solution is needed to replace 1 mL of casualty blood. This amount is needed because approximately two thirds of the infused isotonic crystalloid solution will leave the vascular spaces in about 1 hour.

When replacing lost volume, it is imperative to remember that crystalloid solutions do not have the capability of carrying oxygen. Boluses of 20 mL/kg should be given to maintain perfusion (radial pulses), but not to raise blood pressure. Increasing blood pressure with IV solutions not only dilutes remaining blood volume, thereby decreasing the proportion of hemoglobin, but also may increase internal bleeding by interfering with hemostasis—the body's internal blood-clotting mechanism.

Hextend

Hextend is indicated in the treatment of hypovolemia when plasma volume expansion is desired. It is not a substitute for blood or plasma. Hextend is a formulation of 6% hetastarch combined with a physiologically balanced crystalloid carrier that more closely mirrors the plasma-electrolyte balance than 6% hetastarch in 0.9% sodium chloride does.

The hetastarch component creates oncotic pressure, which is normally provided by blood proteins, and permits retention of intravascular fluid. The crystalloid carrier provides electrolytes necessary for physiologic functions and has a composition resembling that of the principal ionic constituents of normal plasma. Hextend contains a normal physiologic level of calcium. It is the replacement fluid of choice to treat hypovolemia due to hemorrhage in the tactical environment.

Colloid Solutions

Colloid solutions contain molecules (usually proteins) that are too large to pass out of the capillary membranes and therefore remain in the vascular compartment. The very large protein

Field Medical Care TIPS

Colloids are not commonly given by the combat medic. These solutions are only given under the direct supervision of a doctor or physician's assistant.

molecules give colloid solutions a very high osmolarity. As a result, they draw fluid from the interstitial and intracellular compartments into the vascular compartments. Colloid solutions work very well in reducing edema (as in pulmonary or cerebral edema) while expanding the vascular compartment. These fluids could cause dramatic fluid shifts and place the casualty in considerable danger if they are not administered in a controlled setting. Examples of colloids are:

- Albumin
- Steroids
- Whole blood and blood products
- Packed red blood cells
- Fresh frozen plasma
- Plasma protein fraction
- Dextran
- Hetastarch

■ IV Techniques and Administration

Indications for Administering an Intravenous Infusion

The indications for an intravenous infusion include:

- Dehydration when oral replacement is inadequate or impossible
- To replace blood and blood products
- To maintain or replace electrolytes
- To administer medications and dilute poisons in the blood
- To provide a source of nutrients
- To administer water-soluble vitamins

IV Administration

The most important point to remember about IV techniques and fluid administration is to keep the IV equipment sterile. Forethought will help prevent mental and procedural errors while starting the IV.

One way to ensure proper technique is to develop a routine to follow as you assemble the appropriate equipment. A routine will help you keep track of your equipment and the steps necessary to complete a successful IV.

Assembling Your Equipment

To avoid delays or the possibility of IV site contamination, gather and prepare all your equipment before you attempt to start an IV. TABLE 13-2 ▾ shows a logical sequence of steps in assembling your equipment; each will be described in this chapter.

TABLE 13-2 Steps in Assembling IV Equipment

1. Always wear gloves! BSI precautions cannot be emphasized strongly enough.
2. Check the solution for clarity and the expiration date and to ensure it is the correct one.
3. Choose an administration set appropriate for the needs of the casualty.
4. Choose an appropriate IV site.
5. Choose an appropriately sized catheter.
6. Recheck your work before you go any further.
7. Tear tape for securing the IV site.
8. Have a couple of catheters ready for insertion.
9. Open an alcohol wipe.
10. Have 4″ × 4″ gauze pads ready for catching blood.
11. Then, and only then, apply a constricting band. (It is the last thing done before inserting the IV.)
12. Insert the catheter.
13. Hook up the IV tubing and adjust the flow.
14. Secure the site.
15. Adequately dispose of sharps.
16. Document every procedure.

Field Medical Care TIPS

Helpful IV Hints
- Allow the hand or arm to hang.
- Pat or rub the area.
- Apply chemical hot packs.
- If you meet resistance from a valve, elevate the extremity.
- Try sticking without the tourniquet if the vein keeps infiltrating.
- Never pull the catheter back over or through the needle.
- The more IVs you perform, the more proficient you will become.

IV Solution

Each IV solution bag is wrapped in a protective sterile plastic bag and is guaranteed to remain sterile until the posted expiration date. Once the protective wrap is torn and removed, the IV solution has a shelf life of 24 hours. The bottom of each IV bag has two ports: an injection port for medication and an access port for connecting the administration set. A removable pigtail that represents a point-of-no-return line protects the sterile **access port**. Once this pigtail is removed, the bag must be used immediately or discarded.

IV solution bags come in different fluid volumes FIGURE 13-8 ▾ . Volumes commonly used are 1,000 mL, 500 mL, 250 mL, and 100 mL; the more common volumes are 1,000 mL and 500 mL. The smaller volumes (250 mL and 100 mL) more commonly contain D_5W and are used for mixing and administering medication via IV **piggyback administration**.

Choosing an Administration Set

An administration set moves fluid from the IV bag into the casualty's vascular system. As with IV solution bags, IV administration sets are sterile as long as they remain in their protective packaging. Once they are removed from the packaging, their sterility cannot be guaranteed. Each IV administration set has a piercing spike protected by a plastic cover. Again, once the piercing spike is exposed and the seal surrounding the cap is broken, the set must be used immediately or discarded.

There are different sizes of administration sets for different situations and casualties. Most **drip sets** have a number visible on the package FIGURE 13-9 ▸ , which indicates the number of drops it takes for a milliliter of fluid to pass through the orifice and into the **drip chamber**. Drip sets come in two primary sizes: microdrip and macrodrip. **Micro-**

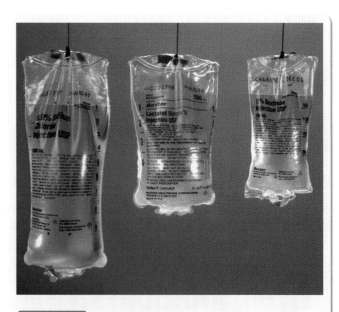

FIGURE 13-8 IV solution bags come in different fluid volumes.

drip sets allow 60 **gtt** (drops)/mL through the small, needle-like orifice inside the drip chamber. Microdrips are ideal for medication administration because it is easy to control their fluid flow. **Macrodrip sets** allow 10 to 15 gtt/mL through a large opening between the piercing spike and the drip chamber. Macrodrip sets are best used for rapid fluid replacement.

A blood set is a special type of macrodrip set designed to facilitate rapid fluid replacement by manual infusion of either multiple IV bags or IV/blood replacement combinations. Most blood sets have dual piercing spikes that allow two bags of fluid to be hung at once on the same casualty FIGURE 13-10 ▾. The central drip chamber has a special filter designed to filter the blood during transfusions.

Choosing a Catheter

A **catheter** is a hollow, laser-sharpened needle inside a hollow plastic tube inserted into a vein to keep the vein open FIGURE 13-11 ▸. The most common types of catheters are butterfly catheters and over-the-needle catheters FIGURE 13-12 ▾. Catheter selection should reflect the need for the IV, the age of the casualty, and the location for the IV.

Catheters are sized by their diameter and referred to by the gauge of the catheter. The larger the diameter of the catheter, the smaller the gauge. Thus, a 14-gauge catheter has a greater diameter than a 22-gauge catheter. The larger the diameter, the more fluid can be delivered through the catheter.

Select the largest-diameter catheter that will fit the vein you have chosen or that will be the most appropriate and comfortable for the casualty. A good rule of thumb to follow is: The more distal the IV site, the smaller the catheter. An 18-gauge catheter is usually a good size for adult casualties who do not need fluid replacement. Metacarpal veins of the hand accommodate 18- to 20-gauge catheters; antecubital veins of the upper arm can accommodate larger 16- to 14-gauge catheters.

Butterfly catheters derive their name from the plastic tabs attached to the sides of the needle. These allow for a stable anchoring platform.

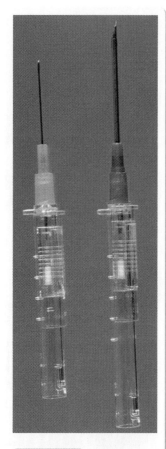

FIGURE 13-11 A catheter is a hollow tube that is inserted into a vein to keep the vein open, allowing a passageway into the vein.

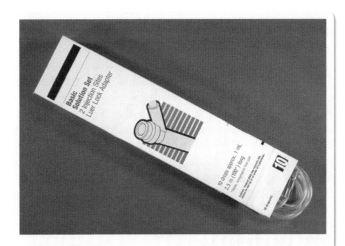

FIGURE 13-9 The number visible on the drip set refers to the number of drops it takes for a milliliter of fluid to pass through the orifice and into the drip chamber.

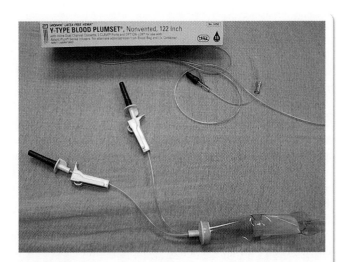

FIGURE 13-10 Most blood sets have dual piercing spikes that allow two bags of fluid to be hung at once on the same casualty.

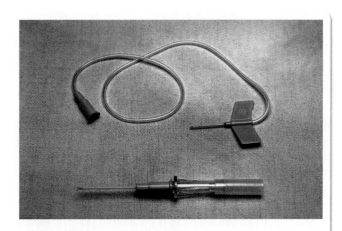

FIGURE 13-12 The most common types of catheters are butterfly catheters and over-the-needle catheters.

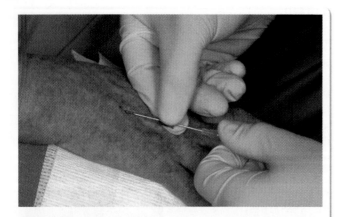

FIGURE 13-13 The over-the-needle sheath slides off the needle during cannulation and remains inside the vein to keep the vein open.

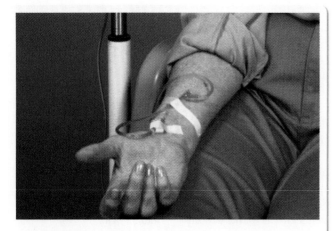

FIGURE 13-14 A cannulated artery can be recognized by the bright red blood quickly seen through the IV tubing due to the pressure that exists in the arteries.

Over-the-needle catheters (angiocaths) can be used for all adults for long-term IV therapy **FIGURE 13-13 ▲**. The plastic catheter allows for greater casualty movement and often does not require immobilizing the entire limb. Over-the-needle catheters come in different gauges as well as in different lengths. The most common lengths are 2½″ and 1¼″. The shorter the catheter, the more fluid can flow through it.

In recent years, an attempt has been made to create over-the-needle catheters that minimize the risk of a contaminated stick. A contaminated stick occurs if you puncture your skin with the same catheter that was used to cannulate the vein of a casualty. Newer over-the-needle catheters use several different methods to protect you from the possibility of a contaminated stick. One of the more common methods is automatic needle retraction after insertion, usually accomplished with a locking slide mechanism or a spring-loaded slide mechanism.

Occasionally, **cannulation** of an artery occurs. Cannulation of an artery is easily recognized because bright red blood is quickly seen in the IV tubing and the IV bag because of the high pressure that exists in the arteries **FIGURE 13-14 ▲**. If

cannulation of an artery occurs, you must stop the IV, remove the catheter, and apply direct pressure to the site until any bleeding is controlled.

Preparing an Administration Set

After choosing the IV administration set and the IV solution bag, verify the expiration date of the solution and check for the solution clarity or leaks. Prepare to spike the bag with the administration set. Remove the infusion set from the box and inspect for any holes, cracks, or other signs of defects. Tighten the clamp 6″ to 8″ below the drip chamber. Inspect the catheter for barbs or nicks. Loosen the catheter by rotating the catheter at the hub. Discard in a sharps container if flawed.

Remove the protective covers from the spike of the drip chamber and from the outlet (long spout) of the IV container without contaminating them. Insert the spike into the container. If using a bag, push the spike firmly into the container's outlet tube. If using a bottle, push the spike firmly through the container's diaphragm. Hang the container at least 2′ above the level of the casualty's heart if possible and squeeze the drip chamber until it is half full of solution.

Remove air from the IV tubing by holding the end of the tubing above the level of the bottom of the IV container. Loosen the protective cover on the needle adapter to allow air to escape. Release the clamp on the IV tubing. Gradually lower the tubing until the solution reaches the end of the needle adapter. If small air bubbles remain in the tubing, tap the IV tubing with your finger from the bottom to the top allowing air bubbles to rise. Then clamp the IV tubing, retighten the protective cover, and loop the IV tubing over the IV stand.

Select the Infusion Site

Choose the most distal and accessible vein of an uninjured arm or hand. Avoid veins that are infected. Also avoid injured and irritated areas. Use the lower extremities only if there is no accessible site in the upper extremity. Avoid sites over joints because the catheter is difficult to stabilize. Dislodgement and infiltration can occur and flow may increase or decrease with joint movement. Use the nondominant hand or arm, whenever possible. Select a vein large enough to accommodate the size of the needle or catheter to be used.

Prepare the Infusion Site

Apply a constricting band to the casualty, about 2″ above the venipuncture site, tight enough to stop venous flow but not so tight that the radial pulse cannot be felt. Do not leave the constricting band in place for more than 2 minutes. Instruct the casualty to open and close his or her fist several times to increase circulation.

Select and palpate a prominent vein. Clean the casualty's skin with an antiseptic sponge (betadine and/or alcohol) in a circular motion from the center outward. If the casualty is allergic to betadine, only use the alcohol pad. Put on sterile gloves to protect yourself against bloodborne pathogens.

Prepare to Pierce the Skin

Hold the catheter with your dominant hand and remove the protective cover without contaminating the needle. Hold the **flash chamber** with your thumb and forefinger directly above the vein or slightly to one side of the vein. Draw the skin below the cleaned area downward to hold the skin taut over the site of venipuncture with your nondominant hand.

Pierce the Skin

Position the needle point, bevel-up, parallel to the vein and about ½″ below the site of venipuncture. Hold the needle at approximately a 20° to 30° angle and pierce the skin. Ensure that the thumb holding the skin taut does not contaminate the catheter or the cleansed skin area. Decrease the angle until almost parallel to skin surface and direct the needle point toward the vein. Continue advancing until the vein wall is pierced. A faint "give" will be felt as the vein wall is pierced, but do not assume you are in the vein wall by feeling the give.

Always check the flash chamber for blood. If blood is not noted in the flash chamber, pull the needle back slightly (but not above skin surface) and attempt to redirect the needle point into the vein. If still unsuccessful, release the constricting band, withdraw the catheter, and use the alcohol swab or sterile gauze to put pressure on the site. If possible, notify your supervisor before attempting a venipuncture at another site.

If you were successful, advance the needle approximately ⅛″ further to ensure the catheter is in the vein. Stabilize the flash chamber with your dominant hand, grasp the catheter hub with your nondominant hand, and thread the catheter into the vein to the catheter hub. Press lightly on the skin over the catheter tip to decrease or stop the blood flow from the catheter hub after the needle is removed.

Remove the flash chamber or needle. Dispose of the needle properly in a sharps container as soon as possible. Never reinsert a stylet needle into a catheter; a portion of the catheter sheath could be sheared off causing an embolus. With your dominant hand, remove the protective cover from the needle adapter on the tubing and quickly connect the adapter into the catheter hub, while maintaining stabilization of the catheter hub with your nondominant hand.

Tell the casualty to unclench his or her fist and then you can release the constricting band. If the constricting band is not released, the casualty will bleed excessively when the needle is removed.

Unclamp the IV tubing and adjust the flow to appropriate drip rate (TKO or per doctor's orders). Maintain at a flow rate of 30 mL/hour. Examine the infusion site for infiltration and discontinue if it is present.

Secure the Site

Clean the area of blood, if necessary, and secure the hub of the catheter with tape, leaving the catheter hub and the tubing connection visible. Do not release your hold on the catheter hub or the catheter connection until it is secured with at least one piece of tape. Apply a sterile dressing over the puncture site or in accordance with (IAW) local standard operating procedure. Loop the IV tubing on the extremity and secure with tape. Splint the arm loosely on a padded splint, if necessary, to reduce movement. The insertion site and catheter hub should always be accessible. Do not splint so tightly to occlude venous flow. Recheck and adjust the flow rate to doctor's orders.

Prepare and place the appropriate labels. Print the date, gauge of the catheter, time the IV was started, and initials of the person initiating the IV on a piece of tape and secure it to the dressing. Print the casualty's identification, drip rate, date, time the IV infusion was initiated, and the initials of the person initiating the IV on another piece of tape and secure it to the IV container. Print the date and time the tubing was put in place and the initials of the person initiating the IV on a third piece of tape and wrap the tape around the tubing, leaving a tab. Re-examine the site for infiltration. Remove your gloves and perform a casualty care handwash. Record the procedure on the appropriate form.

Initiate an Intravenous Infusion

To initiate an intravenous infusion, perform **SKILL DRILL 13-1 ▶**:

1. Obtain a physician's order.
2. Wash your hands.
3. Gather your equipment.
4. Identify the casualty and explain the procedure. Ask about any allergies.
5. Inspect and assemble the equipment.
6. Hang the container at least 2′ above the level of the casualty's heart and squeeze the drip chamber until it is half full of solution (**Step ①**).
7. Remove the air from the IV tubing.
8. Cut several tape strips and hang them in an accessible location (**Step ②**).
9. Select the infusion site.
10. Prepare the infusion site. Apply a constricting band 2″ above the venipuncture site—tight enough to stop venous flow, but not so tight that the radial pulse cannot be felt. Instruct the casualty to open and close his or her fist several times to increase circulation. Select and palpate a prominent vein. Clean the skin with an antiseptic sponge in a circular motion from the center outward (**Step ③**).
11. Put on sterile gloves.
12. Hold the catheter with your dominant hand and remove the protective cover without contaminating the needle.
13. Hold the flash chamber with your thumb and forefinger directly above the vein or slightly to the side of the vein (**Step ④**).
14. Draw the skin below the cleansed area downward to hold the skin taut over the site of the venipuncture.
15. Position the needle point, bevel up, parallel to the vein and about ½″ below the venipuncture site.

16. Hold the needle at approximately a 20° to 30° angle and pierce the skin.

17. Decrease the angle until the needle is almost parallel to the skin surface and direct it toward the vein.

18. Continue advancing the needle until the vein is pierced.

19. Check for blood in the flash chamber.

20. Advance the needle approximately ⅛″ further to ensure the proper catheter placement in the vein (**Step 5**).

21. Stabilize the flash chamber with your dominant hand, grasp the catheter hub with your nondominant hand, and thread the catheter into the vein to the catheter hub.

22. Remove the flash chamber or needle and lay it aside.

23. With your dominant hand, remove the protective cover from the needle adapter on the IV tubing and quickly connect the adapter into the catheter hub, while maintaining stabilization of the hub with your nondominant hand (**Step 6**).

24. Tell the casualty to unclench his or her fist and then you can release the constricting band.

25. Unclamp the IV tubing and adjust the flow rate to the appropriate drip rate.

26. Examine the infusion site for infiltration and discontinue if infiltration is present.

27. Clean the area of blood, if necessary, and secure the hub of the catheter with tape, leaving the hub and tubing connection visible (**Step 7**).

28. Apply a sterile dressing over the puncture site.

29. Loop the IV tubing on the extremity and secure it with tape.

30. Splint the arm loosely on a padded splint, if necessary, to reduce movement.

31. Print the date, gauge of the catheter, time the IV was started, and initials of the person starting the IV on a piece of tape. Secure the tape to the dressing.

32. Print the casualty's identification, drip rate, date and time the IV infusion was initiated, and the person initiating the IV on another piece of tape. Secure the tape to the IV container.

33. Print the date and time the tubing was put in place and the initials of the person initiating the IV on a third piece of tape and wrap the tape around the tubing, leaving a tab.

34. Re-examine the IV site for infiltration.

35. Remove gloves and perform a casualty care handwash.

36. Record the procedure on the appropriate form (**Step 8**).

Saline Locks

<u>Saline locks</u> (buff caps, Hep-locks, INTs) are a way to maintain an active IV site without having to run fluids through the vein. These access devices are used primarily for casualties who do not need additional fluids but may need rapid medication delivery. Saline locks are access ports commonly used with casualties who have disorders such as congestive heart failure (CHF) or pulmonary edema. A saline lock is attached to the end of an IV catheter and filled with approximately 2 mL of normal saline to keep blood from clotting at the end of the catheter **FIGURE 13-15**. Because this is a sealed-access site, the saline remains in the port without entering the vein, thus preventing clotting. These are also known as intermittent or INT sites because they eliminate the need to completely reestablish an IV each time the casualty needs medication or fluid. When the saline lock is not being used at regular intervals for medication administration, it must be flushed to maintain patency.

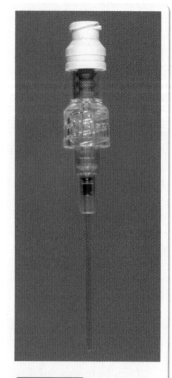

FIGURE 13-15 A saline lock is attached to the end of an IV catheter and filled with approximately 2 mL of normal saline in order to keep blood from clotting at the end of the catheter.

The advantages of the saline lock include:

- Maintains IV access
- Eliminates administration of unneeded IV fluids
- Prevents the need for new venipuncture each time medication is to be given

The equipment needed to perform a saline lock includes:

- IV catheter
- Saline lock adapter plug
- Syringe filled with 5 cc sterile saline for flush
- Alcohol wipes

To establish a saline lock with an existing IV, follow the steps in **SKILL DRILL 13-2**:

1. Verify the physician's order.

2. Gather your equipment.

3. Identify the casualty and explain the procedure.

4. Perform a casualty care handwash and put on sterile gloves.

Initiate an Intravenous Infusion

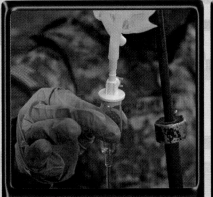

1 Obtain a physician's order. Wash your hands. Gather your equipment. Identify the casualty and explain the procedure. Ask about any casualty allergies. Inspect and assemble the equipment. Hang the container at least 2′ above the level of the casualty's heart and squeeze the drip chamber until it is half full of solution.

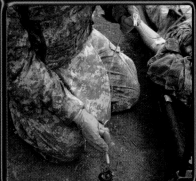

2 Remove the air from the IV tubing. Cut several tape strips and hang them in an accessible location.

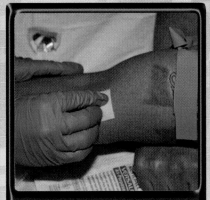

3 Select the infusion site. Prepare the infusion site. Apply a constricting band 2″ above the venipuncture site. Instruct the casualty to open and close his or her fist several times to increase circulation. Select and palpate a prominent vein. Clean the skin with an antiseptic sponge in a circular motion from the center outward.

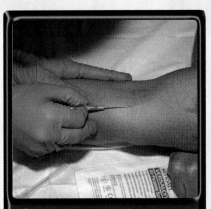

4 Put on gloves. Hold the catheter with your dominant hand and remove the protective cover without contaminating the needle. Hold the flash chamber with your thumb and forefinger directly above the vein or slightly to the side of the vein.

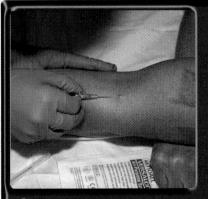

5 Draw the skin below the cleansed area downward to hold it taut over the site of the venipuncture. Position the needle point, bevel up, parallel to the vein and about ½″ below the venipuncture site. Hold the needle at approximately a 20° to 30° angle and pierce the skin. Decrease the angle until almost parallel to the skin surface and direct it toward the vein. Continue advancing the needle until the vein is pierced. Check for blood in the flash chamber. Advance the needle approximately ⅛″ further to ensure catheter placement in the vein.

(continues)

Initiate an Intravenous Infusion (*continued*)

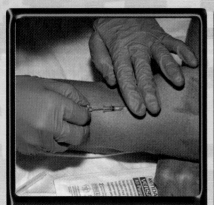

6 Stabilize the flash chamber with your dominant hand, grasp the catheter hub with your nondominant hand, and thread the catheter into the vein to the catheter hub. Remove the flash chamber or needle and set aside. With your dominant hand, remove the protective cover from the needle adapter on the IV tubing and quickly connect the adapter to the catheter hub, while maintaining stabilization of the hub with your nondominant hand.

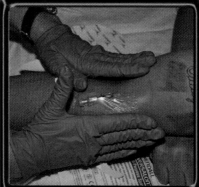

7 Tell the casualty to unclench his or her fist and then you can release the constricting band. Unclamp the IV tubing and adjust the flow rate to the appropriate drip rate. Examine the infusion site for infiltration and discontinue if infiltration is present. Clean the area of blood, if necessary, and secure the hub of the catheter with tape, leaving the hub and tubing connection visible.

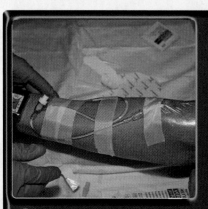

8 Apply a sterile dressing over the puncture site. Loop the IV tubing on the extremity and secure with tape. Splint the arm loosely on a padded splint, if necessary, to reduce movement. Print the date, gauge of the catheter, time IV was started, and initials of the person starting the IV on a piece of tape. Secure the tape to the dressing. Print the casualty's identification, drip rate, date and time the IV infusion was initiated, and the person initiating the IV on another piece of tape. Secure the tape to the IV container. Print the date and time the tubing was put in place and the initials of the person initiating the IV on a third piece of tape and wrap the tape around the tubing, leaving a tab. Re-examine the IV site for infiltration. Remove gloves and perform a casualty care handwash. Record the procedure on the appropriate form.

5. Clean the junction of the tubing and the IV catheter using an alcohol wipe (**Step ①**).

6. Close the roller clamp on the IV tubing to stop the flow (**Step ②**).

7. Loosen the tubing from the hub of the catheter (**Step ③**).

8. Using aseptic technique, quickly remove the tubing from the catheter and connect the adapter plug to the hub (**Step ④**).

9. Clean the rubber diaphragm on the adapter plug (**Step ⑤**).

10. Uncap the needle of the saline syringe and insert it into the rubber diaphragm (**Step ⑥**).

11. Aspirate the syringe to check for blood return.

12. Inject 1 to 5 cc of saline into the lock.

13. Secure the site and cover with a dressing (**Step ⑦**).

■ Calculate an IV Flow Rate

One task you will do in the garrison is determine the flow rate for an intravenous infusion. You must be able to obtain the required information and perform the calculations to keep the IV infusion at the correct rate in order to maintain a safe fluid balance for your patient. The information required to determine the flow rate is:

• Total volume to be infused
• Time period over which it is to be infused

The properties of the administration set (how many drops/mL it delivers) are found on the box containing the administration set.

SKILL DRILL 13-2

Perform a Saline Lock

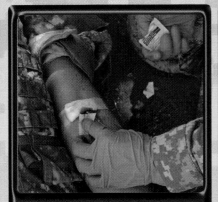

1 Verify the physician's order. Gather your equipment. Identify the casualty and explain the procedure. Perform a casualty care handwash and put on sterile gloves. Clean the junction of the tubing and the IV catheter using an alcohol wipe.

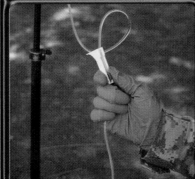

2 Close the roller clamp on the IV tubing to stop the flow.

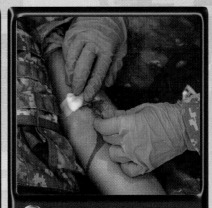

3 Loosen the tubing from the hub of the catheter.

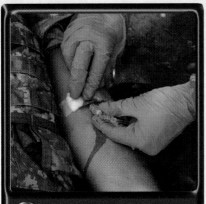

4 Using aseptic technique, quickly remove the tubing from the catheter and connect the adapter plug to the hub.

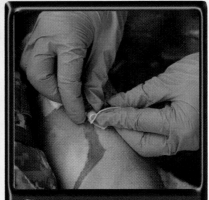

5 Clean the rubber diaphragm on the adapter plug.

(continues)

SKILL DRILL 13-2

Perform a Saline Lock (continued)

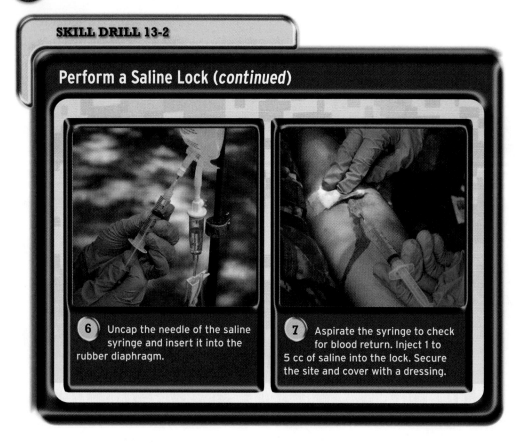

6 Uncap the needle of the saline syringe and insert it into the rubber diaphragm.

7 Aspirate the syringe to check for blood return. Inject 1 to 5 cc of saline into the lock. Secure the site and cover with a dressing.

The formula for calculating IV flow rate is:

$$\frac{\text{Volume to be infused} \times \text{Drops/mL of infusion set}}{\text{Total time of infusion in minutes}}$$

Sample Calculations

SFC Murray received a physician's order to administer an intravenous infusion. The order stated that the total volume of 1,000 mL is to be delivered over a 4-hour period. The IV set that is to be used will deliver 20 drops/mL. How many drops per minute should be administered?

Total volume to be infused = 1,000 mL
Infusion set (drops/mL) = 20
Total time of infusion = 240 min (4 hr × 60 min/hr)
Multiply 1,000 × 20 = 20,000 then divide by 240
= 83.33:

$$\frac{1000 \times 20}{240 \text{ min}}$$

Drops per minute = 83.33; round to 83 gtt/min
CPT Smith's IV is ordered at 150 mL to be delivered over 1 hour. The administration set being used delivers 20 gtt/mL. Calculate the drops/minute to be administered.

$$\frac{150 \times 20}{60} = 50 \text{ gtt/min}$$

Mr. Cadiz has an order for 1,000 mL of D_5W. The administration set delivers 10 gtt/mL. Calculate the flow rate of the fluid to be infused over 4 hours and 2 hours.

4 hr = 41.66 or 42 gtt/min
2 hr = 83.33 or 83 gtt/min

Dimensional Analysis

One of the easiest ways to figure out **drip rates**, dose calculations, weight-based calculations, and drug concentration equations is to use dimensional analysis. Dimensional analysis uses the same simple conversions as equations, and you will not need to memorize the equation! Dimensional analysis allows you to compare seemingly unrelated items by setting up a relationship (that is, a comparison between two items).

An example of a relationship could be a car and the wheels on a car. Every car rides on four wheels, so there are four wheels for every car.

$$\frac{1 \text{ car}}{4 \text{ wheels}} = \frac{4 \text{ wheels}}{1 \text{ car}}$$

Another way to look at these comparisons is as a ratio, which is by nature a relationship. Dimensional analysis uses ratios as conversion factors.

Drip Rates

Use dimensional analysis to solve IV drip rates. For this work you need to know:

• Which administration set to use
• Length of time for the infusion
• Amount to flow

You may need the conversion factor of 1 hour = 60 minutes. Example:

• Order given is for 250 mL normal saline (NS) over 90 minutes.
• Administration set is 5 macrodrip (10 gtt/mL).

Determine how many drops per minute should be given. Set up the equation:

$$\frac{?\ gtt}{min} = \frac{10\ gtt}{1\ mL} \times \frac{250\ mL}{90\ min}$$

Cancel out what you can and reduce the fractions:

$$\frac{?\ gtt}{min} = \frac{\cancel{10}\ gtt}{1\ \cancel{mL}} \times \frac{250\ \cancel{mL}}{\cancel{90}\ min}$$

Multiply and divide:

$$= \frac{250\ gtt}{9\ min} = \frac{27.77\ gtt}{1\ min} = 28\ gtt/min$$

You will need to set the drip rate at 28 gtt/min normal saline to achieve the desired order.

Field Medical Care TIPS

KVO means *keep vein open*; TKO means *to keep open*. Both are abbreviations for rates equal to about 8 to 15 drops per minute that are used to allow just enough fluid through the IV to keep blood from clotting at the end of the catheter.

Drops per Minute

Another useful formula to remember is a simple drip rate calculation that gives you the number of drops per minute:

$$\frac{(volume\ in\ mL) \times (drip\ set)}{time\ in\ minutes} = \frac{gtt}{min}$$

■ Possible Complications of IV Therapy

Peripheral IV insertion carries associated risks. The problems associated with IVs can be categorized as either local or systemic reactions. **Local reactions** include problems such as infiltration and phlebitis. **Systemic complications** include allergic reactions and circulatory overload.

Local IV Site Reactions

Most local reactions require that you discontinue the IV, reestablish the IV in the opposite extremity, and document the event. Some examples of local reactions include:

- Infiltration
- Phlebitis
- Occlusion
- Vein irritation
- Hematoma
- Nerve, tendon, or ligament damage
- Air embolism

Infiltration

Infiltration is the escape of fluid into the surrounding tissue. This escape of fluid causes a localized area of edema. Some of the more common reasons for infiltration include the following:

- The IV has passed completely through the vein and out the other side.
- The casualty is moving excessively.
- The tape used to secure the area has become loose or dislodged.
- The catheter was started at an angle that is too shallow and has only entered the **fascia** surrounding the vein. (This is more common with IVs in larger veins, such as those in the upper arm.)

Some of the associated signs and symptoms of infiltration include the following:

- Edema at the catheter site.
- Continued IV flow after occlusion of the vein above the insertion point.
- Casualty complains of tightness, pain, tenderness, burning, or irritation around the IV site.
- Flow rate may or may not be slow or there may be no flow of the solution.
- Infusion site is cool and hard to the touch.
- Infusion site or extremity is pale and swollen.
- Fluid leaking around infusion site.

To correct the infiltration, discontinue the IV and remove the needle or catheter. Elevate the extremity that had the IV. Apply warm compresses to encourage absorption. If possible, notify your supervisor of infiltration. Document the casualty's observations and actions. Avoid wrapping tape around the extremity for direct pressure because this could create a constricting band. Reestablish the IV in the opposite extremity or at a more proximal location on the same extremity. To prevent this complication, tape the catheter hub and tubing securely to the limb. Stabilize the extremity in use by applying an arm board, if necessary.

Phlebitis

Phlebitis is an inflammation of the wall of the vein. The causes of this complication include injury to the vein during puncture, irritation of the vein as a result of long-term therapy (vein overuse), an irritating or incompatible additive, using large-bore catheters, using lower extremities as IV sites, and infection. The signs and symptoms include:

- Sluggish flow rate
- Swelling around the infusion site
- Casualty complaints of pain and tenderness
- Redness and warmth at the site and along the vein

To correct this complication, stop the IV infusion immediately. Report the casualty observations to your supervisor. Restart the IV in another site, preferably on the opposite extremity, with new tubing and fluids if directed. Document all observations and actions taken. To prevent this complication, keep the infusion flowing at the prescribed rate. Select a large vein when irritating medications or fluids are given. Change the IV tubing every 24 to 48 hours or in accordance with (IAW) local standard operating procedures (SOPs). Change the IV solutions and dressings every 24 to 48 hours or IAW local SOPs. Change the IV site IAW local SOPs.

Air Embolism

An air embolism is an obstruction of a blood vessel (usually occurring in the lungs or heart) by air carried via the bloodstream. The minimum quantity of air that may be fatal to humans is not known. Animal experimentation indicates that fatal volumes of air are much larger than the quantity present in the entire length of IV tubing. The average IV tubing holds about 5 mL of air, an amount not ordinarily considered dangerous.

The causes of this complication include:

- Failure to remove air from the tubing
- Allowing the solution to run dry
- Disconnected IV tubing

The signs and symptoms include:

- Abrupt drop in blood pressure
- Weak, rapid pulse
- Cyanosis
- Chest pain

To correct this complication, notify your supervisor and the physician immediately. Immediately place the casualty on his or her left side with the feet elevated to allow the pulmonary artery to absorb small air bubbles. Administer oxygen.

To prevent this complication, clear all air from tubing before attaching it to the casualty. Monitor solution levels closely and change IV bags before they are empty. Check to see that all connections are secure.

Circulatory Overload

Circulatory overload is an increased volume resulting from excessive IV fluid being infused too rapidly into the vein. Use extreme caution when administering IV fluid to pediatric or geriatric casualties and to casualties experiencing congestive heart failure (CHF), pulmonary edema, or head trauma. All of these types of casualties are at increased risk of circulatory overload. The causes include:

- Fluid delivered too fast
- Reduced kidney function
- Congestive heart failure or cardiac insufficiency

The signs and symptoms include:

- Elevated blood pressure
- Distended neck veins (JVD)
- Rapid breathing, shortness of breath, tachycardia
- Fluid intake is much greater than urinary output (I&O)

To correct this complication, decrease flow rate to keep vein open (KVO). Place the casualty in the semi-Fowler's position to facilitate breathing. Notify your supervisor immediately. Record your observations of the casualty and any actions taken. To prevent this complication, frequently check flow rate to maintain the desired rate.

Infection

The causes of infection include the use of contaminated equipment, poor aseptic venipuncture technique, a contaminated site, and IV equipment that is not changed regularly. The signs and symptoms of infection include:

- Redness, swelling, and soreness around IV site
- Casualty complains of chills, fever, or malaise
- Sudden rise in temperature and pulse
- Drainage from IV site

Notify your supervisor immediately. Discontinue the IV by removing the catheter tip and take a culture of the wound to identify the pathogens present. Local policy will dictate when and how wound cultures will be performed. Some policies require the tubing and catheter to be sent to the lab for analysis in addition to the wound culture. Use strict aseptic technique when cleaning and dressing the wound. If a culture of the site is ordered, it must be done before cleaning the site. Document the wound appearance and all corrective actions taken.

To prevent this complication, use a completely aseptic technique when starting an IV. Clean the site thoroughly when the IV is initiated and then periodically IAW local SOPs to prevent infection. Anchor the catheter and tubing securely. Check the IV site at least daily for signs of inflammation IAW local SOPs.

Occlusion

Occlusion is the physical blockage of a vein or catheter. If the flow rate is not sufficient to keep fluid moving out of the catheter tip and if blood enters the catheter, a clot may form and occlude the flow. The first sign of a possible occlusion is a decreasing drip rate or the presence of blood in the IV tubing. A positional IV site can cause occlusion, which means that fluid flows at different rates depending on the position of the catheter within the vein. Close proximity to a valve is often the reason for positional IVs. Other causes can be related to casualty movement that allows the line to become physically blocked from either resting on the line or crossing the arms. Occlusion may also develop if the IV bag nears empty and the blood pressure overcomes the flow and backs up in the line.

Vein Irritation

Occasionally, a casualty will experience vein irritation in reaction to the fluid used for an IV. Casualties who have this problem often complain immediately that the solution is bothering them. It may tingle, sting, or itch. Note these complaints and observe the casualty closely in case the casualty develops a more serious allergic reaction to the fluid. The vein irritation is usually caused by the infusion being too rapid. If redness develops at the IV site with rapidly developing phlebitis, discontinue the IV and save the equipment for later analysis. Reestablish the

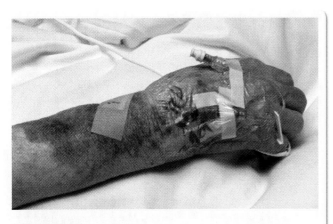

FIGURE 13-16 Hematomas can be caused by the improper removal of a catheter, resulting in the pooling of blood around the IV site, leading to tenderness and pain.

IV in the other extremity with all new equipment in case there were unseen contaminants in the old equipment. Be sure to document the event and the casualty's response.

Hematoma

A hematoma is an accumulation of blood in the tissues surrounding an IV site. Hematomas result from vein perforation or improper catheter removal that allows blood to accumulate in the surrounding tissues. Blood can be seen rapidly pooling around the IV site, leading to tenderness and pain **FIGURE 13-16 ▲**. Casualties with a history of vascular diseases (diabetes) or casualties receiving certain drug therapies (such as corticosteroids) can have a predisposition to vein rupture or a tendency to develop hematomas rapidly on IV insertion.

If a hematoma develops while you are attempting to insert a catheter, stop and apply direct pressure to help minimize bleeding. If a hematoma develops after a successful catheter insertion, evaluate the IV flow and the hematoma. If the hematoma appears to be controlled and the flow is not affected, monitor the IV site and leave the line in place. If the hematoma develops as a result of discontinuing the IV, apply direct pressure with a 4″ × 4″ gauze pad to the site.

Nerve, Tendon, or Ligament Damage

Improper identification of anatomic structures around the IV site can lead to perforation of tendons, ligaments, or nerves. An IV site choice around joints increases the risk for perforation of these structures. Casualties will experience sudden and severe shooting pain when a nerve, tendon, or ligament is perforated. Numbness in the extremity after the incident can be common. Immediately remove the catheter and select another IV site. Be sure to document the event.

Systemic Complications

Systemic complications can evolve from reactions or complications associated with IV insertion. Systemic complications usually involve other body systems and can be life-threatening. If the IV line is established and patent, do not remove it, because it may be needed for treatment of the casualty. Common systemic complications are:

- Allergic reactions
- Air embolus
- Catheter shear
- Vasovagal reactions
- Circulatory overload

Allergic Reactions

Often, allergic reactions are minor, but **anaphylaxis** is possible and must be treated aggressively. Allergic reactions can be related to an individual's unexpected sensitivity to an IV fluid or medication. Such sensitivity could be an unknown condition to the casualty; thus, vigilance must be maintained with any IV for a possible reaction.

Casualty presentation depends on the extent of the reaction. Common signs and symptoms of an allergic reaction include:

- Itching
- Shortness of breath
- Edema of face and hands
- Urticaria
- Bronchospasm
- Anaphylaxis
- Wheezing

If an allergic reaction occurs, discontinue the IV and remove the solution. Leave the catheter in place as an emergency medication route. Notify your supervising medical health care provider immediately and maintain an open airway. Document the event and keep the solution or medication for evaluation.

Air Embolus

Healthy adults can tolerate as much as 200 mL of air introduced into the circulatory system, but casualties who are already ill or injured can be affected if any air is introduced into the IV line. Properly flushing an IV line in advance of insertion will help eliminate any potential of introducing air into a casualty. IV bags are designed to collapse as they empty to help prevent this problem, but collapse does not always occur. Be sure to replace empty IV bags with full ones.

If your casualty begins developing respiratory distress with unequal breath sounds, consider the possibility of an air embolus. Other associated signs and symptoms include:

- Cyanosis (even in the presence of high-flow oxygen)
- Signs and symptoms of shock
- Loss of consciousness
- Respiratory arrest

Treat a casualty with a suspected air embolus by placing the casualty on his or her left side with the head down to trap any air inside the right atrium or right ventricle, and rapidly transport to the closest most appropriate facility. Be prepared to assist ventilations if the casualty experiences increasing shortness of breath or inadequate tidal volume. Document the event.

Catheter Shear

Catheter shear occurs when part of the catheter is pinched against the needle, and the needle slices through the catheter, creating a free-floating segment. This allows the catheter segment to travel through the circulatory system and possibly end up in the pulmonary circulation, causing a pulmonary embolus.

Treatment involves surgical removal of the sheared tip. Catheter hubs are radiopaque (that is, they will appear white in an x-ray) to aid in diagnosing this type of problem. Never rethread a catheter. Dispose of the used one and use a new one.

Casualties who have experienced catheter shear with pulmonary artery occlusion present with sudden dyspnea, shortness of breath, and possibly diminished breath sounds. They will mimic the presentations of an air embolus casualty and can be treated in the same way. Such casualties will need continued IV access, so you must try to obtain an IV site in the other extremity. Fortunately, this complication is extremely rare.

Circulatory Overload

An unmonitored IV bag can lead to circulatory overload. Healthy adults can handle as much as 2 to 3 extra liters of fluid without compromise. Problems occur when the casualty has cardiac, pulmonary, or renal dysfunction. These types of dysfunction do not tolerate any additional demands from increased circulatory volume. A possible cause of circulatory overload is failure to readjust the drip rate after flushing an IV line immediately after insertion. Always monitor IV bags to ensure the proper drip rate.

Casualty presentation includes dyspnea, jugular vein distension (JVD), and increased blood pressure. Crackles are often heard when evaluating breath sounds. Acute peripheral edema can also be an indication of circulatory overload.

To treat a casualty with circulatory overload, slow the IV rate to keep the vein open and raise the casualty's head to ease respiratory distress. Administer high-flow oxygen and monitor vital signs and breathing adequacy. Contact medical control immediately and inform them of the developing problem, because there are drugs that can be given to reduce the circulatory volume. Document the event.

Vasovagal Reactions

Some casualties have anxiety concerning needles or the sight of blood. Such anxiety may cause vasculature dilation, leading to a drop in blood pressure and casualty collapse. Casualties can present with anxiety, diaphoresis, nausea, and **syncopal episodes**.

Treatment for casualties with **vasovagal reactions** (also known as "vagaling down") centers on treating them for shock:

1. Place the casualty in shock position.
2. Apply high-flow oxygen.
3. Monitor vital signs.
4. Establish an IV in case fluid resuscitation is needed.

■ Troubleshooting

Several factors can influence the flow rate of an IV. For example, if the IV bag is not hung high enough, the flow rate will not be sufficient. It is always helpful to perform the following checks after completing IV administration. Also, if there is a flow problem, rechecking these items will help determine the problem.

- **Check your IV fluid.** Thick, viscous fluids such as blood products and colloid solutions infuse slowly and may be diluted to help speed delivery. Cold fluids run slower than warm fluids. If you can, warm IV fluids before administering them in cold weather.
- **Check your administration set.** Macrodrips are used for rapid fluid delivery, whereas microdrips are designed to deliver a more controlled flow.
- **Check the height of your IV bag.** The IV bag must be hung high enough to overcome the casualty's own blood pressure. Hang the bag as high as possible.
- **Check the type of catheter used.** The wider the catheter (the smaller the gauge), the more fluid can be delivered; 14 gauge is the widest catheter size typically available and 27 gauge is the narrowest.
- **Check your constricting band.** One of the most overlooked factors is leaving the constricting band on the casualty's arm after completing the IV.

■ Manage an IV

Every 24 hours when running a slow infusion, the solution container needs to be replaced. Do not allow a solution container to become completely empty before changing containers. To manage an IV, follow the steps in **SKILL DRILL 13-3**:

1. Perform a casualty care handwash.
2. Select or prepare the new solution container by removing the protective cover from the outlet tube.
3. Clamp the IV tubing shut (**Step ①**).
4. Remove the used container from the IV hanger, and remove the spike from it. The old tubing is connected to the catheter. Care must be taken to maintain sterility. To prevent the back flow of blood, keep the spike and tubing elevated.
5. Insert the IV spike into the new IV container (**Step ②**).
6. Hang the new container.
7. Adjust the infusion rate (**Step ③**).
8. Label the solution container and prepare a timing label.
9. Record the amount of solution received from the previous container, and time, type, and amount of new solution (**Step ④**).

Replace the IV tubing every 48 hours or IAW local SOPs. Changing the IV tubing should coincide with the

SKILL DRILL 13-3

Manage an IV

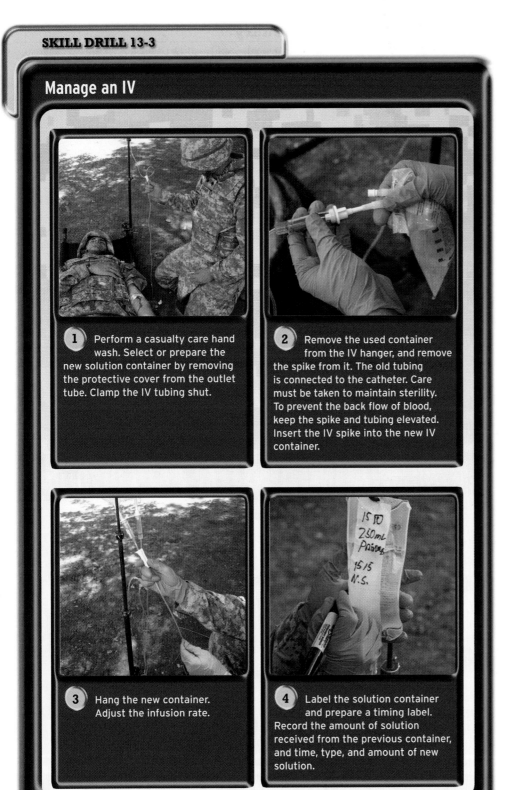

1 Perform a casualty care hand wash. Select or prepare the new solution container by removing the protective cover from the outlet tube. Clamp the IV tubing shut.

2 Remove the used container from the IV hanger, and remove the spike from it. The old tubing is connected to the catheter. Care must be taken to maintain sterility. To prevent the back flow of blood, keep the spike and tubing elevated. Insert the IV spike into the new IV container.

3 Hang the new container. Adjust the infusion rate.

4 Label the solution container and prepare a timing label. Record the amount of solution received from the previous container, and time, type, and amount of new solution.

time the solution container will be changed. To change the IV tubing, follow the steps in **SKILL DRILL 13-4 ▶**:

1. Perform a casualty care handwash.

2. Spike the new tubing into a new solution container and hang it from the IV pole.

3. Prime the tubing and clamp it (**Step ①**).

4. Clamp the old tubing shut (**Step ②**).

5. Wear gloves for self-protection and to protect the casualty against transmission of contaminants whenever coming into contact with body fluids.

6. Loosen the tape on the old tubing without dislodging the catheter.

7. Place a sterile gauze pad under the catheter hub to provide a small sterile field for the hub.

8. Grasp the new tubing between the fingers of one hand.

9. Grasp the catheter hub with a sterile gauze pad and carefully disconnect the old adapter. Press your fingers over the catheter tip to help prevent the back flow of blood (**Step ③**).

10. Remove the protective cap from the new tubing adapter and quickly connect it to the catheter hub. Never remove the protective cap with your teeth (**Step ④**).

11. Remove the gauze pad from under the catheter hub and clean the site, if necessary.

12. Secure the tubing to the arm and reinforce the dressing as necessary.

13. Adjust the infusion rate. If replacing a catheter, discontinue the IV, select a new IV site proximal to the old IV site (if using the same limb), and start a new IV. The IV catheter site is normally changed every 72 hours.

14. Maintain the saline lock. When the saline lock is not being used at regular intervals for medication administration, it must be flushed to maintain patency (**Step ⑤**).

■ Summary

As a combat medic, you will be expected to initiate, manage, and discontinue an intravenous infusion. It is important to remember the principles discussed in this chapter in order to ensure that fluids infuse at the correct rate and that complications of IV therapy are detected and treated promptly.

SKILL DRILL 13-4

Change the IV Tubing

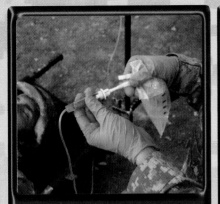

1 Perform a casualty care handwash. Spike the new tubing into a new solution container and hang it from the IV pole. Prime the tubing and clamp it.

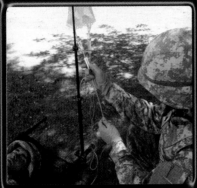

2 Clamp the old tubing shut.

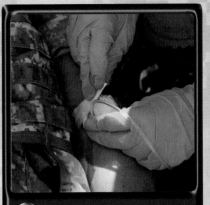

3 Loosen the tape on the old tubing without dislodging the catheter. Place a sterile gauze pad under the catheter hub to provide a small sterile field for the hub. Grasp the new tubing between the fingers of one hand. Grasp the catheter hub with a sterile gauze pad and carefully disconnect the old adapter. Press your fingers over the catheter tip to help prevent the back flow of blood.

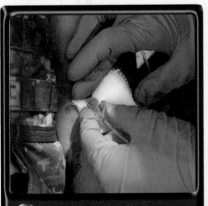

4 Remove the protective cap from the new tubing adapter and quickly connect it to the catheter hub. Never remove the protective cap with your teeth.

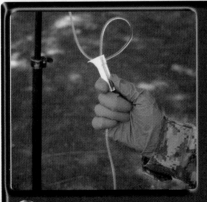

5 Remove the gauze pad from under the catheter hub and clean the site, if necessary. Secure the tubing to the arm and reinforce the dressing as necessary. Adjust the infusion rate. If replacing a catheter, discontinue the IV, select a new IV site proximal to the old IV site (if using the same limb), and start a new IV. The IV catheter site is normally changed every 72 hours. Maintain the saline lock. When the saline lock is not being used at regular intervals for medication administration, it must be flushed to maintain patency.

YOU ARE THE
COMBAT MEDIC

You are assessing casualties following a brief fire fight in neutral territory. The last casualty you triage is a young soldier bleeding from his right arm. Your general impression of this casualty indicates that he is suffering from a gunshot wound to his right arm with a considerable amount of bleeding present. A combat lifesaver (CLS) is with you to assist in rendering care. The situation is safe, the weather is hot and rainy, the closest MTF is 10 miles from your current location, and MEDEVAC is not available.

Assessment

Upon initial assessment of the casualty, you observe that he is lethargic, slightly tachypneic with adequate chest rise and volume; skin is cool, pale, and diaphoretic (despite the weather conditions) with a significant amount of blood flow coming from the right shoulder. His respiratory rate is 26 breaths/min and radial pulses are present but weak. Exposure of the upper extremities and chest discloses a gunshot wound to the right shoulder with a substantial amount of non-arterial bleeding still coming from the wound.

Treatment

Treatment of this casualty includes bleeding control. You determine that the casualty requires immediate evacuation and the squad leader arranges for immediate ground transport. Bleeding control is managed by the CLS who applies a bulky dressing and direct pressure. Meanwhile, you establish a 16-gauge saline lock and hang an intravenous solution of Ringer's lactate. A fluid bolus of 200 mL is in progress when the ground ambulance crew arrives and assumes care of the casualty.

1. LAST NAME, FIRST NAME		RANK/GRADE	X	MALE
Carey, Sam		PFC		FEMALE

SSN	SPECIALTY CODE	RELIGION
000-111-000	00Z	Lutheran

2. UNIT

FORCE				NATIONALITY		
A/T	AF/A	N/M	MC/M			
	BC/BC		NBI/BNC		DISEASE	PSYCH

3. INJURY				
			AIRWAY	
			HEAD	
FRONT	BACK	X	WOUND	
			NECK/BACK INJURY	
			BURN	
			AMPUTATION	
			STRESS	
			OTHER (Specify)	

4. LEVEL OF CONSCIOUSNESS			
ALERT	X	PAIN RESPONSE	
VERBAL RESPONSE		UNRESPONSIVE	

5. PULSE	TIME	6. TOURNIQUET		TIME
140 bpm	1615	X NO	YES	

7. MORPHINE		DOSE	TIME	8. IV	TIME
X NO	YES			RL	1620

9. TREATMENT/OBSERVATIONS/CURRENT MEDICATION/ALLERGIES/NBC (ANTIDOTE)

GSW to the right arm. Direct pressure to wound 16 gauge saline lock of RL, 200 mL fluid bolus

10. DISPOSITION		RETURNED TO DUTY		TIME
	X	EVACUATED		1630
		DECEASED		

11. PROVIDER/UNIT	DATE (YYMMDD)
Green, Manny	

Ready for Review

- Intravenous (IV) therapy is one of the most invasive procedures you will learn. Few procedures require more training or practice.

- A human cell can exist only in a special balanced environment. Understanding how this environment is created and maintained will give you the foundation you need to perform IV therapy.

- The role of water in the body is diverse; it plays a part both in cellular metabolism and in the maintenance of homeostasis. Without the presence of water in the body, people would quickly succumb to illness and disease, cellular function would cease, and body systems would shut down.

- The most important point to remember about IV techniques and fluid administration is to keep the IV equipment sterile. Forethought will help prevent mental and procedural errors while starting the IV.

- One way to ensure proper technique is to develop a routine to follow as you assemble the appropriate equipment.

- Peripheral IV insertion carries associated risks. The problems associated with IVs can be categorized as either local or systemic reactions.

- The solution container needs to be replaced every 24 hours when running a slow infusion. Do not allow the solution container to empty completely before changing containers.

Vital Vocabulary

access port A sealed hub on an administration set designed for sterile access to the IV fluid.

acidosis A pathologic condition resulting from the accumulation of acids in the body.

alkalosis A pathologic condition resulting from the accumulation of bases in the body.

anaphylaxis An extreme, life-threatening systemic allergic reaction that may include shock and respiratory failure.

anion An ion that contains an overall negative charge.

antidiuretic hormone (ADH) A hormone produced by the pituitary gland that signals the kidneys to prevent excretion of water.

ataxia A staggered walk or gait caused by injury to the brain or spinal cord.

buffer A substance or group of substances that controls the hydrogen levels in a solution.

butterfly catheter A rigid, hollow, venous cannulation device identified by its plastic "wings" that act as anchoring points for securing the catheter.

cannulation The insertion of a hollow tube into a vein to allow for fluid flow.

capillary beds The terminal ends of the vascular system where fluids, food, and wastes are exchanged between the vascular system and the cells of the body.

catheter A flexible, hollow structure that delivers fluid.

cation An ion that contains an overall positive charge.

cellular perfusion The ability of a cell to take in oxygen and remove carbon dioxide.

concentration gradient The natural tendency for substances to flow from an area of higher concentration to an area of lower concentration, either within the cell or outside the cell.

crystalloid solution A type of intravenous solution that contains compounds that quickly disassociate in solution and can cross membranes; considered the best choice for prehospital care of injured casualties who need fluids to replace lost body fluid.

D_5W An intravenous solution made up of 5% dextrose in water.

depolarization The rapid movement of electrolytes across a cell membrane that changes the cell's overall charge. This rapid shifting of electrolytes and cellular charges is the main catalyst for muscle contractions and neural transmissions.

diabetes insipidus A form of diabetes characterized by polyuria and polydipsia (excessive thirst) that often results from decreased or absent ADH production.

diffusion A process in which molecules move from an area of higher concentration to an area of lower concentration.

drip chamber The area of the IV administration set where fluid accumulates so that the tubing remains filled with fluid.

drip rate Number of drops per minute.

drip set Another name for an administration set.

electrolyte A charged atom or compound that results from the loss or gain of an electron. These are ions the body uses to perform certain critical metabolic processes.

epinephrine A hormone (adrenaline) produced by the body and a drug produced by pharmaceutical companies to increase pulse and blood pressure; the drug of choice for an anaphylactic reaction.

fascia The fiber-like connective tissue that covers arteries, veins, tendons, and ligaments.

flash chamber The area of a catheter that fills with blood to help indicate when a vein is cannulated.

gtt A measurement that indicates drops.

homeostasis The balance of all systems of the body; also known as homeostatic balance.

hydrophilic Water-loving.

hydrophobic Water-fearing.

hypercalcemia High serum calcium levels.

hyperkalemia High serum potassium levels.

hypertonic solution A solution that has a greater concentration of sodium than does the cell; the increased extracellular osmotic pressure can draw water out of the cell and cause it to collapse.

hypocalcemia Low serum calcium levels.

hypokalemia Low serum potassium levels.

hypotonic solution A solution that has a lower concentration of sodium than does the cell; the increased intracellular osmotic pressure lets water flow into the cell, causing it to swell and possibly burst.

infiltration The escape of fluid into the surrounding tissue.

interstitial Water between the vascular system and the surrounding cells (for example, between the membranes of two cells located outside the vascular compartment in the body).

intravascular The water portion of the circulatory system surrounding the blood cells (for example, in the heart, arteries, or veins).

ion A charged atom or compound that results from the loss or gain of an electron.

ionic concentration The amount of charged particles found in a particular area.

isotonic solution A solution that has the same concentration of sodium as does the cell. In this case, water does not shift, and no change in cell shape occurs.

lactated Ringer's (LR) solution A sterile crystalloid isotonic intravenous solution of specified amounts of calcium chloride, potassium chloride, sodium chloride, and sodium lactate in water.

local reaction Mild to moderate allergic reaction occurring in a localized area.

lysis The rupturing of a cell caused by either the presence of certain enzymes or the uncontrolled influx of material into the cell.

macrodrip set An administration set named for the large orifice between the piercing spike and the drip chamber; allows for rapid fluid flow into the vascular system.

metabolic The breakdown of ingested foodstuffs into smaller and smaller molecules and atoms that are used as energy sources for cellular function.

microdrip set An administration set named for the small orifice between the piercing spike and the drip chamber; allows for carefully controlled fluid flow and is ideally suited for medication administration.

normal saline (NS) 0.9% sodium chloride; an isotonic crystalloid.

occlusion Blockage, usually of a tubular structure such as a blood vessel.

osmolarity The ability to influence the movement of water across a semipermeable membrane.

osmosis The movement of water across a cell membrane from an area of lower to higher solute molecules.

osmotic pressure Pressure created against the cell wall by the presence of water.

over-the-needle catheter The prehospital standard for IV cannulation. It consists of a hollow tube over a laser-sharpened steel needle; also referred to as an angiocath.

pH A measure of the acidity of a solution; potential of hydrogen

phospholipid bilayer The cell membrane's double layer, consisting of a hydrophilic outer layer composed of phosphate groups and a hydrophobic inner layer made up of lipids, or fatty acids. It is this structure and composition that allows the cell membrane to have selective permeability.

piggyback administration The addition of a second IV administration set to a primary line via an access port.

polyuria The passage of an unusually large volume of urine in a given period. In diabetes, polyuria can result from excreting excess glucose in the urine.

postural hypotension Symptomatic drop in blood pressure related to the casualty's body position, detected by measuring pulse and blood pressure while the casualty is lying supine, sitting up, and standing. An increase in pulse rate and a decrease in blood pressure in any one of these positions is considered a positive sign for this condition.

saline lock A special type of IV, also called a buff cap or heparin cap.

selective permeability The ability of the cell membrane to selectively allow compounds into the cell based on the cell's current needs.

sodium/potassium pump The mechanism by which the cell brings in two potassium ions and releases three sodium ions.

syncopal episode Fainting; brief loss of consciousness caused by transiently inadequate blood flow to the brain.

systemic complications Moderate to severe allergic reaction affecting the systems of the body.

tachycardia Rapid heart rhythm, more than 100 beats/min.

tachypnea Rapid respirations.

third spacing The shifting of fluid into the tissues, creating edema.

tonicity The osmotic pressure of a solution, based on the relationship between sodium and water inside and outside the cell, that takes advantage of their chemical and osmotic properties to move water to areas of higher sodium concentration.

tubule A section of the kidney where the filtration of wastes, electrolytes, and water is controlled.

vasovagal reaction A reaction consisting of precordial distress, anxiety, nausea, and sometimes syncope.

COMBAT MEDIC *in Action*

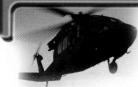

You are called to care for a soldier who was recently assigned to your squad. He was on patrol when he suddenly collapsed. The casualty had been on duty for the past 8 hours wearing full battle gear. Your general impression indicates that the casualty is potentially suffering from a heat-related illness. As you perform your initial assessment, you observe that the casualty is awake and mumbling incoherently with an elevated respiratory rate; skin is hot, flushed, and dry. His respiratory rate is 28 breaths/min with adequate chest rise and volume and radial pulses are rapid and weak. The current temperature is 105°F and humid. A combat lifesaver notes that the casualty's canteen is full.

1. What should you do if you meet resistance against a valve while inserting the catheter into the vein?
   A. Pull the catheter back over the needle.
   B. Elevate the extremity.
   C. Lower the extremity.
   D. Apply the tourniquet tighter.

2. Which of the following statements regarding catheter size is true?
   A. The larger the diameter, the smaller the gauge
   B. The smaller the diameter, the smaller the gauge
   C. The larger the diameter, the larger the gauge
   D. The smaller the diameter, the larger the gauge

3. Constricting bands are frequently used to help identify potential veins for cannulation. Which of the following statements regarding use of a constricting band is true?
   A. Apply the constricting band approximately 6" above the cannulation site.
   B. Tighten the constricting band so that both arterial and venous blood flow are stopped.
   C. Do not leave the constricting band in place for more than 2 minutes.
   D. All of the above statements are true.

4. Prior to piercing the skin, the needle should be held at a:
   A. 20°–30° angle.
   B. 30°–45° angle.
   C. 45°–60° angle.
   D. 60°–90° angle.

5. Information that needs to be documented on a label and placed on the IV bag includes:
   A. the casualty's name.
   B. the date and time that the IV was started.
   C. the name of the person initiating the IV.
   D. all of the above.

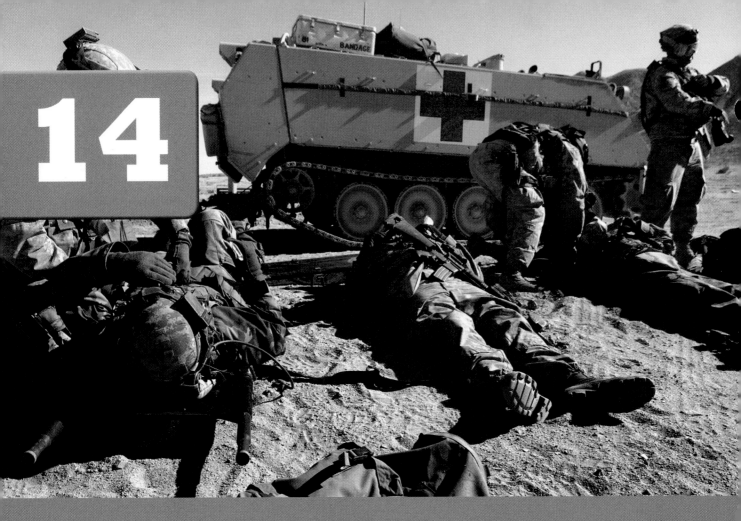

14

Triage

Objectives

Knowledge Objectives

☐ Identify the principles that govern the priorities for treatment and evacuation.

☐ Define the categories of triage.

☐ Identify the four categories of triage for conventional battlefield casualties.

☐ Define the two alternative triage categories.

Introduction

In dealing with multiple casualties during combat, those with the most severe injuries or the greatest threat to life are not necessarily the ones who should receive the first priority. In these situations, consideration must be given to each casualty's likelihood of survival. The predominant principle of casualty triage is to treat and return to duty the greatest number of soldiers in the shortest possible time. This gives the combat commander additional assets to defeat the enemy and accomplish the mission. A familiarity with the principles of casualty triage will assist you in rendering vitally important emergency medical care to casualties in a timely manner and will help reduce the number of casualties who die from their combat wounds.

Treatment and Evacuation Priority Principles

Mass casualty (MASCAL) situations occur when the number of casualties exceeds the available medical capability to rapidly treat and evacuate them. The actual number of casualties required before a MASCAL situation is declared varies from situation to situation, depending upon the availability of medical resources. Technically, a MASCAL situation occurs if you have more than one seriously injured casualty to care for at one time.

Triage is the medical sorting of casualties according to the type and seriousness of the injury, the likelihood of survival, and the establishment of priorities of treatment and evacuation. Triage ensures that medical resources are properly used to provide care for the greatest benefit to the largest number of casualties. Triage affords the greatest number of casualties with the greatest chance of survival. And finally, triage locates the casualties with minor wounds and returns them to duty.

Triage is usually the responsibility of the senior medical person, who establishes the order of treatment and determines whether treatment is not given, regardless of the injury.

Field Medical Care TIPS

Nuclear weapons exposure will not be used as criteria for sorting. Field experience with these injuries does not exist.

Casualties may not always fit into nice, neat, convenient categories. It is incumbent upon the senior medical person to attempt to triage to the best of his or her ability and medical experience, with consideration of the mission and every soldier in the unit.

During triage, the following tactical and environmental situations must be determined:

- Is it necessary to transport casualties to a more secure collection point for treatment?
- What are the number and location of the injured?
- How severe are the injuries?
- Is assistance—buddy-aid, self-aid, or additional medical personnel—available?
- What are the evacuation support capabilities and requirements (eg, air ambulance, ground transportation)?
- Plan for the conservation and utilization of medical supplies. For example, if no medical resupply is possible for 36+ hours do you want to use all your medical supplies in an attempt to save a likely expectant casualty and leave your unit without any medical capabilities?

Triage on the Conventional Battlefield

This chapter focuses on performing triage on the conventional battlefield **TABLE 14-1 ▾**. However, the enemy may use chemical weapons during combat, making the battlefield integrated. Integrated battlefield casualties are covered in **TABLE 14-2 ▸**. We'll discuss each of the casualty types in the following sections.

Field Medical Care TIPS

Triage Principles
- Do the greatest good for the greatest number of casualties.
- Employ the available resources in the most efficient way.
- Return key personnel to duty as quickly as possible.
- Continually reassess and retriage.
- Move quickly.
- Do not second guess.
- The most experienced provider should triage.
- Plan, prepare, and train.

TABLE 14-1 Conventional Battlefield Triage Categories

Triage Category	Description
Immediate	Casualty who needs immediate treatment to save life, limb, or eyesight
Delayed	Casualty who has less risk of losing life or limb
Minimal	Walking wounded, self-aid, or buddy-aid
Expectant	Casualty so critically injured that only complicated and prolonged treatment offers any hope of improving life expectancy

TABLE 14-2 Integrated Battlefield Triage Categories

Triage Category	Description
Immediate	Conventional life threats and no chemical life threats
Chemical Immediate	Severe chemical life threats and no conventional life threats
Delayed	No conventional life threats and mild chemical life threats
Minimal	Minor conventional injuries and no chemical life threats
Expectant	Conventional life threats and severe chemical life threats

Immediate

The **immediate** triage category is for the casualty whose condition demands immediate resuscitative treatment to save his or her life. Casualties in this category present with severe, life-threatening wounds. Generally the procedures used to correct these conditions are short in duration and economical in terms of medical resources. Casualties within this group have a high likelihood of survival. This category has the highest priority.

Approximately 20% of casualties fall into this category. After a casualty with a life-threatening condition has been stabilized, no further treatment will be given until other immediate casualties have been treated. Remember, salvage of life takes priority over salvage of limb. Examples of injuries in the immediate category are:

- Airway obstruction
- Sucking chest wound (with respiratory distress)
- Tension pneumothorax
- Unstable abdominal wounds with shock
- Massive external bleeding (eg, amputation)
- Open fractures of long bones
- Hemorrhagic shock
- Burns of the face, neck, hands, feet, or perineum and genitalia or second- or third-degree burns of 15% to 40% or more of the total body surface area (TBSA)

Cardiorespiratory distress may not be considered to be an immediate condition on the battlefield. It would most likely be classified as expectant, contingent upon the mission, the battlefield situation, the number of casualties, and support. The mission is always a factor when triaging casualties.

Delayed

Delayed casualties have less risk of losing life or limb by treatment being delayed. Casualties in the delayed category can tolerate delay prior to intervention without unduly compromising the likelihood of a successful outcome. When medical resources are overwhelmed, casualties in this category are held until the immediate cases are cared for. Approximately 20% of casualties fall into this category. Examples of injuries in the delayed category are:

- Open chest wound (without respiratory distress)
- Abdominal wounds (without shock)
- Eye injuries
- Soft-tissue wounds requiring debridement (removal of foreign material and dead or damaged tissue); all combat wounds require some form of debridement
- Fractures
- Second- and third-degree burns (not involving the face, hands, feet, genitalia, and perineum) covering 20% or more of TBSA
- Maxillofacial wounds without airway compromise
- Genitourinary tract disruption

Minimal

Minimal (or ambulatory) casualties are considered to be the walking wounded. These casualties can utilize self-aid or buddy-aid. This category is composed of casualties with wounds that are so superficial that they require no more than cleansing, minimal debridement under local anesthesia, administration of tetanus toxoid, and first-aid dressings. They must be rapidly directed away from the triage area to uncongested areas where first aid and nonspecialty medical personnel are available. Approximately 40% of casualties fall into this category. Casualties in this category usually are not evacuated to an MTF. Examples of injuries in the minimal category are:

- Minor lacerations or abrasions
- Contusions
- Sprains and strains
- Minor combat stress problems
- First- or second-degree burns under 15% of TBSA and not involving critical areas such as hands, feet, face, genitalia, or perineum
- Upper extremity fractures without neurovascular compromise
- Behavioral disorders or other obvious psychiatric disturbances
- Suspicion of blast injury (ruptured eardrums)
- Symptomatic but unquantified radiation exposure

Expectant

An **expectant** casualty is so critically injured that only complicated and prolonged treatment offers any hope of improving life expectancy. A casualty in the expectant category has wounds that are so extensive that even if he or she was the sole casualty and had the benefit of optimal medical resources application, his or her survival would be very unlikely. During a MASCAL situation, this type of casualty would require an unjustifiable expenditure of limited resources that are more wisely applied to several other more salvageable casualties. This does not mean "no treatment." Rather, it means that intensive, time-consuming treatment will be withheld until higher-priority casualties are cared for. Comfort care should be given.

The expectant casualties should be separated from the view of other casualties but not abandoned. Above all, attempt

Field Medical Care TIPS

Triage in TC-3: Care Under Fire

Return fire as required or directed. Casualties should return fire if able. Your goal is to keep yourself from being shot. Once the shooting has stopped and it is safe to do so, triage the casualties. To perform triage, state the following loud enough for all casualties to hear:

- "If you can hear my voice and can walk, move to this area now." These casualties are your minimal casualties.
- "If you can hear my voice, but can't walk, raise your hand and let me know." These casualties are your delayed casualties. Request for additional help; call for squad member and/or combat lifesaver (CLS) and direct them to assist you with these casualties.

What remains are the immediate, expectant, or the dead. Determine which casualty is which by using the decision-making algorithm in Figure 14-1 and go to work:

- Stop life-threatening hemorrhage using tourniquets.
- Perform or direct assistant to perform immediate treatment(s) and movement of casualties to a secure area or casualty collection point (CCP).
- Airway and breathing management are best deferred until you are no longer receiving effect fire and have moved off the target.
- Move the casualties to the secure area or CCP and triage these casualties.

to make expectant casualties comfortable by whatever means necessary and provide attendance.

Approximately 20% of casualties are in this category. Examples of injuries in the expectant category are:

- Unresponsive casualties with penetrating head wounds and signs of impending death
- Burns, mostly third-degree, covering more than 60% of TBSA
- Cervical spinal cord injuries
- Mutilating explosive wounds involving multiple anatomic sites and organs
- Profound shock with multiple injuries
- Agonal respiration
- Convulsions and vomiting within 24 hours of radiation exposure
- Without vital signs or signs of life
- Transcranial gunshot would (GSW)
- Open pelvic injury with uncontrolled bleeding (shock with decreased mental status)

■ MEDEVAC Priority Categories

The next step is to establish medical evacuation (MEDEVAC) priorities by precedence category. A minimal casualty should not be evacuated before an immediate casualty. The MEDEVAC priority categories ensure that this does not happen.

Priority I—Urgent

The **Priority I—Urgent** category is assigned to emergency cases who should be evacuated as soon as possible and within a maximum of 2 hours in order to:

- Save life, limb, or eyesight
- Prevent complication of serious illness
- Avoid permanent disability

This category includes casualties whose conditions cannot be controlled and have the greatest opportunity for survival. It also includes those:

- In cardiorespiratory distress
- In shock and not responding to IV therapy
- Suffering prolonged unconsciousness
- With head injuries and signs of increasing intracranial pressure
- Suffering burns covering 20% to 85% of the TBSA

Priority IA—Urgent Surgical

The **Priority IA—Urgent Surgical** category is assigned to casualties who must receive far forward surgical intervention to save life and stabilize them for further evacuation. This category includes casualties with:

- Decreased circulation in the extremities
- Open chest and/or abdominal wounds with decreased blood pressure
- Penetrating wounds
- Uncontrollable bleeding or open fractures with severe bleeding
- Severe facial injuries
- Burns on the hands, feet, face, genitalia, or perineum, even if under 20% of the TBSA

Priority II—Priority

The **Priority II—Priority** category is assigned to sick and wounded casualties requiring prompt medical care. This precedence is used when the casualty should be evacuated within 4 hours or:

- The casualty's medical condition could deteriorate to such a degree that he or she will become an urgent or urgent surgical precedence.
- The casualty's requirements for special treatment are not available locally.
- The casualty will suffer unnecessary pain or disability.

This category includes casualties with:

- Closed chest injuries
- Brief periods of unconsciousness
- Soft-tissue injuries and open or closed fractures
- Abdominal injuries with no decreased blood pressure
- Eye injuries that do not threaten the eyesight
- Spinal injuries

Priority III—Routine

The **Priority III—Routine** category is assigned to sick and wounded casualties requiring evacuation but whose condition is not expected to deteriorate significantly. The sick and wounded in this category should be evacuated within 24 hours. This category includes:

- Casualties with simple fractures
- Casualties with open wounds including chest injuries without respiratory distress
- Psychiatric cases
- Terminal cases

Priority IV–Convenience

The **Priority IV—Convenience** category is assigned to casualties for whom evacuation by medical vehicle is a matter of medical convenience rather than necessity. This category includes casualties with:

- Minor open wounds
- Sprains and strains
- Minor burns under 20% of the TBSA

■ Two Alternative Triage Categories

Two alternative categories are useful in dividing casualties: those requiring further medical or surgical care (emergent) and those who are less injured, still require care, but have little chance of dying (nonemergent).

The **emergent** group requires attention within minutes to several hours to avoid death or major disability. Emergent casualties range from unstable and requiring attention within 15 minutes to temporarily stable but requiring care within a few hours. This group was historically categorized as immediate. The types of wounds include:

- Airway obstruction/compromise (actual or potential)
- Uncontrolled bleeding
- Shock (Systolic blood pressure < 90 mm Hg and mental status change without head injury)
- Unstable penetrating or blunt trauma to the trunk, neck, head, or pelvis
- Threatened loss of limb or eyesight
- Multiple long-bone fractures

Nonemergent casualties do not require the same attention as the emergent group although they may require surgery. Nonemergent casualties also lack significant potential for loss of life, limb, or eyesight. Historically categorized as delayed and minimal; these casualties have wounds, such as:

- Walking wounded
- Single long-bone fractures
- Closed fractures

Field Medical Care TIPS

Remember, triage is an ongoing process that includes reassessment, which may change the casualty's triage category.

- Soft-tissue injuries without significant bleeding (without shock)
- Facial fractures without airway compromise

■ Triage Decision Making

On the battlefield, you must make decisions about whether or not to evacuate casualties from the battlefield and how quickly the evacuation must take place. The following triage tool maybe used in the battlefield as an initial decision-making aid. It is the recommended technique for initial tactical emergency care when resources are scarce FIGURE 14-1 ▶. This modified START (Simple Triage And Rapid Treatment) technique has four key decision points that are based on:

1. Is the casualty able to walk (ambulate)?
2. Is the casualty responsive or unresponsive?
3. Is the casualty breathing?
4. Does the casualty have a palpable radial pulse?

The decision steps are:

- **Step 1:** The combat medic announces that all casualties who can walk should get up and walk to a designated area for eventual secondary triage. Categorize these casualties as nonemergent (minimal). This technique does not work well in situations with no or low light or excess noise.
- **Step 2:** Assess casualties in the order in which they are encountered. Assess responsiveness using the shake and shout method. If the casualty is conscious, proceed to Step 3. If the casualty unconscious, proceed to Step 4.
- **Step 3:** In the conscious casualty, assess the casualty's radial pulse and ease of breathing. If conscious casualty does not have a radial pulse and respiratory distress is emergent; then perform lifesaving interventions now! A conscious casualty with a

palpable radial pulse and comfortable breathing is nonemergent.

- **Step 4:** In the unconscious casualty who is breathing, address the airway with simple maneuvers. An emergent casualty has a patent airway, with or without simple maneuvers, and spontaneous respirations. An unconscious casualty who is breathing, but has a guarded airway who requires a Combitube or cricothyrotomy, is categorized as expectant.

This is a technique for initial triage. All casualties must be continually reassessed for potential change in category. Time, resources, and arrival of evacuation assets and personnel can quickly move an expectant casualty to an immediate category.

■ Establishing Triage, Treatment, and Holding Areas

Depending on the tactical situation or the location of the MASCAL, the triage, treatment, and holding areas may be established in the existing MTF, an available shelter, or outdoors. Regardless of the location, there are general guidelines to establishing a triage site. The initial triage area should be established for all casualties to flow through **FIGURE 14-2 ▶**. Casualties can then be directed to separate areas for treatment. Each area should be clearly identified and the route to that area marked. Ideally, each section will have at least one combat medic. Unidirectional flow is highly recommended in order to prevent clogging the system. No significant treatment should be performed in the triage area; however, fluid replacement may be initiated.

The qualities of an ideal initial triage area are:

- Proximity to the receiving area: landing zone (LZ), ground evacuation, decontamination areas. This will reduce the distance to be traveled by litter bearers. It is important to remember to establish separate triage areas for contaminated casualties.
- One-way flow both into and out of the triage area into treatment areas.

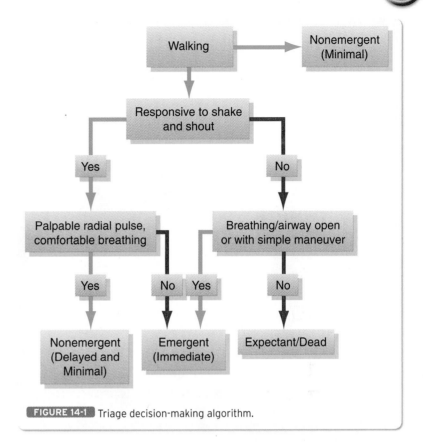

FIGURE 14-1 Triage decision-making algorithm.

- Well-lit, covered, and spacious—significant area for easy access, evaluation, and transport of incoming and outgoing casualties. It must have a designated area and one-way flow for vehicles dropping off and picking up casualties. In some instances, a MASCAL station may be required to be established outdoors. When this occurs, efficient use of overhead cover and available shade is essential. Unless inclement weather occurs, the triage area and the minimal treatment area remain outdoors.
- Casualty recorders to identify, tag, and record initial triage/disposition.
- Sufficient litter bearers controlled by someone other than the designated triage combat medic.

The emergent/immediate treatment area should be close to the initial triage area. It should have room for a three-person team to work with an available advanced trauma life

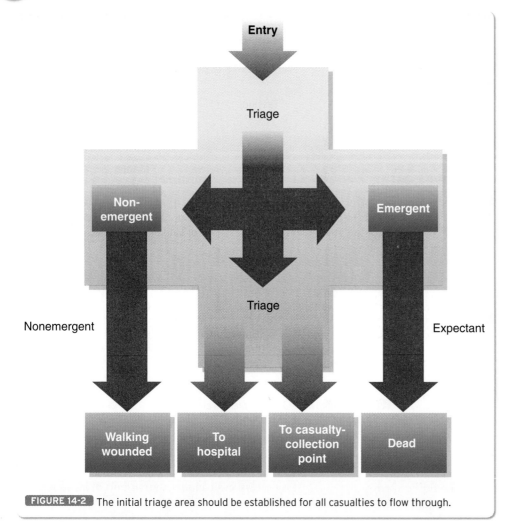

FIGURE 14-2 The initial triage area should be established for all casualties to flow through.

support (ATLS) style set-up. Triaged casualties should be brought inside an improvised shelter as soon as possible. The use of improvised shelters or the use of cover (such as caves) may be required until more appropriate shelters can be obtained or established.

The nonemergent (delayed and minimal) area should be a large area containing all required supplies for minor treatment(s). The expectant area should be established away from all other treatment areas to reduce stress and anxiety among casualties and attending combat medics. A combat medic should be available for pain control. The Chaplain's staff should have quick, easy access. After all other casualties have been treated, a retriage of these casualties should be performed and treatment initiated if appropriate.

Ideally, holding areas for each of the four triage categories should be established. Marking can be accomplished with the use of different color panels or a numbering system. Each area can be designated as a specific color or number and the route to that area marked accordingly. The marking system used should function during times of good visibility as well as times of limited visibility (such as at night or during blackout conditions). Often the acronym "D-I-M-E" or "I-D-M-E" is used for triage "lanes" from the first letter of each category (ie, I for *immediate*). Chemical sticks (chem-lights) have been used for nighttime markings. Whichever system is decided upon, it must be briefed and practiced with all personnel. Casualty triage tags, which correlate with the color or numbering system, can be used. Alternatively, the field medical card (FMC) can be marked with the appropriate color or number.

■ **Disposition of the Dead**

Death is one of the most challenging and emotional experiences you will encounter. Under normal circumstances, the physician, being the best qualified, is responsible for declaring a person dead and is required to sign the death certificate. US laws require that a death certificate be prepared for each soldier who dies on the battlefield. On the battlefield when KIAs are identified, a spot report is generated identifying the location of the remains so that when the battle is over, the remains can be recovered and turned over to mortuary affairs.

The transportation and disposition of remains is a quartermaster function. Air and ground ambulance personnel do not clear the battlefield of remains nor do they carry remains in their dedicated medical vehicles or aircrafts. Medical units do not accept remains or provide temporary morgues in which to hold remains for other units until they can be transferred to mortuary affairs sites/personnel.

The only remains that a medical unit handles are those of its own unit members or of casualties who are dead on arrival (DOA) or who died of wounds (DOW) while in their care. Whenever a medical unit must establish a temporary morgue, it should be established out of sight of the triage and treatment areas. This area can be established behind a natural barrier, such as a stand of trees or it can be set off by using tentage and tarpaulins. This is not an actual morgue, as it has neither the required equipment nor is it staffed; it is only a temporary holding area until the quartermaster can assume custody of the bodies.

■ Summary

A firm understanding of triage will help you to maximize resources and reduce complications. In this chapter, we have identified steps in performing triage. Given this knowledge, you should be able to perform triage on the battlefield and save lives.

YOU ARE THE COMBAT MEDIC

While participating as a member of a small convoy delivering supplies to an outlying medical treatment facility (MTF), the lead HUMMWV strikes an IED. Following a brief exchange of fire, the commander yells, "Medic!" The commander directs you to the driver of the HUMMWV who is lying next to the vehicle. Your general impression indicates that the casualty has an amputation of the left leg up to the knee with significant bleeding. He is your only casualty. A combat lifesaver (CLS) from the convoy is available to assist you with care. The MTF is 35 miles from your current location and air evacuation is available.

Assessment

You note that the casualty is awake, alert, and anxious with an increased respiratory rate; his skin is cool, pale, and diaphoretic, with a considerable amount of blood flow coming from the left lower extremity. The respiratory rate is 26 breaths/min with adequate chest rise and volume. Radial pulses are rapid and weak. Exposure of the left lower leg reveals a large amount of bleeding. The rapid trauma survey reveals no additional injuries.

The casualty has an open airway and a radial pulse, but he is suffering from shock. Treatment of this casualty includes management of bleeding and shock. Without controlling the bleeding, the casualty can rapidly deteriorate due to a significant loss of blood volume. You determine that this casualty requires immediate evacuation and the commander calls in a 9-line MEDEVAC request while you continue caring for the casualty.

Treatment

You instruct the CLS to apply a CAT to the casualty's left lower leg while you establish a large-bore saline lock and begin to deliver an intravenous solution of normal saline. Reassessment of the casualty reveals that he remains awake and alert with a respiratory rate of 22 breaths/min demonstrating adequate chest rise and volume, radial pulse of 106 beats/min and strong, and a blood pressure of 100/68 mm Hg. The MEDEVAC crew arrives and assumes care for the casualty en route to the MTF.

1. LAST NAME, FIRST NAME		RANK/GRADE		MALE ✓
Allen, Nate		PFC		FEMALE
SSN 000-111-0000	SPECIALTY CODE 002			RELIGION Baptist

2. UNIT

FORCE				NATIONALITY
A/T	AF/A	N/M	MC/M	
	BC/BC		NBI/BNC	DISEASE	PSYCH

3. INJURY

	AIRWAY
FRONT BACK	HEAD
	✓ WOUND
	NECK/BACK INJURY
	BURN
	AMPUTATION
	STRESS
	OTHER (Specify)

4. LEVEL OF CONSCIOUSNESS

✓ ALERT	PAIN RESPONSE
VERBAL RESPONSE	UNRESPONSIVE

5. PULSE 106 bpm	TIME 1405	6. TOURNIQUET ☐ NO [X] YES	TIME 1400
7. MORPHINE [X] NO ☐ YES	DOSE	TIME	8. IV NS	TIME 1402

9. TREATMENT/OBSERVATIONS/CURRENT MEDICATION/ALLERGIES/NBC (ANTIDOTE)

Casualty was driver of HMMWV hit by an IED. Leg amputated to left knee. Applied tourniquet & started large-bore saline lock of NS.

10. DISPOSITION	RETURNED TO DUTY		TIME
	X	EVACUATED	1415
		DECEASED	
11. PROVIDER/UNIT Andrews, Justin			DATE (YYMMDD)

Ready for Review

- In combat, the casualties with the most severe injuries or the greatest threat to life are not necessarily the ones who should receive the first priority when dealing with multiple casualties.

- Consideration must be given to the casualty's likelihood of survival.

- The predominant principle of casualty triage is to treat and return to duty the greatest number of soldiers in the shortest possible time.

- Mass casualty (MASCAL) situations occur when the number of casualties exceeds the available medical capability to rapidly treat and evacuate them.

- Triage is the medical sorting of casualties according to the type and seriousness of the injury, the likelihood of survival, and the establishment of priorities of treatment and evacuation.

- Triage ensures that medical resources are properly used to provide care for the greatest benefit to the largest number of casualties.

- Depending on the tactical situation or the location of the MASCAL, the triage, treatment, and holding areas may be established in the existing medical treatment facility (MTF), an available shelter, or outdoors.

- Establish MEDEVAC priorities by precedence category. A minimal casualty should not be evacuated before an immediate casualty. The MEDEVAC priority categories ensure that this does not happen.

Vital Vocabulary

delayed Triage category for casualties who have less risk of losing life or limb due to delayed treatment.

emergent Alternative triage category that denotes a casualty who requires attention within minutes to several hours to avoid death or major disability.

expectant Triage category for casualties so critically injured that only complicated and prolonged treatment would offer any hope of improving life expectancy.

immediate Triage category for casualties whose condition demands immediate resuscitative treatment.

mass casualty (MASCAL) situation When the number of casualties exceeds the available medical capability to rapidly treat and evacuate.

minimal Triage category for casualties with superficial wounds who can utilize self-aid or buddy-aid.

nonemergent Alternative triage category that denotes a casualty who does not require the attention of the emergent group although they may require surgery; also lack significant potential for loss of life, limb, or eyesight.

Priority I—Urgent MEDEVAC category assigned to casualties who should be evacuated as soon as possible and within a maximum of 2 hours.

Priority IA—Urgent Surgical MEDEVAC category assigned to casualties who must receive far forward surgical intervention to save lives and stabilize for further evacuation.

Priority II—Priority MEDEVAC category assigned to sick and wounded casualties requiring prompt medical care.

Priority III—Routine MEDEVAC category assigned to casualties requiring evacuation but whose condition is not expected to deteriorate significantly.

Priority IV—Convenience MEDEVAC category assigned to casualties for whom evacuation by medical vehicle is a matter of medical convenience rather than necessity.

triage The medical sorting of casualties according to the type and seriousness of the injury, likelihood of survival, and establishment of priorities of treatment and evacuation.

COMBAT MEDIC *in Action*

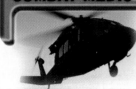

After the casualty is safely transferred to the care of the MED-EVAC crew, you are asked to assess and triage the pas-senger from the impacted HUMMWV who twisted his ankle when he removed the casualty from the vehicle. Your general impression of the casualty shows a soldier who is awake, alert, and oriented, and in no apparent distress. The rapid trauma survey reveals no immediate life threats. The additional assessment demonstrates moderate swelling of the right ankle with no compromise of neurovascular status.

1. Based upon the above findings, how would you categorize this casualty using the triage criteria?
   A. Immediate
   B. Delayed
   C. Minimal
   D. Expectant

2. How does being placed in the minimal triage category affect the care received by the casualty?
   A. Care will be rendered by the combat medic on scene.
   B. Care will be rendered by the physician assistant at the MTF.
   C. Care will be rendered using self-aid or buddy-aid.
   D. Care will be rendered by the command officer.

3. Casualties placed in the minimal category are considered to be:
   A. critically wounded.
   B. walking wounded.
   C. mortally wounded.
   D. uninjured.

4. How would the above casualty be prioritized for MEDEVAC?
   A. Priority I–Urgent
   B. Priority II–Priority
   C. Priority III–Routine
   D. Priority IV–Convenience

5. Which of the following is NOT a primary goal for triage?
   A. Returning the walking wounded to duty as soon as possible
   B. Continually reassessing casualties for changes
   C. Establishing MEDEVAC priorities by precedence category
   D. Providing treatment to the most critical casualties first

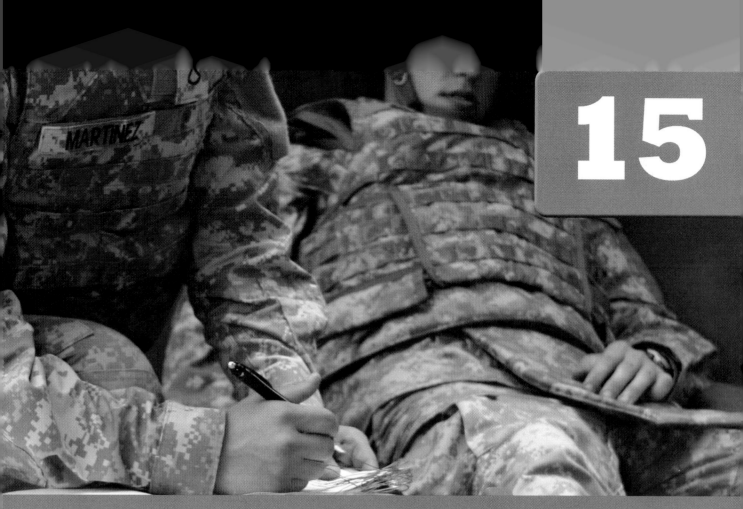

15

Documentation

Objectives

Knowledge Objectives

- [ ] Describe the uses, components, and requirements of the field medical card.

- [ ] List the minimum information required on the field medical card.

- [ ] List the authorized abbreviations for the field medical card.

- [ ] List the steps in initiating the field medical card.

■ Introduction

The DD Form 1380, Field Medical Card (FMC) is part of the official and permanent medical treatment records. It aids the medical treatment staff by creating a record of the casualty care initiated prior to the casualty's arrival to the medical treatment facility (MTF). As a record of events, the FMC may prevent accidental medication overdose, alerts the receiving medical facility to any special care needed for treatment, and provides an accurate record of care already given. It is critical to document all of your actions—if it is not documented, then it did not happen!

■ Field Medical Card Uses, Components, and Requirements

The **Field Medical Card (DD Form 1380)** is about 4″ × 8″ and serves as the medical record for battle injury and illness FIGURE 15-1 ▶. It is designed to provide medical information about the casualty's injury or illness and the medical treatment provided. It records the casualty's entire disposition, including death. In the garrison, it may be used to record outpatient treatment when the medical record is not available. It is used for all US and NATO casualties to document medical care given in a theater of operations.

Components

FMCs are issued as a blue pad of 20 cards FIGURE 15-2 ▶. Each pad contains an original card, a carbon protective sheet, and a duplicate, and has a copper wire to attach to a casualty FIGURE 15-3 ▶.

Requirements

First and foremost, write legibly and concisely. The FMC is the first, and sometimes the only, record of treatment of the casualty, so the accuracy and thoroughness of the information provided is of the utmost importance. The FMC will be reviewed and signed by the supervising Army Medical Depart-

ment (AMEDD) officer. It is critical that the information on the FMC is clear, concise, and complete, so that the AMEDD officer can quickly understand the casualty's condition and the treatment given.

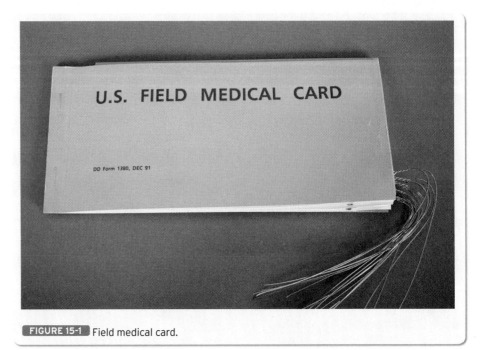

FIGURE 15-1 Field medical card.

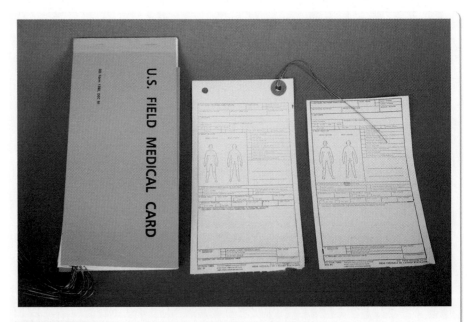

FIGURE 15-2 Each pad holds 20 cards and contains an original card, a carbon protective sheet, and a duplicate.

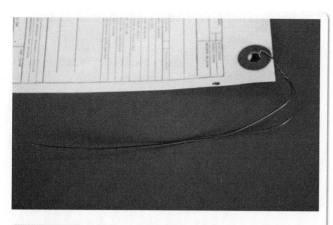

FIGURE 15-3 Each pad has a piece of copper wire attached so that the FMC may be attached to the casualty.

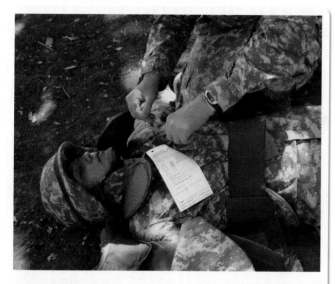

FIGURE 15-4 Attach the completed FMC to the casualty's uniform by twisting the copper wire after threading it through the top buttonhole of the uniform.

The FMC must be attached to the casualty's clothing, where it will remain until one of the following occurs:

- The casualty arrives at the MTF.
- The casualty returns to duty (RTD).
- The casualty dies and is buried.

The completed FMC should be attached to the casualty's uniform by twisting the copper wire after threading it through the top buttonhole of the uniform FIGURE 15-4 ▲. Do not attach the FMC to the casualty's body armor, load carrying equipment (LCE), or light combat vehicle (LCV) because this equipment will be separated from the casualty upon arrival at the MTF.

■ Minimum Information Required

Each block of the FMC provides critical information to subsequent caregivers and must be properly filled in by the attending combat medic. As a minimum, complete blocks 1, 3, 4, 7, 9, and 11. Complete blocks 2, 5, 6, 8, 10, 12, 13, 14, 15, 16, and 17 as time permits.

Required Blocks

In Block 1, enter the casualty's name, rank, and complete Social Security number (SSN). If the casualty is a foreign military person (including prisoners of war), enter his or her military service number. Enter the casualty's military occupational specialty (MOS) or area of concentration for the specialty code. Enter the casualty's religion and sex.

In Block 3, use the figures in the block to show the location of the injury or injuries. Check the appropriate box or boxes to describe the casualty's injury or injuries.

In Block 4, check the appropriate box for level of consciousness. In Block 7, check the yes or no box. Write in the medication dose administered and the date and time it was administered. In Block 9, write in the information requested. If you need additional space, use Block 14. In Block 11, initial the far right side of the block.

Additional Blocks

Complete the other blocks as time permits. Most of these blocks are self-explanatory. Note the following specifics:

- **Block 2:** Enter the casualty's unit and the country whose armed forces he or she is a member of. Check the armed services of the casualty.
- **Block 5:** Write the casualty's pulse rate and the time the pulse was obtained.
- **Block 6:** Check the "yes" or "no" box. If a tourniquet is applied, write the time and date it was applied.
- **Block 8:** Write in the time, date, and type of IV solution administered.
- **Block 10:** Check the appropriate box. Write the date and time of disposition.
- **Block 12:** Write the time and date of the casualty's arrival. Record the blood pressure, pulse, and respirations in the space provided.
- **Block 13:** Document the appropriate comments by the date and time of observation.
- **Block 14:** Document the provider's orders by date and time. Record the dose of tetanus administered and the time it was administered. Record the type and dose of antibiotic administered and the time it was administered.
- **Block 15:** The signature of the provider or medical officer (do not print) and date is written in this block.

- **Block 16:** Check the appropriate box and enter the date and time.
- **Block 17:** This block will be completed by the United Ministry Team. Check the appropriate box of the service provided. The signature of the chaplain providing the service is written in this block.

■ Authorized Abbreviations

In Block 3, use only authorized abbreviations. Abbreviations may not be used for diagnostic terminology. The complete list of authorized abbreviations can be found in TABLE 15-1 ▾ .

TABLE 15-1 Authorized Abbreviations	
Term	**Abbreviation**
Abraded wound	Abr W
Contused wound	Cont W
Fracture (*compound*) open	FC
Fracture (*compound*) open comminuted	FCC
Fracture simple (*closed*)	FS
Lacerated wound	LW
Multiple wounds	MW
Penetrating wound	Pen W
Perforating wound	Perf W
Severe	SV
Slight	SL
Gunshot wound	GSW

■ Initiating the Field Medical Card

To initiate the field medical card, follow these steps:

1. Remove DD Form 1380, Field Medical Card, from the medical aid bag.
2. Remove the protective sheet from the carbon copy.
3. Complete the minimum required blocks.
4. Keep the filled out white sheet (without wire) for your records. If the casualty is RTD, the original copy of the FMC is forwarded to the Battalion Aid Station (BAS) for entry into the journal.
5. Attach the card (top form) to the casualty's uniform by twisting the copper wire after threading it through the top buttonhole of the uniform. Do not attach the FMC to the casualty's body armor or LCE/LCV. In overseas commands, carbon copies (duplicate white sheet) of the FMC are used as the Senior Command Surgeon prescribes. In the United States, the Senior Medical Officer (SMO) prescribes the disposition of the carbon copies through the standard operating procedures (SOPs) or in the Administrative/Logistics order.
6. Keep the FMC in plain view.

■ Summary

The field medical card is a casualty's lifeline when passed from one medical treatment facility to another. Mistakes or omissions on this form can cost lives. Be sure you have mastered this procedure well. The Tactical Combat Casualty Care Card is also being used widely for documentation FIGURE 15-5 ▾ . Please consult your local protocols.

Name/ID: _____

DTG: _____ ALLERGIES: _____

Friendly   Unknown   NBC

TQ
TIME

GSW BLAST MVA Other_____

TIME				
AVPU				
PULSE				
RESP				
BP				

A: Intact Adjuct Cric Intubated
B: Chest Seal NeedleD Chest Tube
C: TQ Hemostatic Packed PressureDx
    IV IO

FLUIDS: NS / LR   500   1000   1500
        Hextend   500   1000

Other:
DRUGS (Type/ Dose/ Route):
PAIN
ABX
OTHER
_____
_____
_____
_____
_____

Medic's Name_____

FIGURE 15-5 The Tactical Combat Casualty Care Card is currently being used for documentation.

YOU ARE THE COMBAT MEDIC

While on foot patrol, your unit enters an abandoned construction site. A gust of wind blows dust and debris around. Some dust lands on a soldier's face. Thinking that it is harmless sand and dirt, the soldier continues on. Later, the soldier feels a burning sensation on his cheeks and nose and notifies the commander, who summons you. Your general impression indicates that the casualty is suffering from a chemical burn to the face from a dry powder that may have been absorbed through the skin. A combat lifesaver (CLS) arrives to assist you to care for the wounded soldier. The closest MTF is 10 miles from your location and air medical evacuation is available.

Assessment

You note that the casualty is alert but very anxious and in pain. He has rapid respirations and his airway is open and clear. He has no external bleeding but his skin is warm, pale, and dry with a lot of dried powder about his face that looks like cement dust. The rapid trauma survey reveals that the soldier was wearing his protective goggles and did not get any of the powder into his eyes. There are additional powder burns on his neck but not on his extremities or other parts of his body. You estimate that the burn involves approximately 4% to 5% of the body surface area.

The eyes have not been affected by the dust and they respond appropriately to light. A complete set of baseline vital signs is obtained and shows a respiratory rate of 24 breaths/min, nonlabored; radial pulse of 100 beats/min and strong; and blood pressure of 126/80 mm Hg.

Treatment

The treatment of this casualty involves brushing off the powder and flushing the skin with copious amounts of sterile saline. You know that injury from exposure to cement dust (calcium oxide) takes time to develop. Cement dust tends to penetrate through clothing and can react with sweat on the surface of the skin. This is why the CLS is helping the casualty remove his shirt and shake as much powder as possible out of the clothing. Cement dust causes a corrosion burn, which can be very painful and this casualty will need an analgesic since he is already in a lot of pain. You determine that this casualty requires immediate evacuation and the commander calls in a 9-line MEDEVAC request while you care for the casualty.

While waiting to evacuate the casualty, you establish a large-bore IV saline lock and administer

morphine for pain according to your protocols. Reassessment reveals an alert casualty with a respiratory rate of 20 breaths/min nonlabored; radial pulse of 100 beats/min and strong; and blood pressure of 122/78 mm Hg. The air medical asset arrives and assumes care for the casualty en route to the MTF.

---

1. LAST NAME, FIRST NAME: Howard, Terry
RANK/GRADE: SGT
MALE: ✓
FEMALE:
SSN: 000-111-0000
SPECIALTY CODE: 002
RELIGION: Methodist
2. UNIT:

FORCE: A/T | AF/A | N/M | MC/M
NATIONALITY:

BC/BC	NBI/BNC	DISEASE	PSYCH

3. INJURY

FRONT   BACK

	AIRWAY
	HEAD
	WOUND
	NECK/BACK INJURY
X	BURN
	AMPUTATION
	STRESS
	OTHER (Specify)

_____

_____

4. LEVEL OF CONSCIOUSNESS

✓ ALERT	PAIN RESPONSE
VERBAL RESPONSE	UNRESPONSIVE

5. PULSE: 100 bpm   **TIME:** 1730
6. TOURNIQUET: X NO   ☐ YES   **TIME:**
7. MORPHINE: ☐ NO   X YES   **DOSE:** 5 mg   **TIME:** 1725
8. IV: NS   **TIME:** 1725

9. TREATMENT/OBSERVATIONS/CURRENT MEDICATION/ALLERGIES/NBC (ANTIDOTE)

Casualty received dry cement powder burns to the face. Dusted & flushed the skin. Administered 5 mg morphine via saline lock large bore IV.

10. DISPOSITION

	RETURNED TO DUTY	TIME
X	EVACUATED	1740
	DECEASED	

11. PROVIDER/UNIT: Fisher, Theo
DATE (YYMMDD):

Aid Kit

Ready for Review

- The DD Form 1380, Field Medical Card (FMC) is part of the official and permanent medical treatment records. It aids the medical treatment staff by creating a record of the casualty care initiated prior to the casualty's arrival to the medical treatment facility (MTF).
- The FMC is about 4" × 8" and serves as the medical record for battle injury and illness.
- In the garrison, the FMC may be used to record outpatient treatment when the medical record is not available.
- The FMC is used for all US and NATO casualties to document medical care given in a theater of operations.
- Each block of the FMC provides critical information to subsequent caregivers and must be properly filled in by the attending combat medic.
- As a minimum, complete blocks 1, 3, 4, 7, 9, and 11. Complete blocks 2, 5, 6, 8, 10, 12, 13, 14, 15, 16, and 17 as time permits.

Vital Vocabulary

Field Medical Card (DD Form 1380) Designed to provide medical information about the casualty's injury or illness and the medical treatment provided; records the casualty's entire disposition.

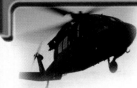

COMBAT MEDIC in Action

While on an evening patrol, a soldier falls down three steps and lands on his left knee. He sustains a painful knee dislocation when his tibia is forced back as it takes the brunt of his weight on a concrete step. The commander calls for you right away. You establish that the scene is safe and that the casualty is alert and did not lose consciousness. It becomes clear that the soldier injured the left knee and leg. He is in severe pain and the joint is deformed and swollen with a developing contusion.

After conducting the rapid trauma survey, it is clear that the casualty sustained a dislocation to the left knee and there is no distal pulse. Baseline vital signs are stable so it is appropriate to consider administering morphine prior to manipulating the joint. With the assistance of a CLS, you carefully manipulate the knee by moving the tibia in an anterior motion and then reassessing the distal pulse. As the pulse returns, the knee is splinted. The time of the manipulation and return of the distal pulse is noted on the FMC.

1. The FMC prepared on this casualty must be attached to his clothing where it will remain until which of the following occurs?
   A. The casualty arrives at the MTF.
   B. The casualty returns to duty.
   C. The casualty dies and is buried.
   D. All of the above are correct.

2. Why is it important to document the time and day for treatments and assessment findings on the FMC?
   A. It is not really important to document the day of the assessment on the FMC.
   B. This is done as a tradition so the record may be complete.
   C. Because time is muscle in terms of the care of the heart, stroke, and potential for reimplantation.
   D. In case the AMEDD officer needs to do a review of the incident.

3. While inspecting the casualty's injury, you should look for all of the following signs, EXCEPT:
   A. deformity, including asymmetry, angulation, shortening, and rotation.
   B. skin changes, including contusions, abrasions, avulsions, punctures, burns, lacerations, and bone ends.
   C. shrinkage or atrophy of the muscle.
   D. increased or decreased range of motion.

4. When you suspect that the casualty has severe pain from a dislocation it should be managed by:
   A. immediate evacuation.
   B. splinting as if it was a fracture and administering pain medication.
   C. multiple attempts to reposition the extremity.
   D. most dislocations are simply popped back into their place in the field.

5. From the authorized abbreviations used to describe assessment findings, which would be used on the FMC for the casualty in this case?
   A. Cont W
   B. LW
   C. Pen W
   D. Perf W

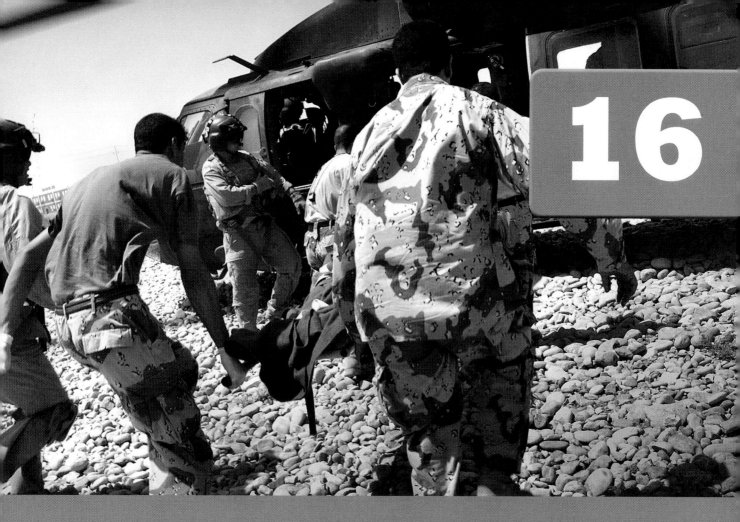

16

Evacuation

Objectives

Knowledge Objectives

☐ Describe the medical evacuation system.

☐ Describe the echelons of medical care.

☐ Give an overview of manual evacuation.

☐ Describe the steps in casualty handling.

☐ Give the general rules for bearers.

☐ Describe how to position the casualty.

☐ Describe the categories of manual carries.

☐ Explain special manual evacuation techniques.

☐ Describe how to make the determination to request medical evacuation and assignment of medical evacuation precedence.

☐ Describe how to collect medical evacuation information.

☐ Know how to prepare and transmit a medical evacuation request.

☐ Describe how to relay requests.

☐ Identify the types of litters.

☐ Describe how to dress a litter.

(continues)

■ Introduction

As a combat medic, you must be familiar with the medical evacuation system so that timely evacuation and definitive care can be rendered to the casualties you treat. **Medical evacuation (MEDEVAC)** is the timely, efficient movement and en route care by medical personnel of the wounded, injured, or ill casualties from the battlefield and other locations to medical treatment facilities (MTFs). Evacuation begins when medical personnel receive the injured or ill casualty.

In previous chapters, you learned how to treat combat injuries. Now it is imperative that you learn how to efficiently evacuate casualties to further enhance their survival and full recovery.

■ Medical Evacuation System

The current medical evacuation doctrine and organizations are the result of an evolutionary process. This process includes both trial and error and the assimilation of lessons learned on the battlefield and in training environments. The purpose of the medical evacuation system is to ensure that casualties are moved quickly into and through the Combat Health Support system. The preponderance of casualties who die in combat do so within minutes due to penetrating trauma and hemorrhage. In order to save lives, prompt localization, resuscitation, and stabilization, followed by timely and rapid evacuation of casualties, is essential.

Medical evacuation encompasses:

- Collecting the wounded
- Triage (sorting) and prioritizing
- Providing an evacuation mode (transportation)
- Providing medical care en route
- Anticipating complications and being ready to perform emergency medical interventions

The increase in the speed and lethality of combat formations has served to increase the importance of medical evacuation as the key link in the continuum of care. The air and

Field Medical Care TIPS

Casualties on the dispersed and nonlinear battlefield are subject to increased evacuation times.

ground evacuation assets currently used to perform battlefield evacuation have both strengths and limitations. To be effective, they must be employed in a synchronized system, each complementing the capabilities of the other. An efficient medical evacuation system:

- Minimizes mortality by rapidly and efficiently moving the sick, injured, and wounded to an MTF
- Quickly clears the battlefield, enabling the tactical commander to continue the mission
- Builds the morale of the soldiers by demonstrating that care is quickly available if they are wounded
- Provides en route medical care that is essential for improving the prognosis and reducing disability of wounded, injured, or ill soldiers

Additional benefits of an efficient medical evacuation system are:

- Provides timely resupply of medical supplies through the backhaul method using returning ambulances
- Acts as a carrier of medical records and resupply requests
- Provides transportation of medical personnel and equipment

The initial decision of the treatment echelon required is made by the treatment element (squad, team, or treatment platoon). Casualties are evacuated by the most expeditious means of evacuation depending on their medical condition and their assigned evacuation precedence **TABLE 16-1**. Refer to Chapter 14, *Triage*, for an in-depth discussion of triage and evacuation precedence.

TABLE 16-1 MEDEVAC Precedence

Priority Level	Description
Priority I: Urgent	• Assigned to emergency cases that should be evacuated as soon as possible. • Casualty requires evacuation within a maximum of 2 hours. • Evacuation required in order to save life, limb, or eyesight. • Used to prevent complications of serious illness or to avoid permanent disability.
Priority IA: Urgent Surgery	• Assigned to casualties who must receive far forward surgical intervention. • Goal is to save life and to stabilize casualty for further evacuation.
Priority II: Priority	• Assigned to sick and wounded personnel requiring prompt medical care. • Used when the casualty should be evacuated within 4 hours. • Medical condition could deteriorate to such a degree that the casualty will become an urgent priority. • Requirements for special treatment are not available locally. • Casualty will suffer unnecessary pain or disability.
Priority III: Routine	• Assigned to sick and wounded casualties requiring evacuation but whose condition is not expected to deteriorate significantly. • Sick and wounded in this category should be evacuated within 24 hours.
Priority IV: Convenience	• Assigned to casualties for whom evacuation by medical vehicle is a matter of medical convenience rather than necessity.

Medical evacuation (MEDEVAC) is performed by dedicated medical vehicles and aircraft that are staffed with medical personnel who provide en route medical care. The provision of en route care on medically equipped vehicles or aircraft enhances casualty survivability. Standard MEDEVAC platforms have no organic capability for defense; therefore, pick-up or transfer points need to be secure or require armed escorts.

Casualty evacuation (CASEVAC) is the use of nonmedical vehicles or aircraft that are available to transport casualties to nearest medical facilities. With CASEVAC, no medical equipment or medical personnel are available to provide care during transit. If these assets are used to transport casualties, they should be augmented with a combat medic or **combat lifesaver (CLS)** if possible.

The decision to request medical evacuation places responsibilities on the requesting unit in the overall evacuation effort. To prepare for and assist during evacuation, the unit must:

- Ensure that the tactical situation permits successful evacuation
- Have an English-speaking representative at the pickup site (PZ) when evacuation is requested for non-US personnel
- Ensure that casualties are ready for pickup when the request is submitted and provide casualty information, as required
- Receive backhauled medical supplies and report the type, quantity, and where they are delivered

Move casualties to the safest aircraft approach and departure point or ambulance exchange point (AXP) if they are to be evacuated by air. Ensure that ground personnel are familiar with the principles of helicopter operations. The ground crew:

- Selects and prepare the landing zone (LZ) site
- Loads and unloads the helicopter according to the aircrew's instructions
- Briefs the aircrew of the enemy troops and directs them to other units in the area, if asked

Medical regulating is the tool used to identify the casualties awaiting evacuation to the next echelon of medical care. It coordinates and controls the movement of casualties through the echelons of care. It also includes the functions of casualty reporting and accountability.

Echelons of Medical Care

Combat health support is arranged in echelons of care. Each echelon (from I through V) reflects an increase in medical capabilities while retaining the capabilities found in the preceding echelon. The medical evacuation system moves casualties into and through each echelon of medical care.

Echelon I

The first medical care that a casualty receives is provided at **Echelon I**. In Echelon I, physician's assistants are the battalion medical officers. Treatment is provided either by designated combat medics or by treatment squads in Battalion Aid Stations (BAS) for conventional forces. This echelon of care includes:

- Immediate far forward care
- Disease and nonbattle injury prevention (DNBI)

Field Medical Care TIPS

Ensure that you are familiar with the type(s) of aircraft that are being utilized for aeromedical evacuation in your area of operations.

- Combat stress control preventive measures
- Casualty collection
- Medical evacuation from supported units to the supporting MTF

Major emphasis is placed on those measures necessary for the casualty to return to duty (RTD), or to stabilize the casualty to allow for his or her evacuation to the next echelon of care. These measures include maintaining the airway, stopping bleeding, preventing shock, protecting wounds, immobilizing fractures, and performing other emergency measures as indicated.

Echelon II

At **Echelon II**, care is provided at the clearing stations, which are operated by the treatment platoons of the medical company. Physician's assistants and physicians are the medical officers here. In this echelon of care:

- Emergency medical treatment, including beginning resuscitation, is continued.
- Additional emergency measures are instituted, but do not go beyond the measures dictated by immediate necessities.
- Group O RBC (red blood cell) is available.
- Limited x-ray, laboratory, and dental capabilities are available.
- Casualties who are nontransportable due to their medical/surgical condition may receive immediate surgical care from a forward surgical team (FST) co-located with a division or corps medical company.

Echelon III

At **Echelon III**, the casualty is treated in an MTF. This MTF is staffed and equipped to provide resuscitation, initial wound surgery, and postoperative treatment.

Echelon IV

At **Echelon IV**, the casualty is treated in a hospital. The hospital is staffed and equipped for general and specialized medical and surgical care. Care is designed to stabilize the casualty for further evacuation or to return the casualty to duty. Echelon IV facilities are located outside the theater of operations.

Echelon V

Echelon V care is provided by support base hospitals. These hospitals are generally located within the Continental United States.

■ Overview of Manual Evacuation

Manual evacuation is the process of transporting casualties by manual carries. It is accomplished without the aid of a litter or other forms of transport. It is intended to end when a litter, vehicle, or other form of conveyance is available.

Casualty Handling

Casualties evacuated by manual means must be handled carefully. Rough or improper handling may cause further injury to the casualty. The evacuation effort should be organized and performed methodically. Each movement made in lifting or moving casualties should be performed as deliberately and gently as possible. Casualties should not be moved before the nature and extent of their injuries are evaluated and the required care is administered.

The exception to this occurs when the situation dictates immediate movement for safety reasons. For example, if a casualty is on the ground near a burning vehicle, it may be necessary to move him or her a safe distance away from the vehicle. This situation dictates that the urgency of casualty movement outweighs the need to administer care. Even when immediate movement of a casualty is required, he or she should be moved only far enough to be out of danger.

Steps Taken Prior to Moving the Casualty

Many lifesaving and life-preserving measures are carried out before evacuating casualties. Except in extreme emergencies, the nature and extent of injuries must be evaluated before any movement of the casualty is attempted. Measures are taken, as needed, to:

- Open the airway and restore breathing and heartbeat
- Stop bleeding and prevent or control shock
- Protect the wound from further contamination

When a fracture is evident or suspected, the injured part must be immobilized. Every precaution must be taken to prevent broken ends of bones from possibly cutting through muscle, blood vessels, nerves, and skin. When a casualty has a serious wound, the dressing over the wound should be reinforced to provide additional protection during manual evacuation.

General Rules for Bearers

In manual evacuation, individuals performing the evacuation are referred to as bearers. Improper handling of a casualty may result in injury to the bearers as well as to the casualty. To minimize disabling injuries such as muscle strain or sprains that could hamper the evacuation effort, the following rules should be followed:

- Use the body's natural system of levers when lifting and moving a casualty.
- Know your physical capabilities and limitations.
- Maintain solid footing when lifting and transporting a casualty.
- Use your leg muscles—not your back muscles—when lifting or lowering a casualty.
- Use your shoulder and leg muscles—not your back muscles—when carrying or standing with a casualty.
- Keep your back straight and use your arms and shoulders when pulling a casualty.
- Work in unison with other bearers using deliberate, gradual movements. Slide or roll, rather than lift, heavy objects that must be moved.
- Rest frequently or whenever possible while transporting a casualty.

Normally, a casualty's individual weapon is not moved through the evacuation chain with the casualty. Weapons are turned in at the first available MTF, BAS, or division clearing station to be returned to the casualty's unit through supply channels. Individual equipment, including protective clothing and mask, remains with the casualty and is evacuated with the casualty.

Manual Carries

Manual carries are tiring for the bearers and involve the risk of increasing the severity of the casualty's injuries. However, in some instances manual carries are essential to save the casualty's life. When a litter is not available or when the terrain or the tactical situation makes other forms of casualty transportation impractical, a manual carry may be the only means to transport a casualty to where a combat medic can treat him or her.

The distance a casualty can be transported by a manual carry depends on many factors, such as:

- Strength and endurance of the bearers
- Weight of the casualty
- Nature of the injuries
- Obstacles encountered during transport
- Terrain and weather

Position the Casualty

The first step in any manual carry is to position the casualty to be lifted. If conscious, the casualty should be told how he or she is to be positioned and transported. This helps to lessen the casualty's fear of movement and gains his or her cooperation. It may be necessary to roll casualties onto their abdomen or back, depending on the position in which they are laying and the particular carry to be used. To roll a casualty onto his or her abdomen, follow the steps in **SKILL DRILL 16-1 ▶**:

1. Kneel at the casualty's uninjured side (**Step ①**).
2. Place the casualty's arms above his or her head, and cross the ankle that is farthest from you over the one that is closest to you (**Step ②**).
3. Place one of your hands on the shoulder that is farthest from you; place your other hand in the area of the casualty's hip or thigh (**Step ③**).
4. Roll the casualty gently toward you onto the abdomen (**Step ④**).
5. To roll a casualty onto his or her back, follow the same procedure, except gently roll the casualty onto the back, rather than onto the abdomen (**Step ⑤**).

Categories of Manual Carries

One-Person Carries

One-person carries should be used when only one bearer is available to transport the casualty. The fireman's carry is one of the easiest ways for one individual to carry another **FIGURE 16-1 ▶**. The arms carry is useful in carrying a casualty for a short distance (up to 50 meters) and for placing a casualty on a litter **FIGURE 16-2 ▶**.

With the supporting carry, the casualty must be able to walk, or at least hop on one leg, using the bearer as a crutch.

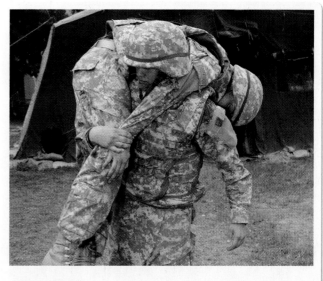

FIGURE 16-1 The fireman's carry.

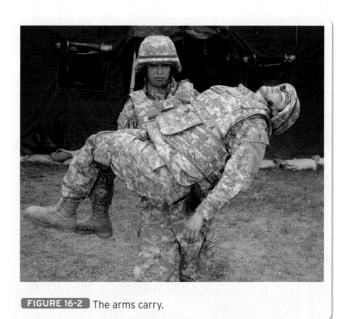

FIGURE 16-2 The arms carry.

This carry may be used to transport a casualty as far as he or she is able to walk or hop **FIGURE 16-3 ▶**. Only a conscious casualty can be transported by the saddleback carry because he or she must be able to hold onto the bearer's neck **FIGURE 16-4 ▶**. With the pack-strap carry, the casualty's weight rests high on your back, making it easier for you to carry the casualty a moderate distance (50 to 300 meters). To eliminate the possibility of injury to the casualty's arms, you must hold the casualty's arms in a palms-down position. Once the casualty is positioned on the bearer's back, the bearer remains as erect as possible to prevent straining or injuring his or her back **FIGURE 16-5 ▶**.

A pistol-belt carry is the best one-person carry for long distances, over 300 meters. The casualty is securely supported

SKILL DRILL 16-1

Position a Casualty

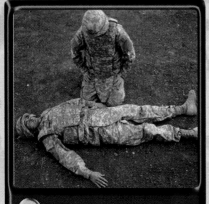

1 Kneel at the casualty's uninjured side.

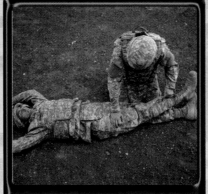

2 Place the casualty's arms above his or her head, and cross the ankle that is farthest from you over the one that is closest to you.

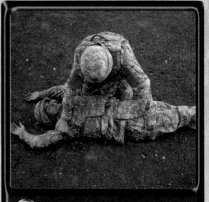

3 Place one of your hands on the shoulder that is farthest from you; place your other hand in the area of the casualty's hip or thigh.

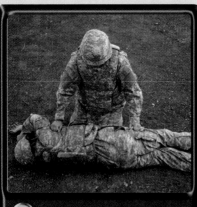

4 Roll the casualty gently toward you onto the abdomen.

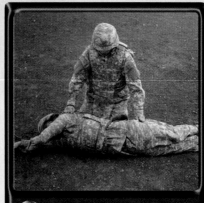

5 To roll a casualty onto his or her back, follow the same procedure, except gently roll the casualty onto the back, rather than onto the abdomen.

upon your shoulders by a belt **FIGURE 16-6**. Both your hands and the hands of the conscious casualty are free for carrying a weapon or equipment, or for climbing obstacles. With your hands free and the casualty secured in place, you are also able to creep through shrubs and under low-hanging branches. If pistol belts are not available for use, other items such as rifle slings, two cravat bandages, two litter straps, or any other suitable material that will not cut or bind the casualty may be used.

The pistol-belt drag, as well as other drags, is generally used for short distances (up to 50 meters). This drag is useful in combat, because both the bearer and the casualty can remain closer to the ground than in other drags.

The neck drag is useful in combat because the bearer can transport the casualty as he or she creeps behind a low wall or shrubbery, through a culvert, or under a vehicle. If the casualty is unconscious, tie his or her hands together. The casualty's head must be protected from the ground **FIGURE 16-7**.

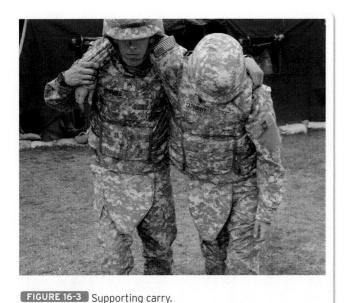

FIGURE 16-3 Supporting carry.

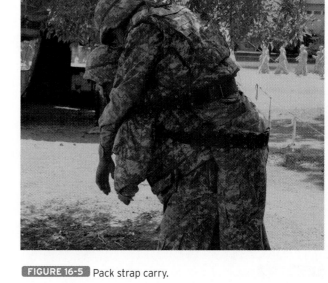

FIGURE 16-5 Pack strap carry.

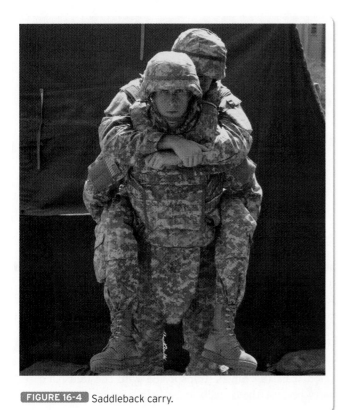

FIGURE 16-4 Saddleback carry.

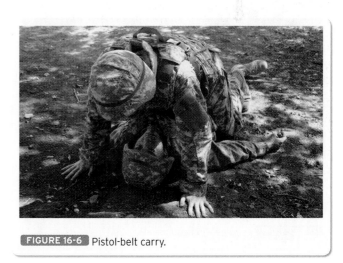

FIGURE 16-6 Pistol-belt carry.

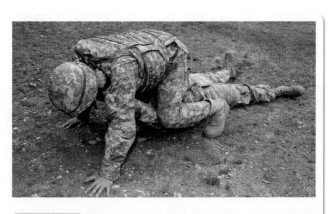

FIGURE 16-7 Neck drag.

The neck drag cannot be used if the casualty has any upper body fractures.

The cradle-drop drag is effective in moving a casualty up or down steps **FIGURE 16-8 ▶**. If the casualty needs to be moved up the steps, you should back up the steps, using the same procedure. The load bearing equipment (LBE) carry using the bearer's LBE can be used with a conscious casualty **FIGURE 16-9 ▶**.

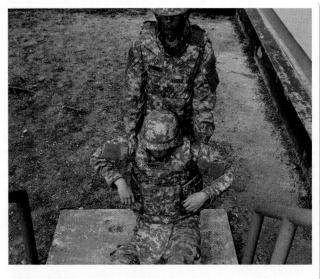

FIGURE 16-8   Cradle-drop drag.

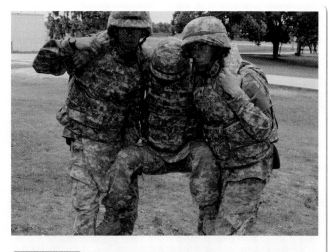

FIGURE 16-10   Two-person supporting carry.

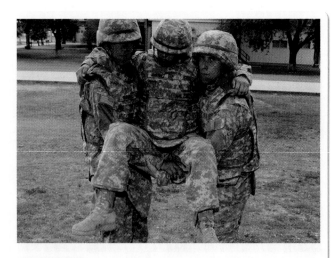

FIGURE 16-9   Load-bearing equipment carry.

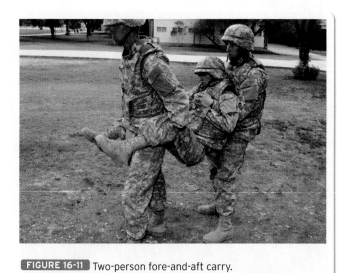

FIGURE 16-11   Two-person fore-and-aft carry.

Two-Person Carries

Two-person carries should be used whenever possible. Two-person carries provide more comfort for the casualty, are less likely to aggravate injuries, and are less tiring for the bearers. Five different two-person carries can be used on the battlefield.

The two-person supporting carry can be used in transporting both conscious and unconscious casualties. If the casualty is taller than the bearers, it may be necessary for the bearers to lift the casualty's legs and let them rest on their forearms. The two-person arms carry is useful in carrying a casualty for a moderate distance, 50 to 300 meters, and placing him or her on a litter   FIGURE 16-10 ▶ . To lessen fatigue, the bearers should carry the casualty high and as close to their chests as possible. In extreme emergencies when there is not sufficient time to obtain a spine board, this carry is the safest way to transport a casualty with a back injury. If possible, two additional bearers should be used to keep the casualty's head and legs in alignment with the body.

The two-person fore-and-aft carry is a useful carry for transporting the casualty over a long distance, over 300 meters   FIGURE 16-11 ▲ . The two-hand seat carry is used when carrying a casualty for short distances, up to 50 meters, and in placing a casualty on a litter   FIGURE 16-12 ▶ . Only a conscious casualty can be transported with the four-hand seat carry because the casualty must help support him- or herself by placing arms around the bearer's shoulders. This carry is especially useful in transporting a casualty with a head or foot injury for a moderate distance, between 50 and 300 meters   FIGURE 16-13 ▶ .

Special Manual Evacuation Techniques

Special techniques may be required to remove injured casualties from tanks, other armored vehicles, motor vehicles, or other limited-access positions. Parking next to a battle-damaged tank can draw anti-tank fire to the ambulance. If there is the potential for enemy fire, approach from the oppo-

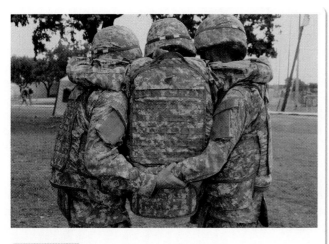

FIGURE 16-12   Two-hand seat carry.

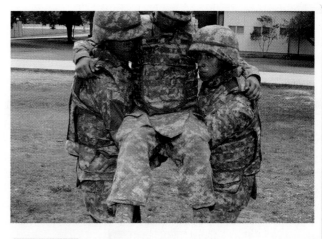

FIGURE 16-13   Four-hand seat carry.

site side of the vehicle, using all available cover and conceal-ment. Ambulance teams should park the vehicle behind pro-tective terrain and dismount with the equipment needed to provide emergency medical treatment, including stabilization of the head and spine, when required.

Observe the vehicle for fire and exercise extreme caution when approaching a burning vehicle. Use fire suppression equipment and any protective measures available. In some cases, attempting to save the crew of a burning vehicle may only result in the injury or death of the rescuer. It must be your decision whether to attempt a rescue from a burning vehicle based on the specific circumstances.

The procedure for extracting a casualty from a vehicle is as follows:

1. Gain access to the casualty.
2. Administer lifesaving measures.
3. Free the casualty from the vehicle or other limited-access positions.
4. Prepare the casualty for removal.
5. Transport the casualty from the site.

Evacuating a Casualty From a Tank

Tanks are assets often targeted by the enemy. The steps in casualty evacuation from a tank are:

1. Observe the tank for fire.
2. Stabilize the head and neck of the casualty, if possible.
3. Extract the casualty from the tank.
4. Check and treat the casualty.
5. Evacuate the casualty.

The main battle tank, the M-1 Abrams, is equipped with three exits. Some of these exits are used to evacuate specific crew members while others are used to evacuate any of the crew. The exits are:

- Commander's hatch
- Loader's hatch
- Driver's hatch

Removing a casualty from the interior of a tank is dif-ficult and requires speed, because there is the potential that a damaged tank may explode or the tank may be more easily acquired or targeted by the enemy. Whenever possible, crew members of the tank should be used to help extract casual-ties because of their experience with these vehicles. Removing casualties from a tank requires at least three crew members or soldiers.

Always attempt to stabilize the casualty's head and neck prior to moving. If a head and/or spine injury are suspected, stabilize the neck as much as possible prior to attempting to extract the casualty. The neck should be stabilized using a cer-vical collar and a Kendrick extrication device (KED). Manual stabilization, using your forearms, is appropriate when no equipment is available. Depending on the tactical situation, these procedures may be abbreviated if the vehicle and its crew are in imminent danger.

Evacuating Casualties in Urban Warfare

There may be instances where casualties need evacuation from open streets during fighting in cities. It is not uncom-mon for casualties to be wounded and exposed to enemy fire and unable to move to cover. While these casualties are exposed to enemy fire, they are at great risk for further inju-ries or even death. Traditionally it has been the role of the combat medic to rescue these casualties. Time and time again this has brought about exposure of additional personnel to enemy fire and has resulted in more wounded or even dead soldiers. If you are wounded or killed, you are no help to your unit.

The Kosmo MOUT Lifeline is a casualty retrieval device designed to be worn by a soldier on his LCE. It is used in urban warfare when a casualty is injured and unable to move to cover. The device consists of a canvas pouch worn on the soldier's shoulder. It contains 30 feet of nylon rope with a tensile strength of 1,100 lbs. The proximal end of the rope is attached to the back cross strap of the soldier's LCE. If the sol-dier is wounded and unable to move to cover, he or she can remove the canvas pouch from the LCE, leaving the proximal end of the rope attached to the back of the LCE, and toss the canvas bag to another soldier who can then drag him or her to safety. This can be accomplished without exposing another soldier to enemy fire. It has proven to be an effective means to extract a casualty from a danger zone while under enemy fire.

■ Establish a Casualty Collection Point

Tactical battle plans will vary depending on the type and number of units incorporated into the plan. The plan for **casualty collection points (CCP)** will vary also. The medical treatment provided on the battlefield is usually accomplished by the unit's combat medics and combat lifesavers. Point-of-wounding care is vital in saving lives on the battlefield. Establishment of a CCP is essential for the rapid treatment and evacuation of the casualty FIGURE 16-14 ▾.

To create a CCP, first, select the site. The location of the CCP will depend on the unit location, the tactical situation, and the number of casualties to be evacuated. This location should decided by the company/platoon medics and the unit first sergeant. Battle drills and tactical standard operating procedures (TSOPs) should be established on how they will get the casualty from the fighting position or vehicle to the CCP. The platoon CCP should be located at the platoon's rear. The company CCP should be located in a covered and concealed position with the company trains. All CCPs are identified with both day and night marking systems and contain a triage area.

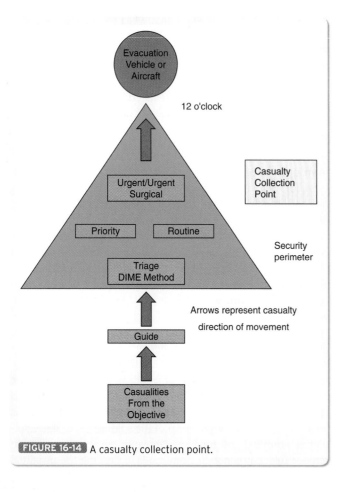

FIGURE 16-14 A casualty collection point.

■ Medical Evacuation Request

The determination to request medical evacuation and assignment of precedence is made by the senior military person present. This decision is based on the advice of the senior medical person at the scene, the casualty's condition, and the tactical situation. Assignment of medical evacuation precedence is necessary to ensure that proper care is given to as many casualties as possible. The precedence assigned to the casualties provides the supporting medical unit and controlling headquarters with information that is used in determining priorities for committing evacuation assets and validated information in controlling the flow so resources will not be strained. The request is made through the medical evacuation request form.

Prepare a Medical Evacuation Request

TABLE 16-2 ▸ lists the lines on the medical evacuation request form. These lines must be completed by the senior medical person. During wartime, brevity codes must be used in preparing all medical evacuation requests, and these requests should be transmitted by secure means only. Use the brevity codes listed in FM 8-10-6, Evacuation Request Procedures. Brevity codes should also be in Signal Operating Instruction (SOI), or using the Automated Net Control Device (ANCD). Locally devised brevity codes are not authorized.

If the use of nonsecure communications is necessary, the request must be transmitted in encrypted form. Information on the form must be encrypted except for:

- Medical evacuation line number identifier, which is always transmitted in clear text
- Call sign and suffix (Line 2), which can be transmitted in clear text

During peacetime, two line number items (Lines 6 and 9) will change. More detailed procedures for use of the peacetime request format must be developed by each local command to meet specific requirements. TABLE 16-3 ▸ lists the differences between wartime and peacetime medical evacuation request formats and procedures.

General Rules of Radio Communications

Transmission Security
The following basic rules are essential to transmission security and are strictly enforced on all military radiotelephone circuits. No transmission will be made if the proper authority

---

Field Medical Care TIPS

Overclassification is the tendency to classify a wound as more severe than it actually is. This is a continuing problem on the battlefield. When properly classified, casualties are picked up as soon as possible and pickup is consistent with available resources and pending missions. Those casualties in greatest need are evacuated first and receive the necessary care required to help ensure their survival.

TABLE 16-2 9-Line MEDEVAC Request

Line 1	Pickup location	• It is not necessary to encrypt grid coordinates when using secure communications equipment or channel skipping equipment. • To preclude misunderstanding, state that grid zone letters are included in the message. • Obtain grid coordinates of the pickup site from the grid map of the operational area. • This information is required so that the evacuation vehicle crew knows where to pick up the casualty and the unit personnel coordinating the evacuation mission can plan the route for the evacuation vehicle (if casualties must be picked up from more than one location).
Line 2	Radio frequency, call sign, and suffix	• Send the frequency of the radio at the pickup site, not a relay frequency. • The call signs (and suffix if used) on the person to be contacted at the pickup site may be transmitted in the clear. • Obtain radio frequency, call sign, and suffix of signal operation instructions from Signal Operating Instruction (SOI), or the Automated Net Control Device (ANCD) or radio supervisor. • This information is required so that the evacuation vehicle crew can contact the requesting unit while en route to obtain additional information (for example, a change in situation, directions, or other information).

Line 3	Number of casualties by precedence (evacuation) category	• Report only the applicable information and use the appropriate amount(s) and brevity code(s) as follows:
		  - The brevity code precedes the description in the line number block under the information column of the Procedure for Information Collection and MEDEVAC Request Preparation.
		    • **A–URGENT** (evacuate as soon as possible or within 2 hours)
		    • **B–URGENT SURGICAL** (evacuate within 2 hours to the nearest surgical unit)
		    • **C–PRIORITY** (evacuate promptly or within 4 hours)
		    • **D–ROUTINE** (evacuate within 24 hours)
		    • **E–CONVENIENCE** (medical convenience rather than necessity)
		  - If two or more categories must be reported in the same request, insert the word "Break" between each category.
		  - These details are obtained as part of the evaluation(s) of the casualties, and provided by the combat medic or the senior person present. This information is required by the unit controlling the evacuation vehicles in order to assist in prioritizing missions when more than one is received.

Line 4	Special equipment required	• Some of the types of equipment and their brevity codes are as follows:
		  - **A:** None
		  - **B:** Hoist
		  - **C:** Extraction equipment
		  - **D:** Ventilator
		• Information on special equipment requirements are determined as part of the evaluation(s) of the casualties by the combat medic or the senior person present. This information is required so the equipment can be placed on board the evacuation vehicle prior to the start of the mission.

Line 5	Number of casualties by type (ambulatory vs. litter)	• Report only applicable information. If requesting MEDEVAC for both types, insert the word "Break" between the litter entry and ambulatory entry:
		  - **L:** (litter) plus the number of casualties
		  - **A:** (ambulatory [sitting]) plus the number of casualties
		• Obtain information on casualties by type, a part of the evaluation(s) of the casualties, and the number of casualties from the combat medic or the senior medical person present. This information is required to determine the appropriate number of evacuation vehicles to be dispatched to the pickup site. The information is also needed to configure the vehicles to carry the casualties requiring evacuation.

(continues)

TABLE 16-2 9-Line MEDEVAC Request (*continued*)

Line 6	Security of pickup site (wartime) or number/ type of wounded, injured, illness (peacetime)	• This information is used during wartime. Use one of the following brevity codes to transmit the information concerning pickup-site security: - **N:** No enemy troops in the area - **P:** Possibly enemy troops in the area (approach with caution) - **E:** Enemy troops in the area (approach with caution) - **X:** Enemy troops in the area (armed escort required) • This information is required to assist the evacuation crew in assessing the situation and determining if assistance is required in accomplishing the mission. More definitive guidance can be furnished to the evacuation vehicle while it is en route (for example, the specific location of the enemy would assist the crew in planning the approach).
Line 7	Method of marking pickup site	• Use the following appropriate brevity code(s) for the method of marking the pickup site: - **A:** Panels - **B:** Pyrotechnic signal - **C:** Smoke signal - **D:** None - **E:** Other • This information is based on the situation and the availability of materials and is provided by the combat medic or senior medical person present. The information is required to assist the evacuation aircraft crew in identifying the specific location of the pickup site. • The color of the panels, smoke, or other markings should not be transmitted until the evacuation vehicle contacts the unit just prior to arrival. For security reasons, the crew should identify the color of the marking(s) and the unit should verify the color.
Line 8	Casualties' nationality and status	• The codes and categories are as follows: - **A:** US military - **B:** US civilian - **C:** Non-US military - **D:** Non-US civilian - **E:** Enemy prisoner of war (EPW) • The number of casualties in each category need not be transmitted. Obtain this information as part of the casualty evaluation(s), from the combat medic or senior medical person present. This information is required in planning for destination of facilities and the need for guards. • The unit requesting evacuation support should ensure that there is an English-speaking representative at the pickup site.
Line 9	NBC contamination (wartime) or terrain description (peacetime)	• Use the appropriate brevity code(s) to indicate contamination: - **N:** Nuclear - **B:** Biological - **C:** Chemical • Obtain NBC contamination situation information from the combat medic or senior medical person present. Include this line only when applicable. This information is required to assist in planning for the mission. • Determine which evacuation vehicle will accomplish the mission and when it will be accomplished (arrive at the pickup site). Information concerning the vehicle to be used and the time of arrival can be obtained from the evacuation unit.

does not authorize it. The following practices are specifically forbidden:

- Violation of radio silence
- Unofficial conversation between operators
- Transmission on a directed net without permission
- Excessive tuning and testing
- Transmission of the operator's personal sign or name
- Unauthorized use of plain language
- Use of other than authorized prowords

- Unauthorized use of plain language in place of applicable prowords or operating signals
- Association of classified call signs and address groups with unclassified call signs
- Profane, indecent, or obscene language

Call signs are used in radio communications to identify a communications facility, a command, an authority, or a unit. There are two forms of call signs: complete call signs and abbreviated call signs. Complete call signs consist of a

TABLE 16-3 Wartime and Peacetime Medical Evacuation Request Formats and Procedures

Line	Wartime	Peacetime
Line 6	Security of pickup site	Number and type of wounds, injury, or illness. If serious bleeding is reported, the casualty's blood type should be given, if known.
Line 9	NBC contamination	Description of terrain (flat, open, sloping, wooded). If possible, include the relationship of the landing area to prominent terrain features.
Requesting procedures	During wartime, the rapid evacuation of casualties must be weighed against the importance of unit survivability. Wartime medical evacuation requests are transmitted by secure means only.	Under all nonwar conditions, the safety of US military and civilian personnel outweighs the need for security. Clear text transmissions (information not encrypted) of medical evacuation requests are authorized.

TABLE 16-4 Types of Call Signs

Complete call sign	A2D28
Abbreviated call sign	D28

Field Medical Care TIPS

To keep voice transmission as short and clear as possible, radio operators use procedure words (prowords) to take the place of long sentences.

TABLE 16-5 Pronunciation of the Phonetic Alphabet

A Alpha (al fah)	**J** Juliet (jewlee ett)	**S** Sierra (see air rah)
B Bravo (brah voh)	**K** Kilo (key loh)	**T** Tango (tang go)
C Charlie (Char lee)	**L** Lima (lee mah)	**U** Uniform (you nee form)
D Delta (dell tah)	**M** Mike (mike)	**V** Victor (vik tah)
E Echo (eck oh)	**N** November (no vem ber)	**W** Whiskey (wiss key)
F Foxtrot (foks trot)	**O** Oscar (oss cah)	**X** X-Ray (ecks ray)
G Golf (golf)	**P** Papa (pah pah)	**Y** Yankee (yang key)
H Hotel (hoh tell)	**Q** Quebec (keh beck)	**Z** Zulu (zoo loo)
I India (indee ah)	**R** Romeo (row me oh)	

letter-number-letter combination and a suffix and are used when you enter a net in which you do not normally operate or you are so requested by the NCS or another station in the net. Abbreviated call signs are used at all other times **TABLE 16-4 ▲**. If no confusion exists as to which operators are on the radio net, no call signs need be used.

Pronunciation of Letters and Numerals

To avoid confusion and errors during voice transmission, special techniques have been developed for pronouncing letters and numerals. The phonetic alphabet is used by the operator to spell difficult words and thereby prevent misunderstanding on the part of the receiving operator **TABLE 16-5 ▶**. The phonetic alphabet is also used for the transmission of encrypted messages. For example, the cipher group CMVVX is spoken, "CHARLIE MIKE VICTOR VICTOR X-RAY."

Numbers are spoken digit by digit, except that exact multiples of thousands may be spoken as such **TABLE 16-6 ▶**. For example, 84 is "AIT FOW-ER," 2,500 is "TOO FIFE ZE-RO ZE-RO," and 16,000 is "WUN SIX TOUSAND." The date-time group is always spoken digit by digit, followed by the time zone indication. For example, 291205Z is "TOO NIN-ER WUN TOO ZE-RO FIFE ZOO-LOO." Map coordinates and call sign suffixes also are spoken digit by digit.

TABLE 16-6 Pronunciation of the Phonetic Numerals

1 One (wun)	**5** Five (fife)	**9** Nine (niner)
2 Two (too)	**6** Six (six)	**0** Zero (ze ro)
3 Three (tree)	**7** Seven (seven)	
4 Four (fow er)	**8** Eight (ait)	

Transmit the Request

The medical evacuation request should be made by the most direct communications means to the medical unit that controls evacuation assets. The communications means and channels used depend on the situation (organization, communication means available, location on the battlefield, and distance between units). The primary and alternate channels to be used are specified in the unit evacuation plan.

Security Transmissions

Under all wartime conditions, requests are transmitted by secure means only. Nonsecure communications dictate that the request is transmitted in encrypted form. Regardless of the type, the transmission must:

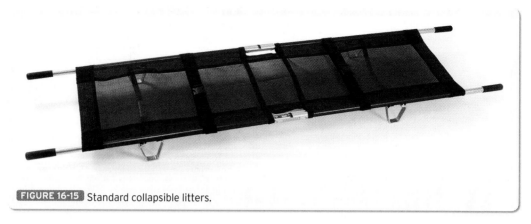

FIGURE 16-15 Standard collapsible litters.

- Make proper contact with the intended receiver
- Use the effective call sign and frequency assignments from the SOI
- Use the proper radio procedure
- Ensure that transmission time is kept to a minimum (25 seconds maximum)
- Provide the opening statement: "I have a MEDEVAC request."

After the appropriate opening statement is made, the transmitting operator breaks for acknowledgment. Authentication by the receiving or transmitting unit should be done in accordance with the tactical standard operating procedures (TSOPs).

Letters and numbers are pronounced according to standard radio procedure. Give the Line Number Identifier followed by applicable information, and then transmit the request. Line numbers 1 to 5 must be transmitted first. This allows the evacuation unit to begin the mission without delay. Lines 6 to 9 should be transmitted as soon as possible. After transmission and authentication, monitor the frequency, wait for additional information, and relay contact information from the evacuation vehicles.

Relay Requests

If the unit receiving the request does not control the evacuation means, it must relay the request to the headquarters that has control or to another relaying unit. When relaying to a unit without secure communications means, transmit in encrypted form. Regardless of the method of transmission, you must ensure that the relay is the exact information originally received. The radio call sign and frequency relayed (Line 2 of the request) should be that of the requesting unit and not that of the relaying unit. If possible, intermediate headquarters or units relaying requests will monitor the frequency specified in Line 2. This is necessary in the event contact is not established by the medical evacuation unit, vehicle, or aircraft with the requesting unit.

■ Litters

Litters are used to transport casualties on the battlefield, and to and from evacuation vehicles. A litter may be prefabricated or may be improvised from available materials. The Armed Forces use several types of standard litters. This standardization allows a casualty to travel in various evacuation vehicles

on the same litter, thereby minimizing the possibility of further injury and saving valuable time.

Standard Litters

The standard collapsible litter is most widely used **FIGURE 16-15 ▲**. It folds along the long axis only. The basic components of the litter include:

- Two straight, rigid, lightweight aluminum poles
- A cover (bed) of cotton duck
- Four wooden handles attached to the poles
- Four stirrups (one bolted near the end of each pole) that support the litter when it is placed on the ground
- Two spreader bars (one near each end of the litter) that are extended crosswise at the stirrups to hold the cover taut when the litter is open
- Two litter securing straps (one attached to each pole at the stirrup bolts) that are used to secure the litter when it is closed
- Accessories such as casualty-securing straps

The dimensions of the standard collapsible litters are:

- Overall length: 90″
- Overall width: 22⅞″
- Bed length: 72″
- Bed width: 227/80
- Weight: 15 lb

The casualty-securing strap is used to hold the casualty in position on the litter and is designed to fit the straight and folding aluminum litters as well as other standard litters **FIGURE 16-16 ▶**. The strap also can be used with an improvised litter as a restraint, if required. The strap is made from a 6′ length of 2″ webbing and a buckle with a locking device and spring. The folding lightweight aluminum poles can be folded to half their length when the litter is not in use.

The poleless semi-rigid litter **FIGURE 16-17 ▶** is useful in evacuating casualties from ships and in mountainous areas. It holds the casualty securely in position and facilitates the movement of the casualty vertically.

The dimensions of this litter are:

- Length: 83¾″
- Width: 22¾″
- Weight: 18¾ lb

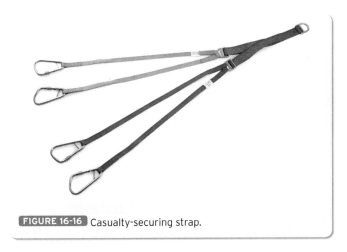

FIGURE 16-16 Casualty-securing strap.

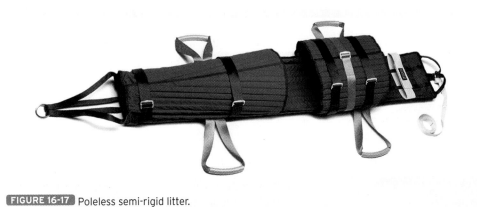

FIGURE 16-17 Poleless semi-rigid litter.

- Has ropes, cables, or steel rings that can be attached to the litter as required for vertical recoveries

The dimensions of the Stokes litter are:

- Length: 84″
- Width: 23″
- Weight: 31½ lb

The SKED litter **FIGURE 16-20 ▶** is a compact and lightweight transport system used to evacuate a casualty over land. It can also be used to rescue a casualty in water.

Improvised Litters

There are times when a casualty may have to be moved and a standard litter is not available. The distance may be too great for manual carries or the casualty may have an injury that would be aggravated by manual transportation. In these situations, litters can be improvised from materials at hand. Improvised litters must be as well constructed as possible to avoid the risk of dropping or further injuring the casualty. Improvised litters are emergency measures and must be replaced by standard litters at the first opportunity.

A satisfactory improvised litter can be made by securing poles inside such items as:

- Blanket
- Poncho

The basic components of the poleless semi-rigid litter are:

- Semi-rigid cotton duck with wooden supports
- Four webbing handles (two at each end) that can be used when the litter is carried by four bearers
- Four loops used to insert the poles for carrying
- A headpiece used to support the casualty's head
- Seven casualty-securing straps used to secure the casualty to the litter

The poleless nonrigid litter **FIGURE 16-18 ▶**:

- Is folded and carried by the combat medic
- Has folds into which improvised poles can be inserted for evacuation over long distances
- Has slings for hoisting, lowering, and carrying, and casualty-securing straps to secure the casualty to the litter

The Stokes litter **FIGURE 16-19 ▶**:

- Affords maximum security for the casualty when the litter is tilted
- Is composed of a steel or aluminum tubular frame supporting a bed of wire mesh netting
- Has wooden slats to support the casualty's back
- Has its lower half divided into two compartments to accommodate the casualty's legs
- Has four webbed casualty-securing straps

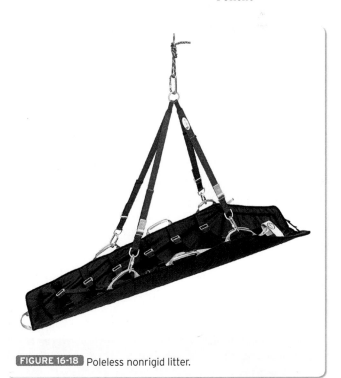

FIGURE 16-18 Poleless nonrigid litter.

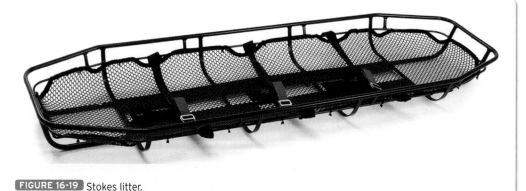

FIGURE 16-19 Stokes litter.

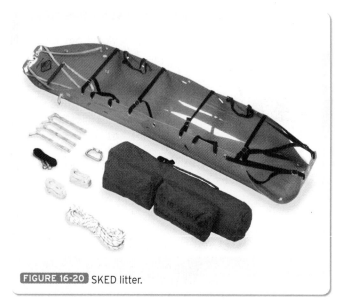

FIGURE 16-20 SKED litter.

- Shelter half
- Tarpaulin material such as waterproof canvas
- Mattress cover
- Jackets
- Shirts
- Bed-ticking
- Bags
- Sacks

Poles can be improvised from:

- Strong branches
- Tent poles
- Skis
- Lengths of pipe

Most flat-surface objects of suitable size can be used as litters:

- Doors
- Boards
- Window shutters
- Benches
- Ladders

- Cots
- Chairs

Dress a Litter

A litter is dressed with one, two, or three blankets to reduce the danger of shock and to afford warmth and comfort to the casualty during transport. To dress the litter with one blanket, follow the steps in **SKILL DRILL 16-2 ▶**:

1. Place the blanket diagonally over the litter (**Step ①**).
2. After the casualty is placed on the litter, bring the sides of the blanket over the casualty and tuck in the edges at the head and feet (**Step ②**).

To dress the litter with two blankets, follow the steps in **SKILL DRILL 16-3 ▶**:

1. Center the first blanket and place it lengthwise across the litter with the blanket edge just beyond head end of the litter.
2. Fold the second blanket into thirds and place in the center of the litter. At the feet end of the litter, open the fold (**Step ①**).
3. After the casualty is placed on the litter, bring the folds of the second blanket up over the casualty's feet. Tuck the blanket around the casualty's feet (**Step ②**).
4. With the first blanket, wrap the casualty with one side and then the other (**Step ③**).

To dress the litter with three blankets, follow the steps in **SKILL DRILL 16-4 ▶**:

1. Fold the first and second blankets into thirds. Place the first blanket lengthwise on the litter so that one edge is even with the litter pole farthest from you.

Field Medical Care TIPS

Chemical litters have specialized features:
- The cover fabric is a honeycomb weave of monofilament polypropylene.
- They will not absorb any agents and are not degraded by decontamination fluids.
- They are flame retardant and rip resistant.
- They are treated to withstand weather and sunlight.
- Their aluminum poles are painted with a chemical agent-resistant coating.
- They conform to all NATO standards and weigh about 15 lb.

2. Place the second blanket lengthwise on top of the first blanket so that one edge is even with the litter pole. (**Step ①**).

3. The third blanket is folded in half and placed over the casualty (**Step ②**).

4. Bring the folds of the first and second blanket up and over the casualty. Tuck the edges of the blankets in securely around the casualty (**Step ③**).

Securing Straps

After the casualty is placed on the dressed litter and covered, the securing straps are used to hold the casualty in position. The number of straps and body parts over which they should be placed depend on the type of terrain over which the casualty is carried. If two straps are necessary,

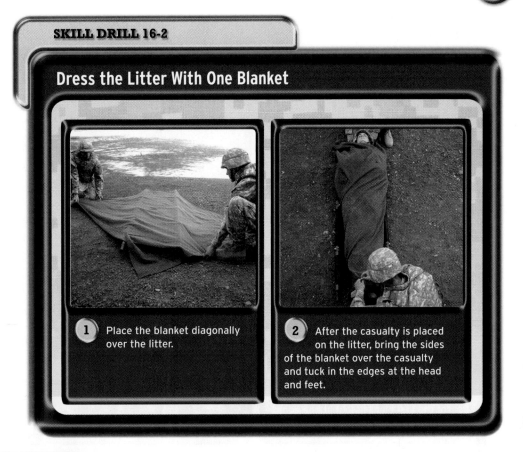

SKILL DRILL 16-2

Dress the Litter With One Blanket

① Place the blanket diagonally over the litter.

② After the casualty is placed on the litter, bring the sides of the blanket over the casualty and tuck in the edges at the head and feet.

SKILL DRILL 16-3

Dress the Litter With Two Blankets

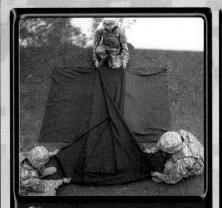
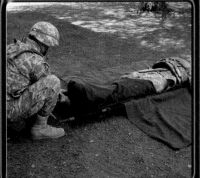
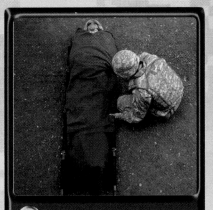

① Center the first blanket and place it lengthwise across the litter with the blanket edge just beyond head end of the litter. Fold the second blanket into thirds and place in the center of the litter. At the feet end of the litter, open the fold.

② After the casualty is placed on the litter, bring the folds of the second blanket up over the casualty's feet. Tuck the blanket around the casualty's feet.

③ With the first blanket, wrap the casualty with one side and then the other.

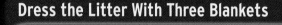

SKILL DRILL 16-4

Dress the Litter With Three Blankets

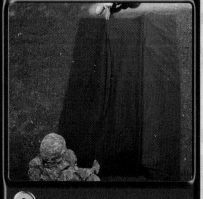

1 Fold the first and second blankets into thirds. Place the first blanket lengthwise on the litter so that one edge is even with the litter pole farthest from you. Place the second blanket lengthwise on top of the first blanket so that one edge is even with the litter pole.

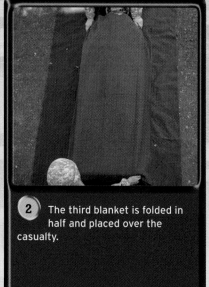

2 The third blanket is folded in half and placed over the casualty.

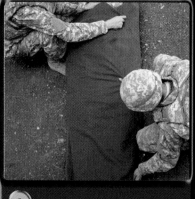

3 Bring the folds of the first and second blanket up and over the casualty. Tuck the edges of the blankets in securely around the casualty.

put one strap across the chest and one across the legs just below the knees. Then extend the straps under the litter and buckle them against the litter pole.

If the terrain is rough, apply two additional straps—one across the waist and the other across the thighs. Then extend the straps under the litter and buckle them against the litter pole. If the casualty is carried either up or down steep slopes, you'll need to use two additional straps to secure each thigh to the litter separately. Take one strap over one thigh, under the other thigh, then under the litter and buckle it against the litter pole. Take the remaining strap and secure the opposite thigh in the same manner.

General Rules for Litter Bearers

In moving a casualty, the litter bearers must make every movement deliberately and be as gentle as possible. The command "Steady" should be used to prevent undue haste. The rear bearers should watch the movements of the front bearers and time their movements accordingly to ensure a smooth and steady action.

The litter must be kept as level as possible at all times, particularly when crossing obstacles, such as ditches. Normally, the casualty should be carried on the litter feet first, except when going uphill or upstairs; his or her head should then be forward. If the casualty has a fracture of a lower extremity, he or she should be carried uphill or upstairs feet

first and downhill or downstairs head first to prevent the weight of the body from pressing upon the injured part.

When the casualty is loaded on the litter, his or her individual equipment is carried by two of the bearers or placed on the litter. For balance and support when lowering a litter, each bearer places their free hand on the knee that remains in an upright position.

Spine Boards and the Kendrick Extrication Device (KED)

Spine boards and the KED aid in rescuing and immobilizing casualties with known or suspected spinal fractures. Spine boards can be prefabricated from plywood or any suitable material.

When a casualty has a fracture or suspected fracture of the neck, use a short spine board FIGURE 16-21 ▶. The short spine board is applied from the waist up to immobilize the upper spine before moving. Bearers assemble the required items:

- Short spine board
- Rigid cervical collar
- Two 6′ casualty-securing straps
- Cravat

If an item is not available, the bearers should improvise it from any available material.

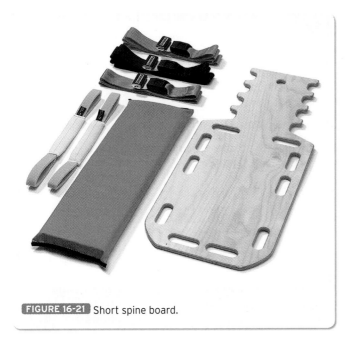

FIGURE 16-21 Short spine board.

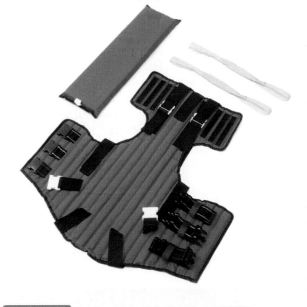

FIGURE 16-22 The Kendrick extrication device (KED) is a prefabricated flexible type of short spine board.

The Kendrick extrication device (KED) is a prefabricated flexible type of short spine board FIGURE 16-22 ▶ . It is useful in extricating a casualty suspected of having spinal injuries, especially if the casualty is in the sitting position. Bearer 1 maintains inline stabilization until the KED is completely applied. Bearer 2 applies a rigid cervical collar, and Bearer 3 ties the casualty's hands together and places the casualty on a long board.

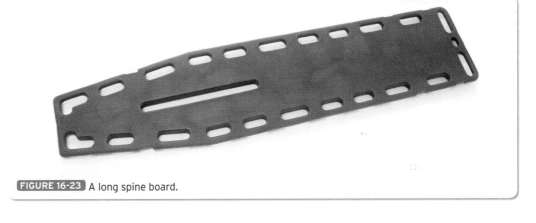

FIGURE 16-23 A long spine board.

A long spine board is used when a casualty has a fracture or suspected fracture of the back as well as the neck FIGURE 16-23 ▲ . Bearers assemble the required items:

- Long spine board
- Four 6′ casualty-securing straps
- Cravat
- Four pieces of padding
- Cervical collar

■ Army Ground Ambulances

A litter can be used to carry casualties to ground ambulances, which are vehicles designed for, or converted for, carrying casualties. They are dedicated assets to be used solely for the medical mission. They may be organic to the combat battalion in which the driver and combat medic are assigned. Ground ambulances are staffed with a driver/medical aidman and an additional combat medic, who are both qualified in EMT-Basic (EMT-B) procedures. These vehicles are equipped with a medical equipment set designed for use in these ambulances, consisting of:

- The combat medic's medical aid bag
- Long and short spine boards, KEDs, and cervical stabilization equipment
- Supplemental oxygen and suction equipment
- Litters, casualty-securing straps, and a blanket set

Track ambulances are staffed with three medical personnel: an ambulance driver, a track commander, and a combat medic. They are co-located with maneuver elements and readily available when needed. With track ambulances, operations are not limited by inclement weather. They possess mobility and survivability comparable to the unit being supported. These vehicles are normally used to evacuate casualties from the front line to the BAS.

Ambulance drivers are military occupational specialty (MOS) qualified combat medics. Their duties and responsibilities include, but are not limited to, the following:

- Responsible for the ambulance at all times
- Driver maintenance of the vehicle and reporting of major deficiencies to their section chief or supervisor
- Providing emergency medical care as necessary
- Providing maximum safety and welfare to the casualties entrusted to their care
- Ensuring the operational readiness and responsiveness of their vehicle and equipment:
  - Litters
  - Blankets
  - Splinting materials
  - Medical expendables
  - Oxygen canisters
  - Flashlights
  - Auxiliary fuel
  - Decontamination equipment
  - Special medical materials and equipment
- Ensuring that they have the required information, tools, and equipment to navigate to the pickup location. These include:
  - Maps
  - Map coordinates
  - Map overlays
  - Compass and position locator equipment such as a GPS
- Preparing the ambulance for loading and unloading
- Assisting litter bearers in the loading and unloading of casualties
- Performing property exchange when casualties are loaded or unloaded
- Providing emergency transport of medical personnel, medical supplies, blood, and blood products
- Acting as a messenger within medical channels

The combat medic's duties and responsibilities include:

- Assistant driver duties
- Familiarity with the condition of each casualty being transported and reviewing the information on the field medical card (FMC)
- Coordination with the individual in charge for any special instructions in the care and treatment of casualties en route
- Providing emergency medical treatment as required
- Making periodic checks of casualties while en route
- Supervising and assisting in loading and unloading of the ambulance
- Assisting the driver with land navigation and guiding the driver when backing or moving off roads, or when under blackout conditions

Current field ambulances are normally used to evacuate casualties from forward units to battalion aid stations. **TABLE 16-7 ▶** lists the current field ambulances in use.

TABLE 16-7 **Current Field Ambulances**

Truck ambulance	4 × 4 utility HMMWV with casualty carrying capacity	M-996	2 litter or 6 ambulatory or 1 litter and 3 ambulatory
Truck ambulance	4 × 4 utility HMMWV with casualty carrying capacity	M-997	4 litter or 8 ambulatory or 2 litter and 4 ambulatory
Armored ambulance	Carrier personnel, full tracked, armored T113E2	M-113	When configured with a litter kit, an NBC kit, and an MES, this is classified as a standard evacuation vehicle. Carrying capacity: 4 litter or 10 ambulatory or a combination of the two.
Light armored vehicle	Stryker M1133 MEV	LAV-III	When configured with a litter kit, CBRN kit, and MES chest, it is classified as a standard evacuation vehicle. Carrying capacity: 4 litter or 6 ambulatory or a combination of the two.

Ambulance Loading and Unloading

When loading and unloading ambulances, litter casualties are moved carefully so as not to cause additional discomfort and/or injury. Procedures may vary depending on the number of litter bearers, the presence or absence of a combat medic, and the type of vehicle used.

Casualties are normally loaded head first for the following reasons:

- They are less likely to experience motion sickness or nausea.
- They experience less noise from doors opening and closing.
- There is less danger of further injury in the event of a rear collision.

When a casualty requires en route care for an injury to one side of the body, it may be necessary to load the casualty feet first to make the injury readily accessible.

For casualties who require IV therapy, a lower berth may be indicated in order to obtain a gravity flow. Casualties with bulky splints may also require a lower berth (if possible). The loading sequence for four litters into an ambulance is: (1) upper right, (2) lower right, (3) upper left, (4) lower left. The most seriously injured are loaded last so they will be the first to be off-loaded. A three-person squad is required to load and unload the ambulance.

■ Aeromedical Ambulances

Aeromedical evacuation is accomplished by both rotary-wing (helicopter) and fixed-wing aircraft **FIGURE 16-24 ▼**. Dedicated aeromedical evacuation assets permit en route casualty care. This care minimizes further injury to the casualty and decreases mortality. The advantages of aeromedical evacuation include the speed with which the casualty can be evacuated by air to an MTF. This ensures timeliness of treatment and contributes to saving lives and reducing permanent disability. It also increases the number of casualties returned to duty.

The range and speed of aircraft make it possible to evacuate casualties over long distances in short periods of time. Helicopters can move casualties over terrain where evacuation by other means would be difficult, if not impossible. Because of the speed, range, flexibility, and versatility of aeromedical evacuation, casualties can be moved to the MTF best equipped to deal with their condition. Fewer specialty treatment teams are required because aeromedical evacuation assets allow the casualty to be evacuated directly and quickly to where the specialists are located. Hospitals are required to

move less often, thereby reducing their periods of noneffectiveness during movement and reestablishment.

It is the responsibility of the senior medical personnel who initiated the evacuation request to have the casualty delivered to the landing site for loading aboard the aircraft. The actual loading is supervised by aeromedical evacuation personnel. The combat medic on the ground will direct litter teams to move casualties in concert with the air ambulance crew member directing the approach to and loading of the aircraft.

Types of Army Rotary-Wing Air Ambulances

Helicopters are rotary-wing aircraft that are capable of:

- Horizontal flight
- Vertical flight
- Lateral flight
- Hovering flight

Their ability to circumvent terrain and obstacles, and the minimum requirements for take-off and landing enable them to operate from areas inaccessible to fixed-wing aircraft or ground vehicles. The helicopter's capability of flight at relatively slow speeds permits operations during periods of reduced ceiling and visibility. Helicopters are organic to the air ambulance units and aviation units of the division and corps. Military helicopters are designated by a combination of letters and numbers that are used to identify their basic mission and type:

- Observation helicopters (OH)
- Utility helicopters (UH)
- Cargo/transport helicopters (CH)
- Attack helicopters (AH)
- Special operations helicopters (MH)

Utility and cargo helicopters also can be used for the air evacuation of litter casualties. The UH-60A Blackhawk is the primary dedicated air ambulance in use today. The normal evacuation configuration is four litter casualties and one ambulatory casualty. The maximum evacuation configuration is six litter casualties and one ambulatory casualty or seven ambulatory casualties.

The UH-1H/V Iroquois is often referred to as a "Huey" and is also used as a dedicated air ambulance **FIGURE 16-25 ▶**.

The normal evacuation configuration is three litter and four ambulatory casualties. The maximum evacuation configuration is six litter or nine ambulatory casualties.

Helicopter Landing Sites

The unit requesting aeromedical evacuation support is responsible for selecting and properly marking the helicopter landing zone (LZ)/pickup zone (PZ). The helicopter LZ and the approach zones to the area should be free of obstructions.

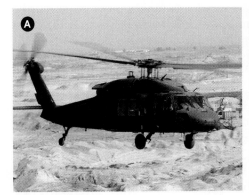
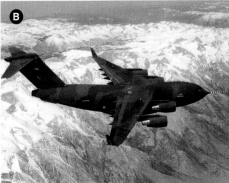

FIGURE 16-24 Aeromedical evacuation is accomplished by both (**A**) rotary-wing (helicopter) and (**B**) fixed-wing aircraft.

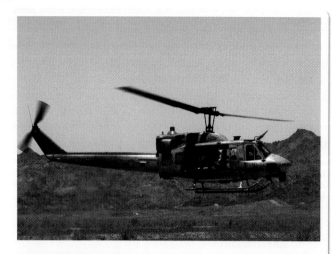

FIGURE 16-25 The UH-1H/V Iroquois is often referred to as a "Huey."

Sufficient space must be provided for the hovering and maneuvering of the helicopter during landing and takeoff. The approach zones should permit the helicopter to land and take off into the prevailing wind whenever possible. Landing sites should afford helicopter pilots the opportunity to make shallow approaches. The minimum requirement for light helicopters is a cleared area 30 m in diameter with an approach and departure zone clear of obstructions. Definite measurements for LZs cannot be prescribed because they vary with:

- Temperature
- Altitude
- Wind
- Terrain
- Loading conditions
- Individual helicopter characteristics

Any objects such as paper, cartons, ponchos, blankets, tentage, or parachutes that are likely to be blown about by the wind from the rotor should be removed from the landing area. Obstacles such as cables, wires, or antennas at or near the LZ that cannot be removed and may not be readily seen by the pilot must be clearly marked. Red lights are normally used at night to mark all obstacles that cannot be easily eliminated within an LZ. In most combat situations, it is impractical for security reasons to mark the tops of obstacles at the approach and departure ends of an LZ. If obstacles or other hazards cannot be marked, pilots should be advised of existing conditions by radio. In a training situation or at a rear area LZ, red lights should be used whenever possible to mark obstructions.

Identifying the LZ

When the tactical situation permits, a landing site should be marked with the letter "H" or an inverted "Y" using identification panels or other appropriate marking material. Special care must be taken to secure panels to the ground to prevent them from being blown about by the rotor wash. Firmly driven stakes will secure the panels tautly; rocks piled on the corners are not adequate. If the tactical situation permits, the wind direction may be indicated by a small windsock or rag tied to the end of a stick in the vicinity of the LZ.

Smoke grenades that emit colored smoke may be used as soon as the helicopter is sighted. Smoke color should be identified by the aircrew and confirmed by ground personnel.

Night Operations

One of the preferred methods to mark an LZ at night for aircrews is to use night optical devices by placing an infrared light source at each of the four corners of the usable LZ. These lights should be colored to distinguish them from other lights that may appear in the vicinity. A particular color can also serve as one element in identifying the LZ. Flare pots or other types of open lights should be used only as a last resort. They usually are blown out by the rotor downwash and often will create a hazardous glare or reflection on the aircraft's windshield.

The LZ can be further identified by using a coded signal flash to the pilot from a ground operator. This signal can be given with the directed beam of a signal lamp, flashlight, vehicle lights, or other means. When using open flames, ground personnel should advise the pilot before approach; burning material must be secured in such a way that it will not blow over and start a fire in the LZ. Precautions should be taken to ensure that open flames are not placed in a position where the pilot must hover over or be within 3 m of them.

Lighting

All lights are displayed for only a minimal time before arrival of the helicopter. These lights are turned off immediately after the aircraft lands. Blue and green light sources should be used only as a last resort; the filters on night optical devices may make them difficult to detect.

When standard lighting methods are not possible, pocket-sized white (for day) or amber (for night) strobe lights are excellent means to aid the pilot in identifying the LZ. During takeoff, only those lights requested by the pilot are displayed and are turned off immediately after the aircraft's departure.

When the helicopter approaches the LZ, the ground contact team can ask the pilot to turn on his or her rotating beacon briefly. This enables the ground personnel to identify the aircraft and confirm its position in relation to the LZ.

Loading Casualties Aboard a Rotary-Wing Aircraft

The pilot is responsible for ensuring that the litter squad follows the prescribed methods for loading and securing litters and related equipment. The final decision regarding how many casualties may be safely loaded rests with the pilot-in-command (PIC).

Litter casualties should be positioned in the helicopter according to the nature of their injuries or condition. Personnel aboard the aircraft supervise the loading and positioning

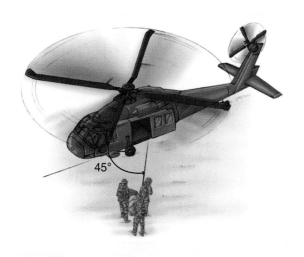

FIGURE 16-26 The litter bearers should approach the aircraft at a 45° angle from the front of the helicopter.

of the casualties. Normally, the medical evacuation helicopter has a crew of four: the PIC, the co-pilot (PI), the crew chief, and the flight medic.

The most seriously injured casualties are loaded last on the bottom pans of the litter support unit; however, if it is anticipated that a casualty's medical condition may require in-flight emergency medical care (such as cardiopulmonary resuscitation) the casualty should be loaded onto either of the top pans to facilitate access. The structuring of the litter support unit allows casualties to receive IV fluids and oxygen in flight. Casualties receiving IV fluids can be placed on any of the litter pans, depending on their injuries or condition. Casualties in traction splints should be loaded last and on a bottom pan.

The UH-60A can be loaded on both sides simultaneously. Casualties should be loaded so that upon rotating the litter support (carousel), the casualty's head will be forward in the cabin. To accomplish this:

- Casualties loaded on the left side of the aircraft should be loaded head first.
- Casualties loaded on the right side of the aircraft should be loaded feet first.

Safety Measures

When loading and unloading a rotary-wing aircraft, certain precautionary measures must be observed. Failure to observe proper safety procedures could cause severe injury or death. Litter bearers must present a low silhouette and must keep clear of the main and tail rotors at all times. The helicopter must not be approached until a crewmember signals to do so. The litter bearers should approach the aircraft at a 45° angle (UH-60A) from the front of the helicopter **FIGURE 16-26 ▲**. If the helicopter is on a slope and conditions permit, loading personnel should approach the aircraft from the downhill side. Directions given by the crew must be

followed and litters must be carried parallel to the ground. Smoking is not permitted within 50′ of the aircraft.

Hoist Operations

A hoist is a motor-driven device with a cable on a spool. It is mounted in two configurations: internal and external. Both configurations require the crewmember to swing the metal boom and casualty into the aircraft. The hoist can be used to extract casualties in areas where the helicopter cannot land. The most common type of hoist used in Army aircraft today is the "high-performance" hoist. It has 250′ (usable) of cable and can lift up to 600 lb. The three most common devices used by the hoist to extract casualties are:

- The Stokes basket
- The jungle penetrator (JP)
- The SKED litter

■ Nonmedical Vehicles Used for Casualty Evacuation

In combat areas, ambulances are often not immediately available, are too few in number, or are incapable of evacuating casualties over certain types of terrain. Many vehicles available to most units can be used to transport casualties with little or no change in their configuration. Some amphibious cargo and personnel vessels can be used for this purpose; however, their casualty carrying capacity varies. When casualties have entered the combat health support (CHS) system, they are classified as patients. Patient evacuation includes providing en route medical care to the casualty being evacuated. A casualty moved on a nonmedical vehicle without en route medical care is considered to be *transported*, not evacuated.

To provide timely and responsive evacuation or casualty transport, combat health planners develop proactive operation plans. These are detailed plans of how the operation is to be conducted to meet the challenges of mass casualty situations. Contingency plans should identify:

- Nonmedical transportation resources
- Nonmedical personnel for litter teams
- Evacuation routes
- Ambulance exchange points
- Medical personnel resources to provide en route
- Medical care on nonmedical vehicles
- Capabilities and locations of MTFs

- Communications frequencies and call signs for command and control (C²)
- Procedures for medical equipment exchanges

All available ground vehicles should be considered for use when medical evacuation assets are overwhelmed in an emergency. Ground nonmedical assets that can be used for casualty transport include:

- Bradley infantry fighting vehicle (BIFV), M2/3
- Truck, cargo, medium tactical vehicle (MTV), long wheelbase (LWB), 5 ton, M-1085
- Truck, cargo 2½ ton, M-35
- Truck, cargo, heavy expanded, mobile tactical truck (HEMTT), 8 × 8, cargo, M-997
- Truck, cargo, MTV, light vehicle air drop/air delivery (LVAD/AD), 5 ton, M-1093
- Truck, cargo, light medium tactical vehicle (LMTV), air drop/delivery, 2½ ton, M-1081
- Semi-trailer, cargo, 2½ ton, M-871
- Armored personnel carrier, M-113
- Medium armored vehicle (Stryker), M-1133
- High mobility, multipurpose wheeled vehicle, M-998

Military medical and nonmedical aircraft include:

- **CH-47 Chinook:** Can carry 24 litters or 33 ambulatory/ 2 crew seats.
- **C-130J Hercules:** Can carry a mix of 74 litters or 92 combat troops.
- **C-17 Globemaster III:** Has a crew of 3 and can carry a mix of 48 litter and 48 ambulatory.
- **UH-60 Black Hawk:** Can carry 11 troops.

■ Recovery of Human Remains

During combat operations, medical personnel are asked to take care of not only the wounded, but also the deceased. The transportation and recovery of the deceased on the battlefield is directed in Army Regulations to be the responsibility of the Quartermaster Corps, more commonly known as Logistic Operations. However on the battlefield, as a combat medic, you will be asked to help in recovering human remains. Human remains recovery is important for the full accounting to family members regarding the circumstances in which their loved ones were killed in action (KIA).

Human remains recovery operations should begin after the area is secure. Treat with all human remains with dignity, reverence, and respect. Prepare a DD Form 1380, mark the form deceased, and attach it to the remains. Do not remove any clothing or any organizational clothing and individual equipment (OCIE). Do not remove any personal effects (PE).

If a casualty dies during treatment, do not remove any IVs or monitor patches. Instead, cut the IV tubes and leave all catheters in place. Prepare DD Form 1380 and attach the form to the remains. List all lifesaving procedures that were performed. Mark the form deceased. Place the remains and any clothing removed from the deceased in the human remains pouch. Place individual body armor in a separate bag marked with deceased's name and date. Evacuate the deceased to nearest mortuary affairs collection point (MACP).

Personal effects that were separated from the deceased during the death event should be individually bagged. Individually bagged disassociated effects may be placed in one plastic bag or in a human remains pouch to facilitate transport. Evacuate to the nearest MACP.

■ Summary

In the battlefield, manual evacuation of casualties is often a challenging task. In this chapter, we have identified steps, procedures, and rules associated with manual evacuation. As a combat medic, it is essential that you have an understanding of manual evacuation in order to prevent injury to yourself and further injury to the casualty in your care.

Medical evacuation is the timely, efficient movement of wounded, injured, or ill persons from the battlefield or other location. In this chapter, we have identified the procedures for requesting medical evacuation support. The same format used to request aeromedical evacuation is also used for requesting ground evacuation. You have been taught the procedural guidance and standardization of request procedures and should now be able to apply the knowledge in the field. Evacuation is essential, especially in a battlefield when life is at stake.

We also have evaluated evacuation platforms available for use. Given this knowledge, you are more than prepared to move casualties by ground or air.

YOU ARE THE
COMBAT MEDIC

While on a morning foot patrol, your unit encounters a series of abandoned shacks. A man and his family are hiding in one of the shacks. The man confronts a soldier with a knife and there is a scuffle. In the middle of the fight, the soldier is stabbed with the knife before the man can be subdued. The closest MTF is 15 miles from your location and air evacuation is available.

Assessment

Upon your initial assessment of the casualty, you note he is alert but very anxious and in pain. The knife is impaled in his right eye. He has rapid respirations and his airway is open and clear. He has a small amount of external bleeding from his eyelid, which will be easily controlled with the immobilization of the impaled object. His skin is cool, pale, and clammy and peripheral circulation is good. The rapid trauma survey reveals some minor contusions on the arms from the fight. The casualty states that he is dizzy and nauseated but is mostly concerned with his sight. A complete set of baseline vital signs is obtained and shows a respiratory rate of 24 breaths/min nonlabored, radial pulse of 100 beats/min and thready, and blood pressure of 120/72 mm Hg.

Treatment

Treatment of this casualty involves bleeding control from the eyelid and applying a bulky dressing to the impaled knife to minimize its movement. The CLS is working with you to accomplish this and utilizes a paper cup to stabilize the impaled object. This casualty needs a fluid infusion of normal saline and an analgesic since he is already in a lot of pain. You determine that he warrants evacuation and the commander calls in a 9-line MEDEVAC request. Due to the potential for permanent disability he is given a Priority I: Urgent status.

While waiting to evacuate the casualty, you establish a large-bore intravenous line and run in 250 mL of normal saline and administer 5 mg of morphine for pain. Reassessment reveals an alert casualty less anxious than before with a respiratory rate of 20 breaths/min, nonlabored; radial pulse of 100 beats/min and thready; and blood pressure of 122/78 mmHg.

---

1. LAST NAME, FIRST NAME: Lopez, Ronaldo
RANK/GRADE: PFC
X MALE / FEMALE
SSN: 000-111-0000
SPECIALTY CODE: 002
RELIGION: Catholic

2. UNIT

FORCE				NATIONALITY			
A/T	AF/A	N/M	MC/M				
	BC/BC		NBI/BNC		DISEASE		PSYCH

3. INJURY

	AIRWAY
	HEAD
X	WOUND
	NECK/BACK INJURY
	BURN
	AMPUTATION
	STRESS
	OTHER (Specify)

FRONT   BACK

4. LEVEL OF CONSCIOUSNESS

X	ALERT		PAIN RESPONSE
	VERBAL RESPONSE		UNRESPONSIVE

5. PULSE: 100 bpm **TIME:** 0800
6. TOURNIQUET: X NO ☐ YES **TIME:**
7. MORPHINE: ☐ NO X YES **DOSE:** 5 mg **TIME:** 0758
8. IV: NS **TIME:** 0758

9. TREATMENT/OBSERVATIONS/CURRENT MEDICATION/ALLERGIES/NBC (ANTIDOTE)

Immobilized impaled knife w/bulky dressing, bleeding control of wound to eyelid, treated for shock, IV NS 250 mL. No allergies, no meds.

10. DISPOSITION

	RETURNED TO DUTY	TIME
X	EVACUATED	0805
	DECEASED	

11. PROVIDER/UNIT: Green, Amanda **DATE (YYMMDD):**

Aid Kit

Ready for Review

- Medical evacuation (MEDEVAC) is the timely, efficient movement and en route care by medical personnel of wounded, injured, or ill casualties from the battlefield and other locations to medical treatment facilities (MTFs).
- The purpose of the medical evacuation system is to ensure that casualties are moved quickly into and through the combat health support system.
- The preponderance of casualties who die in combat do so within minutes due to penetrating trauma and hemorrhage. In order to save lives, prompt localization, resuscitation, and stabilization, followed by timely and rapid evacuation of casualties is essential.
- Manual evacuation is the process of transporting casualties by manual carries.
- The determination to request medical evacuation and assignment of precedence is made by the senior military person present. This decision is based on the advice of the senior medical person at the scene, the casualty's condition, and the tactical situation.
- Assignment of medical evacuation precedence is necessary to ensure that proper care is given to as many casualties as possible.
- Litters are used to transport casualties on the battlefield, and to and from evacuation vehicles.
- A litter may be prefabricated or may be improvised from available materials.
- The US Armed Forces use several types of standard litters to carry casualties to ground or air ambulances.
- Ground ambulances are vehicles designed for, or converted for, carrying casualties.
- Aeromedical evacuation is accomplished by both rotary-wing (helicopter) and fixed-wing aircraft.
- Dedicated aeromedical evacuation assets permit en route casualty care.
- Many vehicles available to most units can be used to transport casualties with little or no change in their configuration.
- Some amphibious cargo and personnel vessels can be used for casualty transport; however, their casualty carrying capacity varies.

Vital Vocabulary

casualty collection point (CCP) Term used to refer to the area where a casualty is collected by a medical evacuation team.

casualty evacuation (CASEVAC) Term used by nonmedical units to refer to the movement of casualties aboard nonmedical vehicles or aircraft.

combat lifesavers (CLS) Nonmedical personnel in the unit who have been trained in bandaging, splinting, and IV initiation.

Echelon I Medical treatment is provided by designated combat medics or by treatment squads in Battalion Aid Stations.

Echelon II Medical treatment is provided at the clearing stations operated by treatment platoons of the medical company.

Echelon III Medical treatment is provided in a medical treatment facility.

Echelon IV Medical treatment is provided in a hospital.

Echelon V Medical treatment is provided by support base hospitals.

medical evacuation (MEDEVAC) The transportation of casualties to medical facilities, performed by dedicated medical vehicles and aircraft staffed with medical personnel who provide care en route.

medical regulating Tool used to identify the casualties awaiting evacuation to the next echelon of medical care.

COMBAT MEDIC *in Action*

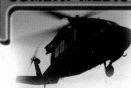

While on a midday patrol, a soldier steps in a large pothole and trips, falling on his outstretched right arm. He was able to break his fall but his right wrist may have sustained a sprain. The commander calls for you to take a look at his arm as another soldier walks the casualty to a nearby safe and secure building. It becomes clear that the injury the casualty sustained is to his right wrist. He is in pain that is tolerable and the joint is already becoming deformed and swollen. After conducting a rapid trauma survey, it is clear that the casualty sustained a bad sprain and possible fracture. With the assistance of a CLS, you carefully splint the right wrist and apply a sling. The time of the splint application is noted on the FMC.

1. Suspecting only a sprain, what priority would you make this casualty?
    A. Priority I: Urgent
    B. Priority II: Priority
    C. Priority III: Routine
    D. Priority IV: Convenience

2. When a nonmedical member of the service provides first aid assistance this is referred to as:
    A. combat medic care.
    B. combat lifesaver care.
    C. buddy-aid.
    D. aide bearer care.

3. Prior to moving a casualty, such as the sprained wrist, you should ensure that measures are taken, as needed, to:
    A. open the airway and restore breathing and heartbeat.
    B. stop bleeding and prevent or control shock.
    C. protect the wound from further contamination.
    D. all of the above.

4. The casualty in this case may just walk but if he gets weak or dizzy a litter may be used, requiring bearers. When a bearer is used during the evacuation it is recommended that the bearer utilize each of the following, EXCEPT:
    A. use your back muscles when carrying or standing with a casualty.
    B. maintain solid footing when lifting and transporting a casualty.
    C. use the body's natural system of levers when lifting and moving a casualty.
    D. rest frequently or whenever possible while transporting a casualty.

5. During combat, if a bearer needs to transport a casualty while creeping behind a low wall or shrubbery, through a culvert or under a vehicle, which manual one-person carry would be most effective?
    A. Supporting carry.
    B. Pistol-belt carry.
    C. Neck drag.
    D. Cradle-drop drag.

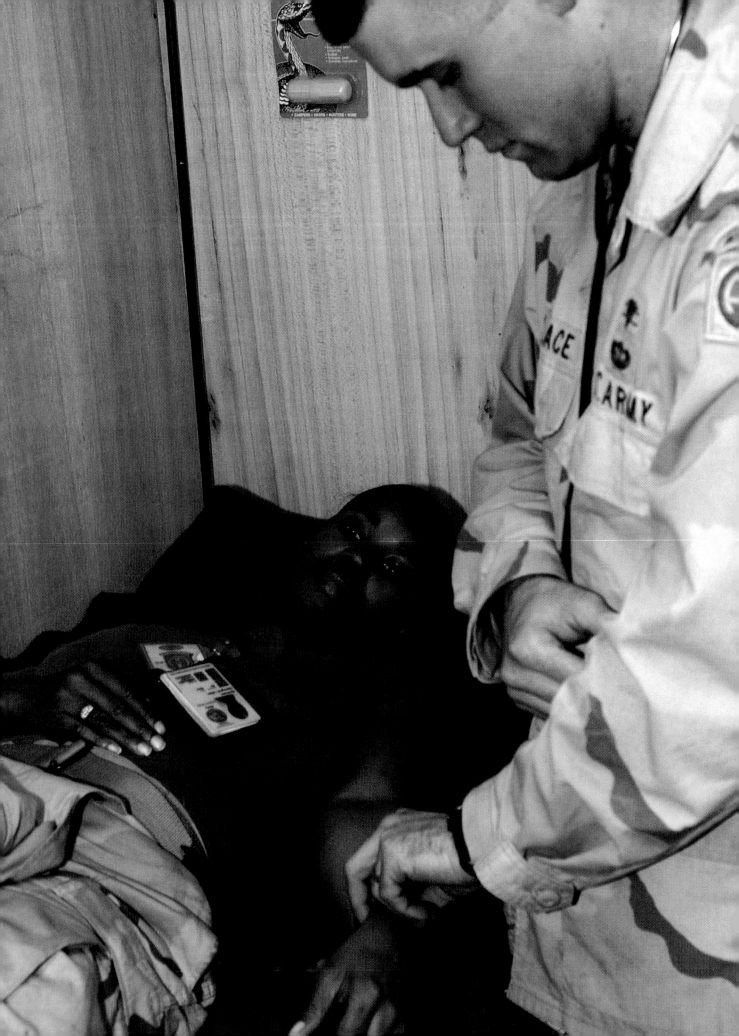

Garrison Care

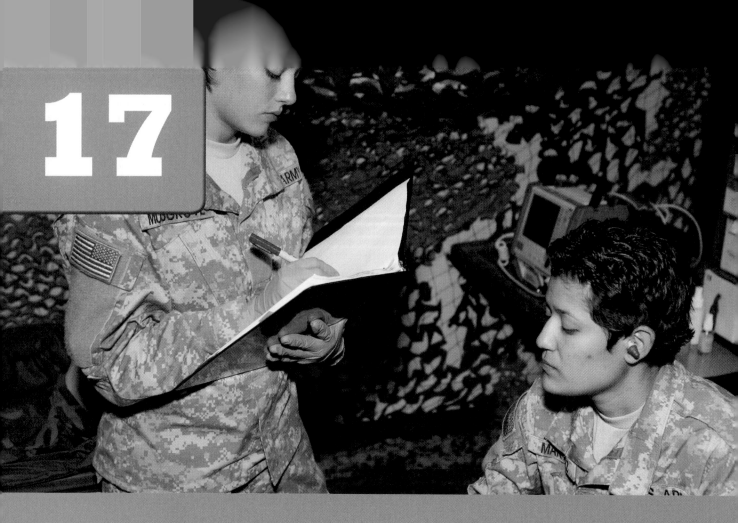

17

Sick Call Procedures and Medical Documentation

Objectives

Knowledge Objectives

- [ ] Describe the sick call (BAS) concept, organization, and tactical use.
- [ ] Know how to record the patient's identification and administrative data/vital signs.
- [ ] Describe how to obtain a patient's history.
- [ ] Explain how to document using the SOAP format.
- [ ] Describe the vital sign parameters.
- [ ] Describe the process for determining disposition and referral.

Introduction

Knowledge of the echelons of care, sick call procedures, and the principles of accurate documentation of patient care is the bedrock of military medical care in the garrison. In the previous section, we referred to injured soldiers as casualties to indicate traumatic injuries from the battlefield. In the *Garrison Care* section, we will refer to ill soldiers as patients.

Accurate documentation of the patient's symptoms and your observations are critical to appropriate treatment and recovery. Entries written in a patient's medical record are part of a legal and permanent written document. If documentation is incomplete or poorly entered into a medical record, a patient may receive improper or potentially harmful care. What you document in a medical record is used by physicians, nursing personnel, and physician's assistants to plan, implement, and evaluate the patient's course of treatment.

This chapter provides an overview of sick call concepts and procedures. It also provides an opportunity to learn and practice a crucial part of medical record documentation that is used when caring for patients and when planning for care.

Battalion Aid Station

The **Battalion Aid Station (BAS)** provides Echelon I Combat Health Support (CHS) for the maneuver battalions of the brigade as a medical platoon and utilizes combat medics in direct support of the maneuver companies of the battalion. The BAS provides evacuation capabilities from forward areas and operates as far forward as combat operations permit while treating and returning the wounded to duty or stabilizing and evacuating them to the next higher echelon of care. The BAS has no patient-holding capacity. The BAS is under the tactical control of the Battalion S-4 (logistics) and is normally deployed in the vicinity of the combat trains (support assets).

Battalion Aid Station Staff

The **battalion surgeon** is a physician who is a special staff officer and advisor to the battalion commander regarding the employment of the medical platoon and the health of the battalion. The battalion surgeon is responsible for all CHS provided by the medical platoon. Officially, the battalion surgeon is the medical platoon leader. Under peacetime conditions, this slot is usually not filled and the physician's assistant serves as the battalion surgeon.

The **physician's assistant (PA)** is a health care professional who performs general technical health care and administrative duties. The PA works under the clinical supervision of the battalion surgeon and serves as the medical platoon leader in the absence of an assigned physician.

The **field medical assistant** is a medical service corps officer who is the operations/readiness officer of the platoon. A field medical assistant is the principle assistant to the battalion surgeon for operations, administration, and logistics. A field medical assistant coordinates CHS operations with the battalion S-3 and S-4 and coordinates patient evacuation with the Brigade Support Medical Company (BSMC) or other echelons of care as the situation may dictate.

The **platoon sergeant** assists the platoon leader and supervises the operations of the platoon. The platoon sergeant also serves as the ambulance section sergeant and requests general supplies and class VIII (medical) supplies. He or she also supervises the activities and functions of the ambulance section including operator maintenance of ambulances and equipment.

Tactical Use of the BAS

When deployed in an operational environment, the BAS is capable of subdividing into two independent and equally functioning aid stations: the Main Aid Station and the Forward Aid Station. The **Main Aid Station (MAS)** consists of the battalion surgeon, combat medics, and ambulances. At this location, casualties are evaluated, treated for immediate life-threatening injuries, and stabilized for transport to a higher level treatment facility. The **Forward Aid Station (FAS)** is identical to the MAS except the primary care provider at the FAS is the battalion PA. The MAS and FAS provide the battalion with two Echelon I medical care facilities. They normally operate in a "leapfrogging" mode—as one is set and ready to receive casualties, the other can be moving forward and following an ongoing operation/battle.

BAS Procedures in a Noncombat Environment

The BAS serves as the primary health care facility for the soldiers of the battalion. Each BAS has established hours of sick call operation. During this time, soldiers present for evaluation of nonemergent complaints, often illnesses as opposed to the injuries seen on the battlefield. Most soldiers who report to sick call are not seriously ill; however, some may present with significant and potentially life-threatening symptoms.

The BAS should be clearly identified in addition to the procedures to obtain emergency care after regular hours of operation. Soldiers are required to obtain a DD Form 689, Individual Sick Slip from their first-line supervisor (section sergeant or platoon sergeant) **FIGURE 17-1 ▶**. This ensures that accountability for the soldier is maintained. The soldier then presents to the BAS or Troop Medical Clinic (TMC) with the DD Form 689. A combat medic is assigned to sign in these individuals into a Daily Disposition Log. The combat medic notes the soldier's name, unit/section, time of arrival, and reason for the visit, and upon departure notes the soldier's disposition (ie, return to duty or any profiles issued).

Soldiers reporting to the BAS follow an accepted routine designed to enhance both the efficiency and quality of medical care. Upon arrival, the soldier proceeds to the front desk where he or she presents a valid ID card and DD Form 689. The soldier's data is entered in the sick call log in accordance with established standard operating procedures (SOPs). Patients generally are seen in order of arrival. It is extremely important for all personnel working in the BAS/TMC to be

INDIVIDUAL SICK SLIP

☐ ILLNESS ☐ INJURY

DATE

LAST NAME - FIRST NAME - MIDDLE INITIAL OF PATIENT

ORGANIZATION AND STATION

SERVICE NUMBER/SSN

GRADE/RATE

UNIT COMMANDER'S SECTION

IN LINE OF DUTY

REMARKS

SIGNATURE OF UNIT COMMANDER

MEDICAL OFFICER'S SECTION

IN LINE OF DUTY

DISPOSITION OF PATIENT ☐ DUTY ☐ QUARTERS ☐ SICK BAY ☐ HOSPITAL ☐ NOT EXAMINED ☐ OTHER *(Specify)*:

REMARKS

SIGNATURE OF MEDICAL OFFICER

DD FORM 689, MAR 63 PREVIOUS EDITIONS ARE OBSOLETE. Reset Adobe Professional 7.0

FIGURE 17-1 DD Form 689.

able to recognize patients who require immediate care. In such cases, the supervising medical officer is immediately notified. Routine sick call patients have their vital signs taken and their complaints reviewed by qualified enlisted medical personnel. Screeners must realize their own personal limitations and seek assistance from the medical officer whenever any doubt exists. All patients may request to be seen by a medical officer.

The combat medic retrieves the soldier's medical record and initiates an entry on an SF 600, Chronological Record of Medical Care FIGURE 17-2. Patients then have their vital signs obtained and the combat medic initiates an entry on the SF 600 in a SOAP format by eliciting the patient's chief complaint and history of the present illness or injury. (The SOAP format is covered in detail later in this chapter.) The supervising medical officer (MO) establishes a protocol for how much of a medical history and physical examination the combat medic elicits prior to the patient being evaluated by the MO.

Most patient encounters during sick call are nonemergent; however, there will be patients who present with signs and/or symptoms that could possibly indicate a serious underlying disease process. As a combat medic, you may decrease the likelihood of overlooking these conditions by maintaining an index of suspicion based on the presenting symptoms and by promptly obtaining accurate vital signs on each and every patient. You must actively look for patients with worrisome symptoms to ensure they are evaluated first. Techniques for identifying acutely ill patients include promptly obtaining the chief complaint from each patient as the soldier arrives to your aid station and identifying patients with signs and symptoms that have increased potential for complications. Examples include, but are not limited to:

- Headaches
- Acute vision changes
- Neck pain/stiffness
- Chest pain
- Shortness of breath (SOB)
- Abdominal pain
- Altered mental status

Promptly obtain vital signs on these patients and alert the supervising MO to the signs and/or symptoms and vital signs results. If the situation permits, examine related body areas to the best of your ability and level of training. Report your findings to the MO. In a garrison environment, you must be familiar with the procedures for activating the Emergency Medical Services (EMS) system.

Patient Records and Confidentiality

It is important to protect medical confidentiality of all patients as fully as possible. Access to medical information may be given to only the patient, patient care personnel, medical researchers, and medical educators. Do not discuss patient information within hearing range of another patient or with unauthorized personnel. Personnel not involved in a patient's care or in medical research do not have access to patient information unless the following situations apply:

- Access is required by law (court order).
- Access is needed for hospital accreditation.
- Access is authorized by the patient.

Unauthorized disclosure of medical information is grounds for Uniform Code of Military Justice (UCMJ) action against the informant. All requests for disclosure must be in writing except in emergency situations. Such disclosure requests should be handled by a patient administrator and should not be provided by the combat medic.

Entries in health records should be legibly handwritten in black or blue-black ink or typed. Entries must be signed by

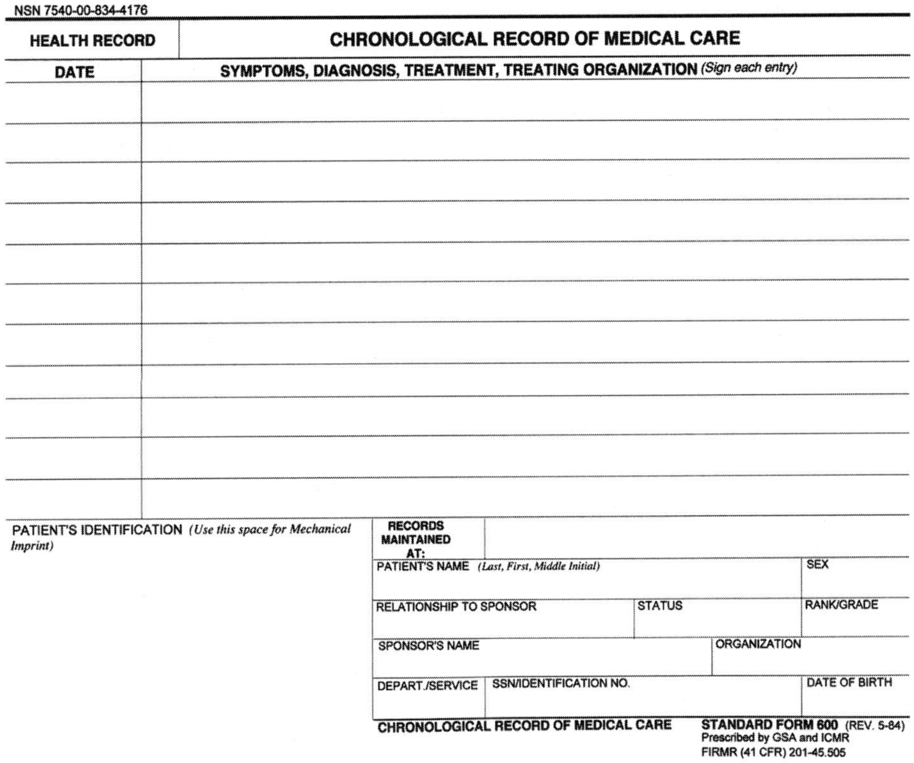
NSN 7540-00-634-4176

HEALTH RECORD	CHRONOLOGICAL RECORD OF MEDICAL CARE
DATE	SYMPTOMS, DIAGNOSIS, TREATMENT, TREATING ORGANIZATION (Sign each entry)

PATIENT'S IDENTIFICATION (Use this space for Mechanical Imprint)

RECORDS MAINTAINED AT:

PATIENT'S NAME (Last, First, Middle Initial) | SEX

RELATIONSHIP TO SPONSOR | STATUS | RANK/GRADE

SPONSOR'S NAME | ORGANIZATION

DEPART./SERVICE | SSN/IDENTIFICATION NO. | DATE OF BIRTH

CHRONOLOGICAL RECORD OF MEDICAL CARE

STANDARD FORM 600 (REV. 5-84)
Prescribed by GSA and ICMR
FIRMR (41 CFR) 201-45.505

FIGURE 17-2 SF 600, Chronological Record of Medical Care.

the individual who made the entry, above the printed name and title. Military personnel sign with full payroll signature, rank, military occupational specialty (MOS), and branch of service. Civilian personnel sign with full payroll signature, title, and pay grade (GS). Entries should be dated with the day-month-year sequence (eg, 25AUG2008). In addition, entries should be capitalized at the beginning, written with present or past tense verbs, and recorded as soon as possible, and must be clear, concise, and objective. Recorders should use only approved abbreviations per IAW AR 40-66. Include patient identification in the patient identification block TABLE 17-1. Use an addressograph or write information legibly. If you need to make a correction, follow the rules listed in TABLE 17-2.

Vital Signs

Vital signs that are accurately obtained and properly recorded are the foundation of quality medical care. All patients reporting for treatment have their vital signs taken and recorded in their charts for each visit to the BAS. It is a generally accepted practice during peak periods of sick call to assign one combat medic to obtain and record designated vital signs. This practice allows for the centralization of equipment and the efficient use of manpower, but may be modified to fit local situations and circumstances. Vital signs should be recorded in the designated area of the SF 600 (Chronological Record of Medical Care).

Abnormal vital signs may be the first clue to a serious illness or injury TABLE 17-3. The combat medic assigned to take vital signs must be aware of their significance and adhere to guidelines.

Temperature

The patient's temperature should be taken orally by using a properly cleansed glass thermometer or disposable probe from an electric thermometer FIGURE 17-3, or by using

TABLE 17-1 Patient Identification

Patient Identification	Administrative Data
• Name (Last, First, MI) • Sex • Two-digit prefix plus SSN (complete nine digits) • Rank • Unit • Unit phone number • Name of treatment facility	• Date • TMC/BAS • Arrival time

TABLE 17-2 Correction Procedures for an Entry Error

Do	Do Not
• Draw a single line through the information. • Write your initials above the line. • Add correct information with the reason for the change and the date and signature/signature block of the person making the change.	• Erase or use correction fluid. • Skip lines. • Write between lines. • Chart for someone else. • Leave blank lines above the signature.

TABLE 17-3 Parameters for Abnormal Vital Signs

Adults at Rest	6- to 12-Year-Olds at Rest	3- to 6-Year-Olds at Rest
Heart rate less than 60 beats/min or greater than 100 beats/min	Heart rate less than 70 beats/min or greater than 120 beats/min	Heart rate less than 80 beats/min or greater than 140 beats/min
Respiratory rate less than 12 breaths/min or greater than 20 breaths/min	Respiratory rate less than 18 breaths/min or greater than 30 breaths/min	Respiratory rate less than 22 breaths/min or greater than 34 breaths/min
Diastolic blood pressure less than 60 mm Hg or greater than 90 mm Hg		
Systolic blood pressure less than 100 mm Hg or greater than 140 mm Hg		
Temperature less than 96°F or greater than 101°F orally		
Pulse oximetry less than 95% while breathing room air		

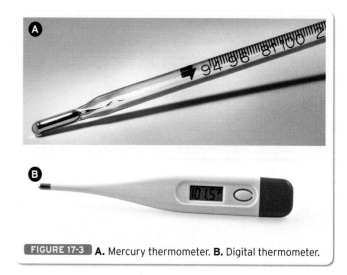

FIGURE 17-3 **A.** Mercury thermometer. **B.** Digital thermometer.

heat-sensitive paper thermometers. In young pediatric patients or unconscious adult patients, a rectal temperature is necessary. Be sure to use the thermometer in its intended orifice (red-tipped for rectal and blue-tipped for oral). In an alert patient, a temperature below 96°F is probably an error and should be repeated. Any temperature greater than 101°F should be brought to a medical officer's attention immediately.

Pulse Rate

The pulse rate is generally taken by counting pulsations at the radial artery on the thumb side of the patient's wrist. Count the number of pulsations felt in 15 seconds and multiply by 4 for the rate per minute. Some electronic machines also count the pulse while obtaining a blood pressure. A quick check of the patient's pulse using your fingers easily determines if there is an irregular pulse. If the pulse seems to have an irregular rhythm, count the number of pulsations in one full minute. Patients with a resting pulse rate greater than 100 per minute

or less than 60 per minute or with an irregular pulse require referral to a medical officer.

Respiratory Rate

A respiratory rate less than 12 breaths/min or greater than 20 breaths/min is abnormal. Respirations may be checked while the temperature is being checked. A normal respiratory rate does not necessarily equate to normal respirations. You must also note the quality of respirations. Patients with any respiratory distress require immediate referral to a medical officer.

Blood Pressure

Routine screening of blood pressures is normally taken in either arm with the patient sitting and the arm supported by the examiner or a table. Clothing that must be rolled up tightly over the arm to allow access to the antecubital space may produce false readings and should be removed. If the first measurement is slightly elevated and the patient has just arrived at the clinic, repeat the measurement after several minutes of rest. The second measurement usually falls within the normal range. Adult patients with a systolic blood pressure above 140 mm Hg or below 100 mm Hg and/or a diastolic blood pressure above 100 mm Hg or below 60 mm Hg require referral to a medical officer.

Blood Oxygen Saturation

A pulse oximeter may sometimes be used to determine how well the blood is saturated with oxygen. This device is placed on the patient's distal fingertip (usually the index or middle finger). It is particularly useful in patients presenting with respiratory symptoms. This device gives you an idea as to the efficiency of the patient's respirations. To guarantee accurate results, it is important to ensure the patient's fingernail is free of nail polish. A patient who is breathing room air (not receiving supplemental oxygen) will normally have an oxygen saturation of 95% or higher.

Patient History

The medical history gives you an idea of the patient's problem before you perform a physical examination. Your observations or examination findings are *not* documented in this section. Record the age, sex, and race of the patient. If the patient is a female, document the first day of last menstrual period (FDLMP); for example, "FDLMP: 3 days ago." This date raises or lowers your degree of suspicion for the possibility of pregnancy in the female patient.

Then, using direct quotes from the patient and avoiding diagnostic terms, record the patient's **chief complaint**. This is the reason for the patient's visit and is typically one sentence in length; for example, "My throat hurts."

Next, record the patient's history of present illness/injury (HPI). Use OPQRST as it applies to the patient's chief complaint. These are the characteristics of the symptoms that you were previously eliciting as the "S" in the history. OPQRST stands for:

- **Onset:** The setting in which an event occurs; for example, "My eyes and nose always get watery and runny when the pollen count is high."
- **Provoking/palliative factors:** What makes the problem worse and what makes it better; for example, "Eating spicy foods makes my abdominal pain worse and taking Maalox makes it better."
- **Quality:** What the pain feels like; for example, "It feels like an elephant is sitting on my chest!"
- **Radiation:** Does the pain travel to other areas; for example, "The pain radiates from my right lower back down the back of my right leg to the bottom of my foot and tips of my toes."
- **Severity/symptoms associated with:** The pain graded on scale of 1 to 10 (1 being minimal pain and 10 being severe, debilitating pain). "Symptoms associated with" refers to symptoms that accompany the chief complaint; for example, a patient with the chief complaint of abdominal pain may have associated nausea and vomiting.
- **Timing:** The frequency and duration that an event occurs and what, if anything, triggers the event; for example: occasional, constant, intermittent, "Only when I do this [activities or foods]."

You also need to note:

- **Associated symptoms:** Any other symptoms the patient reports that are secondary in importance to the patient. For instance, a patient complaining of abdominal pain may also complain of associated nausea and vomiting or fever and chills, and so on.
- **Past history:** Use the SAMPLE method. This contains information that may be helpful in determining possible causes of the patient's chief complaint or ruling out possible causes. This information may also impact your treatment decisions.
- **Symptoms:** A further explanation of the chief complaint. This information is essentially the same as the completed OPQRST. If the patient is complaining of pain, note the location of the pain. If the chief complaint is abdominal pain an example might be, "Patient complains of (c/o) right-lower quadrant (RLQ) abdominal pain."
- **Allergies:** Allergies to medications and the reaction experienced after taking them; for example: "When I take penicillin (PCN) I break out in hives and I have difficulty breathing." A positive history should be annotated by using the phrase "Allergic to:" followed by the medication concerned. The entry may be circled to emphasize it. The use of colored ink is encouraged. A patient with no history of allergies may be annotated by using the common abbreviation no known allergies (NKA) or no known drug allergies (NKDA). Failure to adequately establish and document a history of an allergic condition may result in the patient suffering a severe allergic or a potentially fatal anaphylactic reaction. Each combat medic involved with patient care must be aware of the potential for allergic reactions and repeatedly check for allergies before administering, prescribing, or dispensing *any* medication. Do not rely on the patient's health record or SF 600.
- **Medications:** All medications currently taken, whether by prescription or over-the-counter (OTC); include dosage and frequency taken.

The patient's **past medical history (PMH)** notes significant past or ongoing medical conditions, such as hypertension (HTN), diabetes, high cholesterol, or lumbar disk disease. Any illness or injury that has not improved with prior treatment should be considered chronic, and consultation with, or referral to, a medical officer is required. The patient's **past surgical history (PSH)** lists any surgeries that the patient has had; common examples include appendectomy, hernia repair, vasectomy, and tonsillectomy.

The patient's social history (Soc. Hx) includes the use of recreational (illegal) drugs, alcohol, and tobacco. A smoking history should be documented in pack-years. You can calculate pack-years by multiplying the number of cigarette packs smoked per day times the number of years the patient has been smoking. For example, a 30-year-old female who smokes two packs of cigarettes a day for 10 years would have a 20 pack-year smoking history. Patients who chew tobacco should also have this history documented. The patient's last oral intake indicates what the last food or beverage ingested was and when the soldier had it. The patient's events refers to the events leading up to the illness or injury. It is commonly synonymous with the "O" in onset from the OPQRST.

History-Taking Techniques

Efficient history-taking techniques incorporate developing and using a systematic method and approach to each patient encounter. Observation should begin as soon as the patient walks through the door. Listen carefully; this will help guide you to the cause of the problem. Open-ended questions help you to get more complete and accurate information, "What does the pain feel like?" is more useful than asking, "Does the pain feel like an elephant is sitting on your chest?"

A potential obstacle may be your attitude or predetermination, which may prevent you from making an accurate judgment. A patient seen repeatedly in your BAS who rarely has identifiable problems is a challenge. You must assume that every patient has a legitimate complaint on each visit, until proven otherwise, to ensure you do not miss a significant illness or injury. Patients also have obstacles to overcome. They must have confidence in you. Patients seeking medical evaluation and treatment have certain expectations that may or may not be realistic. For instance, patients without medical training will very often request specific diagnostic studies such as x-rays, blood tests, and referrals to specialists in situations where these are not warranted.

■ Documentation Procedures

The SOAP method is the allowed standard for documentation in medical treatment records. This reference is designed to allow the experienced combat medic to make detailed notes and assists the less experienced combat medic in making adequate documentation. The SOAP method is designed to allow easy reference for follow-up care. This method follows the standard and natural flow of a patient interview, beginning with the *subjective* data, proceeding to the *objective* findings, arriving at an *assessment*, and formulating a treatment *plan*. When obtaining a patient's history, keep in mind the patient history comprises the "S" or subjective component of the SOAP method.

Subjective

The subjective portion of SOAP includes all information of a historic nature; that is, what the patient tells you the trouble is, how long it has been bothering him or her, and other important aspects of the patient's medical history. Note that this portion of the patient interview may well be the most significant contribution in providing quality patient care. The existence of certain complaints, circumstances, or methods of injury can often lead the examiner to concentrate on a special part of the physical examination and may greatly influence the final assessment and the treatment plan. Some subjective findings will require the patient to be referred to a medical officer. An appropriate subjective note will contain the following information:

- Age
- Race
- Sex
- First day of last menstrual period (FDLMP)
- Chief complaint(s)
- History of present illness/injury (HPI)
- Past history

Objective

The objective portion includes all of the examiner's observations and physical findings. It may also include the results of pertinent laboratory and x-ray studies. Remember that a medical record is a legal document and that good intentions do not make good medical notes. A basic rule of thumb to remember is that, if you did not do it, do not chart it. Likewise remember that, if it is not charted, then it is assumed you did not perform that part of the examination. An appropriate objective note demonstrates that the care provider has performed at least those parts of the physical examination that are relevant to the chief complaint. Some objective findings will require the patient to be referred to a medical officer. A complete objective note will contain the following information:

- Vital signs
- General impression
- Pertinent physical findings by body area (HEENT, neck, lungs, etc.)
- Relevant laboratory results
- Relevant x-ray/imaging studies

Assessment

The assessment portion of the notes is frequently given the most attention and concern by many care providers and by most patients. It is, however, the least important in the process of providing safe, quality patient care. It should be remembered that what we label a disease or condition is nowhere near as important as the process of first recognizing the patient's problem and then ensuring that the problem is treated or referred in a timely and successful manner. It is assumed that the art of arriving at more specific assessments will develop with experience. The assessment is either your diagnosis or, if you are not sure, a restatement of the chief complaint; for example, "A. Headache, rule out migraine." Some assessments will require referral to a medical officer.

Plan

The plan portion of the notes includes all medications prescribed, treatments given, special instructions, diets, physical limitations imposed, disposition, and plans for follow-up. Number your plan. Immediately following the plan should be the care provider's identification data, either stamped or printed, including:

- Rank
- Name
- MOS
- Signature

Many plans require consultation with a medical officer. An adequate plan contains the following information:

- Medication (with strength, dosage schedule, and duration)
- Special instructions
- Disposition (duty, profile, quarters, referrals)
- Follow-up plans

■ Disposition and Referral

Unless specifically authorized by the supervising medical officer and local SOP, screeners are not authorized to issue profiles or quarters/bed rest. Remember, profiles should be written in nonmedical language and should be specific concerning physical limitations. Profiles should have a specific expiration date; for example, "No running until 15 April" or "Quarters for 24 hrs then return to BAS at 0630 on 15 April." Profiles that contain such terms as ($\times$ 14 hrs) or ($\times$ 3 days) may be misunderstood, particularly if the patient was seen in the afternoon or on a Friday.

Quarters means restriction and rest within the patient's place of domicile (ie, barracks) and should allow the patient freedom of movement within the living space. In other words, the patient may be free to use the day room and the like. Patients on quarters may not perform military duties. Quarters do not normally exceed 72 hours. **Bed rest** means the patient is restricted to bed, with allowances for necessary travel to the dining facility and latrine. Patients on bed rest *may not perform any military duties.* **Duty** means the patient is returned to his or her unit for full duty without any restrictions. It should also be remembered that profiles and duty limitations are only strong suggestions issued to command channels by medical authorities. Commanders may decide that the successful completion of a mission requires that a soldier "break" profile. In such an instance, the commander takes responsibility for the patient's actions. Medical personnel must continue to support and follow the concerned soldier's health.

■ Summary

Accurate documentation of the patient's symptoms and your observations are critical to appropriate treatment and recovery. Entries written in a patient's medical record are part of a legal and permanent written document. If documentation is incomplete or poorly entered into a medical record, a patient may receive improper or potentially harmful care. What you document in a medical record is used by physicians, nursing personnel, and physician's assistants to plan, implement, and evaluate the patient's course of treatment.

YOU ARE THE
COMBAT MEDIC

You are staffing an evening sick call at the Battalion Aid Station. A soldier arrives with a signed DD Form 689 and says, "I am having one of the worst headaches of my life!" Thus the initial entry on the SF 600 is for a chief complaint of a severe headache. The initial assessment reveals no immediate life threats to be managed, so you proceed with an elaboration of the chief complaint and obtain a full set of baseline vital signs. He has a respiratory rate of 16 breaths/min with normal quality, a radial pulse rate of 88 beats/min and strong, and a blood pressure of 140/84 mm Hg. His mental status is alert. His color is pale with cool and clammy skin and his oxygen saturation is 99%. His core body temperature is slightly elevated at 99.8°F. You alert your supervisor who asks you to obtain additional information.

The soldier complains that the bright lights bother him, so you take him into a quiet examining room and turn down the lights as you complete the patient assessment process. It seems that he has not been feeling well all day and he says that the headache was accompanied by nausea and vomiting. At first, he thought that he just was not keeping up with his fluids but when the headache continued to worsen, he decided to get checked out.

The soldier says that he is usually very fit and takes no medications. He states that he has an allergy to penicillin. You learn from questioning that the onset of the headache was this morning but has been getting progressively worse all day. He states that nothing provokes the pain and describes the pain as throbbing. He further describes the pain as, "located in the center of my head." On the quality scale of 1 to 10, he rates the pain at a 7. He is not sure how to answer a question about timing of the headache since this is his first experience with one so severe.

Next you proceed to ask about his past medical history. He had his appendix removed about 5 years ago but has no other remarkable injuries or illnesses. When asked about his social history, he states, "I gave up cigarettes when I was in the hospital for my appendix. I drink a few beers on the nights we are off duty." On physical examination he denies any trauma, yet has a sore neck as well as pain upon lying supine and flexing his knees.

After reporting your findings to the MO, it is agreed that although this patient may seem nonemergent, further testing may be necessary to determine if he may have a dangerous and potentially life-threatening infection (ie, meningitis). Simply based on the fever of unknown origin combined with the stiff neck, you should wear the appropriate personal protective equipment when managing this patient. The treatment for this patient will also involve some rest, some pain medication, an IV with normal saline, some blood testing, and possibly some medication for the nausea. You will definitely keep an eye on him until the results of the blood tests come back. The supervising MO will make the decision on the need for a spinal tap to test for meningitis. It is agreed to isolate him from other patients until the cause of the fever is determined. Documentation of the patient's assessment and treatment should be accurately completed in the SOAP format on the medical record.

Aid Kit

Ready for Review

- Knowledge of the echelons of care, sick call procedures, and the principles of accurate documentation of patient care are the bedrock concepts of military medical care in the garrison.
- The Battalion Aid Station (BAS) provides Echelon I Combat Health Support (CHS) for the maneuver battalions of the brigade as a medical platoon and utilizes combat medics in direct support of the maneuver companies of the battalion.
- The BAS serves as the primary health care facility for the soldiers of the battalion.
- Each BAS has established hours of sick call operation.
- The SOAP method is the allowed standard for documentation in medical treatment records. This reference is designed to allow the experienced combat medic to make detailed notes, and assists the less experienced combat medic in making adequate documentation.
- Unless specifically authorized by the supervising medical officer and local SOP, screeners are not authorized to issue profiles or quarters/bed rest.
- Profiles should be written in nonmedical language and should be specific concerning physical limitations.

Vital Vocabulary

Battalion Aid Station (BAS) Provides combat health support for the maneuver battalions of the brigade as a medical platoon and utilizes combat medics in direct support of the maneuver companies of the battalion.

battalion surgeon Physician who is a special staff officer and advisor to the Battalion Commander regarding the employment of the medical platoon and the health of the battalion.

bed rest The patient is restricted to bed, with allowances for necessary travel to the dining facility and latrine.

chief complaint Reason for the patient's visit; typically one sentence in length.

duty Patient is returned to his or her unit for full duty without any restrictions.

field medical assistant Medical service corps officer who is the operations/readiness officer of the platoon; the principle assistant to the battalion surgeon for operations, administration, and logistics.

Forward Aid Station (FAS) At this location, patients are evaluated, treated for immediate life-threatening injuries, and stabilized for transport to a higher level treatment facility. The primary care provider is the battalion physician assistant.

Main Aid Station (MAS) Consists of the battalion surgeon, combat medics, and ambulances. At this location, patients are evaluated, treated for immediate life-threatening injuries, and stabilized for transport to a higher level treatment facility.

past medical history (PMH) Significant past or ongoing medical conditions.

past surgical history (PSH) Any surgeries the patient has had.

physician's assistant (PA) Health care professional who performs general technical health care and administrative duties.

platoon sergeant Assists the platoon leader and supervises the operations of the platoon.

quarters Restriction and rest in the patient's place of domicile with freedom of movement within the living space.

COMBAT MEDIC *in Action*

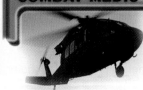

During sick call, a soldier arrives with a signed DD Form 689. He tells you, "I have a headache and feel like I am burning up!" The initial assessment reveals no immediate life threats. The patient's vital signs are obtained: he has a respiratory rate of 24 breaths/min and nonlabored; a radial pulse rate of 90 beats/min and bounding; and a blood pressure of 136/74 mm Hg. His mental status is alert. His skin color is pale with hot and dry skin and his oxygen saturation is 98%. His core body temperature is elevated at 105°F.

You alert the supervising MO right away that you are interviewing a soldier with heat symptoms. It seems that he was performing rigorous exercise most of the day in the direct sunlight and may not have been keeping up on his fluid intake. He said that he was trying to rest but the headache did not go away and he has not been able to keep any fluids down.

The soldier says that he is basically healthy and usually the heat does not bother him. He states that he has been taking a NSAID for knee pain that he has had for some time. He also states that he has exercise-induced asthma that has not bothered him in a long time. He denies any known allergies.

Next you proceed to ask about his past medical history and aside from the asthma it is unremarkable. When asked about his social history he states, "I have never smoked and, well, everyone has a few beers when off duty." On physical examination he denies any trauma, yet is weak and a little shaky on both sides.

After reporting your findings to the MO it is agreed that this patient has more than a headache going on and his problem may actually be mild heat stroke. He is moved to a cool room and asked to remove most of his clothing. The treatment for this patient will also involve cooling, an IV for fluids, possibly some pain medication, some medication for the nausea, and oxygen therapy.

1. What is the advantage of asking "open-ended" questions as a part of your history taking technique?
   - A. Open-ended questions are quicker to ask the patient.
   - B. Closed-ended questions are more accurate and easier to ask.
   - C. Open-ended questions are easier to document on the record.
   - D. Open-ended questions help you obtain more complete and accurate information.

2. When assessing a patient, you should be aware of which "potential obstacle" that can prevent making an accurate judgment?
   - A. The age of the patient.
   - B. Your attitude or predetermination.
   - C. The number of patients in the clinic.
   - D. The time of day that the patient is seen.

3. Your observation of the patient who walks into your BAS should begin:
   - A. as soon as he walks through the door.
   - B. once he is placed onto a stretcher.
   - C. after he is told to remove some of his clothing.
   - D. after a complete set of baseline vitals have been taken.

4. The best clinicians, in assessing nonemergent patients, have perfected the art of:
   - A. diagnosis.
   - B. treatment.
   - C. listening to patients.
   - D. ordering tests and interpreting results.

5. If appropriately authorized by the supervising medical officer to issue a profile or quarters/bed rest to a soldier it should include:
   - A. a specific expiration date.
   - B. specific nonmedical language.
   - C. specific physical limitations.
   - D. all of the above.

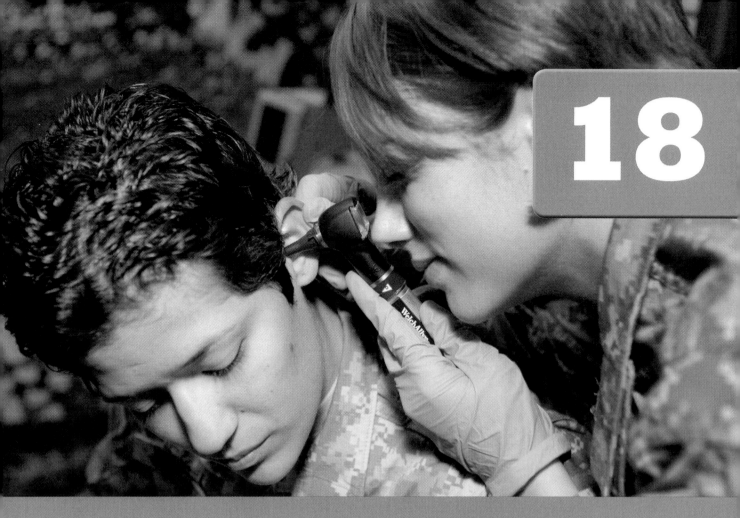

Force Health Protection

Objectives

Knowledge Objectives

- ☐ Discuss the importance of the field sanitation team.
- ☐ List the four major components of the medical threat to field forces.
- ☐ List the differences between being in the garrison and being in the field.
- ☐ Discuss the role of the combat medic in preventive medicine.
- ☐ Discuss the role of the combat medic in hearing conservation.
- ☐ Describe the hearing conservation program (HCP).

Skills Objective

- ☐ Fit a soldier with preformed earplugs.

■ Introduction

As a combat medic, you will be called upon to establish and provide assistance to your unit's preventive medicine programs, such as training and assisting your unit's field sanitation teams, educating soldiers about force health protection measures, and assisting with your unit's hearing conservation program. The effectiveness with which you accomplish this responsibility will have a far-reaching effect on the health and performance of your fellow soldiers, and in turn, the success of your unit's mission. As a combat medic, you must understand that preventive medicine and force health protection measures are only effective when you are capable of adapting them to the existing medical threat elements of a particular environment.

■ Importance of the Field Sanitation Team

The field sanitation team (FST) is responsible for the preventive medicine measures (PMM) that affect units. A unit's effectiveness depends on the health of its soldiers. The role of the combat medic in respect to sanitation is:

- To perform and maintain field hygiene and sanitation
- To promote good personal hygiene by setting a good personal example
- To disinfect water supplies
- To prevent and eliminate deficiencies in food service sanitation
- To supervise and inspect the construction of garbage and soaking pits
- To construct sufficient field latrines and urinals
- To supervise routine maintenance of field latrines and urinals

■ Medical Threats

The impact of casualties caused by disease nonbattle injuries (DNBI) during military campaigns has been a prominent and continuous feature of military operations throughout history. Armies have had immense problems with heat, cold, and communicable diseases. In all US conflicts, three times as many soldiers have been lost to DNBI as have been lost to enemy action. The ultimate objective of a military force is success in battle, and this requires that troops be maintained in a constant state of good health.

There are four major components of the medical threat to field forces: heat, cold, arthropods, and diarrheal diseases. The most lethal category of all is heat. During the 1967 Arab-Israeli conflict, the Israelis enveloped the Egyptians, severing their lines of support **FIGURE 18-1 ▶**. The Egyptians suffered 20,000 deaths due to the heat while the Israelis had no deaths and only 128 cases of heat injury. This demonstrates that health hazards, such as heat, can be as effective as tactical weapons.

The effects of heat can be minimized by ensuring that soldiers drink adequate amounts of water. Remember that

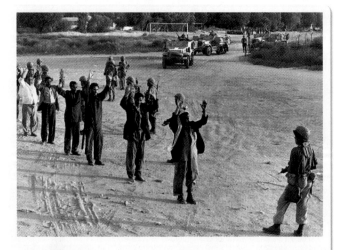

FIGURE 18-1 Heat injury was devastating to the Egyptian army during the 1967 Arab-Israeli conflict.

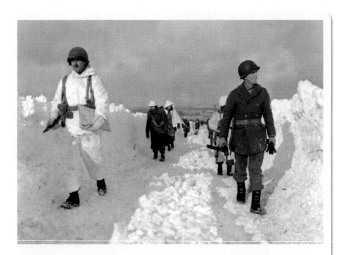

FIGURE 18-2 In World War II, during the winter of 1944 to 1945 in the European theater, more than 54,000 US soldiers were admitted to hospitals with cold injuries.

thirst is a poor indicator of the body's need for water. Ensure that soldiers consume three meals a day to replace lost electrolytes, and when the tactical situation permits, follow correct work/rest cycles.

Cold also can be very incapacitating on the battlefield. In World War II, during the winter of 1944 to 1945 in the European theater, more than 54,000 US soldiers were admitted to hospitals with cold injuries **FIGURE 18-2 ▲**. More than 90,000 US soldiers were admitted with cold injuries throughout World War II. In the 24 days that the British were in combat on the Falkland Islands, they sustained 777 total casualties—109 (14%) were cold injuries.

The risk of cold injuries can be reduced by:

- Incorporating weather data into operations planning
- Enforcing the proper wearing of the uniform

- Frequently changing wet or damp socks or gloves
- When the tactical situation permits, providing warming areas

Many species of arthropods (insects, ticks, mites, spiders, scorpions, and the like) transmit diseases that can seriously affect military operations. Napoleon's Grand Armée numbered over 500,000 when it crossed the Russian border in June 1812. Although he reached Moscow in the winter as the Russians pulled back, disease and cold injury decimated Napoleon's troops as his army retreated to Paris, returning with fewer than 20,000 men. There were approximately 70,000 combat losses and 400,000 DNBI losses. It is estimated that more than 100,000 of Napoleon's soldiers were lost to louse-borne typhus.

Ensure that your unit uses the Department of Defense (DOD) Insect Repellent System (33% DEET on skin, permethrin on uniforms, and proper wearing of the uniform), uses bed nets when appropriate, and consumes prescribed prophylactic medications when necessary.

Diarrheal diseases can be contracted from contaminated water or food; in either case, they can have a catastrophic impact on the fighting force. Rommel's situation in North Africa during World War II is a superb example. Not one of Rommel's original highly successful generals was available to help him when he needed them the most—at El Alamein—because they had all been evacuated for illness. Rommel himself was not present when the battle began; he was in Germany recovering from hepatitis. His chief of staff and his intelligence officer were evacuated just before the battle, and his operations officer was evacuated during the battle—all three for amebic dysentery.

In Operation Bright Star in 1980, the US commander rewarded his troops for a job well done by allowing them to go into town the evening before redeployment. Thirty percent of his command contracted shigellosis and were simultaneously vomiting and defecating in the aircraft on the flight back to the states. These examples are just as relevant to you today.

As the combat medic, you must protect the health of the soldiers in your unit. Ensure that soldiers only consume food and water from approved sources. You can also prevent disease by ensuring that waste disposal and handwashing devices are constructed and used. It is also your responsibility to ensure that unit dining facilities are operated under sanitary conditions.

Soldier Health

The direct relationship between soldier health and success in battle cannot be overemphasized. With sound preventive medicine measures (PMM), an army can maintain its fighting strength and exploit that strength when the enemy expects weakness.

In the field, soldiers have increased vulnerability to DNBI because of numerous factors. The operational environment may be infested with mosquitoes, sand flies, or other disease-carrying pests; it may be a hot, dusty desert or a cold, windy plain. Soldiers and their leaders must be prepared to live and fight in such places.

The human body has an excellent capacity to protect itself against disease and climatic injury; however, the efficiency of these mechanisms depends on an individual's overall well-being. Deploying soldiers halfway around the world disrupts their personal biological rhythms. The addition of heat or cold, meals served at irregular hours, and sleep deprivation soon result in soldiers who are more susceptible to illness and combat stress. Additionally, because soldiers have not been exposed to the diseases present in many deployment areas, they are more susceptible to becoming seriously ill from these diseases than the native population. Vectorborne disease may present a hidden threat to deploying units. Immunologically naïve soldiers may be at more risk from vectorborne disease than the local populace due to the local populace's relatively higher immunity to them. There may be the mistaken impression that the disease threat is low when it is high for deployed units; therefore, PMM are essential on all deployments.

Breakdowns in basic sanitation can occur. Potable water and proper waste disposal are examples of things taken for granted in garrison. Using the latrine or changing your socks becomes a challenge when one is living in a muddy foxhole. Also, do not allow your unit to consume unauthorized rations, including locally procured and scavenged food.

■ Soldiers in the Field Environment

Ordinarily, the US soldier has a high standard of personal hygiene when in an environment with convenient facilities. In the field, however, where proper sanitation requires coping with the elements of nature, a problem arises: The soldier is suddenly faced with inconveniences.

In garrison, soldiers readily conduct daily personal hygiene. Routine acts of personal hygiene are performed in a conveniently located latrine that is warm and has hot and cold water. However, upon arising in the field, a soldier may feel too cold to change into clean underwear. Even in the summer, a cold-water shower is uncomfortable. Usually the toilet in the field is not as pleasant as the one in the garrison. An ordinarily well-groomed soldier may become dirty and unkempt. Filth and disease go hand in hand. Dirty, sweaty socks may cause feet to be more susceptible to disease. Dirty clothing for prolonged periods of time and unwashed hair are open invitations to lice. In addition to keeping uniforms clean, treating them with clothing repellent will prevent body louse infestations.

You can promote the personal hygiene of soldiers by arranging for facilities such as handwashing and showering devices, hot water for shaving, and a heated place to dress. Handwashing devices should be provided outside latrine enclosures and in the food service area. They may also be set up at other points in the bivouac area. These devices are constructed so that they operate easily and must be kept filled with water at all times. All handwashing and showering devices must have a soakage pit underneath them to prevent water from collecting and forming pools.

Ensure that soldiers understand and receive guidance as needed concerning the hazards involved when personal hygiene is neglected. Inspect soldiers to ensure adequate personal hygiene, including body, hair, and teeth; airing sleeping bags; wearing clean clothes (including socks); and disposing of refuse. Enforcement of sanitary control measures pertaining to all camp facilities encourages soldiers to have more pride in their personal hygiene.

■ The Role of the Combat Medic

Medical Intelligence

Another aspect to preventive care is gathering **medical intelligence** to perform a medical threat assessment. Medical intelligence is the process of gathering essential medical information before an operation begins. It allows unit leaders and combat medics to tailor their operational plans. Medical intelligence should continue to be gathered during an operation and should be followed by an assessment after an operation has ended. It is your duty to gather information on medical facilities, assess evacuation assets, and report intelligence findings to your unit leaders.

Field Hygiene and Proper Sanitation

As stated previously, you must perform and maintain field hygiene and proper sanitation. Arrange for facilities such as handwashing and showering devices, hot water for shaving, and heated dressing areas. Through your own personal example, promote good personal hygiene.

Waterborne Diseases

Water is essential to the army in the field. Safe water ranks in importance with ammunition and food as a unit of supply in combat and often has an important bearing on the success or failure of a mission. When in the field, soldiers must be supplied with sufficient potable water to drink and for personal hygiene (such as shaving, brushing teeth, helmet baths, and comfort cleaning). The water for these purposes must be safe for human consumption and should be reasonably free of objectionable tastes, odors, turbidity (cloudiness), and color. For showering, disinfected nonpotable fresh water should be used. However, only potable water should be used for showering, bathing, or bodily contact in the following locations:

- Where diseases such as schistosomiasis and leptospirosis are endemic and prevalent
- Where chemical agents may be present

Water can also be a vehicle in disease transmission. Waterborne disease organisms are a primary source of illness to soldiers. Common waterborne diseases include hepatitis, typhoid and paratyphoid fever, bacillary and amebic dysentery, cholera, common diarrhea, leptospirosis, and schistosomiasis (snail fever). No direct method has been developed for detecting the minimum infectious quantities of these organisms in water; therefore, it is necessary to resort to an indicator test to determine the bacteriologic acceptability of water. The water is tested for the presence of coliform bacteria, which are found in great numbers in the excreta (feces) of humans and warm-blooded animals, and in the soil. Also, many of the diseases mentioned earlier are spread through feces. Although the presence of coliform bacteria in water may not prove fecal contamination, it is an indication that pathogenic (disease-carrying) organisms may be present. The indicator test is the best sign that contamination exists; therefore, you must assume that pathogens are present. Many military units in the field do not have the capability to determine the presence of coliform bacteria in water, however; hence, all water must be thoroughly treated and disinfected before use.

The quantity of water required for soldiers varies with the season of the year, the geographic area, and the tactical situation. In a cold climate, only 2 gallons of water per soldier per day may be required when soldiers are engaged in only sedentary duty. Additional amounts of water are required for personal hygiene and cooking. A guide for meeting the water requirements in an arid zone is to plan for 3 to 6 gallons per individual per day unless improvised showering facilities are made available. In this case, the requirement should be increased to 15 gallons or more.

Food Sanitation

Factors that create a high risk for foodborne diseases include poor food inspection and sanitation, poor personal hygiene habits, inadequate refrigeration, and lack of eradication programs for foodborne diseases such as hepatitis A and brucellosis. Food transportation, storage, preparation, and service have direct bearing on the success or failure of a mission. Dining facility sanitation is a chronic operational problem. The prospect of disease outbreaks, particularly dysentery and food poisoning, is always present and must be recognized as a constant threat to unit health.

Potentially hazardous foods (PHFs) are any food that contains milk, milk products, eggs, meat, poultry, fish, shellfish, or other ingredients in a form capable of supporting the rapid growth of infectious or toxic microorganisms. PHFs are typically high in protein and have a water content greater than 85% and a pH greater than 4.5. The following factors most often cause foodborne disease outbreaks:

- Failure to keep PHFs cold (below 40°F [4.4°C] internal temperature)
- Failure to keep PHFs hot (above 145°F [62.8°C] internal temperature)
- Preparing foods one day or more before serving
- Allowing sick employees who practice poor personal hygiene to handle food

Field Medical Care TIPS

Consider a Lyster bag for disinfecting water.

Food contamination can be classified into three categories:

- **Biologic:** Contamination by pathogenic micro-organisms (protozoa, bacteria, fungus, virus) or unacceptable levels of spoilage. This category is the major threat to personnel.
- **Chemical:** Contamination with chemical warfare agents, industrial chemicals, and/or other adulterating chemicals (zinc, copper, cadmium, pesticides, etc.).
- **Physical:** Contamination by arthropods, debris, radioactive particles, and the like.

Bacteria that multiply at temperatures between 60°F (15.5°C) and 125°F (52°C) cause most foodborne illnesses. Maintain the internal temperature of cooked foods that will be served hot at 145°F (63°C) or above. Maintain the internal temperatures of foods that will be served cold at 40°F (4.4°C) or below to control any bacteria that may be present in the food. The high food temperatures (160°F to 212°F [71°C to 100°C]) reached in boiling, baking, frying, and roasting will kill most bacteria that can cause foodborne illness. Prompt refrigeration to 40°F (4.4°C) or below in containers less than 2″ deep inhibits growth of most (but not all) of these bacteria. Freezing at 0°F (−18°C) or below essentially stops bacteria growth but will not kill bacteria that are already present.

Thorough reheating to an internal temperature of 165°F (74°C) or above will kill bacteria that may have grown during storage. However, foods that have been improperly stored or otherwise mishandled cannot be made safe by reheating. Ensure that everything that touches food during preparation and serving is clean to avoid introducing illness-causing bacteria.

Procurement of Food

The order of preference for food acquisition is:

- US military rations brought with unit or previously cached
- Local food procured from sources approved by supporting Veterinary and Environment Science Officers
- Local food procured from unapproved sources

Special Operations Forces will probably have to procure food from unapproved sources during real-world contingencies, presenting a serious medical threat to the team and the mission. The following guidelines should be used.

Avoid local street vendors because their personal hygiene habits tend to be poor, which results in contaminated food (eg, through fecal–oral contamination). Consider all ice to be contaminated, because it is often made from nonpotable water, and freezing will not kill disease-causing organisms. Anything with ice in it or on it should be considered contaminated (eg, alcohol in a drink does not make the ice in it safe). Semi-perishable rations (canned and dried products) are relatively safe and should be chosen over fresh food.

Protect canned and dried foods from extreme heating and freezing. Do not use swollen or leaking cans. Do not use moldy grain or grain contaminated with insect larvae.

Be aware that raw fruit and vegetables may be grown in areas where "nightsoil" (human fecal matter) is used as ferti-

TABLE 18-1 **Bleach Solutions**	
Clorox	4.84 oz in 32 gallons = 50 ppm
	9.68 oz in 32 gallons = 100 ppm
	1 Tbsp per gallon = 200 ppm
70% calcium hypochlorite	0.32 oz in 32 gallons = 50 ppm
	0.64 oz in 32 gallons = 100 ppm

lizer or where gastrointestinal or parasitic diseases are prevalent. Wash raw fresh fruits and vegetables in potable water and disinfect with one of the following methods:

- **Dip in boiling water for 15 seconds.** Place small amounts of produce in net bags, completely submerge items for 15 seconds, and then remove and allow them to cool. This method is not recommended for leafy vegetables.
- **Disinfect with chlorine.** Immerse for at least 15 minutes in a 100 parts per million (ppm) solution of chlorine or for 30 minutes in a 50 ppm solution `TABLE 18-1 ▲`. Rinse the produce thoroughly with potable water before cooking or eating. Break apart "head" produce such as lettuce, cabbage, or celery before disinfection.

Always cook eggs to prevent salmonellosis. Blood and meat spots are acceptable, but cracked and rotten eggs are not acceptable and should be discarded. Boil unpasteurized dairy products for at least 15 seconds to prevent tuberculosis, brucellosis, Q fever, and other diseases. Avoid cheese, butter, and ice cream made from unpasteurized milk, which can carry these diseases.

Cook all seafood to prevent hepatitis, tapeworms, flukes, cholera, and so forth. Avoid shellfish because cooking does not degrade some toxins (eg, red tide). Certain saltwater fish also have heat-stable toxins that are not destroyed during cooking. Do not eat any species that the native population does not eat. Avoid large predatory reef fish, such as barracuda, grouper, snapper, jack, mackerel, and triggerfish, which may accumulate toxins (eg, ciguatera). Be aware of geographic areas where toxins may occur in seafood.

Eat carcass or muscle meat rather than visceral meat (liver, heart, kidney, etc.). Muscle flesh is less likely to be contaminated. Fresh meat from healthy animals is safe if cooked thoroughly:

- Perform an antemortem examination (before slaughtering), use correct field slaughter methods, and perform a postmortem examination (after slaughtering).
- The color of beef should be red to slightly red-brown. Do not consume green or brown beef if possible. Avoid meat with off odors, such as sour or sweet, fruity smells.
- Cook meat until it is well done: Do not eat rare, medium, or bloody meat. Sausages and meat products should be well cooked.

Food Storage and Preservation

Protect canned and dried foods from extreme heat and freezing. Store and preserve perishables such as meat, poultry, and fish by refrigerating at or below 40°F (4.4°C). Because refrigeration or potable ice is often not available, slaughter what you need, cook it thoroughly, and then consume it immediately. Meat can be preserved by methods other than refrigeration (eg, by smoking, curing, making jerky or pemmican, salting, or pickling) if time and resources are available. Semi-perishable foods such as potatoes and onions should be stored in a dry place off the ground, allowing air to circulate around then to retard decay and spoilage. Store staple products (flour, sugar, etc.) in metal cans with tight-fitting lids. To prevent zinc poisoning, do not store acidic foods or beverages such as tomatoes or citric juices in galvanized cans.

Preparing and Serving Food

Use pesticides according to the directions on the container. Limit residual sprays to crack and crevice treatment only. Protect all foods and food contact surfaces when applying pesticides. Coordinate food preparation and consumption to eliminate unnecessary lapses of time.

Leftover food presents a problem. Always plan meals to reduce the amount of leftovers. Discard items held at unsafe temperatures (45°F to 140°F [7.2°C to 60°C]) for 3 or more hours. Never save potentially hazardous foods such as creamed beef, casseroles, or gravies.

Meat may contain disease-producing agents that cannot be detected by inspection. Follow cooking procedures strictly to ensure that heat penetrates to the center of the meat and that all the meat is cooked to at least 165°F (74°C). This applies to poultry, pork, beef, and any stuffing or other foods containing these meats.

Cleaning and Disinfecting Utensils

Cooking utensils and mess kits should be cleaned, disinfected, and properly stored after each use. They must be scraped free of food particles, washed in hot (120°F to 130°F [49°C to 54°C]) soapy water, rinsed in boiling water, sanitized for at least 10 seconds in another container of boiling water, and allowed to air dry. They must be stored in clean, covered containers that are protected from dust and vermin. When it is impossible to heat the water, utensils must be washed in soapy water, rinsed in two cans of clear water, and then immersed in a fourth container of chlorine sanitizing solution for at least 30 seconds. Chemical sanitizing solutions are prepared as followed (methods are listed in the order of preference):

- Use disinfectant, food service (NSN: 6840-01-035-5432) as specified on the label.
- Use 1 level mess kit spoonful of calcium hypochlorite for every 10 gallons of water (250 ppm solution).
- Use 1 canteen cup of 5% liquid bleach in 32 gallons of water (250 ppm solution).

If mess kits become soiled or contaminated between meals, they should be rewashed prior to use as described previously. A prewash of boiling water should be available for use prior to all meals.

Heat Injury

As a combat medic, it is your responsibility to prevent heat injury in your unit. (Chapter 30, *Environmental Emergencies*, covers treating heat injuries in greater detail.) It is important to be able to recognize hazardous heat conditions, including:

- Increasing temperature and humidity
- Direct sunlight

Identify the strategies you will use to protect your unit against heat injury:

- Drink plenty of fluids (water).
- Enforce work/rest cycles.
- Stay in shade when possible.
- Choose evening or morning for strenuous work.
- Avoid tight, nonbreathable clothing.
- Maintain physical fitness.
- Avoid medications that increase heat injury risk (antihistamines, antihypertensives).

Cold Injury

As a combat medic, it is your responsibility to prevent cold injuries in your unit. (Chapter 30, *Environmental Emergencies*, covers cold injuries and their care in greater detail.) As the combat medic in charge of preventive medicine for your unit, it is important to be able to recognize hazardous cold conditions, including:

- Decreasing temperature
- Moisture
- Wind speed

Identify the strategies you will use to protect your unit against cold injury:

- Avoid cold, wind, and moisture.
- Wear multiple layers of loose-fitting clothing.
- Wear a water-repellent but "breathable" shell.
- Change socks frequently.
- Drink plenty of fluids.
- Get plenty of rest and eat all meals.
- Avoid alcohol and tobacco.

Provide additional guidance in the use of PMM to prevent specific cold injuries. Hypothermia or frostbite may be prevented by:

- Wearing several layers of warm, loosely fitting clothing
- Protecting your face from the wind
- Exercising face, fingers, and toes to keep them warm

Immersion (trench) foot, which results from standing in cold water or slush when the temperature is between 32°F and 50°F; may be prevented by the use of protective footgear and dry socks. Snow blindness, which occurs when the sun shines brightly on unbroken ice or snow, can be prevented by:

- Wearing sunglasses or an improvised device made of cardboard or cloth
- Blackening the areas around the eyes

Arthropods

Arthropods and Diseases

Arthropods make up over 75% of all animal species; however, fewer than 1% of the 750,000 species of arthropods are

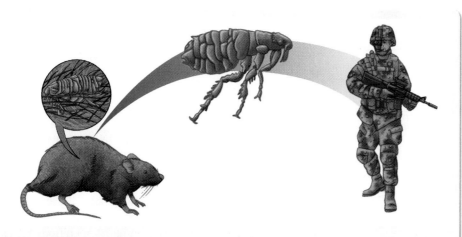

FIGURE 18-3 The chain of infection for arthropod-borne diseases involves a pathogenic organism in an infected person or animal (the reservoir), an arthropod to transmit the disease (the vector), and a susceptible person (the host).

potentially dangerous to humans. The impact of all arthropods is significant because of their high numbers and the negative results of their infestation of stored products and wooden structures. Still, many species are beneficial as pollinators, predators of other pests, scavengers of waste, and manufacturers of food and are a part of the natural balance of nature. However, the economic damage and medical disorders caused by a few arthropods make some pest management practices necessary to control the problem pests.

Historically, arthropod-borne diseases have caused more casualties than combat injuries. Arthropod-borne diseases alone were responsible for the loss of 15,576,000 man-days among the US Armed Forces during World War II. Today, harmful arthropods represent one of the greatest environmental hazards to soldiers in the field. Protection of the soldier from arthropods and arthropod-borne diseases is essential to mission accomplishment. See the Preventive Medicine (PVNTMED) team for effective arthropod control measures.

The chain of infection for arthropod-borne diseases involves a pathogenic organism in an infected person or animal (the reservoir), an arthropod to transmit the disease (the vector), and a susceptible person (the host) **FIGURE 18-3 ▲**. The efficiency of the vector in transmitting disease from a reservoir to a host is related to many factors. Some of the factors are species related, such as vector reproductive capacity, physiology, morphology, and genetics. Other factors that affect the vector's ability to transmit disease are physical and related to environmental conditions, such as temperature, moisture, rainfall, pH, weather, geographic and topographic location, photoperiod, and wind. Soldiers in a field environment must break the chain of infection for arthropod-borne disease or arthropod injury by limiting arthropod pest exposures.

Direct Arthropod Effects on Human Health

In addition to disease transmission, arthropods can cause direct injuries to people. Bites, stings, and allergic reactions are three major categories of injuries caused by arthropods.

Arthropods also affect humans by annoying and disturbing them. The sound of a single mosquito buzzing around your head while you are trying to sleep is annoying. Standing guard with gnats buzzing around your face can be disturbing. Finding cockroaches or other insects or parts of insects in your food is disturbing. The problems of arthropod injury and the exaggerated fear of arthropods can even result in psychiatric problems.

Arthropod-borne Diseases

The diseases transmitted to man by arthropods are some of the most serious. Uncontrolled, these illnesses can cripple or destroy military forces. The effect of these diseases on humans can range from a very mild illness to a severe illness or death. For examples of arthropod-borne diseases and their vectors, see **TABLE 18-2 ▶**.

House flies and other flying insects that are attracted to human wastes or other organic material can spread disease organisms to food and water. By employing individual PMMs, soldiers can stop arthropod-borne diseases from being a factor in their lives and in their unit's mission accomplishment.

Arthropod Control

Bivouac (camp) sites are selected according to well-defined guidelines. The ideal location for a bivouac site is on high, well-drained ground at least 1 mile from breeding sites of flies and mosquitoes and 1 mile from native habitations. It is not always possible to bivouac in the ideal location. A unit commander may be faced with unusual arthropod control problems in the vicinity of the campsite. An effective program for arthropod-borne disease prevention should consist primarily of sanitation measures, but may include the use of individual PMMs, such as bed nets, as well as the application of pesticides. Essential to the operation of an effective control program is an understanding of the life cycles of medically important arthropods and knowledge of where they can be found in nature. For more information, refer to FM 4-25.12 (FM 21-10-1), or see the unit preventive medicine team.

Preventive Medicine Measures for Arthropods

Individual PMMs are those measures that must be used by each soldier. Often they are the only preventive measures available for soldiers in the field. These PMMs can be accomplished by the soldier at work and at rest.

The best strategy for defense against insects and other disease-bearing arthropods is use of the DOD Insect Repellent System. This system includes the application of extended-duration 33% DEET repellent to exposed skin, the application of

TABLE 18-2 Arthropod-borne Diseases and Their Vectors

Disease	Vector
Malaria	Mosquito
Chagas disease	Kissing bug (reduviid)
Leishmaniasis	Sand fly (phlebotomine)
Yellow fever	Mosquito
Dengue fever	Mosquito
Encephalitis	Mosquito
Sandfly fever or phlebotomus fever	Sand fly (phlebotomine)
Typhus fever (epidemic)	Body louse
Typhus fever (murine)	Flea
Scrub typhus	Larval mite
Bubonic plague	Flea
Dysentery	Filth flies (particularly the house fly)
Typhoid fever	Flies and cockroaches (by food contamination)
Spotted fever	Tick
Filariasis (elephantiasis)	Mosquito
Onchocerciasis	Black fly
Rickettsial diseases	Ticks
Streptococcus, Staphylococcus	Housefly
Trypanosomiasis	Tsetse fly

Field Medical Care TIPS

Additional hazards pose a threat to the health of your unit, including:
- Communicable diseases endemic to the area of operations
- Toxic industrial materials in the area of operations
- Noise hazards
- Plants and animals (flora and fauna)

permethrin to the field uniform, and a properly worn uniform. When used correctly, the DOD Insect Repellent System can provide nearly complete protection from arthropod-borne disease.

It is important to note that not all arthropod species are equally repelled by a particular repellent, so a soldier should not discontinue using repellents if some bites are received, because other species that are present are still likely to be repelled. Further, some insect species bite primarily during the day, whereas others do so only at night. This is true even within a pest group like mosquitoes; therefore, a lack of bites during the day does not mean that protective measures will not be needed at night.

Diarrhea

Diarrhea is caused by contaminated food and water. If an outbreak occurs in your unit, consider food preparation and handling as a source of contamination, as well as field sanitation.

Combat Stress

Chapter 29, *Mental Health*, discusses combat stress concerns in depth. During actual combat, military operations continue around the clock at a constant pace, often under severe weather conditions. Terrible things happen in combat. During such periods the soldier's mental and physical endurance will be pushed to the limit. Psychological first aid will help sustain the soldier's mental and physical performance during normal activities, and especially during military operations under extremely adverse conditions and in hostile environments.

Battle Fatigue and Other Combat Stress Reactions

Battle fatigue is a temporary emotional disorder or inability to function experienced by a previously normal soldier as a reaction to the overwhelming or cumulative stress of combat. By definition, battle fatigue gets better with reassurance, rest, physical replenishment, and activities that restore confidence. Physical fatigue, or sleep loss, although commonly present, is not necessary for a diagnosis of battle fatigue. All combat and combat support troops are likely to feel battle fatigue under conditions of intense and/or prolonged stress. They may even become battle fatigue casualties, unable to perform their mission roles for hours or days.

Other negative behaviors may be combat stress reactions (CSRs), but are not called battle fatigue because they require treatment other than simple rest, replenishment, and restoration of confidence. These negative CSRs include drug and alcohol abuse, committing atrocities against enemy prisoners and noncombatants, looting, desertion, and self-inflicted wounds. These harmful CSRs can often be prevented by good psychological first aid; however, some of these negative actions require disciplinary action instead of reassurance and rest.

Preventive Measures to Combat Battle Fatigue

As a combat medic, there are some preventive measures that you can take to combat battle fatigue:
- Welcome new members into your team and get to know them quickly.
- Be physically fit (strength, endurance, and agility).
- Practice rapid relaxation techniques.
- Help out other soldiers when things are tough at home or in the unit.
- Keep informed; ask your leader questions, and ignore rumors.
- Work together to give everyone food, water, shelter, hygiene, and sanitation.
- Sleep when mission and safety permit; let everyone get time to sleep.
  - Sleep only in safe places and by standard operating procedure.
  - If possible, sleep 6 to 9 hours per day.

- Try to get at least 4 hours sleep per day.
- Get good sleep before going on sustained operations.
- Catnap when you can, but allow time to wake up fully.
- Catch up on sleep after going without.

Assess the Hazards

As a combat medic, it is your responsibility to estimate the level of risk for each identified hazard and estimate the overall risk for the operation. Use the assessment tools and ratings in **TABLE 18-3, 18-4, 18-5 ▾**. Be sure to report your findings to your commanders so they can adjust their operational plans if needed.

Develop Controls and Conduct Risk Assessments

To keep your unit healthy, you need to develop educational controls and physical controls. Educational controls are based on the knowledge and skills of units and individuals and implemented through individual and collective training; for example, training soldiers in your unit to always change into a fresh pair of socks every morning. Physical controls may take the form of barriers and guards, signs to warn individuals and units, and special controller or oversight personnel responsible for locating specific hazards; for example, placing a warning sign next to a trench.

Criteria for controls include suitability, feasibility, and acceptability. Suitability means that you must remove the hazard or mitigate residual risk to an acceptable level; for example, spraying a food preparation area with pesticide. Feasibility means that the unit must have the capability to implement the control(s); for example, having the pesticide available. Acceptability means that the benefit gained by implementing control(s) must justify the cost in resources and time. In the case of spraying a pesticide, you are preventing arthropod-borne diseases from infecting the unit. Assessment of acceptability is largely subjective. Make a risk decision and determine whether the risk is justified.

Field Medical Care **TIPS**

Identify the operational threats to the unit, including:
- Sleep deprivation for evacuation drivers
- PMCS of medical equipment/vehicles
- Regulated/medical waste management

TABLE 18-3 Assess the Hazards

Frequent	(A)
Likely	(B)
Occasional	(C)
Seldom	(D)
Unlikely	(E)

TABLE 18-4 Severity of Each Hazard

Catastrophic	(I)
Critical	(II)
Marginal	(III)
Negligible	(IV)

TABLE 18-5 Level of Risk

Extremely high risk (E)	• Loss of ability to accomplish the mission. • A frequent or likely probability of catastrophic loss or critical loss.
High risk (H)	• Significant degradation of mission capabilities in terms of required mission standard. • Inability to accomplish all parts of the mission. • Inability to complete the mission to an acceptable standard. • Occasional to seldom probability of catastrophic loss. • Likely to occasional probability of a critical loss. • Frequent probability of marginal loss.
Moderate risk (M)	• Expected degraded mission capabilities in terms of required mission standard. • Reduced mission capability. • Unlikely probability of catastrophic loss. • Probability of a critical loss is seldom. • Marginal losses occur with likely or occasional probability. • Frequent probability of negligible loss.
Low risk (L)	• Expected losses have little or no impact on accomplishing the mission. • Probability of critical loss is unlikely. • Marginal loss is seldom. • Probability of negligible loss is likely or less.

Ensure that controls are integrated into standard operating procedures (SOPs), written and verbal orders, mission briefing, and staff estimates, and that they are converted into clear, simple execution orders that can be understood at all levels.

Supervise and evaluate to ensure that controls are in place. Supervise the following:

- Spot checks
- Inspections
- Situation reports (SITREPs)
- Brief backs
- Buddy checks

Monitor the controls to ensure they remain effective, and continually assess variable hazards.

Evaluate the following:

- Determine methods to ensure successes continue.
- Capture and disseminate lessons learned.
- Consider the effectiveness of risk assessment in identifying and accurately assessing probability and severity.
- Determine whether the level of residual risk of each hazard and overall mission was accurately estimated.
- Evaluate the effectiveness of each control in mitigating or eliminating the risk.

■ Hearing Conservation

Background

Due to the scope of current operations, hazardous noise exposure is the greatest it has been for over 30 years. Noise-induced hearing loss is on the rise among US soldiers. One in three postdeploying soldiers report acute acoustic trauma (damage to the outer, middle, or inner ear due to excessive noise such as explosions or close weapons fire) to unprotected ears. One in four postdeploying soldiers reports some hearing loss and/or hearing complaints. Between March 2003 and July 2004, 736 US soldiers in Operation Iraqi Freedom (OIF) and Operation Enduring Freedom (OEF) sustained blast-related injuries. This type of injury accounts for 47% of all wounded in action (WIA) evacuations from Iraq and 31.5% of those from Afghanistan. During the same time frame, Walter Reed Army Medical Center treated over 600 soldiers for blast-related injuries. Of those, 123 had traumatic blast injuries to the ear and an additional 110 experienced hearing loss. Among all postdeploying personnel who received hearing evaluations, 28% had some hearing loss.

Mission Impact

Sound is often the first source of information a soldier has before making direct contact with enemy forces. Unlike visual cues, information carried by sound comes to us from all directions, through darkness and over or through many obstacles. It is likely you will hear the enemy before you see them. High intensity, impulse, and impact noise can cause permanent hearing loss for many soldiers who are consistently exposed to them. Soldiers who are routinely exposed to hazardous noise can have progressive, and sometimes unnoticed, hearing

loss that will degrade his or her performance and can threaten combat readiness.

During tactical operations on the battlefield, a soldier's hearing can become permanently disabled in an instant. It is important to remember that noise-induced hearing loss is permanent but preventable, even in combat. The role of the combat medic in hearing conservation is to prevent hearing loss injury among the soldiers in the unit. This is achieved by:

- Educating soldiers about noise-induced hearing loss
- Ensuring that all soldiers have properly fitted hearing protection
- Making certain that soldiers maintain their hearing readiness
- Most importantly, setting a good example!

Symptoms Associated With Hearing Loss

Individuals with a noise-induced hearing loss may be unaware of the loss and may not have any communication problems when in quiet listening situations; however, frequently some symptoms exist:

- Tinnitus (ringing sensation)
- Temporary muffling of sound after exposure to noise
- Sensation of "fullness" in the ear(s)
- Increased stress and fatigue

Soldiers with a high-frequency, noise-induced hearing loss may complain that although they hear people speak, they can't always understand what is being said; often these individuals will experience problems talking on the telephone or communicating by radio. A marked loss in the ability to communicate may ensue as the hearing loss progresses into the middle and lower frequencies. Noise-induced hearing loss is usually painless, progressive, and permanent.

Hearing Conservation Program

Army Regulation 40-5, Preventive Medicine, requires a hearing conservation program (HCP). Department of the Army Pamphlet 40-501, *Hearing Conservation Program* provides the guidance for implementing it. There are seven basic components of a good hearing conservation program:

1. **Noise hazard identification:** Assessing the hazard potential of noise sources in the environment where the soldiers are living or working.

2. **Engineering controls:** Reducing noise at the source.

3. **Hearing protectors:** The most important part of the hearing conservation program.

4. **Routine hearing (audiometric) examinations:** All military personnel receive a reference audiogram (DD Form 2215) during basic training prior to noise exposure. Audiograms are required annually for all soldiers and are placed in their medical records.

5. **Health education:** Ensuring noise-exposed personnel have annual training in hearing conservation, are educated on the effects of noise on their hearing, and understand the benefits of hearing protectors.

TABLE 18-6 **Approved Earplugs**

	TYPE	SIZE (COLOR)	NSN
	Single-flange earplugs	Extra small (White)	6515-00-442-4765
		Small (Green)	6515-00-467-0085
		Medium (Orange)	6515-00-467-0089
		Large (Blue)	6515-00-442-4807
		Extra large (Red)	6515-00-442-4813
	Triple-flange earplugs	Small (Green)	6515-00-442-4821
		Medium (Orange)	6515-00-442-4818
		Large (Blue)	6515-00-467-0092
	Quad-flange earplugs	Medium	
Disposable	Polyvinyl foam earplugs, 400s	Yellow	6515-00-137-6345
Disposable	Silicon (rubber) earplugs, 48s (blister pack)		6515-00-135-2612
Disposable	Silicon (rubber) earplugs, 200s (blister pack)		6515-00-133-5416
	Earplug carrying case and seating device		6515-01-100-1674

6. **Enforcement:** Use of hearing protection is mandatory according to IAW AR 40-5 and DA PAM 40-501; enforcement of this mandatory requirement is a leadership challenge at all levels.

7. **Program evaluation:** AR 40-5 requires commanders to appoint a Unit Hearing Conservation Manager.

Hearing Protection

As stated, the most important component of a good hearing program is the use of hearing protectors. You must ensure that all soldiers in your unit have access to properly fitted hearing protection. According to Department of the Army guidance, all deploying personnel must have a pair of preformed earplugs, and medically trained personnel must examine the fit and condition of preformed and custom earplugs at least annually. Establish a unit policy that an earplug case containing properly fitted earplugs will be worn on the field uniform. The earplug case should not be worn on the LBE/LCV or attached to body armor.

Even during combat operations, soldiers should wear hearing protectors when firing weapons or riding in noisy vehicles or aircraft. Up until recently, soldiers were not able to wear hearing protectors because they impair necessary hearing, such as during the conduct of dismounted infantry operations. The newly developed **combat arms earplug (CAEP)** is a double-ended earplug designed for two different types of hearing protection for use in military environments. The CAEP enhances communication by blocking the harmful hazardous noise that causes hearing loss but allows sound in the speech frequency range to pass through the earplug to the ear.

The green (olive drab) end of the earplug is inserted into the ear canal to protect hearing when operating in or around steady-state noises (aircraft, watercraft, and vehicles). The yellow side is inserted for weapons fire to protect hearing and to hear between firings (such as dismounted patrolling or operating in a high risk IED environment). Over 372,000 pairs of combat arms earplugs were issued as standard equipment to combatants from October 2004 through April 2005.

There is also a single-ended version of the CAEP for weapons and explosive noise, but it also can be used to protect against nonweapon/nonexplosive noise. This type of earplug is used for soldiers who cannot wear the double-ended CAEP. **TABLE 18-6 ▲** lists approved earplugs to protect soldiers' hearing. Other approved hearing protection devices include:

- Noise muffs (Type II, high performance) **FIGURE 18-4 ▼**
- Ear canal caps **FIGURE 18-5 ▶**
- Noise-attenuated helmets
- Aviator and combat vehicle crewmen helmets **FIGURE 18-6 ▶**
- Other types of preformed earplugs **FIGURE 18-7 ▶**

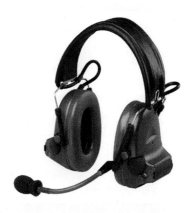

FIGURE 18-4 Noise muffs (Type II, high performance).

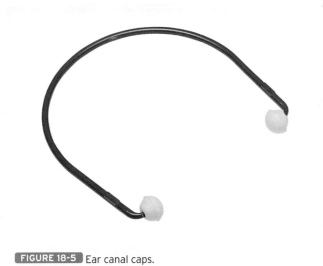

FIGURE 18-5 Ear canal caps.

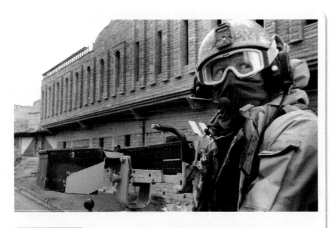

FIGURE 18-6 Aviator and combat vehicle crewmen helmets.

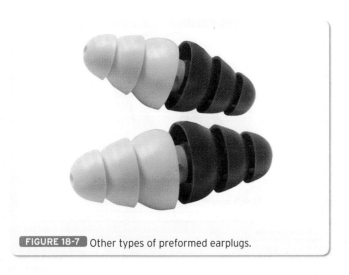

FIGURE 18-7 Other types of preformed earplugs.

Fitting Earplugs

Medically trained personnel must examine the fit and condition of preformed and custom earplugs for all deploying personnel and reexamine personnel at least annually. You must ensure that all individuals examined for earplug fitting have had an **otoscopic examination** within the last year before attempting to insert an earplug into the ear canal. This is especially true for soldiers who have never been fitted for preformed earplugs in the past. Perform an otoscopic examination if the soldier has not had one performed in the previous year or the soldier has complaints of discomfort or pain in either ear FIGURE 18-8 ▾ . Examine the tympanic membrane (TM) and the external auditory canal (EAC) of each ear.

Contraindications to fitting preformed earplugs are:

- Cerumen impaction
- Irritated or swollen EAC FIGURE 18-9 ▸
- Discolored or perforated TM FIGURE 18-10 ▸
- Active drainage FIGURE 18-11 ▸

If, while performing an otoscopic examination, you detect injury, see signs of infection or inflammation, or determine a congenital abnormality exists, do not proceed with the earplug fitting. Refer the soldier to the medical officer or physician's assistant for further evaluation and appropriate medical treatment.

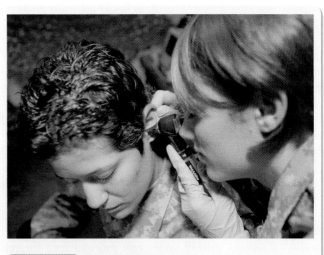

FIGURE 18-8 An otoscopic examination.

To fit a soldier with a preformed earplug, follow the steps in **SKILL DRILL 18-1**▶ :

1. After explaining the procedure to the soldier, inspect the soldier's EAC and determine whether the CAEP can be fitted into the EAC. If the EAC opening

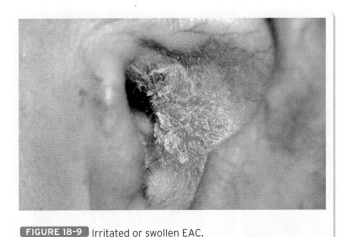

FIGURE 18-9 Irritated or swollen EAC.

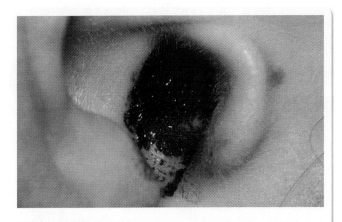

FIGURE 18-10 Discolored or perforated TM.

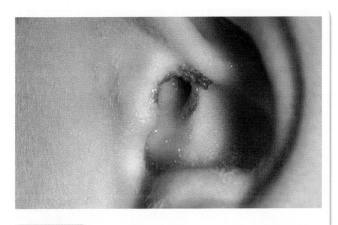

FIGURE 18-11 Active drainage.

appears to be too small, try fitting the single-ended CAEP (**Step ①**).

2. Pull up and back on the external ear. Insert the CAEP into the EAC. (**Step ②**).

3. Gently pull on the inserted earplug; a slight tension should be felt. Ask the soldier if the earplug is comfortable. Fit the soldier's other ear.

4. If the CAEP cannot be fitted to the soldier, attempt to fit the triple-flange earplug into the ear canal. Select the size earplug that closely approximates the EAC. Remove the lid of the earplug case and place the earplug in the seating device on the lid of the carrying case. Pull up and back on the external ear, and attempt to insert the earplug until the largest flange is flush with the opening of the EAC. If unable to fit the outer flange of the triple-flange flush with the EAC, repeat the above steps with a different size triple-flange earplug.

5. If the stem of the triple-flange earplug is bent by contact with the tragus, or the recipient states the triple-flange earplug is uncomfortable, do not fit this ear with the triple-flange earplug. This is done to avoid pressure points in the EAC and the tragus. Pressure points cause pain; soldiers will not wear earplugs that are painful.

6. If the triple-flange on the first ear is a good fit, repeat the above steps in fitting the other ear.

7. If not, attempt to fit the quad-flange earplug. Some individuals may not be able to fit all four flanges into the EAC; for smaller ear canals, at least the first two flanges should fit into the EAC. The seating device cannot be used to fit the quad-flange earplug (**Step ③**).

8. Assess the fit of inserted earplugs. Slight tension should be felt when pulling on the stem of the earplug. The earplug should be comfortable to the soldier. An individual's voice will sound low-toned or muffled (triple-flange/quad-flange). With the CAEP (yellow end) inserted, the individual should still be able to hear speech. Instruct the soldier to count to five; ask how his or her voice sounds.

9. Have the soldier remove one earplug, and then click a noisemaker or snap your fingers. There should be a noticeable difference between the ear with the earplug properly seated and the one without an earplug (**Step ④**).

10. Ask the soldier how the earplug feels; if the earplug is ineffective or uncomfortable, remove the earplug and refer the soldier to the audiology clinic. Only an earplug that is inserted correctly will be effective; therefore, it is critical that soldiers be fitted with the earplug that is correct for them.

11. Train the soldier to insert the earplugs properly. Demonstrate how to insert the earplugs by inserting an earplug into your own ear (**Step ⑤**).

Fitting a Soldier With a Preformed Earplug

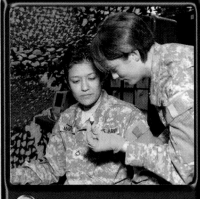

1 After explaining the procedure to the soldier, inspect the soldier's EAC and determine whether the CAEP can be fitted into the EAC. If the EAC opening appears to be too small, try fitting the single-ended CAEP.

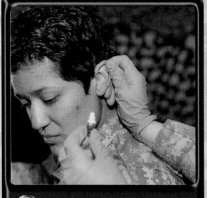

2 Pull up and back on the external ear. Insert the CAEP into the EAC.

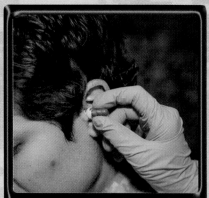

3 Gently pull on the inserted earplug; a slight tension should be felt. Ask the soldier if the earplug is comfortable. Fit the soldier's other ear. If the CAEP cannot be fitted to the soldier, attempt to fit the triple-flange earplug into the ear canal. If the triple-flange earplug does not fit, attempt to fit the quad-flange earplug.

12. Observe the soldier inserting the earplug and coach him or her as necessary to ensure that he or she is inserting the earplugs properly (**Step** ⑥).

13. Document the fitting (type and size of earplug) on an SF-600 and place the document in the soldier's medical record (**Step** ⑦).

■ Summary

The success or failure of any army, the outcome of a war, and the fate of a nation may rest upon how well diseases are prevented through effective field sanitation and preventive medicine measures. The extent to which diseases and disabilities are prevented in your unit area depends on the effectiveness with which you, a member of the field sanitation team or a member of a hearing conservation program, perform your role. Remember, you set the example as the combat medic. Hearing conservation is based on education and prevention. Noise-induced hearing loss is permanent but preventable, even in combat.

SKILL DRILL 18-1

Fitting a Soldier With a Preformed Earplug (*continued*)

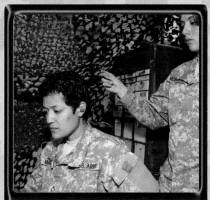

4 Have the soldier remove one earplug, and then click a noisemaker or snap your fingers. There should be a noticeable difference between the ear with the earplug properly seated and the one without an earplug.

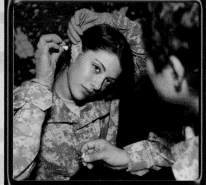

5 Train the soldier to insert the earplugs properly. Demonstrate how to insert the earplugs by inserting an earplug into your own ear.

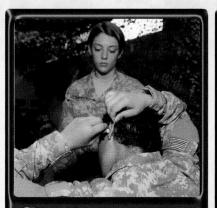

6 Observe the soldier inserting the earplug and coach him or her as necessary to ensure that he or she is inserting the earplugs properly.

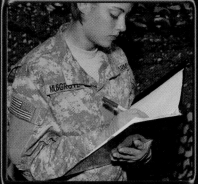

7 Document the fitting (type and size of earplug) on an SF-600 and place the document in the soldier's medical record.

YOU ARE THE
COMBAT MEDIC

During sick call, a member of your unit shuffles into the Battalion Aid Station (BAS). He says that his stomach feels, "wicked bad." You lead him to a more private area of the BAS to begin your examination. His abdominal pain is a red flag that you should obtain his vital signs and history as quickly as possible. The supervising medical officer is going to need this information to help make a swift and accurate diagnosis.

His temperature is 100°F, pulse rate is 90 beats/min, respiration rate is 15 breaths/min and nonlabored, blood pressure is 120/90 mm Hg, and his blood oxygen saturation level is 95%. His vital signs do not present any red flags, so you continue on by taking his patient history. His chief complaint is that his stomach hurts, but you need to know more information, so you use the OPQRST method. His stomach began to hurt 2 days ago. He admits that he's also been suffering from a bout of the runs.

You zero in on this information and ask him when the diarrhea began. His bout began 3 days ago and has been getting worse each day. At this point, his stomach feels bloated and flatulence does not relieve the internal pressure. Today he woke up and felt faint as he got up out of bed. When you palpate his abdomen, it feels protuberant. It's time to bring your findings to the supervising medical officer.

Ready for Review

- As a combat medic, you will be called on to establish and provide assistance to your unit's preventive medicine programs, such as training and assisting your unit's field sanitation teams, educating soldiers about force health protection measures, and assisting with your unit's hearing conservation program.

- The effectiveness with which you accomplish this responsibility will have a far-reaching effect on the health and performance of your fellow soldiers, and in turn, the success of your unit's mission.

- The field sanitation team (FST) is responsible for the preventive medicine measures (PMMs) that affect units.

- A unit's effectiveness is dependent upon the health of its soldiers.

- The impact of casualties caused by disease nonbattle injuries (DNBI) upon military campaigns has been a prominent and a continuous feature of military operations throughout history.

- Ordinarily, the US soldier has a high standard of personal hygiene when in an environment with convenient facilities. In the field, however, where proper sanitation requires coping with the elements of nature, a problem arises: The soldier is suddenly faced with inconveniences.

- Part of preventive care is verifying that all medical records for soldiers in your unit are current for immunizations.

- Due to the scope of current operations, hazardous noise exposure is the greatest it has been for over 30 years.

- Noise-induced hearing loss is on the rise among US soldiers.

Vital Vocabulary

battle fatigue Temporary emotional disorder or inability to function experienced by a previously normal soldier as a reaction to the overwhelming or cumulative stress of combat.

combat arms earplug (CAEP) Double-ended earplug designed for two different types of hearing protection; for use in military environments.

medical intelligence The process of gathering essential medical information before an operation begins, allowing unit leaders and combat medics to tailor their operational plans.

otoscopic examination Medical examination of the inner ears.

COMBAT MEDIC *in Action*

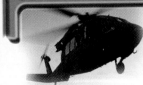

You are the combat medic staffing the Battalion Aid Station during sick call. Three soldiers from the same unit enter the BAS. They are all complaining of upset stomach and one soldier has been vomiting. You call in your supervising medical officer. It turns out that all three soldiers are suffering from food poisoning after eating from a roadside vendor. The first soldier thought he was safe because his food was cooked thoroughly; in fact, the meat was burned. The second soldier had an apple that he rinsed off with some canteen water. The third soldier had a cold soda, which he thought was safe because it came from a can. Unfortunately, it was poured into a glass with a few cubes of ice.

1. True or false? Freezing water instantly kills all disease-causing organisms.

   A. True

   B. False

2. Washing fruit with potable water may not be enough. What should you add to the water?

   A. Chlorine

   B. Heat

   C. Chlorine or heat

   D. Iodine

3. Unpasteurized dairy products should be:

   A. avoided.

   B. frozen.

   C. boiled.

   D. refrigerated.

4. Certain precautions should be taken when preparing fish, including:

   A. avoiding shellfish.

   B. avoiding large, predatory reef fish.

   C. cooking all seafood thoroughly.

   D. all of the above.

5. Bacteria that multiply at temperatures between _____ and _____ cause most foodborne illnesses.

   A. 60°F, 125°F

   B. 30°F, 60°F

   C. 75°F, 125°F

   D. 125°F, 145°F

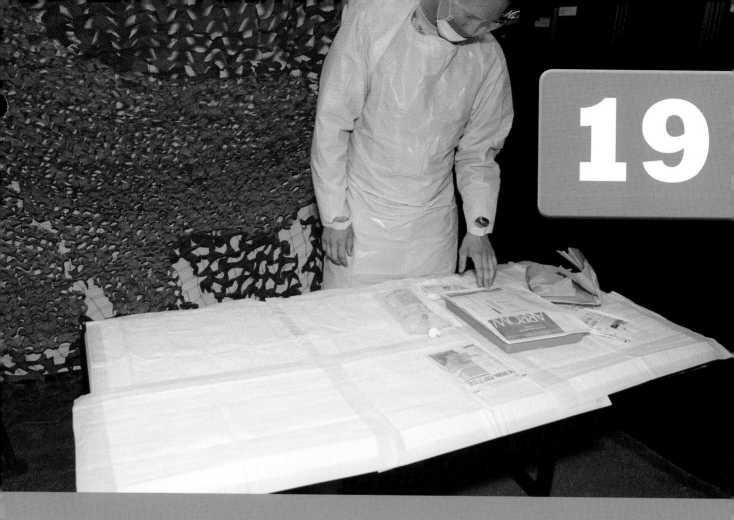

19

Infection Control

Objectives

Knowledge Objectives
- Define microorganisms.
- List the most useful and effective means of breaking the chain of infection.
- Describe the body's response to infection.
- Discuss the conditions that increase the risk for nosocomial infection.
- Describe medical asepsis.
- Describe surgical asepsis.
- Describe infection control.

Skills Objectives
- Establish a sterile field.
- Perform a patient care handwash.
- Don sterile gloves.
- Remove gloves.

■ Introduction

It is important to understand how disease spreads and how to break the chain of infection. Preventing infections is vital. Practicing techniques of medical and surgical asepsis will help protect you, your patients, and your unit from infection.

In ancient times, demons and evil spirits were thought to be the causes of pestilence and infection. Hippocrates (460–ca. 377 BCE), the great healer of his time, irrigated wounds with wine or boiled water, foreshadowing asepsis. Galen (129–ca. 200 AD), a Greek who practiced medicine in Rome, was the most distinguished physician after Hippocrates. He boiled the surgical instruments he used to care for wounded gladiators. In the early to mid-1800s, people like Louis Pasteur introduced us to the world of microorganisms. Since that time, we have witnessed the invention of the first steam sterilizer (1886), the practice of passive and active immunization, and the use of antibiotics.

■ Microorganisms

Microorganisms are microscopic living cells found almost everywhere in the environment. Thousands of species of microorganisms exist in nature. Microorganisms can be beneficial (eg, mold for cheese) or harmful (eg, HIV, which causes AIDS). Understanding the role of microorganisms in disease transmission has helped create technology and personal protective equipment for disease prevention.

Microorganisms: Structure and Function

Microorganisms have similar cell structures to animals and plants. Many microorganisms (such as **bacteria**) take in oxygen, burn food for energy and growth, and excrete wastes in a process called metabolism. They also can increase in size, divide, and mutate. They react in different ways to environment changes. Many microorganisms are able to move on their own. Some microorganisms form protective capsules.

A relatively small percentage of microorganisms cause diseases and disorders. Most microorganisms are helpful. All human beings contain microorganisms in and on their bodies, such as in the digestive system. Most microorganisms do not produce disease under normal conditions. However, pathogenic microorganisms have the potential to negatively affect a person's health.

At the beginning of a **bacterial infection**, a condition in which pathogens invade the body, a group of bacterial cells may number only a few hundred. As the bacteria reproduce, they form groups of many millions of individual cells called *colonies*. The greater the number of pathogens, the greater the opportunity to cause disease.

> ### Field Medical Care **TIPS**
>
> You may be caring for patients who have an infectious or a communicable disease.

The following are environmental factors that affect the growth of microorganisms:

- **Oxygen:** Most require oxygen for growth, whereas others cannot survive in the presence of oxygen.
- **Nutrients:** Organic nutrients are a key ingredient for growth. Parasites live on or within hosts.
- **Temperature:** Most microorganisms grow at normal body temperature. Cold temperatures often slow their growth. High temperatures usually kill most microorganisms. Steam sterilization and boiling water are two common techniques used to kill pathogenic microorganisms.
- **Moisture:** All microorganisms require water or moisture to grow (eg, blood).
- **pH:** The acidity or alkalinity must be at the correct levels for microorganisms to grow.
- **Light:** Some microorganisms need light for growth and some microorganisms flourish in darkness.

Types of Microorganisms

Algae resemble plant cells and are found in sunlit water and rarely cause human disease. Fungi are yeasts and molds. A common yeast is *Candida albicans*, which causes thrush and vaginitis. A common mold is tinea pedis or athlete's foot FIGURE 19-1 ▶. **Protozoa** are microscopic single-cell organisms; for example, *Trichomonas vaginalis* causes vaginal infection in women and urinary tract infection in men.

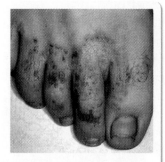

FIGURE 19-1 A common mold is tinea pedis or athlete's foot.

Bacteria are single-celled organisms without a nucleus. Spores protect certain bacteria and making them resistant to the environment and able to survive extreme conditions of light, drying, and chemicals. Bacteria are difficult microorganisms to control and destroy. Pathogenic bacteria include:

- *Neisseria*, which causes gonorrhea, upper respiratory infections, and infectious meningitis
- *Pseudomonas*, which causes pus-forming infections
- *Staphylococcus aureus*, which produces toxins causing infections in postsurgical patients
- *Streptococcus*, which cause strep throat, pneumonia, and scarlet fever

Drug-resistant bacteria are resistant to antibiotic therapy. These include:

- Methicillin-resistant *Staphylococcus aureus* (MRSA)
- Vancomycin-resistant enterococci (VRE)
- *Clostridium difficile*

Viruses must use the host's ability to make protein and energy. Some viruses, such as HIV, affect every system and tissue of the body. Immunization is the most effective means for preventing viral infections such as polio and measles. As discussed in Chapter 18, *Force Health Protection*, soldiers are required to be up-to-date with certain immunizations. Viruses can be spread from person-to-person contact or from animal-to-person contact.

Infectious Diseases

Infectious diseases are caused by pathogenic microorganisms. Communicable diseases, such as HIV, can spread from one person to another. Contagious diseases are communicable diseases that are transmitted to many individuals quickly and easily (eg, SARS). Some diseases can cause an epidemic where a large number of people in the same area are infected in a relatively short time (eg, influenza).

Chain of Infection

Infectious diseases will spread if the chain of infection remains unbroken. A **reservoir** is any place where a microorganism can multiply or survive:

- People
- Domesticated or wild animals
- Insects
- Inanimate objects (eg, air, soil, food, fluids, bedding, and utensils)

The **portal of exit** is where the microorganism leaves the reservoir:

- All body orifices
- Skin discharges
- Natural discharges (eg, mucus, semen, sputum, saliva, urine, and feces)
- Vomitus, drainage, or blood from breaks in the skin

The **vehicles** to transmit the microorganism are:

- **Direct contact:** Touching, shaking hands, kissing, and sexual intercourse
- **Indirect contact:** Bedding, tissues, used syringes, drinking cups, and dressings
- **Human carrier:** Does not exhibit the symptoms of a disease but carries the pathogens and transmits them to others
- **Airborne transmission:** Dust particles carrying microbes or spores that blow from place to place
- **Waterborne transmission:** Public water such as pools and lakes contaminated with feces
- **Foodborne transmission:** Spoiled or uncooked food or food contaminated with feces or soil
- **Bloodborne transmission:** Blood transfusions, kidney dialysis, and injections
- **Disease vectors:** Rodents, mosquitoes, flies, fleas, ticks, and lice

The **portals of entry** through which the microorganism can enter the host include:

- Respiratory tract
- Gastrointestinal tract
- Urinary tract
- Reproductive organs
- Open wounds
- Incisions
- Puncture sites from injections
- Body orifices into which catheters or tubes are inserted

The **susceptible hosts** in which the microorganism can find a reservoir include:

- Hospitalized patients
- Ill or inactive people
- Patients with chronic fatigue
- People with poor nutrition
- Infants, young children, and older adults
- Patients with injury, wounds, shock, and trauma
- Patients suffering from the side effects of some medications
- Patients with emotional factors such as anxiety

As the combat medic, you can break the chain of infection by following the measures listed in TABLE 19-1 ▸.

Asepsis

Asepsis refers to practices that minimize or eliminate microorganisms that can cause infection and disease. There are two types: medical asepsis (clean technique) and surgical asepsis (sterile technique).

Medical Asepsis

Medical asepsis refers to practices that minimize the number of microorganisms or that prevent the transmission of microorganisms from one person to another. Components of medical asepsis include handwashing, using barrier techniques, and keeping the environment clean and controlled.

Personal Protective Equipment

The use of personal protective equipment (PPE) is critical in medical asepsis. PPE keeps organisms from entering or leaving the respiratory tract, eyes, or breaks in skin. PPE includes:

- **Gloves:** Provide a protective barrier when you must touch blood or body fluids FIGURE 19-2 ▸.
- **Eye protection:** Can be goggles/glasses with side/forehead shields FIGURE 19-3 ▸. Eye protection is worn if a patient's body fluids may splash or spray onto you. Always use disposable goggles when caring for patients in isolation.

Field Medical Care TIPS

Proper handwashing is the single most useful and effective means of breaking the chain of infection.

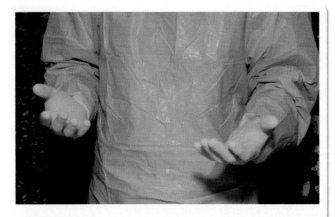

FIGURE 19-2 Gloves provide a protective barrier when you must touch blood or body fluids.

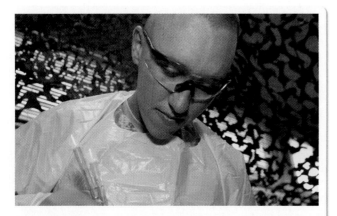

FIGURE 19-3 Eye protection is worn if a patient's body fluids may splash or spray onto you.

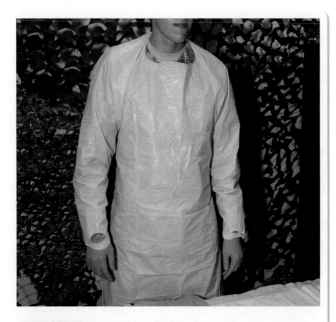

FIGURE 19-4 Gowns or aprons keep your clothing clean if a patient's body fluids splash onto your clothing.

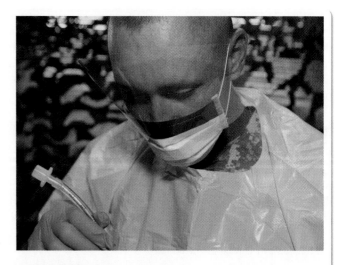

FIGURE 19-5 Masks are used when giving care to patients with communicable diseases that are transmitted through the respiratory tract.

Field Medical Care **TIPS**

If a patient has a respiratory communicable disease, like tuberculosis (TB), a mask is a must. Everyone who comes into contact with the patient, including visitors, should wear a mask. Only the patient should wear a mask when outside of the room.

Field Medical Care **TIPS**

When leaving a patient's room, take special care not to spread any communicable diseases to others. Discard your gown and mask properly. Wash your hands after leaving the patient's room.

- **Gowns or aprons:** These are resistant to fluids, and keep your clothing clean if a patient's body fluids splash onto your clothing **FIGURE 19-4 ◄**.
- **Masks:** Used when giving care to patients with communicable diseases that are transmitted through the respiratory tract **FIGURE 19-5 ▲**. Masks are disposable to reduce the risk of cross-contamination. When you are not using the mask, dispose of it properly.

Disinfectants and Sterilization

Disinfectants destroy most pathogens but not necessarily their spores. **Sterilization** destroys all microorganisms and spores by exposing articles to heat or to chemical disinfectants long enough to kill all microorganisms and spores. One method of sterilization is the use of a pressure steam sterilizer called an **autoclave**. Never touch sterile articles with unsterile articles. Do not risk using a contaminated article.

Sterile Protective Measures

When entering sterile environments, such as an operating room, you must wear clean clothing to prevent contaminating

TABLE 19-1 Breaking the Chain of Infection

Reservoir	• Wash your hands! • Sterilize instruments and dressings used in the operating room. • Disinfect floors and equipment. • Clean thermometers and bedpans after use. • Give baths using soap and water to remove drainage/dried secretions. • Discard disposable equipment after use. • Change dressings when they are wet. • Place contaminated needles and syringes in the appropriate moisture-resistant, puncture-proof container. • Make sure drainage tubes and collection bags drain properly and empty according to standard operating procedures (SOPs).
Portal of exit	• Wash your hands! • Use the appropriate waste disposal method. • Carefully manage secretions and drainage. • Avoid talking, sneezing, or coughing directly over open wounds or a sterile field. • Always wear gloves when the potential for contact with body substances exists. • Patients who have airborne infections may need to wear masks or receive ordered medications that prevent coughing.
Vehicle	• Wash your hands! • Burn all trash in nonresidue incinerators. • Remove linen without shaking it or allowing it to touch your clothing. • Patients should have their own set of personal care items. • Carefully cover all infected wounds. • Properly handle and prepare food. • Isolate patients with contagious diseases. • Control airflow. • Sterilize. • Use syringes and needles safely. • Do not recap or attempt to break needles.
Portal of entry	• Wash your hands! • Keep the patient's skin clean and dry; apply moisturizers to dry skin. • Avoid positioning patients against objects that could cause skin breaks. • Reposition patients who have impaired mobility. • Provide clean, dry, wrinkle-free linen. • Make sure urine collection bags are lower than the patient. • Disinfect tubes and ports before collecting specimens from drainage tubes or IV lines. • Wear gloves, protective eyewear, masks, gowns, and shoe covers to protect yourself appropriately. • Keep wounds that are draining and skin breaks covered. • Use sterile technique when performing invasive procedures.
Susceptible host	• Wash your hands! • Practice infection control measures. • Treat the patient's underlying condition. • Provide adequate rest and skin care. • Give nutritional support. • Encourage adequate fluid intake. • Help to reduce anxiety. • Help with coughing and deep breathing when the patient is immobilized. • Encourage proper immunization of children and older adults who are at high risk for communicable disease.

the area with microorganisms that reside on the skin, hair, and clothing. All hair coverings should cover all hair on the head. The surgical mask should completely cover the mouth and the nose. Touch only the inside of the gown; the back of the gown is considered contaminated.

■ Infection Control

Standard Precautions

Standard precautions are a combination of universal precautions and **body substance isolation**. Universal precautions are designed to reduce the risk of transmission of bloodborne pathogens. Body substance isolation is designed to reduce the transmission of pathogens from moist body substances. Standard precautions apply to blood, all body fluids, secretions, excretions (except sweat), nonintact skin, and mucous membranes. They are designed to reduce the risk of transmission of microorganisms from both known and unknown sources of infection. Standard precautions consider all patients to be infected with bloodborne pathogens. You must use standard precautions in the care of all patients.

Wear gloves when in contact with blood, body fluids containing blood, secretions, excretions, nonintact skin, mucous membranes, or contaminated items. Change gloves after each contact with a patient. Wash your hands and skin surfaces immediately and thoroughly if you are contaminated with blood or body fluids, after each patient contact, and after removing gloves to prevent transfer of microorganisms between patients or between patients and the environment.

Wear a gown or apron when your clothing could become soiled. Wear a mask, eye protection, and face shield if splashing or spraying of blood or body fluids is possible. Place all contaminated linens in a leak-proof bag.

Do not recap or break needles. Place needles and sharp objects in a special, puncture-resistant container after use

FIGURE 19-6 ▸. Use the needless system or safety syringes, if available. Report any exposure to blood or body fluids to your supervisor immediately.

Transmission-Based Precautions

Transmission-based precautions for treating patients with a suspected or known infectious disease are based on the disease's route of transmission. These precautions are designed to interrupt the transmission of pathogens. Airborne precautions are taken when tiny microorganisms from

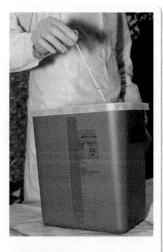

FIGURE 19-6 Place needles and sharp objects in a special, puncture-resistant container after use.

evaporated droplets remain suspended in the air or are carried on dust particles and inhaled. Diseases transmitted this way include tuberculosis (TB), measles, and chickenpox. The patient may be placed in a private room that has monitored negative air flow pressure (air discharged outdoors or specially filtered before circulating to other areas). Doors to these rooms are to be kept closed. Wear a high-filtration particulate respirator when caring for TB patients **FIGURE 19-7** ▾.

Droplet precautions are taken when microorganisms are propelled through the air from an infected person and depos-

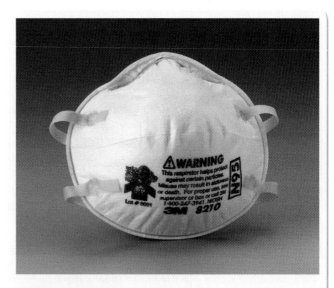

FIGURE 19-7 Specially designed respirator masks, such as the N95 respirator, protect against infection from tuberculosis bacteria.

ited on the host's eyes, nose, or mouth. Transmission can occur through sneezing, coughing, talking, or suctioning. Diseases transmitted in this manner include meningitis, pneumonia, diphtheria, streptococcal pharyngitis, influenza, mumps, and rubella. These patients require a private room or need to share a room with a similarly infectious patient. The doors to this room may remain open. Wear a mask when working within 3′ of the patient. Have the patient wear a mask if you must transport him or her to an area outside the room.

Direct contact is the most frequent mode of disease transmission. Direct contact occurs between a susceptible host's body surface and an infected person. It can also occur between a susceptible host and a colonized person (in whom the microorganism is present but who shows no clinical signs or symptoms of infection). Indirect contact occurs when a susceptible host comes into contact with an intermediate contaminated object like a dirty instrument, needle, or hands. Diseases transmitted by these routes include drug-resistant gastrointestinal, respiratory, skin, and wound infections; hepatitis A; herpes simplex virus; acute diarrhea; draining abscess; impetigo scabies; and pediculosis.

These patients require a private room or need to share a room with a similarly infectious patient. The door may remain open. Wear gloves when entering the room and remove them before leaving. Change gloves after contact with a patient's infective material (eg, fecal matter, wound drainage). Wash your hands with an antimicrobial/waterless antiseptic agent. Wear a gown into the room if you anticipate contact with infectious matter and remove the gown before leaving the room. Try to restrict the use of noncritical equipment to one patient only. Clean and disinfect equipment before using it on other patients.

Additional Standard Precautions

Each health care facility has its own SOPs. Specific procedures for an individual patient will often be prescribed, depending on the reason for precautions **TABLE 19-2 ▶**.

■ Patient Care Handwash

Handwashing reduces the number of bacteria from the hands and prevents the transfer of microorganisms. Wash your hands before and after patient contact. Also wash your hands after contact with dirty or contaminated materials (eg, used linens, used thermometers). To perform a patient care handwash, follow the steps in **SKILL DRILL 19-1 ▶**:

1. Remove all jewelry. Wearing rings in a patient care area should be minimized in order to reduce possible bacteria locations. If rings are worn, they should be plain and washed when the hands are washed **(Step ①)**.

2. Stand in front of the sink and avoid leaning against it. Turn on the water and adjust the temperature. Knee or

foot pedals may be available on some sinks. Warm water is preferable to cold because it avoids chapping the skin and removing skin oils **(Step ②)**.

3. Wash your hands. Thoroughly wet your hands and forearms under running water, keeping your hands lower than your elbows **(Step ③)**.

4. Apply the soap. Wash your hands, wrists, and lower forearms, using a circular scrubbing motion **(Step ④)**.

5. Interlace your fingers and rub your hands back and forth. Give particular attention to the creases and folds in the skin where microorganisms are difficult to dislodge.

6. The duration of the patient care handwash should be a minimum of 10 to 15 seconds. It can range from 10 seconds to as long as 2 minutes, depending on the potential for contamination with microorganisms **(Step ⑤)**.

7. Insert your fingernails from one hand under those of your other hand using a sweeping motion **(Step ⑥)**.

8. Repeat with your other hand. Repeat the procedure if your hands are very dirty.

9. Rinse your hands, wrists, and forearms. Do not touch any part of the contaminated sink or faucets.

10. Rinse thoroughly with your hands and wrists lower than your elbows, so water flows from your elbows to your fingers (Step ⑦).

11. Dry your hands, wrists, and forearms. Dry thoroughly using clean paper towels. Dispose of the towels properly without dropping the hands below waist level. Dispose of drying material in accordance with (IAW) local SOP—use a trash container **(Step ⑧)**.

■ Purpose and Indications for Donning Sterile Gloves

Sterile gloves establish a barrier to microorganisms transferring from combat medic to patient and from patient to combat medic. Sterile gloves are required to maintain a sterile field during hands-on procedures. Indications are invasive procedures such as surgery, sterile procedures, and when sterility must be maintained (eg, changing sterile dressings and irrigating wounds). To don sterile gloves, follow the steps in **SKILL DRILL 19-2 ▶**:

1. Select and obtain the proper size package of sterile gloves.

2. Inspect the glove package for signs of contamination. Discard if you find any of the following: water spots or moisture, tears, and any other evidence of damage or contamination.

TABLE 19-2 Sample Additional Standard Precautions

Administering medications	• Unwrap medications before going into the patient's room. • Use disposable medication trays and cups. • Do not take medication cards into the room. • Wash your hands. • Place needles and syringes in the sharps container in the patient's room. • Use and discard IV bags in the patient's room. • Dispose of all materials in the patient's room.
Sending a specimen to the laboratory	• Before collecting the specimen, label the container. • Place it on a clean paper towel in the anteroom and carefully scrub once outside the room. • Place the specimen into a bag identified with the standard "Biohazard" label. • Wash your hands.
Taking vital signs	• Use the equipment in the room. • Wear gloves and whatever other PPE is indicated. • Use the clock in the room, not your watch. • Use a disposable temperature system.
Double bagging	• Two personnel are needed. • Personnel inside the room are contaminated and the one outside is clean. • Clean personnel fold the top of the clean bag down to make a collar or cuff; the clean personnel keep their hands outside this cuff. • Contaminated personnel touch only the inside of the clean bag; the clean personnel touch only the outside of the clean bag. • Clean personnel fold over the top of the clean bag, seal it carefully, and label it, touching only the outside of the bag.
Transporting the patient to other departments	• Wear PPE as needed. • Have the patient wear PPE as needed. • Control and contain any of the patient's drainage. • Drape the wheelchair/stretcher with a clean sheet/bath blanket; wrap the patient with a clean sheet/bath blanket. • Escort ambulatory patients. • Notify others of the patient's special precautions. • Disinfect transportation devices.
Caring for the patient's body after death	• Take special precautions to prevent the spread of infection. • Use protective (reverse or neutropenic) isolation. • Provide protection from the outside environment.
For weakened immune response patients	• Diseases or injuries of concern include burns or bone marrow transplants, HIV, or a patient undergoing chemotherapy, or experiencing low resistance from another cause.

3. Perform a patient care handwash.

4. Place the package on a flat, clean, dry surface in the area where the gloves are to be worn. Peel the outer wrapper open to completely expose the inner package (**Step ①**).

5. Remove the inner package, touching only the folded side of the wrapper. Position the package so that the cuff end is nearest to you (**Step ②**).

6. Unfold the inner package. Open the package to a fully flat position without touching the gloves.

7. Expose both gloves by grasping the lower inside corners or designated areas on the folder. Pull gently to the side without touching the gloves (**Step ③**).

8. Put on the first glove. Grasp the cuff at the folded edge and remove it from the wrapper with one hand. Step away from the table or tray.

SKILL DRILL 19-1

Patient Care Handwash

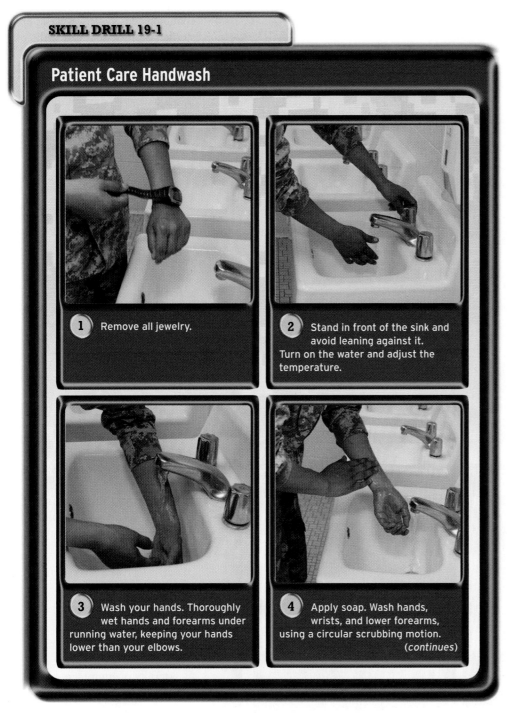

1. Remove all jewelry.

2. Stand in front of the sink and avoid leaning against it. Turn on the water and adjust the temperature.

3. Wash your hands. Thoroughly wet hands and forearms under running water, keeping your hands lower than your elbows.

4. Apply soap. Wash hands, wrists, and lower forearms, using a circular scrubbing motion.
(continues)

9. Keeping your hands above your waist, insert the fingers of your other hand into the glove. Pull the glove on, touching only the exposed inner surface of the glove. If you have difficulty getting your fingers fully fitted into the glove fingers, make any adjustments after both gloves are on (**Step 4**).

10. Put on the second glove. Insert the fingertips of the gloved hand under the edge of the folded over cuff.

The gloved thumb may be kept up and away from the cuff area or may be inserted under the edge of the folded over cuff with the fingertips.

11. Keeping your hands above your waist, insert the fingers of your ungloved hand into the glove. Pull the glove on. *Do not* contaminate either glove by dropping your hands below waist level (**Step 5**).

12. Adjust the gloves to fit properly. Grasp and pick up the glove surfaces on the individual fingers to adjust them. Pick up the palm surfaces and work your fingers and hands into the gloves.

13. Interlock the gloved fingers and work the gloved hands until the gloves are firmly on the fingers. Avoid dropping your hands below waist level once your gloves are on (**Step 6**).

To remove dirty gloves, follow the steps in **SKILL DRILL 19-3** ▶:

1. Grasp one glove at the heel of the hand with the other gloved hand (**Step 1**).

2. Peel off the glove, retaining it in the palm of the gloved hand (**Step 2**).

3. Reach under the cuff of the remaining glove with one or two fingers of the ungloved hand (**Step 3**).

4. Peel off the glove over the glove being held in the palm. Do not contaminate yourself. Discard the gloves according to local SOP.

5. Perform a patient care handwash (**Step 4**).

Surgical Asepsis

Dirty is a term for any object or person that has not been cleaned or sterilized for removal of microorganisms. A

SKILL DRILL 19-1

Patient Care Handwash (*continued*)

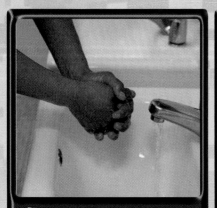

5 Interlace fingers and rub hands back and forth. Pay particular attention to creases and folds in the skin. The handwash duration will be from 10 seconds to as long as 2 minutes or longer, depending on the potential for contamination with microorganisms.

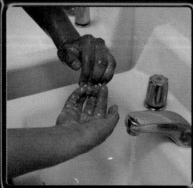

6 Insert your fingernails from one hand under those of your other hand using a sweeping motion. Repeat with your other hand. Repeat the procedure if your hands are very dirty.

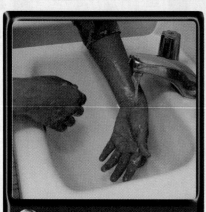

7 Rinse your hands, wrists, and forearms. Do not touch any part of the contaminated sink or faucets. Rinse thoroughly with your hands and wrists lower than your elbow, so water flows from elbows to fingers.

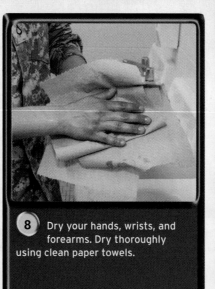

8 Dry your hands, wrists, and forearms. Dry thoroughly using clean paper towels.

contaminated object was clean or sterile before it touched a dirty object. *Clean* implies that many or the most harmful microorganisms have been removed and can be used on the skin, mouth, GI tract, and upper respiratory tract. *Sterile* means that the item is free of all microorganisms and spores and can be used on the abdominal cavity, urinary bladder, or the ovary.

The sterile technique (surgical asepsis) means that no organisms are carried to the patient. The sterile technique destroys microorganisms before they can enter the body. This technique is used when making dressing changes, administering parenteral (outside the digestive tract) medications, and performing surgical and other procedures such as urinary catheterization.

With the sterile technique, articles are sterilized and then they are prevented from making contact with any unsterile articles. When a sterile article touches an unsterile article, it becomes contaminated and is no longer sterile. To establish a sterile field, follow the steps in SKILL DRILL 19-4 ▶:

1. Select a clean work surface above waist level.

2. Assemble all necessary equipment.

3. Check dates, labels, and condition of packaging for sterility of equipment.

4. Perform a patient care handwash (see Skill Drill 19-1).

5. Place the pack containing the sterile drape directly on the work surface and open to ensure its sterility.

SKILL DRILL 19-2

Don Sterile Gloves

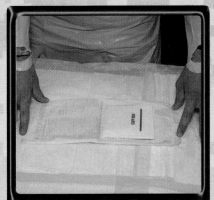

1. Select and obtain the proper size package of sterile gloves. Inspect the glove package for signs of contamination. Perform a patient care handwash. Place the package on a flat, clean, dry surface in the area where the gloves are to be worn. Peel the outer wrapper open to completely expose the inner package.

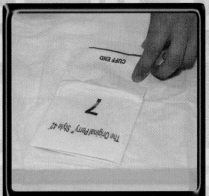

2. Remove the inner package, touching only the folded side of the wrapper. Position the package so that the cuff end is nearest to you.

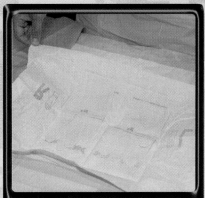

3. Unfold the inner package. Open the package to a fully flat position without touching the gloves. Expose both gloves by grasping the lower inside corners or designated areas on the folder. Pull gently to the side without touching the gloves.

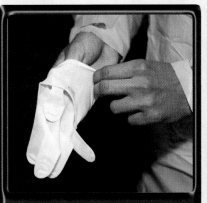

4. Put on the first glove. Grasp the cuff at the folded edge and remove it from the wrapper with one hand. Step away from the table or tray. Keeping your hands above your waist, insert the fingers of your other hand into the glove. Pull the glove on, touching only the exposed inner surface of the glove. If you have difficulty getting your fingers fully fitted into the glove fingers, make any adjustments after both gloves are on.

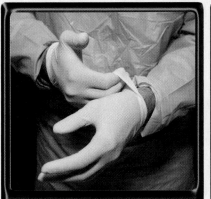

5. Put on the second glove. Insert the fingertips of your gloved hand under the edge of the folded over cuff. The gloved thumb may be kept up and away from the cuff area or may be inserted under the edge of the folded over cuff with your fingertips. Keeping your hands above your waist, insert the fingers of your ungloved hand into the glove. Pull the glove on. Do not contaminate either glove by dropping your hands below waist level.

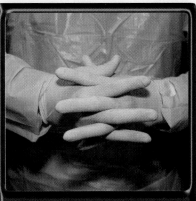

6. Adjust the gloves to fit properly. Grasp and pick up the glove surfaces on the individual fingers to adjust them. Pick up the palm surfaces and work your fingers and hands into the gloves. Interlock the gloved fingers and work your gloved hands until the gloves are firmly on the fingers. Avoid dropping your hands below waist level once your gloves are on.

SKILL DRILL 19-3

Remove Gloves

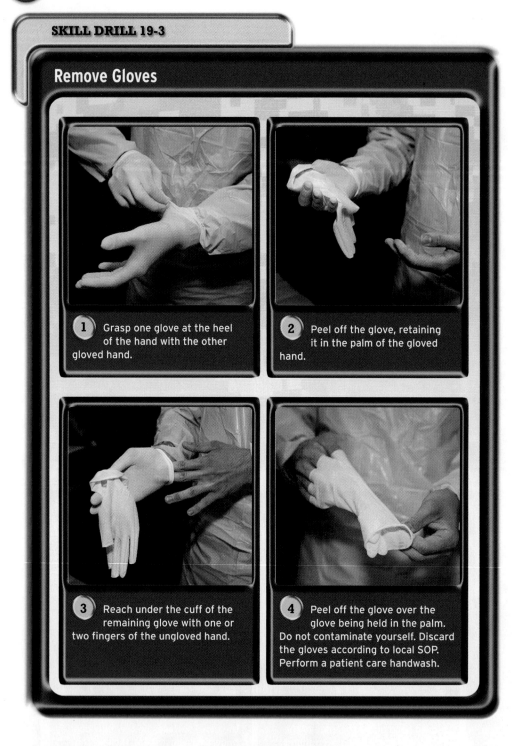

1 Grasp one glove at the heel of the hand with the other gloved hand.

2 Peel off the glove, retaining it in the palm of the gloved hand.

3 Reach under the cuff of the remaining glove with one or two fingers of the ungloved hand.

4 Peel off the glove over the glove being held in the palm. Do not contaminate yourself. Discard the gloves according to local SOP. Perform a patient care handwash.

Field Medical Care **TIPS**

Sterile to sterile remains sterile. Sterile to clean becomes contaminated. Think before you touch anything.

6. Gently lift the drape up from its outer cover and let it unfold by itself without touching any object. Discard the outer cover with your other hand (**Step ①**).

7. Grasp the adjacent corner of the drape and hold it straight up and away from the body; now the drape can be placed properly using two hands. The drape must be held away from any unsterile surface (**Step ②**).

8. Holding the drape, first position the bottom half over the intended work surface (**Step ③**).

9. Allow the top half of the drape to be placed over the work surface last.

10. Perform the procedure using sterile technique (**Step ④**).

■ Response to Infection

Whether or not a pathogen produces an active infection depends on both the organism and the host. The first phase is the incubation period, which lasts from when the pathogen enters the body up to the appearance of the first symptoms of illness. The second phase is the prodromal stage, which lasts from the onset of initial symptoms such as fatigue or low-grade fever to more severe symptoms. The third phase is the full stage of illness when symptoms are acute and specific to the type of infection, such as lesions covering the body or high fever. The final stage is the convalescence stage when acute symptoms of the infection subside and the patient recovers.

SKILL DRILL 19-4

Establish a Sterile Field

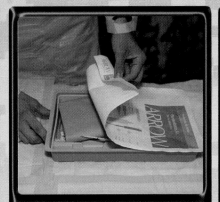

1 Select a clean work surface above waist level. Assemble all necessary equipment. Check the dates, labels, and condition of packaging for sterility of equipment. Perform a patient care handwash. (See Skill Drill 19-1) Place the pack containing the sterile drape directly on the work surface and open to ensure its sterility. Gently lift the drape up from its outer cover and let it unfold by itself without touching any object. Discard the outer cover with your other hand.

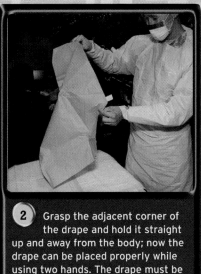

2 Grasp the adjacent corner of the drape and hold it straight up and away from the body; now the drape can be placed properly while using two hands. The drape must be held away from any unsterile surface.

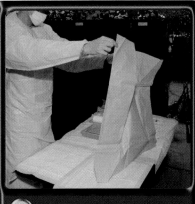

3 Holding the drape, first position the bottom half over the intended work surface.

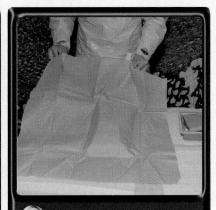

4 Allow the top half of the drape to be placed over the work surface last. Perform the procedure using sterile technique.

The Factors That Influence Infection

Microorganisms cause disease only if they gain access to the body through a specific portal of entry. For example, *Streptococcus* pneumonia causes pneumococcal pneumonia only when it enters the body through the respiratory system. **Virulence** is the pathogen's ability to cause disease. Some bacteria form protective capsules that increase their virulence. Other bacteria produce enzymes that destroy blood cells, stop normal blood clotting, or consume muscle fibers, all of which increase their virulence.

Host resistance is where some naturally occurring body floras have an antibiotic relationship with pathogens and contribute to an individual's health. If the patient has host resistance, the patient's body will be able to fight off the pathogens and resist infection.

Nosocomial Infection

Nosocomial infection is a serious problem in garrison care. These are infections that patients acquire while in the medical care facility. The reasons for nosocomial infections include:

- The number of disease-causing microorganisms present in the facility.
- Many microorganisms are resistant to antibiotics.
- There are many potential reservoirs for pathogenic growth:
  - IV fluids
  - Foods
  - Biological materials
  - Equipment

The conditions that increase the risk for nosocomial infections include:

- Broad-spectrum antibiotics are used frequently.
- Personnel fail to use appropriate techniques.
- Multiple personnel are providing care for a patient.
- Patient has lowered resistance to diseases.

■ Summary

Sterility should never be taken for granted and there should be no compromise. Your responsibility is to ensure that aseptic and sterile techniques are maintained. Infection control is a consideration in any patient care environment, and every individual is accountable. Proper gloving and handwashing techniques will protect you and your patients from contamination and possible infections.

YOU ARE THE
COMBAT MEDIC

It is a hot and dusty afternoon. Your unit is on patrol in a residential, urban area. While carefully exiting a narrow and dark alleyway, shots ring out. Your battle buddy immediately spots the sniper and renders the sniper helpless. Once establishing that the need to return fire is over, you perform a quick triage. "If you can hear my voice, but can't walk, raise your hand and let me know." One soldier is on the ground, holding his bleeding upper left thigh.

Assessment

The casualty can answer you when you ask, "Were you hit?" so you know that his airway is patent. He seems to be controlling the bleeding on his own through direct pressure with his hands. You evacuate the casualty to your armored HMMWV. Once safely inside the vehicle, you don a pair of sterile gloves and expose the wound. Once the casualty removes his hands and you cut through his trousers, the bleeding really starts. There is a clean entry and exit wound on the upper left thigh. The bleeding is getting heavier and heavier. You apply direct pressure with your gloved hands and gauze, but it is not slowing down.

You need to apply a tourniquet before you can continue your assessment and care. After applying the tourniquet, you obtain the casualty's vital signs. His pulse is 130 beats/min weak and regular, respirations are 22 breaths/min and nonlabored.

Treatment

After the large amount of blood loss and now that you have stabilized the casualty by applying a tourniquet, you start an IV and have the HMMWV driver call for a MEDEVAC.

1. LAST NAME, FIRST NAME		RANK/GRADE	X	MALE
Lowe, John		SGT		FEMALE

SSN	SPECIALTY CODE	RELIGION
000-111-0000	002	Presbyterian

2. UNIT

FORCE				NATIONALITY	
A/T	AF/A	N/M	MC/M		
	BC/BC		NBI/BNC	DISEASE	PSYCH

3. INJURY

	AIRWAY
	HEAD
X	WOUND
	NECK/BACK INJURY
	BURN
	AMPUTATION
	STRESS
	OTHER (Specify)

FRONT   BACK

GSW

4. LEVEL OF CONSCIOUSNESS

	ALERT		PAIN RESPONSE
X	VERBAL RESPONSE		UNRESPONSIVE

5. PULSE	TIME	6. TOURNIQUET			TIME
130 bpm	1705	☐ NO	☒ YES		1702

7. MORPHINE		DOSE	TIME	8. IV	TIME
☒ NO	☐ YES			NS	1708

9. TREATMENT/OBSERVATIONS/CURRENT MEDICATION/ALLERGIES/NBC (ANTIDOTE)

GSW to the upper left thigh. Applied tourniquet and established an IV for fluid loss.

10. DISPOSITION	RETURNED TO DUTY		TIME
	X	EVACUATED	1712
		DECEASED	

11. PROVIDER/UNIT	DATE (YYMMDD)
Kelly, John	

Aid Kit

Ready for Review

- Microorganisms are microscopic living cells found almost everywhere in the environment. Microorganisms can be beneficial (eg, mold for cheese) or harmful (eg, HIV, which causes AIDS).
- Infectious diseases are caused by pathogenic microorganisms.
- Communicable diseases can spread from one person to another (eg, HIV).
- Contagious diseases are communicable diseases that are transmitted to many individuals quickly and easily (eg, SARS).
- Whether or not a pathogen produces an active infection depends on both the organism and the host.
- Medical asepsis refers to the practices that minimize the number of microorganisms or prevent the transmission of microorganisms from one person to another.
- The sterile technique means that no organisms are carried to the patient.
- Standard precautions are a combination of universal precautions and body substance isolation.
- Handwashing reduces the number of bacteria on your hands and prevents the transfer of microorganisms.
- Wash your hands before and after patient contact.
- Sterile gloves establish a barrier to microorganisms transferring from combat medic to patient and from patient to combat medic.

Vital Vocabulary

asepsis Practices that minimize or eliminate microorganisms that can cause infection and disease.

autoclave A pressure steam sterilizer.

bacteria Single-celled organisms without a nucleus.

bacterial infection When bacterial pathogens invade the body.

body substance isolation An infection control concept and practice that assumes that all body fluids are potentially infectious.

disinfectants Destroy most pathogens but not necessarily their spores.

host resistance Some naturally occurring body flora have an antibiotic relationship with pathogens and contribute to a person's health.

medical asepsis Practices that minimize the number of microorganisms or prevent the transmission of microorganisms from one person to another.

microorganisms Microscopic living cells found almost everywhere in the environment.

nosocomial infection An infection that patients acquire while in a medical care facility.

portal of exit Where the microorganism leaves the reservoir.

portals of entry Where the microorganism can enter the host.

protozoa Single-celled microscopic microorganisms.

reservoir Any place where a microorganism can multiply or survive.

sterilization Destroys all microorganisms and spores by exposing articles to heat or to chemical disinfectants long enough to kill them all.

susceptible hosts Where the microorganism can reside.

vehicles Ways that microorganisms are transmitted.

virulence A pathogen's strength to cause disease.

COMBAT MEDIC in Action

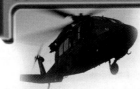

You are the combat medic on duty during the sick call at the Battalion Aid Station. A soldier comes in complaining of night sweats, fever, and a bad cough. During the patient assessment process, he suffers a violent coughing fit and coughs up blood-tinged sputum. The medical officer immediately suspects TB and calls for the proper airborne precautions to be taken to ensure that this patient does not infect the other patients or any of the health care personnel. What precautions should you take? How should the patient be isolated?

1. In addition to your standard personal protective equipment, you should don a:
   A. BVM device.
   B. high-filtration particulate respirator.
   C. surgical mask.
   D. cotton mask.

2. Airborne precautions are taken when patients present with:
   A. measles.
   B. chickenpox.
   C. TB.
   D. all of the above.

3. With airborne precautions, doors to the infected patient's room should remain:
   A. closed.
   B. open.
   C. guarded.
   D. ajar.

4. Droplet precautions are taken when a patient presents with:
   A. meningitis.
   B. mumps.
   C. rubella.
   D. all of the above.

5. With droplet precautions, you should wear a mask when working:
   A. on the same floor as the patient.
   B. in the patient's room.
   C. within 3' of the patient.
   D. with noninfected patients.

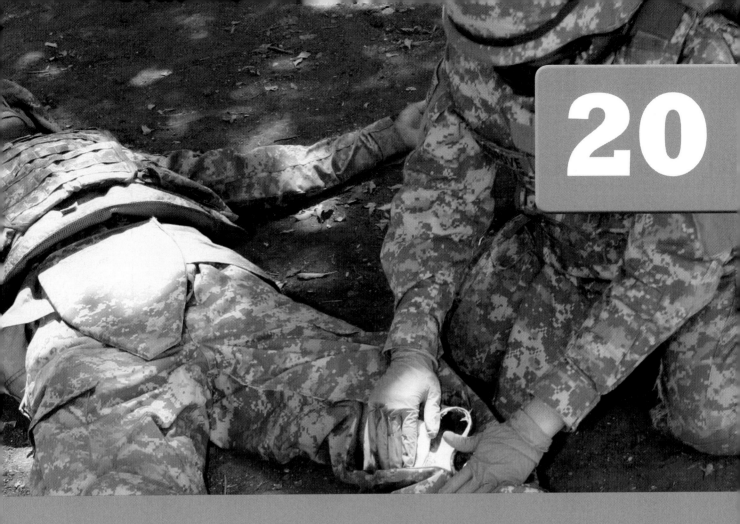

20

Wound Care

Objectives

Knowledge Objectives

☐ Identify the type of wound injury.

☐ Identify forms of wound healing.

☐ Describe assessment considerations.

☐ Describe the emergency treatment of specific wound types.

☐ Describe care for a wound.

☐ Discuss drainage and drainage systems.

☐ Describe how to assist with ongoing casualty management.

Skill Objective

☐ Change a patient's gauze dressing.

■ Introduction

As a combat medic, you will likely encounter a casualty needing wound care. Understanding the wound healing process and proper wound care management for a variety of wounds is essential knowledge basic to any health care setting. Good wound care management includes assessing the soldier's current nutritional status, identifying abnormal wound healing processes, identifying a wound infection, and applying the appropriate dressing for the wound that you are managing.

■ Structure and Function of the Skin

The human skin is much more than a wrapping. Rather, skin, or **integument**, is a complex organ with a crucial role in maintaining the constancy of the internal environment (**homeostasis**):

- The skin protects the underlying tissue from injury, including that caused by extremes of temperature, ultraviolet radiation, mechanical forces, toxic chemicals, and invading microorganisms.
- The skin aids in temperature regulation, preventing heat loss when the core body temperature starts to fall and facilitating heat loss when core temperature rises.
- As a watertight seal, the skin prevents excessive loss of water from the body and drying of tissues, thereby helping maintain the chemical stability of the internal environment.
- The skin serves as a sense organ, keeping the brain informed about the external environment. Changes in temperature, touch, and body position and sensations of pain are mediated through the sense receptors in the skin.

Significant damage to the skin may make the body vulnerable to bacterial invasion, temperature instability, and major disturbances of fluid balance—precisely what happens when an injury results in an opening in the skin.

Epidermis and Dermis

The skin is composed of two layers: the epidermis and the dermis **FIGURE 20-1 ▶**. The **epidermis**, or outermost layer, is the body's first line of defense, the principal barrier against water, dust, microorganisms, and mechanical stress. Underlying the epidermis is a tough, highly elastic layer of connective tissues called the **dermis**.

Subcutaneous Tissue

The layer of tissue beneath the dermis—that is, the **subcutaneous** layer—consists mainly of **adipose** tissue (fat). Blood vessels, lymph vessels, and hair follicle roots also are found in this layer. Subcutaneous fat insulates the underlying tissues from extremes of heat and cold. It also provides a cushion for underlying structures and an energy reserve for the body.

Deep Fascia

Below the subcutaneous tissue is a thick, dense layer of fibrous tissue known as the **deep fascia**. The deep fascia is composed of tough bands of tissue that ensheath muscles and other internal structures. It supports and protects underlying structures from injury. Muscles and bones are found below this layer.

Skin Tension Lines

The skin is arranged over the body structures in a manner that provides tension. This tautness varies by body region but occurs in patterns known as **tension lines**. Static tension develops over areas that have limited movement, such as the scalp. Lacerations occurring parallel to the skin tension lines may remain closed with little or no intervention. Larger wounds may be pulled open by the normal tension and require closure with sutures, staples, or a biodegradable "glue." Even small lacerations that lie perpendicular to the tension lines result in a wound that remains open. Healing occurs more slowly in an open wound, and abnormal scar formation is more likely.

Dynamic tension is found in areas that lie over muscle. The tension varies according to the contraction of the underlying muscle and subsequent movement of the skin. Open injuries to dynamic tension lines interfere with healing because they disrupt the clotting process and the tissue repair cycle, resulting in slowed healing and a tendency toward abnormal scar formation.

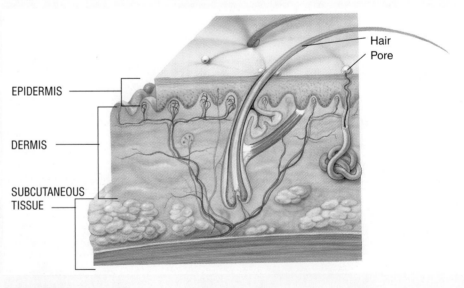

FIGURE 20-1 The skin is composed of a tough external layer called the epidermis and a vascular inner layer called the dermis.

Type of Wound Injury

Closed Wounds

In a **closed wound**, soft tissues beneath the skin surface are damaged, but there is no break in the epidermis. The characteristic closed wound is a **contusion** or bruise FIGURE 20-2 ▾, in which the skin is intact, but damage has occurred beneath the epidermis. Trauma to the nerve endings produces pain, and leakage of fluid into spaces between the damaged cells produces swelling (edema). If small blood vessels in the dermis are disrupted, a black-and-blue mark (**ecchymosis**) will cover the injured area; if large blood vessels are torn beneath the contused area, a **hematoma**—a collection of blood beneath the skin—will be evident as a lump with a bluish discoloration FIGURE 20-3 ▾.

Open Wounds

An **open wound** is characterized by a disruption in the skin. Open wounds are potentially much more serious than closed wounds for two reasons. First, they are vulnerable to infection. An open wound is **contaminated**—that is, microorganisms enter it. Whether the contamination produces infection depends in large measure on how the wound is managed. Second, open wounds have a greater potential for serious blood loss. When the skin is unbroken, bleeding from a disrupted blood vessel is limited. Although a significant volume of blood—up to about two units—can be lost into the soft tissues of the leg, eventually the increasing pressure within the leg will prevent further bleeding. In an open wound, the patient's entire blood volume may be lost.

Abrasions

An **abrasion** FIGURE 20-4 ▸ is a superficial wound that occurs when the skin is rubbed or scraped over a rough surface and part of the epidermis is lost. So-called road rash is a good example of an abrasion. Abrasions typically ooze small amounts of blood and may be quite painful. They may also be contaminated with dirt and debris. Because the skin has been disrupted, infection is a danger.

Lacerations

A **laceration** FIGURE 20-5 ▸ is a cut inflicted by a sharp instrument, such as a knife or razor blade, that produces a clean or jagged incision through the skin surface and underlying structures. Sometimes the word *laceration* is reserved for jagged or irregular cuts, and **incision** is used to refer to a clean (linear) cut. Incisions tend to heal better than lacerations because of their relatively even wound margins. The seriousness of a laceration will depend on its depth and the structures that have been damaged. Lacerations may be the source of significant bleeding if they disrupt the wall of a blood vessel, particularly in regions of the body where major arteries lie close to the surface (as in the wrist). The first priority in treating a laceration is to control bleeding, initially by applying direct manual pressure over the wound. Laceration of a major artery can be fatal due to the severe bleeding that can occur.

Puncture Wounds

A **puncture wound** FIGURE 20-6 ▸ is a stab from a pointed object, such as a nail or a knife. Technically speaking, a bullet wound also is a puncture wound. Most puncture wounds do not cause significant external bleeding, but they may produce extensive—even fatal—internal bleeding and wreak other havoc that cannot be seen from the outside of the body.

A special type of puncture wound is an impaled foreign object FIGURE 20-7 ▸. When the instrument that caused the injury remains embedded in the wound, immobilize the object.

Avulsions

An **avulsion** occurs when a flap of skin is torn loose, partially FIGURE 20-8 ▸ or completely. Depending on where the avulsion occurs, it may or may not be accompanied by profuse bleeding. The principal danger in this type of injury—besides blood loss and contamination—is loss of the blood supply to the avulsed flap. If the part of the flap that connects it to the body (the **pedicle**) is folded back or kinked, circulation to the

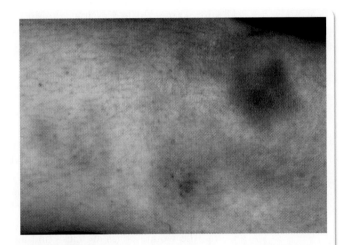

FIGURE 20-2 A contusion, or bruise, produces characteristic black-and-blue discoloration (ecchymosis).

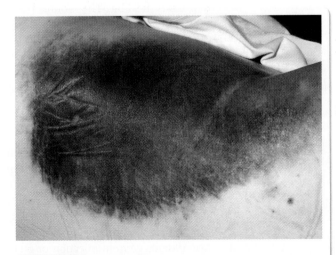

FIGURE 20-3 A hematoma.

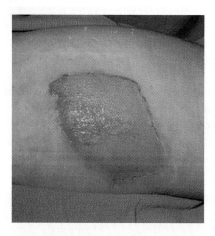

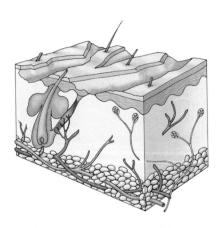

FIGURE 20-4 Abrasions usually do not penetrate completely through the dermis, but blood may ooze from the capillaries. These wounds are typically superficial and result from rubbing or scraping across a hard, rough surface.

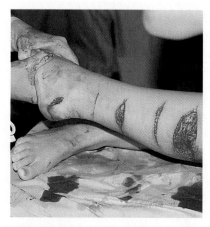

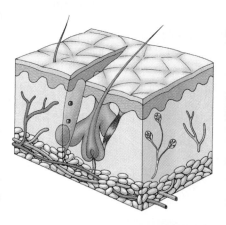

FIGURE 20-5 Lacerations can vary in depth and can extend through the skin and subcutaneous tissue to the underlying muscles, nerves, and blood vessels. These wounds can be smooth or jagged as a result of a cut by a sharp object that tears the tissue.

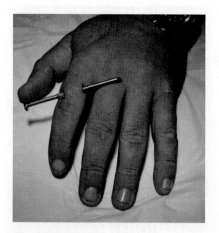

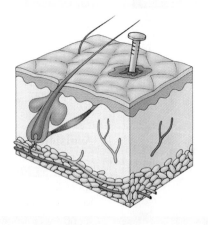

FIGURE 20-6 Penetrating wounds may cause very little external bleeding but can damage structures deep within the body.

flap will be compromised and that piece of skin will die if the circulation is not restored quickly.

Amputations

An **amputation** is an avulsion involving the complete loss of a body part, typically one or more of the extremities. If the amputation was produced by a sharp object, blood loss is often much less than expected because the blood vessels retain the ability to constrict. In contrast, a crushing or tearing amputation can result in **exsanguination** (excessive blood loss due to hemorrhage) if you do not intervene rapidly.

Wound edges in an amputation are commonly jagged, and sharp bone edges may protrude **FIGURE 20-9 ▶**. During wound care, be aware of any sharp bone protrusions that may lead to an exposure. Large, thick dressings should be used to cover the site. In some cases, the body part will be completely detached. In a partial amputation, soft tissues remain attached.

■ Wound Healing

The types of wound healing are primary healing, secondary intention, and delayed primary closure. **Primary healing** refers to wound closure immediately following an injury and prior to the formation of granulation tissue. With primary healing, the wound edges are clean and are directly next to one another. There is little if any tissue loss and minimal scarring occurs. Most surgical wounds heal by primary healing. The wound edges are well-defined and are generally closed with sutures, staples, or adhesives at the time of initial evaluation.

Secondary intention refers to a strategy of allowing a high-risk wound to heal on its own without surgical closure. The wound is treated with only cleaning and minimal debridement and is allowed to granulate and fill in with eventual epithelialization. Granulation tissue must extend from the edges inside the wound toward the center and results in a broader scar. This healing process is slow and can be prolonged by the presence of drainage from infection or other wound debris. Wound care on these wounds must be performed frequently (sometimes several times per day) to encourage wound debris removal and to allow for granulation tissue formation.

Delayed primary closure or DPC (tertiary intention) is a combination of the first and secondary intentions. The wound is initially cleaned, debrided, irrigated, and observed for a period of time (typically 4 or 5 days) before closure. The wound is purposely left open by placing dressing material in the wound to keep the edges apart. It is used for wounds that would have a poor cosmetic appearance if treated by secondary intention.

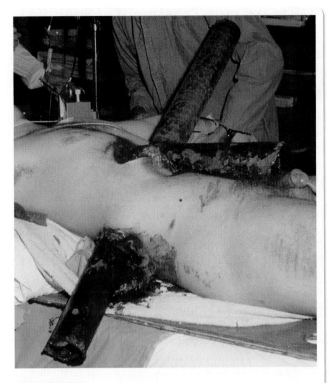

FIGURE 20-7 An impaled object remains embedded in the wound.

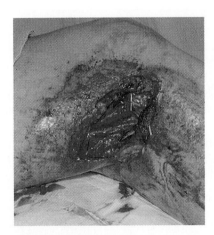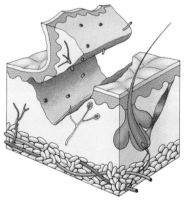

FIGURE 20-8 Avulsions are characterized by complete separation of tissue or tissue hanging as a flap. Significant bleeding is common.

Factors That Complicate the Wound Healing Process

Factors that complicate the wound healing process include:

- **The extent of the injury**
- **The type of injury**
- **The patient's nutritional status:** Malnutrition affects all phases of wound healing. Stress from burns or severe trauma increases the patient's nutritional requirements. The patient's diet should include protein, carbohydrates, lipids, vitamins A and C, and minerals.
- **The age of the patient:** Vascular changes impair circulation to the wound site. Reduced liver function alters the synthesis of clotting factors. The formation of antibodies and lymphocytes is also reduced. Collagen tissue is less pliable in an older patient.
- **Obesity:** Fatty tissue lacks adequate blood supply to aid in decreasing infection and delivering nutrients and cellular elements. Observe the obese patient for signs of wound infection, dehiscence, and evisceration.
- **Impaired oxygenation:** If local circulating blood flow is poor, tissues fail to receive needed oxygen. Decreased hemoglobin (anemia) reduces arterial oxygen levels in capillaries and interferes with tissue repair.
- **Smoking:** Reduces the amount of functional hemoglobin in the blood, thus decreasing tissue oxygenation. Smoking also interferes with normal cellular mechanisms that promote release of oxygen to tissue.
- **Infection:** Infection complicates the healing process.
- **Drugs:** Anti-inflammatory drugs suppress protein synthesis, epithelialization, and the inflammatory response (steroids). Prolonged antibiotic use may increase the risk of superinfection. Chemotherapeutic drugs can depress bone marrow function, the number of leukocytes, and the inflammatory response.
- **Diabetes mellitus:** Causes small blood vessel disease that impairs tissue perfusion. Diabetes also causes hemoglobin to have a greater affinity for oxygen, so it fails to release oxygen to the tissues. It also alters the ability of leukocytes to perform phagocytosis.

■ Assessment Considerations

Obtain the wound injury history from the patient. Find out:

- How did the wound occur?
- What type of object caused the injury?
- How long ago did the wound occur?

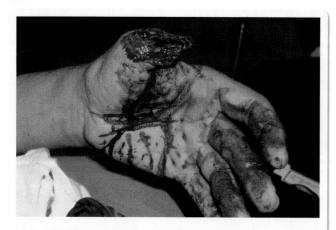

FIGURE 20-9 An amputation involving the thumb.

The neurovascular status of the affected extremity must be assessed prior to wound treatment. You must assess:

- Pulse quality, location, and rate (distal from the wound)
- Capillary refill (distal from the wound)
- Skin color/temperature of area surrounding wound
- Sensation/motor function of the affected extremity, distal to the wound or injury

Next, you need to assess the actual wound. Assessment includes:

- **Color of the wound bed tissue:** Pink tissue usually indicates healthy, granulating, and viable tissue. Black tissue indicates necrotic tissue. White/yellow tissue can indicate infectious process.
- **Wound size:** Length × width × depth. Depth can also be described by stating the tissue that is seen; for example, to subcutaneous tissue, to muscle, to bone. Document the measurements (eg, 1 × 3 × 2) or use a commonly known object for comparison, such as "dime-sized" wound.
- **Wound boundaries:** Are the edges of the wound smooth or irregular?
- **Drainage:** Color (sanguineous, serosanguineous, serous, purulent); amount (small, moderate, copious); and odor (a foul smell can indicate an infection).

Next, assess the patient's tetanus immunization status. Tetanus is an acute, often fatal disease that occurs worldwide. The bacterium that causes tetanus exists as a spore in the soil. The spore gains access through a cut or wound. Germination occurs and the tetanus bacteria begin producing a toxin, which causes muscle contractions. Due to widespread immunization, tetanus is now a rare disease in the United States and developed countries. The tetanus immunization status must be assessed and documented for *any* patient with an open wound.

A primary series of tetanus-diptheria toxoid (Td) is given to all recruits lacking a reliable history of previous immunization. Recruits with a tetanus immunization history receive a booster dose of toxoid on entering active duty. All adults should receive booster doses of toxoid every 10 years. In tetanus-prone wounds (dirty wounds) administer 0.5 mL of Td if more than 5 years has elapsed since the last dose. If the patient's medical records are not available or the patient cannot remember the date of his or her last toxoid booster, administer a booster dose.

Document the tetanus immunization status and tetanus immunization, if administered, for all patients with open wounds. Finally, assess for pain control. Note the sensation function of the affected extremity.

■ Emergency Treatment of Specific Wound Types

Always remember to manage the patient's airway, breathing, and circulation prior to applying wound care treatment.

Contusion

The assessment of a contusion begins with identifying damage to underlying vessels, nerves, and bony structures. Assess the patient's peripheral pulses and sensation. Assess the patient's motor function and strength. Determine whether the patient needs pain control or a tetanus prophylaxis. Treatment of a contusion begins with the elevation of the contused area or extremity. Apply ice packs within the first 24 hours.

Crush Injury

Manage the crush injury as if there is internal bleeding and care for shock if you believe that there is any possibility of internal injuries. Assess for the level of consciousness (LOC). Then determine the neurovascular status of the extremity: pulse quality, location, and rate; capillary refill (considered an unreliable perfusion indicator in adults); and skin color. Assess for pain control and the need for tetanus prophylaxis.

Treatment of a crush injury begins with controlling the bleeding, if an open wound, through either direct pressure or a pressure dressing. Apply a dry, sterile dressing to the wound. Elevate the extremity, if possible. Splint extremities that are painful, swollen, or deformed.

Abrasion

The assessment of an abrasion begins by looking for dirt and other substances in the wound bed tissue. Assess the patient's functional capabilities and the need for tetanus prophylaxis.

Treatment of an abrasion begins with cleaning the wound. Clean the wound surface by manually removing large pieces of foreign matter; do not scrub the wound bed tissue. Irrigate debris from the wound using a 30- to 60-mL syringe filled with normal saline or sterile water. Apply a sterile dressing to the wound after bleeding has been controlled.

Laceration

Assessment of a laceration begins by assessing the depth of the wound. Assess for the presence of and the control of bleeding and for any associated injuries. Determine the neurovascular status of the affected extremity as appropriate: pulse quality, location, and rate; capillary refill; skin color and temperature; sensation; and motor function. Assess for pain control and the need for tetanus prophylaxis.

Treatment of a laceration begins by controlling the bleeding with direct pressure and elevation of an extremity. Cleanse and irrigate the wound thoroughly using a 30- to 60-mL syringe filled with normal saline or sterile water. For minor lacerations, use a butterfly bandage and cover with a gauze dressing. For major lacerations, consider the need for sutures, staples, or surgery. Consult with the supervising medical officer about the appropriate closure technique for the patient.

Avulsion

Assessment of an avulsion begins by assessing the amount of tissue loss and the depth of injury. Assess for pain control and the need for tetanus prophylaxis. Treatment of an avulsion begins by controlling the bleeding. Clean the wound surface. If the skin is still attached, fold the skin back to its normal position after cleaning the wound. Dress the wound using a bulky pressure dressing. If the skin is torn away from the body, dress the wound using a bulky pressure dressing. Save the avulsed part by wrapping it in a dry sterile gauze dressing and placing it in a plastic bag, if available. Keep the avulsed part as cool as possible; however, do not immerse the avulsed part.

Amputations

Assessment of amputations begins by assessing for blood loss and the source of the bleeding. Assess for neurovascular status: pulse quality, location, and rate; capillary refill; skin color and temperature; sensation; and motor function. Assess for pain control and the need for tetanus prophylaxis. Treatment of amputations begins by controlling the bleeding. The amputated part should be rinsed off with saline and wrapped in moist sterile gauze or a towel and placed in a plastic bag or plastic container. The amputated part should then be placed in another container containing ice.

Punctures and Penetrations

Assessment of punctures and penetrations begins by looking for foreign bodies or materials and impaled objects. Assess the depth of penetration for underlying structural damage. Determine the type and degree of contamination. Assess for pain control and the need for tetanus prophylaxis.

Do not remove any impaled object during the treatment phase. The only exception is an impaled object to the cheek causing airway compromise. Removal of the object may cause further injury to nerves, muscles, and soft tissues as well as possible severe hemorrhaging when the object is removed. Expose the wound. Control profuse bleeding by applying pressure on either side of the impaled object and pushing downward. Stabilize the impaled object with a bulky dressing.

■ Wound Care

Dressings

The types of dressings used to care for a wound include:

- **Gauze dressings:** These are highly absorbent and ideal for wounds that are fresh and likely to bleed or have significant drainage. Unless moist, these dressings can remove granulation tissue when allowed to become dry FIGURE 20-10 ▼.
- **Transparent dressings:** The chief advantage of these dressings is that they facilitate wound assessment without removing the dressing. These dressings are less bulky than gauze dressings and do not require tape. These are not absorbent and should not be used on wounds that are bleeding or having significant drainage FIGURE 20-11 ▼.
- **Hydrocolloid dressings:** Self-adhesive, opaque, air- and water-occlusive wound coverings. These dressings cause less pain from air exposure and provide more rapid healing. They require fewer dressing changes and provide better protection from bacteria FIGURE 20-12 ▼.

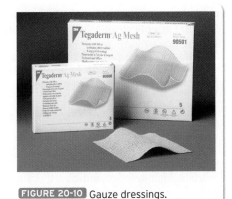

FIGURE 20-10 Gauze dressings.

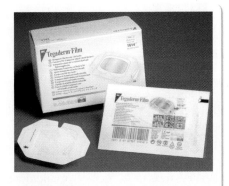

FIGURE 20-11 Transparent dressings.

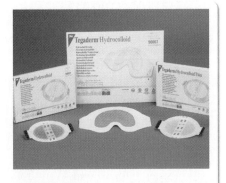

FIGURE 20-12 Hydrocolloid dressings.

Changing a Gauze Dressing

Dressings are changed as per a doctor's order, when the wound requires assessment or care, and/or when the dressings become loose or saturated with drainage. The supplies and equipment needed include:

- Clean gloves
- Individually packaged gauze dressings
- Adhesive tape
- Small basin or container
- Normal saline or sterile water
- 30- to 60-mL syringe for irrigation
- Waterproof pad

To change a gauze dressing, follow the steps in **SKILL DRILL 20-1 ▸** :

1. Wash your hands.
2. Explain the procedure to the patient. Position the patient and expose the area(s) to be redressed.
3. Put on clean nonsterile examination gloves.
4. Place a waterproof pad (chuck) underneath the patient (**Step ①**).
5. Gently loosen the tape toward the wound while supporting the skin around the wound (**Step ②**).
6. Remove the dressing, being careful not to tear the wound or dislodge any drains. Use sterile saline to moisten the dressing if it is sticking to the wound, to prevent discomfort to the patient, and/or to maintain the integrity of the sutures.
7. Assess for the amount, color, odor, and consistency of drainage on the old dressing.
8. Dispose of the old dressing in a trash receptacle.
9. Begin inspecting and cleaning the wound (**Step ③**).
10. To prevent contamination and to clean the bottle rim, pour a small amount of the irrigating liquid into a waste receptacle. If the seal of the bottle has not been broken, this step is not necessary.
11. Pour the irrigating solution (normal saline or sterile water) into the basin.
12. Fill the 30- to 60-mL syringe with solution from the sterile basin (**Step ④**).
13. Hold the tip of the syringe just above the top end of the wound and force fluid into the wound slowly and continuously. Use enough force to flush out debris but do not squirt or splash the fluid.
14. Irrigate all portions of the wound. Do not force solution into wound pockets. Continue irrigating until the solution draining from the bottom end of the wound is clear (**Step ⑤**).
15. Using sterile gauze, gently pat dry the edges and tissues of the wound. Work from the cleanest areas to the most contaminated areas.

16. Begin to dress the wound. Lay the inner dressing over the wound, ensuring that the dressing extends past the edges of the wound. All other dressings will overlap each other and cover the entire wound (**Step ⑥**).
17. Cover all inner dressings with a larger outer dressing. Some wounds (eg, abdominal evisceration) must be kept moist, and will require the use of wet to dry dressings. The inner dressings that touch the wound directly will be dampened with a solution (usually normal saline) before application. The outer dressings are applied dry. During combat conditions, the combat medic does not remove an existing dressing but only reinforces it with additional dressings.
18. Apply tape to ensure that the dressing is secured into place. Tape should not form a constricting band around the wound or extremity (**Step ⑦**).
19. Remove the gloves and place in a trash receptacle.
20. Reposition and cover the patient.
21. Close and dispose of the plastic bag with used supplies in accordance with (IAW) local protocol.
22. Wash your hands.
23. Document wound care and all wound assessments on the appropriate form. Enter the date and time of the procedure and a description of the wound's color, odor, consistency, and amount of drainage. Document all wound assessments to include dimensions and wound appearance (**Step ⑧**).

■ Drainage and Drainage Systems

Exudate is fluid that has penetrated from blood vessels into the surrounding tissues due to inflammation. A **drain** is a device used to remove excess fluid from a wound or body part. Types of drainage (exudate) include:

- **Serous:** Clear, watery drainage that has been separated from its solid elements (eg, the exudate from a blister)
- **Sanguineous:** Drainage that contains blood
- **Serosanguineous:** Drainage that contains serum and blood

Exudate (drainage) greater than 300 mL in the first 24 hours after injury should be treated as abnormal. When the patient first ambulates, a slight increase in drainage may occur. If sanguineous drainage continues, small blood vessels may be oozing. Not all surgical wounds drain.

The following characteristics are important to note and chart in wound documentation:

- Color
- Amount
- Odor

Wound drainage systems include open and closed drains. **Open drains** allow drainage to pass through an open-ended

SKILL DRILL 20-1

Change a Gauze Dressing

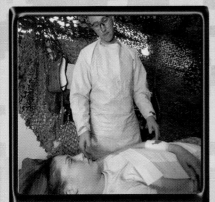

1 Wash your hands. Explain the procedure to the patient. Position the patient and expose the area(s) to be redressed. Put on clean nonsterile examination gloves. Place a waterproof pad (chuck) underneath the patient.

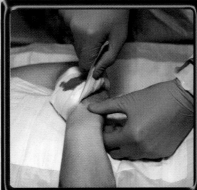

2 Gently loosen the tape toward the wound while supporting the skin around the wound.

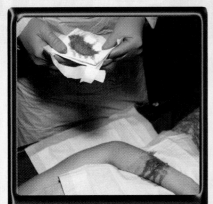

3 Remove the dressing, being careful not to tear the wound or dislodge any drains. Use sterile saline to moisten the dressing if it is sticking to the wound, to prevent discomfort to the patient, and/or to maintain the integrity of the sutures. Assess for the amount, color, odor, and consistency of drainage on the old dressing. Dispose of the old dressing in a trash receptacle. Begin inspecting and cleaning the wound.

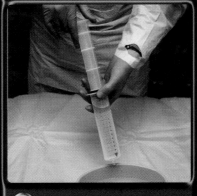

4 To prevent contamination and to clean the bottle rim, pour a small amount of the irrigation liquid into a waste receptacle. If the seal of the bottle has not been broken, this step is not necessary. Pour the irrigating solution (normal saline or sterile water) into the basin. Fill the 30- to 60-mL syringe with solution from the sterile basin.

(continues)

tube into a receptacle or out onto the dressing FIGURE 20-13 ▶. A **Penrose drain** is a soft tube that may be advanced or pulled out in stages as the wound heals from the inside out FIGURE 20-14 ▶. **Closed (suction) drains** are self-contained suction units that connect to drainage tubes within the wound FIGURE 20-15 ▶. Closed drains are more effective than open drains because they pull fluid by creating a vacuum or negative pressure and prevent environmental contaminates from entering the wound or cavity.

Two types of drainage devices that are portable and provide constant low-pressure suction to remove and collect drainage without wall suction are the Jackson-Pratt drain and the Hemovac. **Jackson-Pratt** is used when small amounts, 100 to 200 mL, of drainage is anticipated FIGURE 20-16 ▶. **Hemovac** is a drainage system used for larger amounts, up to 500 mL, of drainage FIGURE 20-17 ▶.

■ Assist With Ongoing Casualty Management

The evaluation of wound healing is performed after:

- Each dressing change
- Application of heat and cold therapies
- Wound irrigation
- Stress to the wound site

Evaluation measures include:

- Assess the condition of the wound and dressing.
- Ask whether the patient notes any discomfort during the dressing change procedure.
- Inspect the condition of dressings at least every shift.

During the evaluation, document the location, size (length ×

SKILL DRILL 20-1

Change a Gauze Dressing (*continued*)

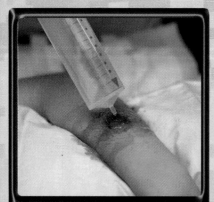

5 Hold the tip of the syringe just above the top end of the wound and force fluid into the wound slowly and continuously. Use enough force to flush out debris but do not squirt or splash the fluid. Irrigate all portions of the wound. Do not force solution into wound pockets. Continue irrigating until the solution draining from the bottom end of the wound is clear.

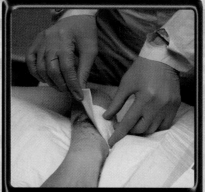

6 Using sterile gauze, gently pat dry the edges and tissues of the wound. Work from the cleanest areas to the most contaminated areas. Begin to dress the wound. Lay the inner dressing over the wound, ensuring that the dressing extends past the edges of the wound. All other dressings will overlap each other and cover the entire wound.

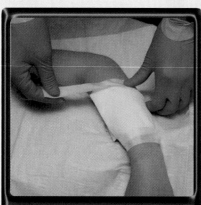

7 Cover all inner dressings with a larger outer dressing. Some wounds must be kept moist, and will require the use of wet to dry dressings. Apply tape to ensure that the dressing is secured into place. Tape should not form a constricting band around the wound or extremity.

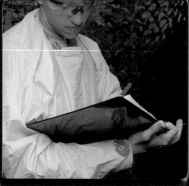

8 Remove the gloves and place in a trash receptacle. Reposition and cover the patient. Close and dispose of the plastic bag with used supplies IAW local protocol. Wash your hands. Document wound care and all wound assessments on the appropriate form. Enter the date and time of the procedure and a description of the wound's color, odor, consistency, and amount of drainage. Document all wound assessments to include dimensions and wound appearance.

width × depth), drainage type and amount, odor, and neurovascular (NV) status. The wound care assessment includes:

- Monitor vital signs.
- Monitor distal peripheral pulses.
- Monitor skin color, sensation, and temperature.
- Monitor motor function.
- Monitor IV fluids.
- Provide pain control.

Wound Complications

The following are terms associated with wound complications:

- **Adhesion:** Band of scar tissue that binds together two anatomical surfaces that are normally separated; most commonly found in the abdomen FIGURE 20-18 ▶.
- **Cellulitis:** Infection of the skin characterized by heat, pain, redness, and edema FIGURE 20-19 ▶.
- **Dehiscence:** Separation of a surgical incision or rupture of a wound closure FIGURE 20-20 ▶.
- **Evisceration:** Protrusion of an internal organ through a wound or surgical incision FIGURE 20-21 ▶.
- **Extravasation:** Passage or escape into the tissues, usually of blood, serum, or lymph FIGURE 20-22 ▶.
- **Hematoma:** Collection of extravasated blood trapped in the tissues or in an organ resulting from incomplete hemostasis.
- **Compartment syndrome:** A progressive ischemic injury to tissue and muscle that results from increased pressure within a closed compartment. Symptoms include pain with pressure over the compartment area and

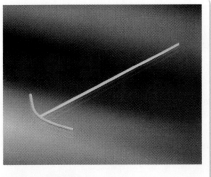

FIGURE 20-13 Open drains.

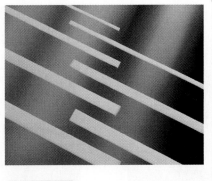

FIGURE 20-14 Penrose drain.

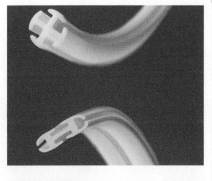

FIGURE 20-15 Closed or suction drains.

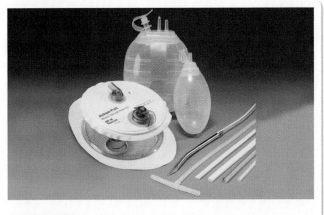

FIGURE 20-16 Jackson-Pratt.

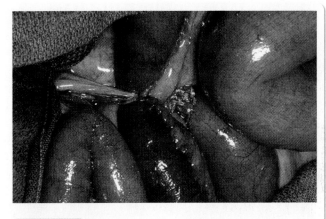

FIGURE 20-18 Adhesion.

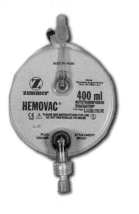

FIGURE 20-17 Hemovac.

decreased urinary output; and cool, clammy skin.

- The patient's abdomen will become rigid and distended.

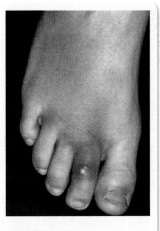

FIGURE 20-19 Cellulitis.

If internal bleeding proceeds undetected, hypovolemic shock can result, causing the circulatory system to collapse, leading to death.

With dehiscence, the patient may say that something has "given way." It may result after periods of sneezing, coughing, or vomiting. Evidence of new or increased serosanguineous drainage on the dressing is an important sign to assess. The patient should remain in bed. Keep the patient NPO (nothing by mouth). Tell the patient not to cough. Reassure the patient. Place a sterile dressing over the area until the physician evaluates the site.

To treat evisceration, the patient is to remain in bed. The wound and contents should be covered with warm, sterile saline dressings. A surgeon must be notified immediately because this is a true medical emergency.

diminished sensation distal to the compartment area. A late symptom is diminished to absent pulses distal to the injury **FIGURE 20-23** ▸.

The wound and dressing aids are inspected in order to detect an increase in drainage or changes in the color of the drainage. If bleeding occurs internally:

- The dressing may remain dry while the abdominal cavity collects blood.
- The patient will have increased thirst; restlessness; a rapid, thready pulse; decreased blood pressure;

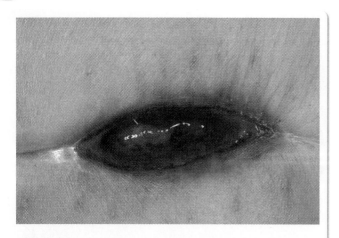

FIGURE 20-20 Dehiscence.

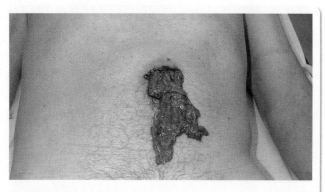

FIGURE 20-21 Evisceration.

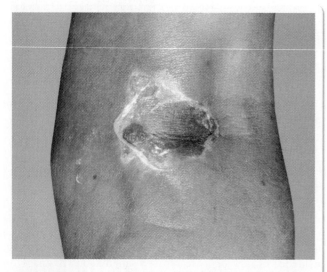

FIGURE 20-22 Extravasation.

Field Medical Care **TIPS**

Wound bleeding may indicate a slipped suture, dislodged clot, coagulation problem, or trauma to blood vessels or tissues.

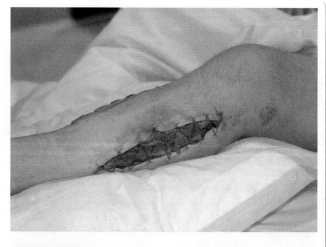

FIGURE 20-23 Compartment syndrome.

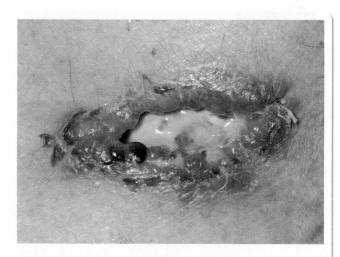

FIGURE 20-24 Purulent drainage has a foul odor and is brown, yellow, or green, depending on the associated pathogen.

Wound Infection

The CDC labels a wound infected when it contains purulent (pus) drainage. A patient with an infected wound will often have a fever, tenderness and pain at the wound site, edema, and an elevated WBC (white blood cell count). Purulent drainage has a foul odor and is brown, yellow, or green, depending on the associated pathogen FIGURE 20-24 ▲.

■ Summary

You will care for all types of wounds throughout your time in the Army. You may scrub a wound in the ER, irrigate a wound on a hospital ward, or change a dressing in a Battalion Aid Station. A combat medic must be knowledgeable about wounds and wound care to prevent infection and facilitate wound healing. These practices will minimize the time that a soldier must be away from his or her unit due to illness or injury. This is one of the best ways "to conserve the fighting strength."

Dusk is settling on the neighborhood that your unit is patrolling. The heat of the day is beginning to dissipate and you can feel the neighborhood begin to unwind. However, you remain on your guard, because it only takes a second for the situation to change completely. As your unit heads up the road, the roar of engines starts up from an alleyway. Two motorcycles tear out of the alleyway, one rider begins shooting with a pistol while the other zig zags behind him. Your unit takes out the attacking rider and focuses on capturing the second rider. The neighbors are beginning to come to their windows. The second rider grabs one soldier's protective vest and begins to drag him down the road. Your unit cuts off the rider and surrounds the motorcycle. The rider is taken into custody and you focus your attention on the casualty.

Assessment

The casualty was dragged about 15′ over a dusty gravel surface. The right side of his trousers looks like it has been dragged up and down a cheese grater. The casualty has a patent airway, normal breathing, and a strong pulse. You expose the wound and find light bleeding up and down the entire side of the right leg. Dirt and debris are embedded up and down the casualty's thigh. You need to evacuate this casualty to a safer area and clean this wound. Your base camp is about three blocks away from your position. With the help of a combat lifesaver (CLS), you evacuate the casualty to your base camp.

Treatment

Once safely at base camp, you begin to clean the casualty's abrasion. With sterile tweezers, you remove the larger pieces of gravel from the wound. You then irrigate the wound to remove the remainder of the debris with a 60-mL syringe of normal saline. Once the wound is clear of debris, you apply direct pressure until the bleeding stops. A sterile dressing is applied and you give the casualty an oral antibiotic to prevent infection.

1. LAST NAME, FIRST NAME Franklin, Curtis | **RANK/GRADE** SGT | **X MALE / FEMALE**
SSN 000-111-0000 | **SPECIALTY CODE** 002 | **RELIGION**
2. UNIT
FORCE A/T AF/A N/M MC/M BC/BC NBI/BNC | **NATIONALITY** | DISEASE | PSYCH
3. INJURY FRONT BACK — AIRWAY / HEAD / **X WOUND** / NECK/BACK INJURY / BURN / AMPUTATION / STRESS / OTHER (Specify)
4. LEVEL OF CONSCIOUSNESS X ALERT / VERBAL RESPONSE / PAIN RESPONSE / UNRESPONSIVE
5. PULSE 65 bpm **TIME** 1835 | **6. TOURNIQUET** X NO / YES **TIME**
7. MORPHINE X NO / YES | DOSE | TIME | **8. IV** No | TIME
9. TREATMENT/OBSERVATIONS/CURRENT MEDICATION/ALLERGIES/NBC (ANTIDOTE) Casualty was dragged 15 ft by motorcycle. Abrasions filled with debris which was cleaned and irrigated moxifloxacin given PO 400 mg
10. DISPOSITION RETURNED TO DUTY / X EVACUATED / DECEASED | **TIME** 2015
11. PROVIDER/UNIT Christensen, Chris | DATE (YYMMDD)

Aid Kit

Ready for Review

- Understanding the wound healing process and proper wound care management for a variety of wounds is essential knowledge basic to any health care setting.
- In a closed wound, soft tissues beneath the skin surface are damaged, but there is no break in the epidermis.
- An open wound is characterized by a disruption in the skin. Open wounds are potentially much more serious than closed wounds for two reasons: Open wounds are vulnerable to infection and they have a greater potential for serious blood loss.
- The types of wound healing are primary healing, secondary intention, and delayed primary closure (tertiary intention).
- Obtain the wound injury history from the patient.
- Always remember to manage the patient's airway, breathing, and circulation prior to applying wound care treatment.
- A drain is a device that is used to remove excess fluid from a wound or body part.
- The evaluation of wound healing is performed after each dressing change, application of heat and cold therapies, wound irrigation, or stress to the wound site.

Vital Vocabulary

abrasion An injury in which a portion of the body is denuded of epidermis by scraping or rubbing.

adhesion A band of scar tissue that binds together two anatomical surfaces normally separated.

adipose Referring to fat tissue.

amputation An injury in which part of the body is completely severed.

avulsion An injury that leaves a piece of skin or other tissue partially or completely torn away from the body.

cellulitis Infection of the skin characterized by heat, pain, redness, and edema.

closed (suction) drains Self-contained suction units that connect to drainage tubes within the wound.

closed wound An injury in which damage occurs beneath the skin or mucous membrane but the surface remains intact.

compartment syndrome A progressive degeneration of tissue and muscle that results from a severe interruption of blood flow.

contaminated Containing microorganisms.

contusion A bruise; an injury that causes bleeding beneath the skin but does not break the skin.

deep fascia A dense layer of fibrous tissue below the subcutaneous tissue; composed of tough bands of tissue that ensheath muscles and other internal structures.

dehiscence Separation of a surgical incision or rupture of a wound closure.

delayed primary closure (tertiary intention) A combination of the primary and secondary intentions. The wound is initially cleaned, debrided, and irrigated, and then is observed for a period of time before closure.

dermis The inner layer of skin, containing hair follicle roots, glands, blood vessels, and nerves.

drain A device that is used to remove excess fluid from a wound or body part.

ecchymosis Extravasation of blood under the skin to produce a "black-and-blue" mark.

epidermis The outermost layer of the skin.

evisceration Protrusion of an internal organ through a wound or surgical incision.

exsanguination Excessive blood loss due to hemorrhage.

extravasation Passage or escape into the tissues, usually of blood, serum, or lymph.

exudate Fluid that has penetrated from blood vessels into the surrounding tissues resulting from inflammation.

hematoma A localized collection of blood in the soft tissues as a result of injury or a broken blood vessel.

Hemovac A drainage system used for larger amounts, up to 500 mL, of drainage.

homeostasis The tendency to constancy or stability in the body's internal environment.

incision A wound usually made deliberately, as in surgery; a clean cut, as opposed to a laceration.

integument The skin.

Jackson-Pratt A drainage device that is used when small amounts (100 to 200 mL) of drainage is anticipated.

laceration A wound made by tearing or cutting tissues.

open drains Drainage that passes through an open-ended tube into a receptacle or out onto the dressing.

open wound An injury in which there is a break in the surface of the skin or the mucous membrane, exposing deeper tissue to potential contamination.

pedicle A narrow strip of tissue by which an avulsed piece of tissue remains connected to the body.

Penrose drain A soft tube that may be advanced or pulled out in stages as the wound heals from the inside out.

primary healing Wound closure immediately following the injury and prior to the formation of granulation tissue.

puncture wound A stab injury from a pointed object, such as a nail or a knife.

sanguineous Drainage that contains blood.

secondary intention A strategy of allowing a wound to heal on its own without surgical closure.

serosanguineous Drainage that contains serum and blood.

serous Clear, watery discharge that has been separated from its solid elements.

subcutaneous Beneath the skin.

tension lines The pattern of tautness of the skin, which is arranged over body structures and affects how well wounds heal.

COMBAT MEDIC in Action

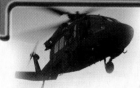

You are the combat medic assisting at the Battalion Aid Station. You are changing the dressing on a patient confined to a hospital bed, who is healing from an open wound to the abdomen. Before receiving his wound, the patient had been on antibiotics for a prolonged period to clear up a stubborn sinus infection. You collect the proper equipment: clean gloves, gauze dressing, adhesive tape, a small basin, normal saline, a 60-mL syringe, and a waterproof pad.

After washing your hands and donning sterile gloves, you place the waterproof pad underneath the patient and then gently loosen the adhesive tape around the wound. You carefully remove the dressing, taking care not to damage the fragile skin underneath the dressing. When you reveal the wound, you find that the tissue is yellow.

1. Which known factors could be complicating the healing process in this patient?
   A. Prolonged antibiotic use
   B. Obesity
   C. Diabetes mellitus
   D. Age

2. Is the patient displaying any signs that you should bring to the attention of the MO?
   A. Yes, the open abdominal wound.
   B. Yes, the yellow tissue around the wound.
   C. No, this patient is healing nicely.
   D. No, you can handle this patient on your own.

3. Assessment of the wound includes the following four categories:
   A. Airway, breathing, circulation, exposure
   B. Pulse, capillary refill, skin color, skin temperature
   C. Color of the wound bed tissue, wound size, wound boundaries, drainage
   D. Drainage, skin color, pulse, skin temperature

4. The types of dressings used to care for a wound include:
   A. gauze dressings.
   B. transparent dressings.
   C. hydrocolloid dressings.
   D. all of the above.

5. Wound complications include:
   A. adhesion.
   B. cellulitis.
   C. compartment syndrome.
   D. all of the above.

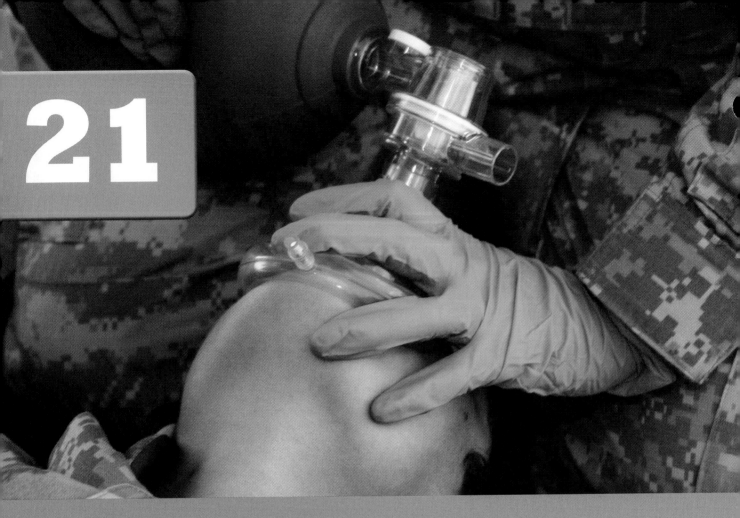

21

Shock

Objectives

Knowledge Objectives
- [ ] Identify the types of shock.
- [ ] Describe how to assess shock.
- [ ] Describe how to assess and treat anaphylactic shock.
- [ ] Describe how to assess and treat cardiogenic shock.
- [ ] Describe how to assess and treat septic shock.
- [ ] Describe how to assess and treat neurogenic shock.

Introduction

Shock is a life-threatening condition that may result from any number of primary causes. As a combat medic, you must be aware of the physiologic effects of shock. Correct management of a patient in shock involves treating the underlying cause of shock and the abnormalities associated with the shock state.

Anatomy and Physiology

Shock is a state of inadequate tissue perfusion resulting in a decreased amount of oxygen to vital tissues and organs. Blood flow is insufficient to provide the nutritional requirements of cells and to remove the waste products of metabolism. Management of patients in shock involves treating both the cause of shock and the abnormalities associated with the shock state. Although shock may have a number of different origins, it is usually caused by one or more major mechanisms: fluid loss, significant vasodilatation, and/or cardiac pump failure.

Perfusion is the circulation of blood within an organ or tissue in adequate amounts to meet the cells' current needs for oxygen, nutrients, and waste removal. Blood enters an organ or tissue first through the arteries, then the arterioles, and finally the capillary beds FIGURE 21-1 ▾ . While passing through the capillaries, the blood delivers nutrients and oxygen to the surrounding cells and picks up the wastes they have generated. Then the blood leaves the capillary beds

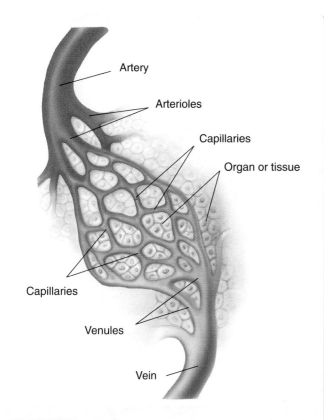

FIGURE 21-1 Perfusion occurs when blood circulates through tissues or an organ to provide the necessary oxygen and nutrients and remove waste products.

through the venules and finally reaches the veins, which take the blood back to the heart. Oxygen and carbon dioxide exchange takes place in the lungs.

Blood must pass through the cardiovascular system at a speed that is fast enough to maintain adequate circulation throughout the body and slow enough to allow each cell time to exchange oxygen and nutrients for carbon dioxide and other waste products. Although some tissues, such as the lungs and kidneys, never rest and require a constant blood supply, most require circulating blood only intermittently, especially when active. Muscles are a good example. When you sleep, they are at rest and require a minimal blood supply; however, during exercise, they need a very large blood supply. The gastrointestinal tract requires a high flow of blood after a meal. After digestion is completed, it can do quite well with a small fraction of that flow.

The autonomic nervous system, the part of the nervous system that regulates involuntary functions such as digestion and sweating, monitors the body's needs from moment to moment and adjusts the blood flow as required. During emergencies, the autonomic nervous system automatically redirects blood away from other organs to the heart, brain, lungs, and kidneys. Thus, the cardiovascular system is dynamic, constantly adapting to changing conditions. At times, the system fails to provide sufficient circulation for every body part to perform its function. This condition is called hypoperfusion, or shock.

Knowing which organs need adequate perfusion is the foundation on which your treatment of patients is based. Emergency medical care is designed to support the following systems:

- The heart (cardiovascular system)
- The brain and spinal cord (central nervous system)
- The lungs (respiratory system)
- The kidneys (renal system)

The heart requires constant perfusion, or it will not function properly. The brain and spinal cord cannot go for more than 4 to 6 minutes without perfusion, or the nerve cells will be permanently damaged. It is important to remember that cells of the central nervous system do not have the capacity to regenerate. The kidneys will be permanently damaged after 45 minutes of inadequate perfusion. Skeletal muscles cannot tolerate more than 2 hours of inadequate perfusion. The gastrointestinal tract can exist with limited (but not absent) perfusion for several hours. These times are based on a normal body temperature (98.6°F [37.0°C]). An organ or tissue that is considerably colder is much better able to resist damage from hypoperfusion because of the slowing of the metabolism. As metabolism decreases, so does the need for oxygen and nutrients. This also decreases the production of waste products that can be damaging if not promptly removed.

Classifications of Shock

The major problem in hypovolemic shock is a loss of intravascular volume, which may occur from blood, plasma, or fluid loss. Severe vomiting and/or diarrhea, and internal or external blood losses are examples of causes that may result in the loss of intravascular volume. Hypovolemic shock is addressed in detail in Chapter 4, *Controlling Bleeding and Hypovolemic Shock*.

Anaphylactic shock is a severe response to a foreign substance (antigen) entering the body. Antigens may enter through the skin, by injections, by inhalation, or by ingestion. In anaphylaxis, a reaction between the antigen and antibody triggers a series of events in the body, which leads to hypoperfusion. Responses may be mild to severe, sometimes causing swelling of the airway, severe vasodilation, and bronchial constriction. If left untreated, anaphylactic shock will lead to death.

Cardiogenic shock is caused by a failure of the heart pumping mechanism. In cardiogenic shock, there is adequate blood volume and no vessel dilation, but the heart is not pumping properly.

Septic shock is caused by an infection (usually bacterial) that leads to vasodilation. The blood vessels dilate due to toxins released into the bloodstream. The blood available for circulation is decreased because it is pooled in dilated veins. In addition, plasma seeps through the blood vessel walls, creating additional fluid losses.

Neurogenic shock is seen in spinal injuries. With neurogenic shock, the spinal nervous system is no longer able to control the diameter of the blood vessels. Without this control, the blood vessels dilate, increasing the volume of the cardiovascular system. Venous return to the heart decreases, and shock results.

■ Stages of Shock

Shock occurs in three successive stages. Your goal as a combat medic is to recognize the signs of the early stages of shock and begin immediate treatment before permanent damage occurs. To accomplish this, you must be aware of the subtle signs exhibited in shock and treat the patient aggressively. Anticipate the potential for shock from the situational assessment. Recognize the signs of poor perfusion that precede hypotension, and do not rely on any one sign or symptom to determine the degree of shock. Always err on the side of caution when treating a potential shock patient.

Compensated (Nonprogressive) Shock

Although you cannot see shock, you can see its signs and symptoms. The earliest stage of shock, while the body can still compensate for blood loss, is called **compensated shock** or **nonprogressive shock**.

The autonomic nervous system releases chemical mediators as it recognizes a potential catastrophic event, which causes the arterial blood pressure to remain normal or slightly elevated. There is also an increase in the rate and depth of respirations to bring in more oxygen and remove more carbon dioxide. This helps to maintain the acid–base balance by creating respiratory alkalosis to offset the metabolic acidosis. At this stage, the blood pressure is maintained; however, there is a narrowing of the **pulse pressure**, which is the difference between the systolic and diastolic pressures. The pulse pressure reflects the tone of the arterial system and is more sensitive to changes in perfusion than the systolic or diastolic blood pressure alone. Treatment at this stage will typically result in recovery.

Decompensated (Progressive) Shock

The next stage, when blood pressure is falling, is called **decompensated shock**, also called uncompensated shock or progressive shock. It occurs when blood volume drops more than 15% to 25%. The compensatory mechanisms are beginning to fail, and signs and symptoms are much more obvious. Cardiac output falls dramatically, leading to further reductions in blood pressure and cardiac function. The signs and symptoms become more obvious as blood is shunted to the brain, heart, and kidneys. At this point, vasoconstriction can have a disastrous effect if allowed to continue. Cells in the nonperfused tissues become hypoxic, leading to anaerobic metabolism. Treatment at this stage will sometimes result in recovery.

Irreversible Shock

The last stage, when shock has progressed to a terminal stage, is called **irreversible shock**. Arterial blood pressure is abnormally low. There is a rapid deterioration of the cardiovascular system that cannot be reversed by compensatory mechanisms or medical interventions. There are life-threatening reductions in cardiac output, blood pressure, and tissue perfusion. Blood is shunted away from the liver, kidneys, and lungs to keep the heart and brain perfused. Cells begin to die, and, even if the cause of shock is treated and reversed, vital organ damage cannot be repaired, and the patient will eventually die. Even aggressive treatment at this stage does not usually result in recovery.

■ Anaphylactic Shock

Anaphylaxis occurs when a person reacts violently to a substance to which he or she has been sensitized. **Sensitization** means becoming sensitive (allergic) to a substance. An allergic reaction typically does not occur, or occurs in a milder form, during sensitization. Do not be misled by a patient who reports no history of allergic reaction to a substance following a first or second exposure. Each subsequent exposure after sensitization tends to produce a more severe reaction.

In anaphylactic shock, there is no loss of blood, no vascular damage, and only a slight possibility of direct cardiac muscular injury. Instead, there is widespread vascular dilation, resulting in relative hypovolemia. In other words, relative to the now-larger container, the normal blood volume is less. Additionally, immune system chemicals result in severe bronchoconstriction (difficulty in breathing).

Anaphylaxis is the most severe of allergic reactions. It is important to remember that even mild allergic reactions may progress to severe anaphylaxis. The most common causes of serious anaphylaxis are antibiotics (such as penicillin and its derivatives) and IV contrast dyes. Penicillin is estimated to cause 100 to 500 deaths annually in the United States. The next most common cause of anaphylaxis is bee, wasp, and yellow jacket stings. Other causes include:

- **Medications:** Aspirin, nonsteroidal anti-inflammatory drugs, sulfa drugs
- **Foods:** Shellfish, nuts, milk, wheat, eggs, MSG (monosodium glutamate)
- **Plants:** Poison oak, poison ivy, and sumac
- **Latex:** Gloves

Cardiogenic Shock

Cardiogenic shock develops when the heart muscle can no longer generate enough pressure to circulate blood to all organs or when the regularity of the heartbeat is so disrupted that the volume of blood within the system can no longer be circulated efficiently. Filling is impaired because of a lack of pressure to return blood to the heart, or outflow is obstructed by lack of pumping function. In either case, direct pump failure is the cause of shock. The same process occurs as a result of a cardiac tamponade or tension pneumothorax in which the heart is physically obstructed and cannot pump effectively. The causes of cardiogenic shock include:

- Aneurysm of the left ventricle wall
- Cardiac tamponade or cardiac contusions resulting from blunt trauma
- Cardiac dysrhythmias (abnormal heartbeat)

Septic Shock

Septic shock is a complex problem. First, there is an insufficient volume of fluid in the container, because much of the blood has leaked out of the vascular system (hypovolemia). Second, the fluid that has leaked out often collects in the respiratory system, interfering with ventilation. Third, there is a larger-than-normal vascular bed to contain the smaller-than-normal volume of intravascular fluid. The blood vessels dilate due to toxins released into the bloodstream. The blood available for circulation is decreased because it is pooled in dilated veins. In addition, plasma seeps through the blood vessel walls, creating additional fluid losses.

Sepsis is the body's systemic response to an infection. Septic shock is sepsis with hypotension plus decreased urine output and altered mental status. Sepsis is the 13th leading cause of death in the United States, with two thirds of the deaths occurring in hospitalized patients.

The most frequent sites of infection are the lungs, abdomen, and urinary tract. Bacterial infections are the cause of the majority of septic infections in patients. Factors that predispose patients to sepsis are trauma, diabetes, burns, indwelling catheters, cancer chemotherapy, and cirrhosis. Sepsis starts as a local infection (eg, urinary tract infection, pneumonia), and then the infection releases toxins and moves through the blood system.

Neurogenic Shock

Damage to the spinal cord, particularly at the upper cervical levels, may cause significant injury to the autonomic nervous system, which controls the size and muscular tone of the blood vessels. Neurogenic shock, or spinal vascular shock, is usually the result. In neurogenic shock, the muscles in the walls of the blood vessels are cut off from the nerve impulses that cause them to contract. Therefore, all vessels below the level of the spinal injury dilate widely, increasing the size and capacity of the vascular system FIGURE 21-2 ▾ and causing blood to pool. The available 5 to 6 L of blood in the body can no longer fill the enlarged vascular system. Even though no blood or fluid has been lost, perfusion of organs and tissues becomes inadequate, and shock occurs; therefore, the patient experiences relative hypovolemia. The skin is pink, warm, and dry. There is no release of the chemical mediators, epinephrine and norepinephrine, to produce the classic pale, cool, diaphoretic skin. A characteristic sign of this type of shock is the absence of sweating below the level of injury.

With an injury that results in spinal shock, many other functions that are under the control of the sympathetic nervous system are also lost. The most important of them, in an acute injury setting, is the ability to control body temperature. Body temperature in a patient with neurogenic shock can rapidly fall to match that of the environment. In many situations, significant hypothermia occurs, severely complicating the situation. **Hypothermia** is a condition in which the internal body temperature falls below 95°F (35°C), usually after prolonged

> **Garrison Care TIPS**
>
> Sepsis is more common in older adults because they are more likely to have conditions that predispose them to bacterial infections, such as diabetes, surgical procedures, and cancer.

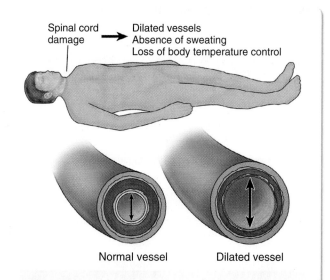

Spinal cord damage → Dilated vessels
Absence of sweating
Loss of body temperature control

Normal vessel   Dilated vessel

FIGURE 21-2 If muscles in the blood vessels are cut off from their impulses to contract, the vessels dilate widely, increasing the size and capacity of the vascular system.

exposure to cool or freezing temperatures. Maintenance of body temperature is always an important element of treatment for a patient in shock.

Acute spinal cord injury is usually due to blunt trauma. Motor vehicle accidents, falls, and sports injuries are the most common causes of spinal cord injury from blunt trauma. The cervical spine region is the most commonly injured area, followed by the lumbar and thoracic segments. The higher the spinal cord injury, the more likely or more severe the resulting neurogenic shock will be. Approximately 10,000 people annually in the United States sustain a significant spinal cord injury.

■ Assess the Patient in Shock

In the garrison, the combat medic has more time and less dangers than those posed on the active battlefield. For these reasons, in the garrison, you should follow the traditional patient assessment that you learned during EMT-Basic training. Here is a short review of the patient assessment process FIGURE 21-3 ▼ .

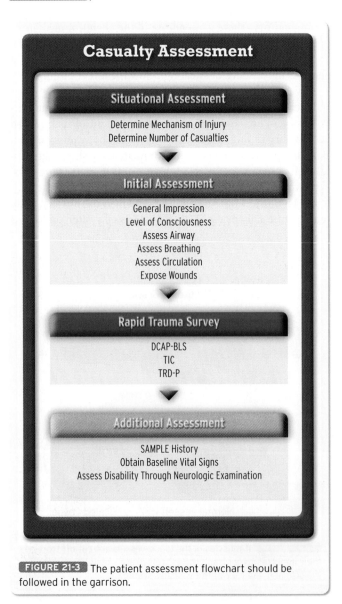

FIGURE 21-3 The patient assessment flowchart should be followed in the garrison.

Focused History

Getting the history of the patient in shock is vital to the establishment of the correct diagnosis. Remember that the goals of the focused history and physical exam are:

- Identify the patient's chief complaint. What happened to this patient?
- Understand the specific circumstances surrounding the chief complaint. What circumstances were associated with the event?
- Direct further physical examination. What problems can be identified through the physical exam?

Often the presence or the history of shock will be instantly apparent along with the underlying cause, such as a history of a bee sting or serious infection. Some patients in shock may have few symptoms other than weakness or altered mental status. Examples of typical questions to ask the patient are:

- Is there a history of trauma (which would make you suspect internal or external hemorrhage)?
- Is there a history of cardiac problems, such as prior heart attack?
- Is there a history of infection? Are you on antibiotics, and if so, for what?
- Have you had any trauma to your spinal cord?
- Have you been in contact with known allergic substances, such as wasps, bees, new foods or medications, or latex?
- Are you taking any new medications, either prescribed, over-the-counter, or recreational?

Garrison Care **TIPS**

Identify patients at increased risk for shock: trauma patients, pregnant women, and the elderly.

Physical Exam

No single vital sign will tell you that a patient is in shock. Do not rely on any one sign or symptom to judge the degree of shock. You must have a high index of suspicion with every patient. Determine level of consciousness (LOC). Report and record, using the AVPU scale: Alert, awake, and oriented; responds to Verbal stimuli; responds to Painful stimuli; Unresponsive to any stimuli.

The signs of early shock include minimum tachycardia, which is caused by epinephrine's effect on the heart. No measurable changes occur in blood pressure, pulse pressure, or respiratory rate. The progression of shock is indicated by a decrease in systolic blood pressure and an increase in diastolic blood pressure. Other signs include:

- Increased tachycardia
- Increased respiratory rate (tachypnea), caused by epinephrine's effect on the respiratory system and hypoxia

- Pale, cool, clammy skin caused by vasoconstriction and loss of circulating blood
- Sweating caused by epinephrine's effect on the sweat glands
- Cyanosis in the nail beds or lips
- <u>Oliguria</u> (decreased urine output) caused by hypovolemia, hypoxia, and circulating epinephrine
- Listlessness, stupor, and loss of consciousness as the condition worsens, caused by cerebral hypoperfusion and epinephrine stimulation

Assessment and Treatment of Anaphylactic Shock

Clinical Features

Anaphylaxis can include any of the following signs along with low blood pressure and airway compromise:

- **Upper airway:** Hoarseness, stridor, edema, rhinorrhea
- **Lower airway:** Bronchial constriction and spasm, wheezing, diminished breath sounds
- **Cardiovascular system:** Tachycardia, hypotension, cardiac arrhythmias, chest pain, chest tightness
- **Gastrointestinal system:** Nausea, vomiting, abdominal cramping, diarrhea
- **Neurologic system:** Apprehension, dizziness, weakness, progressing to coma
- **Skin:** Swelling (edema) of the face, neck, and extremities; itching; hives (urticaria); skin flushing; swelling; and tearing of the eyes and lids

Diagnosis

In most patients, the signs and symptoms of anaphylactic shock begin 15 to 60 minutes after exposure. Anaphylaxis may not occur after the first dose of a medication. In general, the faster the onset of symptoms, the more severe the reaction. Patients treated for anaphylaxis are at risk for a recurrence of symptoms within 12 hours. Many cases of anaphylaxis can be diagnosed easily by a history of exposure (eg, bee sting) combined with the symptoms listed above. However, some cases of anaphylaxis are more difficult to diagnose, for example, food allergies.

Treatment

Securing the patient's airway is the first priority. Give supplemental oxygen by nonrebreathing mask, at a rate of 15 L/min. If the patient is not breathing, perform positive-pressure ventilations until a Combitube or an endotracheal tube can be inserted. Exposure to the causative agent, if identified and ongoing, must be terminated (eg, remove the stinger). Position the conscious patient in a comfortable position (usually seated); position the unconscious patient in a supine or Trendelenburg position.

See Chapter 12, *Battlefield Medications*, for an in-depth discussion on administering medication. Give epinephrine at 0.3 to 0.5 mg (0.3 to 0.5 mL of 1:1,000 solution) subcutaneously (SC) for an adult. Epinephrine may be repeated every 5 to 10 minutes if symptoms continue or recur. Repeat doses may be required. Additional doses should be given according to initial patient response. Monitor the stabilization of blood pressure, pulse, mental status, skin perfusion, and respira-

tions. Briskly massage the site of the SC injection to hasten the medication response.

Antihistamines also may be administered. Administer diphenhydramine (Benadryl) 25 to 50 mg intramuscularly (IM) or by intravenous (IV) bolus. Corticosteroids will be administered to a patient by a medical officer, if needed. A typical dose is 125 mg IV of methylprednisolone (Solu-Medrol). It is given by inserting a large-bore IV and infusing a normal saline 500 cc bolus over 30 minutes. Fluids are continued according to the initial patient response (stabilization of blood pressure, pulse, mental status, skin perfusion, and respirations).

Perform cardiac monitoring, if available. Take the patient's pulse oximetry, if available. Evacuate the patient as soon as possible to a medical treatment facility. Recurrent episodes of anaphylaxis may occur 12 to 24 hours after the initial episode. Patients with severe anaphylaxis should be hospitalized for observation and possible retreatment. Patients with mild symptoms (like urticaria or hives) that resolve with treatment may be discharged at the higher level medical treatment facility.

Patients with minor allergic reactions who do not have hypotension or respiratory symptoms do not need epinephrine. These patients should be given diphenhydramine 25 to 50 mg by mouth (PO), IM, or IV and observed for a response for at least 1 hour. A medical officer must see all patients with an allergic reaction.

Prevention of Anaphylaxis

Inquire carefully about any history of drug allergies before giving any medication. In patients who are drunk, unconscious, or have an altered mental status, search for a card, bracelet, or necklace specifying drug allergies or particular problems (diabetes) that may require special attention. Be cautious when administering immunizations and IV/IM medications. Observe patients for at least 20–30 minutes after injections. Patients with a history of anaphylaxis or severe allergic reactions should carry an Ana-Kit, a self-administration epinephrine kit. Soldiers should carry these kits when out in the field and in garrison.

Assessment and Treatment of Cardiogenic Shock

Clinical Features

The signs and symptoms of cardiogenic shock may include:

- Chest pain
- Shortness of breath
- Weakness
- Cool, clammy skin
- Hypotension
- Tachycardia/tachypnea
- Anxiety and confusion
- Sweating
- Rales (crackles)
- Peripheral edema (swelling of legs)

Diagnosis

Cardiogenic shock can be suspected from the focused history and physical exam; however, additional testing inside a higher level medical treatment facility is needed for confirmation.

Treatment

Securing the patient's airway is the first priority. Give the patient supplemental oxygen by nonrebreathing mask, at a rate of 15 L/min. If the patient is not breathing, perform positive-pressure ventilations until a Combitube or an endotracheal tube can be inserted. Position the patient in a supine or Trendelenburg position. Start a large-bore IV catheter and begin infusing normal saline at a to keep vein open (TKO) rate. Use a cardiac monitor, if available. Take the patient's pulse oximetry, if available. Evacuate the patient as soon as possible to a higher level medical treatment facility. Aspirin may be given en route to the hospital or in hospital, according to standard operating procedures.

Assessment and Treatment of Septic Shock

Clinical Features

The clinical features of shock and infection include:

- Fever (or hypothermia)
- Rigors (shaking chills)
- Petechiae (small, purple hemorrhagic spots on the skin)
- Hypotension
- Tachycardia
- Tachypnea
- Mental status changes—may range from confusion or agitation to lethargy and coma
- Localized signs such as abdominal tenderness, rectal tenderness, or extensive pneumonia

Diagnosis

Septic shock may be suspected from the focused history and physical exam; however, additional testing inside a higher level medical treatment facility is needed for confirmation.

Treatment

Securing the patient's airway is the first priority. Give supplemental oxygen by nonrebreathing mask, at a rate of 15 L/min. If the patient is not breathing, perform positive-pressure ventilations until a Combitube or an endotracheal tube can be inserted. Position the patient in a supine or Trendelenburg position. Start a large-bore IV and begin infusing a normal saline bolus at a rate of 1 to 2 L given over 30 to 60 minutes. After providing initial fluids, decrease the IV rate according to initial patient response (stabilization of blood pressure, pulse, mental status, skin perfusion, and respirations). Assess the patient via a cardiac monitor, if available. Assess the patient via pulse oximetry, if available.

Empiric antibiotics may be given to patients who have a prolonged evacuation time. Use of empiric antibiotics must be cleared by medical direction. Empiric antibiotics is the usage of an antibiotic prior to the establishment of the type of bacteria causing the illness. Evacuate the patient as soon as possible to a higher level medical treatment facility.

Assessment and Treatment of Neurogenic Shock

Clinical Features

The clinical features of neurogenic shock include:

- History of spinal trauma
- Hypotensive
- Usually bradycardic—different than other types of shock
- Warm, dry skin—different than other types of shock

Diagnosis

Neurogenic shock may be suspected from the focused history and physical exam; however, additional testing inside a higher level medical treatment facility is needed for confirmation.

Treatment

Securing the patient's airway and protecting the patient's c-spine are your first priorities. Give the patient supplemental oxygen by a nonrebreathing mask, at a rate of 15 L/min. If the patient is not breathing, perform positive-pressure ventilations until a Combitube or an endotracheal tube can be inserted. Position the patient in a level position.

Start a large-bore IV and begin infusing a normal saline bolus at a rate of 1 to 2 L given over 30 to 60 minutes. After administering initial fluids, decrease the IV rate according to initial patient response (stabilization of blood pressure, pulse, mental status, skin perfusion, and respirations). Place the patient on a spine board. Assess the patient via a cardiac monitor, if available. Assess the patient via pulse oximetry, if available. Corticosteroids will be given by a medical officer, if needed. Evacuate the patient as soon as possible to a higher level medical treatment facility. Any patient with neurogenic shock has suffered a severe traumatic injury and needs to be admitted to the hospital.

■ Summary

Shock is a very serious condition that requires early detection and prompt medical intervention. As a combat medic, you must monitor those casualties susceptible to shock and be prepared to assist with the appropriate medical management. Early identification and treatment of shock is imperative in preventing serious injury and death. Management of patients in shock involves treating both the cause of shock and the abnormalities associated with the shock state.

YOU ARE THE
COMBAT MEDIC

Your unit is on foot patrol in a quiet rural village. It is midmorning and the heat is beginning to rise. While passing by a house, you see a mud-colored bump on the wall. When you get closer, you realize what it is—a wasp nest. You give the stinging critters' home a wide berth and breathe a sigh of relief when you've safely passed by. A minute later, you hear the sound of a hand slapping against skin and a low mutter. As you head down a side road, a soldier calls out in a hoarse voice, "Medic!"

Assessment

You approach the soldier and find him red-faced and out of breath. He is sweating and there is an angry welt on his left cheek. "Damn wasp," he mumbles. He then complains that his throat is closing up.

Treatment

Your first priority is securing this soldier's airway. You ease the soldier into a sitting position, leaning against a wall. Then you apply a nonrebreathing mask and begin to give supplemental oxygen at 15 L/min. You now need to administer epinephrine. Via subcutaneous injection, you give the soldier 0.3 mg of epinephrine. You briskly massage the injection site to hasten the medication response.

You monitor his vital signs to see if the medication is effective in treating his anaphylactic reaction. His pulse is 130 beats/min, but that is to be expected after the administration of epinephrine. His breathing is 50 breaths/min and he seems to be taking less effort to breathe now. His blood pressure is 88/40 mm Hg. It's time to get this soldier to a medical treatment facility for further evaluation and care.

1. LAST NAME, FIRST NAME		RANK/GRADE	X	MALE
Mitchell, Mike		PFC		FEMALE
SSN 000-11-0000	SPECIALTY CODE 002			RELIGION

2. UNIT

FORCE				NATIONALITY		
A/T	AF/A	N/M	MC/M			
	BC/BC		NBI/BNC		DISEASE	PSYCH

3. INJURY		X	AIRWAY
			HEAD
FRONT BACK			WOUND
			NECK/BACK INJURY
			BURN
			AMPUTATION
			STRESS
		X	OTHER (Specify)

Wasp bite

4. LEVEL OF CONSCIOUSNESS			
X	ALERT		PAIN RESPONSE
	VERBAL RESPONSE		UNRESPONSIVE

5. PULSE 130 bpm	TIME 1005	6. TOURNIQUET X NO ☐ YES	TIME
7. MORPHINE X NO ☐ YES	DOSE	TIME	8. IV No	TIME

9. TREATMENT/OBSERVATIONS/CURRENT MEDICATION/ALLERGIES/NBC (ANTIDOTE)

Stung by a wasp on the left cheek. Anaphylactic reaction occurred about 20 minutes after sting. Admin 0.3 mg epinephrine. Breathing 50 breaths/min. Admin O_2.

10. DISPOSITION	RETURNED TO DUTY		TIME
	X	EVACUATED	1030
		DECEASED	

11. PROVIDER/UNIT Gold, Todd	DATE (YYMMDD)

Aid Kit

Ready for Review

- Correct management of a patient in shock involves treating the underlying cause of shock and the abnormalities associated with the shock state.
- Shock is a state of inadequate tissue perfusion resulting in a decreased amount of oxygen to vital tissues and organs.
- In the garrison, the combat medic has more time and fewer dangers than what is posed on the active battlefield. For these reasons, in the garrison, you should follow the traditional patient assessment that you learned during EMT-Basic training.

Vital Vocabulary

anaphylactic shock An unusual or exaggerated allergic reaction to foreign protein or other substances.

autonomic nervous system The part of the nervous system that regulates involuntary functions, such as digestion and sweating.

cardiogenic shock Shock caused by inadequate function of the heart, or pump failure.

compensated shock The early stage of shock, in which the body can still compensate for blood loss.

decompensated shock The late stage of shock, when blood pressure is falling.

empiric antibiotics The usage of an antibiotic prior to the establishment of the type of bacteria causing the illness.

hypothermia A condition in which the internal body temperature falls below 95°F (35°C), usually as a result of prolonged exposure to cool or freezing temperatures.

hypovolemic shock A condition in which low blood volume, due to massive internal or external bleeding or extensive loss of body fluids, results in inadequate perfusion.

irreversible shock The final stage of shock, resulting in death.

neurogenic shock Circulatory failure caused by paralysis of the nerves that control the size of the blood vessels, leading to widespread dilation; seen in spinal cord injuries.

nonprogessive shock A synonym for compensated shock.

oliguria Decreased urine output.

perfusion The delivery of oxygen and nutrients to the cells, organs, and tissues of the body. Also involves the removal of wastes.

pulse pressure The difference between the systolic and diastolic pressures.

sensitization Developing sensitivity to a substance that initially caused no allergic reaction.

septic shock Shock caused by severe bacterial infection.

shock A condition in which the circulatory system fails to provide sufficient circulation to enable every body part to perform its function; also called hypoperfusion.

COMBAT MEDIC *in Action*

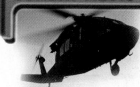

You are the combat medic on duty during sick call. A soldier is brought into the Battalion Aid Station, assisted by two members from his unit. The soldier is weak and has a fever. Upon removing his boots, you find a puncture wound on the bottom of his right foot that appears red and swollen. A small amount of pus is oozing from the middle of the wound. You immediately contact the medical officer.

1. Which type of shock is this soldier at risk of?
   A. Neurogenic
   B. Septic
   C. Cardiogenic
   D. Anaphylactic

2. What is the first priority in treating this soldier, regardless of the type of shock?
   A. Secure the airway
   B. Administer IV fluids
   C. Administer oxygen
   D. Administer antibiotics

3. Clinical features of septic shock include:
   A. fever.
   B. hypotension.
   C. mental status changes.
   D. all of the above.

4. Clinical features of neurogenic shock include:
   A. hypotension.
   B. cold skin.
   C. tachycardia.
   D. hives.

5. Treatment of septic shock includes administration of:
   A. morphine.
   B. epinephrine.
   C. empiric antibiotics.
   D. CO_2.

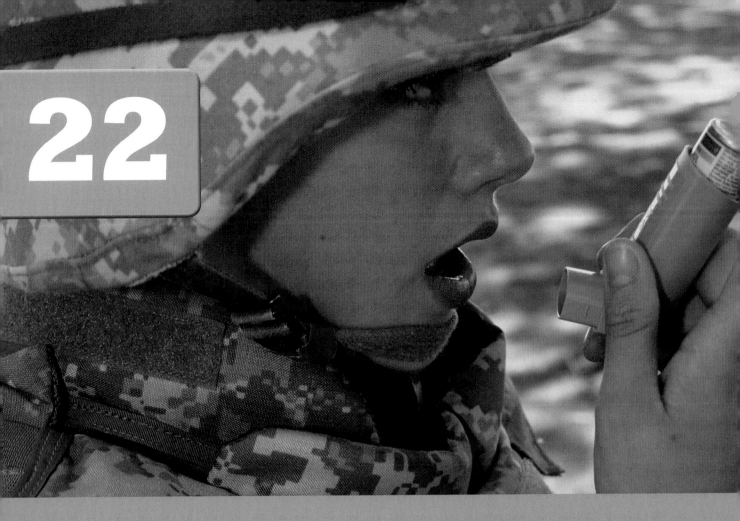

22

Medication Administration

Objectives

Knowledge Objectives

- Discuss the combat medic's role in administering medications.
- Discuss the considerations to take before administering medications.
- List the five rights of medication administration.
- Identify the appropriate medications for use by the combat medic.
- Perform basic computations with whole numbers.
- Work with fractions and decimals.
- Identify the parts of a needle and syringe.
- Inspect equipment for contamination or deterioration.
- Draw up medications.

Skills Objectives

- Assemble a needle and a syringe.
- Reconstitute powdered medication.
- Administer an intradermal injection.

Introduction

As a combat medic, you will perform tasks that involve a basic knowledge of mathematics; for example, determining the correct dosage of a prescribed medication. In Chapter 12, *Battlefield Medications*, mathematics for combat medics was covered in-depth. In this chapter, we will be reviewing important mathematical skills. One task that you will perform in the garrison is to determine the flow rate for an intravenous infusion. You must be able to obtain the required information and perform the calculations to keep the IV infusion at the correct rate in order to maintain a safe fluid balance for your patient.

In the garrison, you will be required to administer injections. Thorough knowledge of this skill is necessary for administering various medications and immunizations as well as sensitivity tests. As a combat medic, you will be dealing with a number of medications to treat various conditions. In order to provide the patient with useful information and to protect the patient, you must understand how drugs affect the body.

Scope of Practice

The combat medic works under the supervision of a licensed health care provider—a doctor, nurse, or physician's assistant. You will dispense certain prescription and nonprescription medications on the order of a supervising health care provider (HCP). You will, at times, dispense medications from an approved formulary in accordance with local protocols and in a manner consistent with the level of medical training of a combat medic.

Roles and Responsibilities

As a combat medic, you are responsible for knowing which medications you are authorized to dispense. You must be thoroughly familiar with the indications, contraindications, and proper dosages of the medications you are authorized to dispense. This responsibility remains even when you administer a medication on the direction of your HCP. You are accountable for errors in dispensing medications even if given on the order of an HCP.

Considerations Before Administering Medications

Right Patient

Many medication errors can be prevented simply by confirming the identity of the patient before you dispense a medication. In particular, patients with common last names may be misidentified if you fail to confirm their first name and perhaps even their Social Security number and/or birth date. For patients in a hospital setting (inpatients), verify the right patient before administering medication by checking the patient name on the medical record; checking the patient name on the HCP's orders, like those found on an SF 600 Chronological Record of Medical Care or Medication Administration Record; or asking the patient to state his or her name **FIGURE 22-1**.

For patients in an outpatient setting (Troop Medical Clinic, Battalion Aid Station, etc.) verify the right patient before administering medication by asking the patient to state his or her name, or by viewing his or her ID card. Patient identification should be checked each and every time you

PREVIOUS EDITION IS USABLE
AUTHORIZED FOR LOCAL REPRODUCTION
MEDICAL RECORD | CHRONOLOGICAL RECORD OF MEDICAL CARE
DATE | SYMPTOMS, DIAGNOSIS, TREATMENT, TREATING ORGANIZATION *(Sign each entry)*
HOSPITAL OR MEDICAL FACILITY | STATUS | DEPART./SERVICE | RECORDS MAINTAINED AT
SPONSOR'S NAME | SSN/ID NO. | RELATIONSHIP TO SPONSOR
PATIENT'S IDENTIFICATION: *(For typed or written entries, give: Name - last, first, middle; ID No or SSN; Sex; Date of Birth; Rank/Grade.)* | REGISTER NO. | WARD NO.
CHRONOLOGICAL RECORD OF MEDICAL CARE
Medical Record
STANDARD FORM 600 (REV. 6-97)
Prescribed by GSA/ICMR
FIRMR (41 CFR) 201-9.202-1

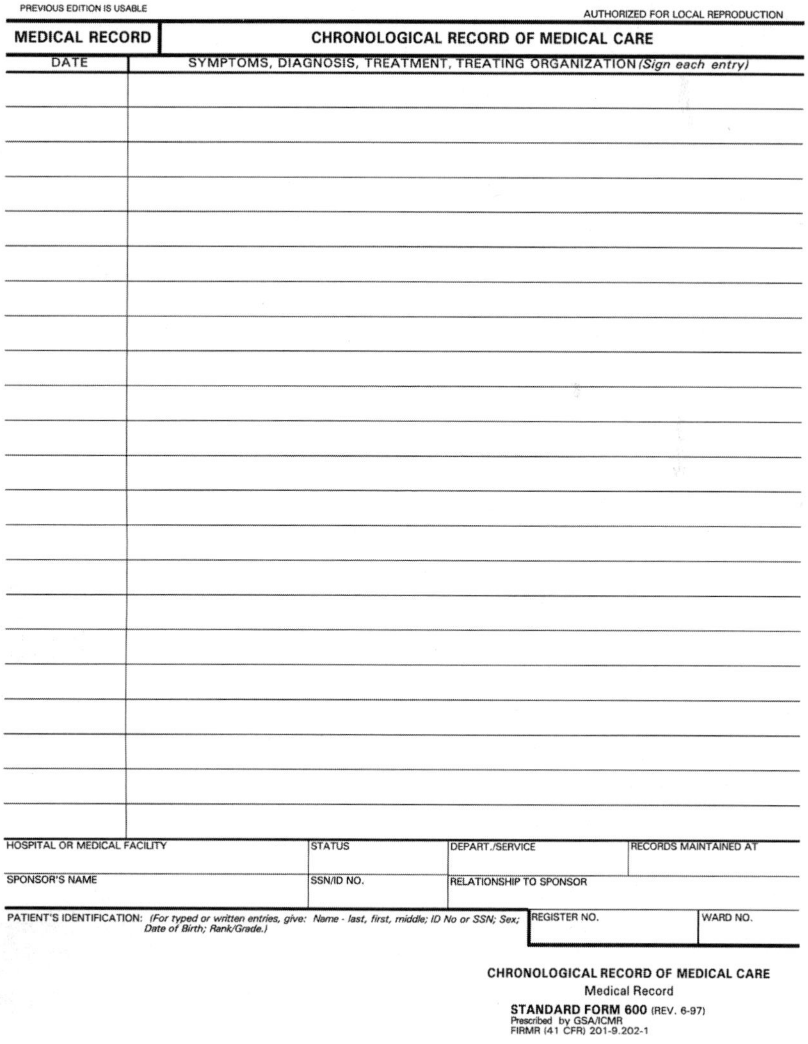

FIGURE 22-1 An SF 600 Chronological Record of Medical Care or Medication Administration Record.

administer any medication, even if this is not the first time you have managed this patient on this day.

Right Medication

Verify the medication a minimum of three times:

1. **When removing the medication or container from the storage area.** For example, the HCP ordered Motrin 800 mg tablets but you have no brand name Motrin on hand. You verify that ibuprofen is the generic equivalent of Motrin, and this is what you obtain from the storage area.

2. **When preparing the medication dose.** For example, acetaminophen (Tylenol) 650 mg is the dose ordered. What you have on hand is acetaminophen 325 mg tablets. Therefore, you realize two tablets are required to fulfill the ordered dose.

3. **When returning the container to the storage area.**

Be familiar with the medications being dispensed, including the brand name, generic name, usual dosages, indications, contraindications, common side effects, and other considerations. If you are dispensing a medication ordered by an HCP, you should not assume the HCP has ensured that the medication is the right medication for the patient. You have the same responsibility as the ordering HCP to prevent medication errors.

Ensure the patient is not allergic to the medication. When a patient states he or she is allergic to a medication, document what the reaction is when he or she takes the medication. Some reported allergies are simply side effects. A patient with a known allergy to one medication is commonly allergic to others. A patient allergic to ibuprofen (Motrin), for example, may be allergic to most if not all of the other anti-inflammatory medications including aspirin. Have a resource available to answer your medication questions when your supervising HCP is not available. When in doubt, look it up. Remember, thousands of Americans die every year as a result of medication errors.

Right Dose

Be familiar with customary medication dosages for the patient population you are most likely to encounter. Imagine reading the written order of an HCP and it appears to you that the order is for Motrin 8,000 mg every 6 hours by mouth for pain. If you were not familiar with the usual dose of 800 mg you can see the potential disaster that could result.

Medications are prescribed and dispensed based on concentration (ie, milligrams per the military) and never by volume (milliliters alone) or quantity (eg, number of tablets). An order to administer 2 cc or mL of a medication does not give a dose, but only a volume of fluid. Most medications for injection, for example, come in various concentrations, with concentration defined as the number of mg per cc or mL. For instance, morphine is available in either 10 mg per cc or 20 mg per cc. It should be easy to see from this example how an order to give 1 cc of morphine to a patient can result in two different doses depending on which concentration you have on hand.

Right Time

You must ensure that it is the right time to administer the medication. Giving a medication too early could lead to an overdose and undesired effects such as toxicity, sedation, and even death. Giving a medication too late could result in other undesired effects such as loss of pain or infection control. Proper documentation in medical records will help ensure correct intervals between doses of medications.

Right Route

The route chosen to administer a medication matters for a number of reasons, chiefly because the onset of action of a medication varies widely from one route of administration to another. Generally speaking, a medication administered orally will have a much slower onset than the same medication given by injection. Most medications, regardless of the route administered, eventually enter the bloodstream. The more quickly the medication enters the bloodstream, the more quickly it will exert its action. There are times when quick onset of action is desired and times when it is not.

Not all medications are available for use in each of the usual methods of administration. If a patient is going to have an adverse reaction to a medication, it will also rapidly appear. For example, an allergic reaction to an antibiotic given by injection will invariably be more severe and more rapid in onset as compared to the same medication given orally.

Use the appropriate route of administration to suit a given situation. Use the least invasive route of administration that will accomplish the desired goal of medication therapy. Translation: do not give a medication by injection if you can accomplish the same desired effect by administering the medication orally. Be aware that the route of administration greatly affects the onset of action of the medication given. Typically speaking, the onset of action is as follows, from fastest to slowest:

- Intravenous (IV)
- Intramuscular (IM)
- Subcutaneous (SQ)
- Orally (PO)
- Topically

Pregnancy and Medications

Many medications, both prescription and over-the-counter (OTC), are either contraindicated in pregnancy or should be used only under limited circumstances. This is one reason why you are taught to determine the first day of last men-

Garrison Care TIPS

You must also consider the form of medication you have on hand for administration. If you are ordered to administer a medication intravenously (IV) you must ensure that the medication form you have on hand is approved for IV use.

strual period (FDLMP) of female patients, to raise or lower your suspicion of pregnancy in your patient. As with any situation where you have doubts, check with your supervising HCP if you have any doubts about the suitability of any medication for any patient. A good rule of thumb to live by is to assume that all teenage and adult females are pregnant until reasonably proven otherwise. Your supervising HCP will help you to determine what reasonably proven otherwise means.

■ Relevant Terms and Definitions

Medication administration requires you to be familiar with a variety of terms and definitions. **Therapeutic effects** include the expected positive effects of medication. A single medication may have several therapeutic effects; for example, aspirin, which is an analgesic, reduces inflammation, reduces fever, and reduces clot formation. Some medications have very specific effects; for example, antihypertensive medications have a therapeutic effect of lowering blood pressure, and antibiotics (ATB) are used to treat bacterial infections.

Mechanism of Action

The **mechanism of action** is a predictable chemical reaction or how the medication works. The medication changes the physiologic activity of the body as the drug bonds chemically at a specific site called a receptor site. An example of this is albuterol (Proventil) for inhalation, which acts on beta receptors in the lung tissue resulting in the dilation of constricted bronchioles (as seen in asthma attacks). Conversely, a certain class of antihypertensive medications known as beta-blockers has the potential to cause bronchial constriction in asthma patients. The same medication causes dilation of blood vessels and lowers blood pressure. Because of its adverse effects on lung tissue in asthma patients, it would be contraindicated to use beta-blockers in this patient population.

Indications and Contraindications

Indications are the acceptable reasons for which a medication may be given. This is guided by the conditions being treated. **Contraindications** are the reasons for not using a particular medication or class of medication. Pre-existing conditions often present contraindications for use. Most, if not all, medications have at least one documented contraindication for use. This includes over-the-counter (OTC) medications such as aspirin, which is contraindicated for patients with a known or suspected stomach ulcer. A true allergy to a medication, although rare, is a contraindication to using it in a given patient.

Allergic Reactions

Allergic reactions are an unpredictable response to a medication. They may be mild, moderate, or severe. Always ask patients about allergies to medications before administering or dispensing a medication. Ask what medications (prescription and over-the-counter, including supplements) they are allergic to as well as the specific reaction experienced. For

instance, if a patient states he is allergic to penicillin, inquire what happens when he takes it. Many patients confuse side effects with allergies. Check unconscious patients for a medical alert bracelet or a medal indicating a medication allergy prior to administering medications. Not all allergic reactions progress to anaphylaxis; some stop with pruritus. However, keep in mind that an allergic reaction may progress rapidly to anaphylaxis without warning. Signs include:

- **Pruritus:** Itching following the administration of a medication.
- **Urticaria:** The formation of hives following the administration of a medication.
- **Angioedema:** Diffuse swelling following the administration of a medication, which may start with the lips, hands, feet, or mucous membranes and may progress to involve swelling of the airway.
- **Anaphylaxis:** A life-threatening allergic reaction, often an acute/rapid onset of the above signs progressing to respiratory distress and shock. This is a true medical emergency that requires immediate diagnosis and appropriate treatment.

Side Effects

Most medications affect more than one system of the body. For instance, ibuprofen may be taken for a muscle strain but it may also upset the stomach, especially if taken without food. **Side effects** should not be confused with allergic reactions. Some side effects are minor and tolerable whereas others may result in the patient discontinuing the medication. Every medication, OTC and prescription, has numerous potential side effects. Some side effects are more likely and common than others. Unintended secondary effects may or may not be harmful to the patient. The side effects of a medication may outweigh the benefits. Patients may stop taking a medication because of unpleasant side effects (eg, codeine prescribed to control coughing but that causes constipation).

Toxic Effects

Toxic effects are caused by intake of high doses of medications; by ingestion of medications not intended to be ingested, such as topical medications; or when a medication accumulates in the system due to impaired metabolism or excretion. Toxic effects may be lethal, depending on the action of the medication. These effects are usually seen in accidental poisonings and intentional medication overdoses (eg, intentional ingestion or accidental administration of a large amount of a narcotic may cause severe respiratory depression and death).

Drug Dependence

Psychological dependence is when the patient is convinced that he or she has a need for the medication. **Physiologic dependence** is when the body has developed a physical need for the medication. This occurs commonly in patients being treated for chronic pain syndromes with narcotics or other controlled substances. **Drug tolerance** is a progressive decrease in effectiveness of a medication. This occurs when the patient receives the same medication for a long period of time and requires higher doses to produce the same effect.

Drug Interactions

<u>Drug interactions</u> occur when one medication modifies the action of another medication. Drug interactions are common in patients who take many medications. A medication may potentiate (enhance) or diminish the action of other medications and may alter the way a medication is absorbed, metabolized, or eliminated from the body. Drug interactions may or may not be desirable. For example, combining alcohol with other central nervous system depressants (narcotics) is not desirable; however, combining diuretics (water

pills) and vasodilators is a way to lower blood pressure in a desirable way.

■ Common Medications

TABLE 22-1 ▾ presents a list of medications according to the frequency with which you will encounter them. Focus on the following aspects of each medication listed:

- Generic name
- Brand name
- Indications
- Considerations

TABLE 22-2 ▸ provides the standard measurement equivalents for medications.

TABLE 22-1 Common Medications

Generic Name	Brand Name	Commonly Supplied	Indications	Usual Dosage	Considerations
Acetaminophen	Tylenol	325-mg or 500-mg tablets	Mild pain, headaches, fever	650 mg to 1,000 mg PO Q6H prn	Overdose and/or consumption with alcohol cause liver toxicity; maximum dose of 4,000 mg daily.
Aspirin (acetylsalicylic acid)	Bayer	325-mg tablets	Mild pain, headache, fever, inflammation	325 mg to 650 mg PO Q4H prn	May cause GI upset; take with food; prolongs blood clotting time.
Bacitracin	various	Topical ointment	Topical infections, abrasions, cuts, minor burns or wounds	Apply a thin film daily to tid based on severity and condition	Not typically used for longer than a week.
Bisacodyl	Dulcolax	5-mg tablets	Constipation	10 mg to 15 mg PO prn	For occasional use only; not for use in patient with abdominal pain.
Bismuth subsalicylate	Pepto-Bismol	Tablets, suspension	Mild, uncomplicated diarrhea; indigestion	Chew 2 tablets PO Q30 minutes to 1 hour up to 8 doses or 30 mL Q30 minutes to 1 hour up to 8 doses	May cause darkening (black discoloration) of tongue and stools; may interfere with many oral medications; shake well before using; reevaluate patients with persistent or worsening diarrhea.
Clotrimazole	Mycelex	1% cream	Superficial fungal infections of the skin	Apply bid to affected areas for at least 2 weeks	Keep affected areas clean and dry.

TABLE 22-1 Common Medications (*continued*)

Generic Name	Brand Name	Commonly Supplied	Indications	Usual Dosage	Considerations
Dextromethorphan with guaifenesin	Robitussin DM	Syrup	Cough due to upper respiratory infection (URI), sinus infection, bronchitis, and pneumonia; guaifenesin is an expectorant (liquefies secretions); dextromethorphan is a cough suppressant	1 to 2 tsp PO Q4-6H prn cough	This is only symptomatic treatment of the cough; the underlying cause may need to be treated.
Diphenhydramine	Benadryl	12.5-mg, 25-mg, and 50-mg capsules; 50 mg per mL injection	Allergic reactions, motion sickness, pruritus	25 mg to 50 mg PO, IM, or IV bid to qid prn	May cause sedation and dry mouth.
Epinephrine	EpiPen	0.3-mg auto-injector	Severe allergic reactions, developing anaphylaxis, severe asthma attack if albuterol is not helping	0.3 mg IM or SC (total dose of auto-injector), may repeat Q10-15 minutes if not improving (for total of three injections)	May cause nervousness, tremor, palpitations, nausea, or vomiting.
Hydrocortisone	Cortaid	1% cream	Inflammation and pruritus; not for use in suspected skin infections	Apply up to qid prn	Discontinue if skin condition persists or worsens during use.
Ibuprofen	Motrin	200-mg, 400-mg, or 800-mg tablets	Arthritis, musculoskeletal pain, menstrual cramps	1,200 mg to 3,200 mg PO daily in 3 to 4 divided doses	Take with food, can cause GI upset; do not take with aspirin.
Kaolin and pectin	Kaopectate	Suspension	Treatment of diarrhea	60 mL to 120 mL (4 to 8 Tbsp) PO after each loose stool or Q3-4H prn	Shake well before using; reevaluate patient with persistent or worsening diarrhea.
Lindane	Kwell	1% cream, lotion, and shampoo	Head lice, crab lice, scabies	Cream/lotion: apply thin layer after bathing and leave in place 24H Shampoo: apply 30 mL and develop lather with warm water for 4 minutes; comb out nits	Caution with overuse, may be absorbed into the blood.

TABLE 22-1 Common Medications (*continued*)

Generic Name	Brand Name	Commonly Supplied	Indications	Usual Dosage	Considerations
Loperamide	Imodium	2-mg capsules	Uncomplicated diarrhea	4 mg PO initially, then 2 mg after each loose stool, up to 16 mg/day	Not for use in cases of suspected infectious diarrhea (abdominal pain, fever, persistent and worsening or bloody diarrhea) because loperamide is a mild narcotic that slows intestinal transit time.
Magnesium hydroxide	Milk of Magnesia	8% suspension	Constipation, hyperacidity (indigestion)	Antacid: 5 mL to 10 mL PO prn Laxative: 15 mL to 30 mL PO prn	Do not use in patients with severe abdominal pain; shake well before using.
Oxymetazoline	Afrin	0.05% nasal spray	Nasal congestion	2 to 3 sprays in each nostril bid prn	Do not use for more than 3 to 5 days.
Phenylephrine	Sudafed	10 mg	Nasal congestion	10 mg PO	Do not use in patients with diabetes or high blood pressure.
Silver sulfadiazine	Silvadene	1% cream	Prevention of sepsis in partial- and full-thickness burns	Aseptically cover affected area with $\frac{1}{16}$" coating bid	Can have systemic absorption with extensive application; not for use in patients with sulfonamide (sulfa) allergy.
Tolnaftate	Tinactin	1% powder and cream	Superficial fungal infection of the skin such as tinea pedis/cruris	Apply bid to affected areas for at least 2 weeks	Keep affected areas clean and dry.

TABLE 22-2 Medication Equivalents

1 teaspoon (tsp)	5 milliliters (mL)	5 cubic centimeters (cc)
1 tablespoon (Tbsp)	15 milliliters (mL)	15 cubic centimeters (cc)
1 fluid ounce (oz)	30 milliliters (mL)	30 cubic centimeters (cc)
1 gram (g)	1,000 milligrams (mg)	
1 milliliter (mL)	1 cubic centimeter (cc)	

■ Mathematics Review

Basic Computations With Whole Numbers

The addition of whole numbers is one of the most basic mathematics skills. Line up the numbers exactly and carry the numbers from one column to the next FIGURE 22-2 ▾.

Solve the following problems:

34 + 17 =
65 + 43 =
89 + 31 =

To subtract whole numbers, line up the numbers correctly. The larger number always goes on top, then subtract FIGURE 22-3 ▾.

Solve the following problems:

34 − 17 =
65 − 43 =
89 − 31 =

To multiply whole numbers, line up the columns correctly. Carry the numbers as you multiply FIGURE 22-4 ▸.

Solve the following problems:

22 × 11 =
13 × 9 =
14 × 56 =

To divide whole numbers, be accurate and be aware of zeros FIGURE 22-5 ▾. In division, the divisor is the number following the $)$ symbol and is placed outside the box. The dividend is the number to be divided and is placed inside the box. The answer is also referred to as the quotient. When rounding, if the number is 5 or greater, round up; if the number is less than 5, then round down.

Solve the following problems:

65 ÷ 5 =
78 ÷ 3 =
871 ÷ 3 =

Fractions

With proper fractions, the numerator (top number) is less than the denominator (bottom number). For example: ¾, ½, ⁷⁄₈. The rule for solving a proper fraction is to reduce it to its

$$\begin{array}{r} 17 \\ +29 \\ \hline 46 \end{array} \qquad \begin{array}{r} 36 \\ +48 \\ \hline 84 \end{array} \qquad \begin{array}{r} 73 \\ +47 \\ \hline 120 \end{array}$$

FIGURE 22-2 To add whole numbers, line up the numbers exactly and carry the numbers from one column to the next.

$$\begin{array}{r} 15 \\ -\ 4 \\ \hline 11 \end{array} \qquad \begin{array}{r} 98 \\ -73 \\ \hline 25 \end{array} \qquad \begin{array}{r} 45 \\ -38 \\ \hline 7 \end{array}$$

FIGURE 22-3 To subtract whole numbers, line up the numbers correctly. The larger number always goes on top, then subtract.

$$\begin{array}{r} 15 \\ \times\ 6 \\ \hline 90 \end{array} \qquad \begin{array}{r} 11 \\ \times 42 \\ \hline 462 \end{array} \qquad \begin{array}{r} 14 \\ \times 12 \\ \hline 168 \end{array}$$

FIGURE 22-4 To multiply whole numbers, line up the columns correctly. Carry the numbers as you multiply.

$$6\overline{)42} = 7 \qquad 8\overline{)56} = 7 \qquad 7\overline{)70} = 10$$

FIGURE 22-5 To divide whole numbers, be accurate and be aware of zeros.

$$\frac{5}{10} \quad \left(5\overline{)5} \;,\; 5\overline{)10} \right) \quad \frac{1}{2}$$

$$\frac{9}{27} \quad \left(9\overline{)9} \;,\; 9\overline{)27} \right) \quad \frac{1}{3}$$

FIGURE 22-6 The rule for solving a proper fraction is to reduce a proper fraction to its lowest term by dividing the numerator and denominator by the same number.

$$\frac{25}{3} = 8\frac{1}{3}$$

FIGURE 22-7 With improper fractions, the numerator is greater than the denominator.

lowest term; to do so you divide the numerator and denominator by the same number **FIGURE 22-6 ▲**.

With improper fractions, the numerator is greater than the denominator; for example, $^6/_5$, $^{11}/_5$. The rules for solving improper fractions are **FIGURE 22-7 ▲**:

- Divide the denominator into the numerator.
- The remainder becomes the new numerator.
- Place the numerator over the denominator.
- Reduce to the lowest term.

A mixed number is a combination of a whole number and a fraction; for example, 1½, 5⅞. The rules for solving mixed fractions are **FIGURE 22-8 ▶**:

- Multiply the whole number by the denominator.
- Add the result to the numerator. This sum is the new numerator.
- Place the new numerator over the denominator.
- Reduce to the lowest term.

Decimals

A decimal number expresses less than a whole number. The decimal point is a dot. All numbers to the left of the decimal are whole numbers. All numbers to the right of the decimal are decimal numbers. The first number to the right of the decimal is tenths, the second is hundredths, and the third is

$$3\frac{5}{6} \;(3 \times 6 + 5) = \frac{23}{6} = 3.833$$

FIGURE 22-8 A mixed number is a combination of a whole number and a fraction.

thousandths; for example, 5.125 is read as 5 (whole number), point, 1 (tenths), 2 (hundredths), 5 (thousandths). If there isn't a whole number in a decimal answer, place a zero to the left of the decimal; for example, 0.75, 0.2. Zeros at the end of a decimal number do not add value and may be eliminated; for example, 2.0 may be written as 2.

■ Needles and Syringes

The parts of a needle include:

- **Lumen:** Hollow cavity inside of the needle
- **Bevel:** Cutting edge of the needle (slanted)
- **Hub:** Point of attachment to the syringe
- **Cannula (shaft):** Needle length
- **Protective cover**

Needles are generally made of stainless steel and are sharp and shiny. Disposable, needleless systems are popular now. The standard needle lengths are from ½″ to 5″. The length is determined from the tip of the point to the junction of the shaft and hub. The gauge (diameter) of the needle varies from 14 to 28. The larger the number, the smaller the needle's diameter. The length and gauge of the needle chosen depend on the type of medication given, the route, the site of injection, and the patient's weight.

The parts of a syringe include:

- **Barrel:** Clear plastic or glass that has calibrated scales on it. The inside of a barrel is sterile.
- **Plunger:** Movable portion inside of barrel. The rubber portion and the shaft are sterile.
- **Needle adapter:** Portion of the syringe where the needle attaches. This part also is sterile.
- **Calibrated scales:** Markings that vary from 0.01 mL on 1-cc syringes to 0.2 mL on 3–5-cc syringes to 0.5 mL on 10-cc and larger syringes. Always check the calibrated markings.
- **Safety syringes:** Prevent needlesticks.

Inspecting Equipment for Contamination and/or Deterioration

Before you use any piece of medical equipment on a patient, you must inspect it for potential contamination or deterioration. Check paper wrappers for tears, water spots, and signs of deterioration or contamination. If any of these signs are present, discard and replace. Plastic caps on needles and syringes should not have been opened prior to use. If the needle or syringe covers appear to be loose, then discard and replace.

Assemble a Needle and Syringe

To assemble a needle and syringe, follow the steps in **SKILL DRILL 22-1 ▶**:

1. Remove the syringe from the package without contaminating the sterile parts (needle adapter or plunger). If the syringe is packaged in a flexible wrapper, peel the sides of the wrapper apart to expose the rear end of the syringe barrel. If the syringe is packaged in a hard plastic container, press down and twist the cap until a distinct "pop" is heard. If you don't hear a pop, the seal has been broken previously, and the equipment must be discarded.

2. Ensure the plunger of the syringe moves freely by grasping the flared end of the syringe and pulling the plunger back and forth. If the syringe does not move freely, replace it with another sterile syringe. *Caution:* The shaft of the plunger is sterile. Contamination could cause infection in the patient. Touch only the end of the plunger when testing for free movement. Do not pull the plunger out of the syringe barrel (**Step ①**).

3. Remove the needle from the package without contaminating the sterile parts (needle hub or shaft). If the needle is packaged in a flexible wrapper, peel the sides of the wrapper apart to expose the needle hub. If the needle is packaged in a hard plastic container, twist the cap until a pop is heard. Remove the cap to expose the needle hub. If you don't hear a pop, the seal has been previously broken, and the equipment must be discarded. *Caution:* All parts of the needle are sterile. Be careful not to touch the hub to prevent contamination. Only the outside of the needle cover may be touched.

4. Join needle and syringe by inserting the needle adapter of the syringe into the needle hub, without contaminating either part.

5. Tighten the needle by turning one fourth of a turn to ensure it is securely attached. If the syringe has threads, you may need to turn more than a quarter turn (**Step ②**).

6. Hold the needle and syringe upright and remove the protective cover from the needle by pulling it straight off. *Caution:* Do not twist the protective cover because it may pull the needle off the hub.

7. Visually inspect the needle for burrs, barbs, damage, and contamination. If the needle has any defects or damage, replace the needle with another sterile needle (**Step ③**).

8. Place the protective cover back on the needle, being careful not to stick yourself or to contaminate the

needle. Place the assembled needle and syringe on the work surface. When you assemble a needle and syringe, you are responsible for maintaining sterility and security of the equipment (**Step ④**).

■ Steps to Utilize Prior to Drawing Up Medications

As discussed in detail earlier in this chapter and in Chapter 12, *Battlefield Medications*, prior to giving any medications, verify the five rights of medication administration. In addition:

- Compare the medication name on the container with the doctor's orders.
- Compare the medication concentration with the doctor's orders.
- Check the expiration date on the medication container.
- Verify the medication label three times:
  - When obtaining the medicine container from its place of storage
  - When withdrawing medication from the container
  - When returning the medication container to storage
- If any of the following defects are noted on a vial, follow directions in accordance with (IAW) local standard operating procedures (SOPs) or return the medication to the pharmacy. *Caution:* If using a multi-dose vial, the protective metal cap may have been removed.
  - Examine the rubber stopper for defects, such as small holes resulting from wear and tear.
  - Hold the vial to the light to check for foreign particles and changes in color and consistency of the medication to be drawn.
- Check the expiration date; for a multi-dose vial, check the date the medication was opened. *Warning:* Refer to the manufacturer's instructions for determining the expiration of medication prior to and after opening a vial. Follow local SOP if discrepancies are noted between SOP and manufacturer's instructions. If in doubt, consult your supervisor, the nurse on duty, or the pharmacy.
- Determine whether the medication is stored properly (eg, shelf or room temperature vs. refrigeration).
- Refer to the manufacturer's instructions for proper storage of medication.

Prepare and Draw Medication

First, select the appropriate needle. The length will depend on the following factors:

- Type of injection to be given (intramuscular, subcutaneous, intradermal)
- The size of the patient (thin, obese)
- The site of injection

The choice of the needle gauge depends on the viscosity (thickness) of the medication. The gauge of the needle is indicated by the numbers 14 through 28. The higher the

Assemble a Needle and Syringe

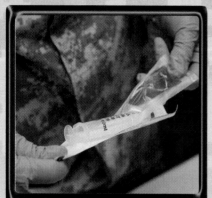

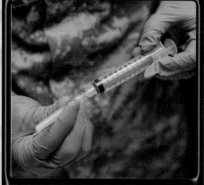

1 Remove the syringe from the package without contaminating the sterile parts (needle adapter or plunger). Ensure the plunger of the syringe moves freely by grasping the flared end of the syringe and pulling the plunger back and forth. If the syringe does not move freely, replace it with another sterile syringe.

2 Remove the needle from the package without contaminating the sterile parts (needle hub or shaft). Join the needle and syringe by inserting the needle adapter of the syringe into the needle hub, without contaminating either part. Tighten the needle by turning one fourth of a turn to ensure it is securely attached. If the syringe has threads, you may need to turn more than a quarter turn.

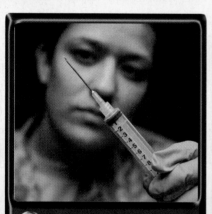

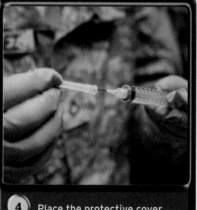

3 Hold the needle and syringe upright and remove the protective cover from the needle by pulling it straight off. Visually inspect the needle for burrs, barbs, damage, and contamination. If the needle has any defects or damage, replace the needle with another sterile needle.

4 Place the protective cover back on the needle, being careful not to stick yourself or to contaminate the needle. Place the assembled needle and syringe on the work surface.

number, the smaller the diameter (bore) of the needle. Small-bore needles are indicated for thin medications (watery medications) or slow infusion rates. Large-bore needles are indicated for thick medications or rapid infusion rates. Drawing medication from an ampule is covered in detail in Skill Drill 12-1 in Chapter 12, *Battlefield Medications*. Drawing medication from a stoppered vial that contains a prepared solution is covered in detail in Skill Drill 12-2 in Chapter 12.

Reconstitution of Powdered Medication

To reconstitute a powdered medication, follow the steps in **SKILL DRILL 22-2** ▸:

1. Receive the doctor's orders (medication, route, dosage).

2. Select the correct medication from the storage area.

3. Peel back the protective plunger cap (**Step 1**).

4. Depress the top of the vial to dislodge the diluent into the powdered medication (**Step 2**).

5. Invert the vial several times until all of the powdered medication is dissolved (**Step 3**).

6. Open an alcohol prep pad (**Step 4**).

7. Clean the stopper on the vial with an alcohol prep pad (**Step 5**).

8. Insert the appropriate-sized needle into the reconstituted medication. Withdraw the predetermined medication amount into the syringe (**Step 6**).

9. Withdraw the needle from the vial and verify the correct dosage (**Step 7**).

Intramuscular Injections

This skill is covered in detail in Skill Drill 12-4 in Chapter 12, *Battlefield Medications*. **Intramuscular (IM) injections** are utilized when a rapid absorption/rate of onset (10–20 minutes) and a long duration (hours to weeks) are desired. It is used when administering viscous or irritating medications. It is also used when a large volume of medication is needed for a stronger effect.

Absorption of medications administered by the intramuscular route relies on adequate blood flow to the muscles, so IM injections should not be used in individuals with poor circulation or symptoms of shock.

The needle for an IM injection should not be less than 1″ for an adult. You may use a smaller size if the patient is thin and you may need up to a 2″ needle for obese patients. The needle must be long enough to reach the muscle. Using a needle that is too short will cause the medication to be injected into subcutaneous tissue, potentially reducing absorption and effectiveness. The needle gauge (diameter) range is 20 to 22.

The primary IM injection site is the deltoid muscle. This site is used for medication volumes up to 2 mL in an adult. The deltoid muscle provides faster absorption than other IM injection sites. The deltoid muscle is located in the outer one third of arm between the shoulder bone (acromion process) and axilla. This injection site is approximately three finger-widths below the shoulder bone, in the middle of the deltoid muscle mass.

The gluteus maximus is used for larger medication volumes, up to 5 mL. It may require a long needle (2″ or longer in large adults). This site is located by dividing one buttock into four imaginary quadrants. The injection area is in the upper, outer quadrant. An injection given in an area outside this site could cause damage to the sciatic nerve or puncture the superior gluteal artery, causing either paralysis or severe bleeding. Use care when identifying the gluteus maximus site.

The vastus lateralis is one of the safest IM injection sites due to the absence of major nerves and blood vessels; however, it may be more painful due to a number of small nerve endings. It is used to administer medication volume up to 5 mL in adults. The muscle mass is on the lateral thigh. The injection site extends from the middle of the anterior thigh to the middle of the lateral thigh, and from one hand's width

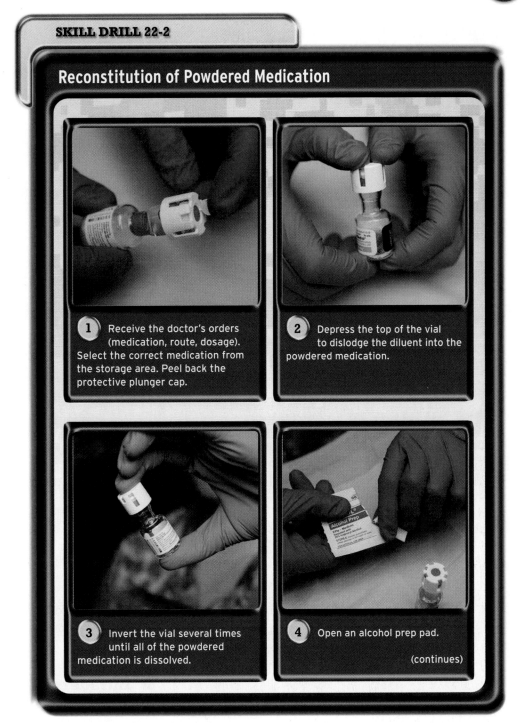

SKILL DRILL 22-2

Reconstitution of Powdered Medication

1. Receive the doctor's orders (medication, route, dosage). Select the correct medication from the storage area. Peel back the protective plunger cap.

2. Depress the top of the vial to dislodge the diluent into the powdered medication.

3. Invert the vial several times until all of the powdered medication is dissolved.

4. Open an alcohol prep pad.

(continues)

SKILL DRILL 22-2

Reconstitution of Powdered Medication (*continued*)

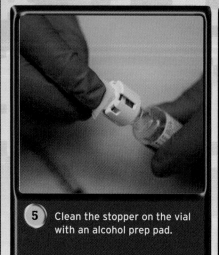

5 Clean the stopper on the vial with an alcohol prep pad.

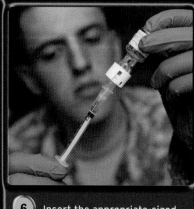

6 Insert the appropriate-sized needle into the reconstituted medication. Withdraw the predetermined medication amount into the syringe.

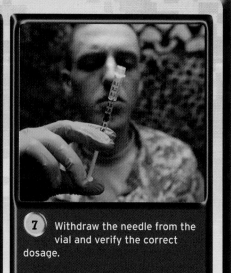

7 Withdraw the needle from the vial and verify the correct dosage.

below the hip joint to one hand's width above the knee. The length and gauge of the needle selected will vary depending on the amount of muscle mass, age, size, and condition of the patient.

■ Subcutaneous Injections

This skill is covered in detail in Skill Drill 12-3 in Chapter 12, *Battlefield Medications*. The **subcutaneous (SQ) injection** is utilized when the absorption rate desired is slower than the IM route. The absorption rate for SQ injection is 15 to 30 minutes. The duration is comparable to the IM route, and repeat injections may be given over hours to weeks. This route is used for small amounts of watery and nonirritating medications. The needle length is between ½″ and 1″ and the gauge ranges from 23 to 25. The selection of needle length and gauge will vary depending on the amount of subcutaneous tissue, age, size, and condition of the patient. The injection sites include:

- **The upper arm, on the rear lateral aspect:** The injection area is approximately one hand's width down from the shoulder and one third of the way around laterally. The medication volume should not exceed 0.5 mL.
- **Vastus lateralis:** The injection site extends from the middle of the anterior thigh to the middle of the

lateral thigh, and from one hand's width below the hip joint to one hand's width above the knee. The medication volume should not exceed 2 mL.
- **Abdomen:** Medications such as insulin and heparin are administered in the subcutaneous tissue of the abdomen. The amount of medication given will vary according to the needs of the patient. A physician will prescribe the dosage to be given in the abdomen.

■ Intradermal (ID) Injections

The purpose of giving an **intradermal (ID) injection** is to test sensitivity (allergy testing) to environmental allergens or medications. It is also used to test for exposure to diseases (eg, tuberculosis, mumps) and to evaluate the immune system (eg, AIDS and cancer patients). The equipment required to give this type of injection are:

- Needle, ¼″ to ½″ in length, 25 to 27 gauge
- Tuberculin or other 1.0-mL syringe

The injection sites must be:

- Free of hair, tattoos, and scars
- Not over a vein or bony area

The inner flat portion of the forearm is the primary injection site for ID injections. This is the preferred site for tuberculin testing and most other routinely given ID injections. Other sites include:

- Back of upper arm
- The back below the shoulder blades

To administer an ID injection, follow the steps in
SKILL DRILL 22-3 :

1. Identify the patient.
2. Verify the injection.
3. Verify the compatibility of the medications if multiple injections are ordered.
4. Ensure the availability of emergency equipment and personnel.
5. Gather the equipment and prepare the medication.
6. Wash your hands.
7. Don sterile gloves.
8. Position the patient with the injection site exposed. For the inner forearm, the patient should be standing, sitting, or supine with the palm up and the arm relaxed and supported. For the back of the upper arm, the patient should be standing or sitting. For the back, the patient should be prone or seated and leaning forward with the body supported by a stable object.
9. Select the injection site.
10. Clean the area with an alcohol prep pad or acetone in a spiral motion; clean outward 3″.
11. Pull the needle cover/cap straight off and dispose of it in a waste receptacle.
12. Using the thumb of your nondominant hand, pull the skin below the injection site downward and hold it taut.
13. Position the syringe with the needle bevel up, at a 15° to 20° angle to the skin surface.
14. Insert the needle just until the bevel is under the skin surface.
15. Gently release the skin tension held by your nondominant hand.

16. Do not aspirate. Push the plunger slowly forward until all medication has been injected and a wheal (a round or elongated elevation of the skin caused by the injection of fluid under the dermis) appears at the site of the injection. The appearance of a wheal indicates that the medication has entered the area between the tissues.
17. If a wheal does not appear, withdraw the needle completely from the arm at the angle of insertion, dispose of the needle and syringe in a sharps container, prepare a new set, and repeat the procedure in another site. If a wheal does appear, continue the procedure.
18. Quickly withdraw the needle at the same angle that it was inserted.
19. Without applying pressure to the skin surface, cover the injection site with dry sterile gauze.
20. Instruct the patient not to scratch, rub, or wash the injection site.
21. If appropriate, instruct the patient when and where to have the test read IAW local SOPs.
22. Discard the needle and syringe into the sharps container without recapping the needle.
23. Check the site for bleeding and observe the patient for allergic reactions.
24. Record the procedure on the appropriate form. If this injection was given to determine sensitivity (PPD), follow local SOPs for patient care and the instructions for reading of the results in 48–72 hours.

■ Summary

The administration of medications requires strict attention to detail and an acute awareness of the effects certain medications can have. Always review the five rights of medication administration before dispensing or administering any medication.

YOU ARE THE
COMBAT MEDIC

You are the combat medic on duty at the Battalion Aid Station. It is the beginning of your shift. The medical officer (MO) assigns you to check on the vital signs of every patient recovering in the BAS. There are three patients occupying the beds. One patient is recovering from an open abdominal wound. The doctors are stabilizing his condition before moving him on to the next level of care. To prevent infection, he is receiving doses of ertapenem (Invanz) via intravenous (IV) administration.

Assessment

As you approach this patient, you notice that his skin looks flushed. His brow is knotted and he looks concerned.

"How are you feeling tonight, sir?" you ask.

He makes eye contact with you and you see that his eyes are tearing up. He opens his mouth to speak, but just a rasp comes out. You quickly check his documentation; his last dose of medication was given very recently, at the end of the previous shift.

You look up from the paperwork. The patient's eyes are now closed and his breathing is labored. This patient is having an allergic reaction to the ertapenem and needs immediate care.

Treatment

You don sterile gloves, and then quickly secure the patient's airway by inserting a Combitube and administering oxygen. Now that the patient's airway is secure, you stop the IV of ertapenem.

Now it is time to administer epinephrine. You fill a syringe with 0.5 mL of epinephrine and administer the injection on the upper arm. After briskly rubbing the injection site, you reassess the patient's condition to determine the effect of the epinephrine. His blood pressure is 106/70 mm Hg; his pulse is 110 beats/min; his mental status is alert; his skin is warm, pink, and dry with some hives; and his respirations are 36 breaths/min. You notify the MO of the patient's situation and he takes over the patient's care.

Ready for Review

- The combat medic works under the supervision of a licensed health care provider—a doctor, nurse, or physician's assistant.
- You will dispense certain prescription and nonprescription medications on the order of a supervising health care provider (HCP).
- You will dispense medications from an approved formulary in accordance with local protocols and in a manner consistent with the level of medical training of a combat medic.
- Medication administration requires you to be familiar with the terms and definitions of medication administration.
- Prior to giving any medications, verify the five rights of medication administration:
  - Right patient
  - Right medication
  - Right dose
  - Right time
  - Right route
- Intramuscular injections are utilized when a rapid absorption/rate of onset (10-20 minutes) and a long duration (hours to weeks) are desired.
- Subcutaneous (SQ) injections are utilized when the absorption rate desired is slower than the intramuscular route.
- The purpose of giving an intradermal (ID) injection is to test sensitivity (allergy testing) to environmental allergens or medications. It is also used to test for exposure to diseases (eg, tuberculosis, mumps) and to evaluate the immune system (eg, AIDS and cancer patients).

Vital Vocabulary

allergic reaction An unpredictable response to a medication.

anaphylaxis A severe hypersensitivity reaction that involves bronchoconstriction and cardiovascular collapse.

angioedema Diffuse swelling following the administration of a medication; may start with the lips, hands, feet, or mucous membranes and may progress to the airway.

contraindications Situations in which a medication should not be given because it would not help or may actually harm.

drug interaction When one medication modifies the action of another medication.

drug tolerance A progressive decrease in the effectiveness of a medication.

indications Therapeutic uses for a specific medication.

intramuscular (IM) injection A method of delivering a medication into the muscle of the body by placing a needle into a muscle space and injecting the medication into the tissue.

intradermal (ID) injection A method of delivering a medication into the skin.

mechanism of action A predictable chemical reaction or how the medication works.

physiological dependence When the body has developed a physical need for the medication.

pruritus Itching following the administration of a medication.

psychological dependence When the patient is convinced that he or she has a need for the medication.

side effects Any effects of a medication other than the desired ones.

subcutaneous (SC) injection Injection into the tissue between the skin and muscle; a medication delivery route.

therapeutic effect The expected positive effect of the medication.

toxic effect Caused by the intake of high doses of medications, ingestion of medications not intended for ingestion, or when a medication accumulates in the system.

urticaria The formation of hives following the administration of a medication.

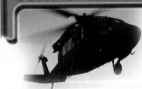

COMBAT MEDIC *in Action*

You are the combat medic assigned to sick call duty at the Battalion Aid Station. A soldier comes in with a headache. After assessing the soldier, you determine that this headache is just a headache, and not a sign of a more serious condition. You need to administer an effective pain medication to give this soldier some relief. What pain medication do you administer?

1. After obtaining the medication, what is the first question you should ask this soldier?
   A. "Can I see your ID card?"
   B. "How old are you?"
   C. "Would you prefer a pill or an injection?"
   D. "What is your middle name?"

2. A patient's identification only needs to be verified:
   A. once per shift.
   B. once per day.
   C. once.
   D. each and every time you administer a medication.

3. Before administering a medication, you should verify the medication a minimum of:
   A. four times.
   B. three times.
   C. two times.
   D. one time.

4. Typically speaking, the onset of the action of a medication is as follows, from fastest to slowest:
   A. topical, oral, subcutaneous, intramuscular, intravenous
   B. subcutaneous, oral, topical, intramuscular, intravenous
   C. intravenous, intramuscular, subcutaneous, oral, topical
   D. oral, topical, intramuscular, intravenous, subcutaneous

5. Administering another dose of a medication can lead to:
   A. documentation errors.
   B. overdose.
   C. You can never give an additional dose of medication too early.
   D. overdose and undesired effects such as toxicity, sedation, and even death.

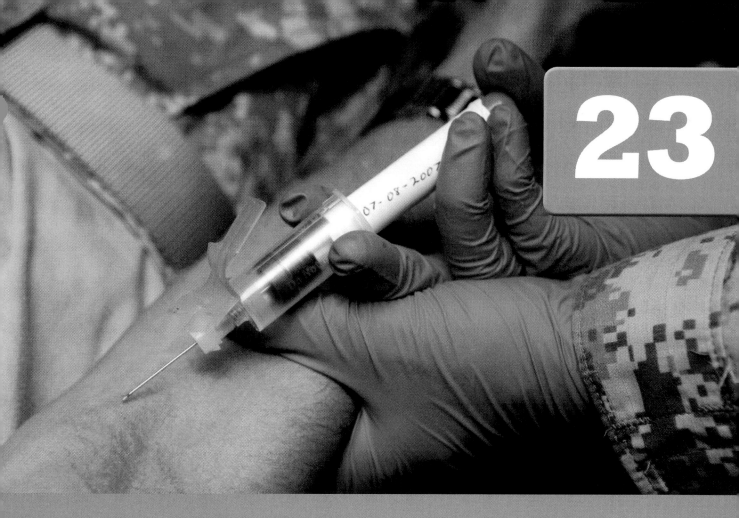

23

Venipuncture

Objectives

Knowledge Objectives
- [ ] Describe the general considerations of venipuncture.
- [ ] List the steps and procedures to perform a venipuncture.

Skills Objective
- [ ] Perform a venipuncture.

■ Introduction

Blood can reveal a great deal of information that will assist a physician in making an accurate diagnosis and creating an effective treatment plan. If blood samples are needed, it is usually at the request of a doctor for laboratory analysis. Blood samples are not taken on the battlefield; this is solely a procedure for the garrison.

■ Venipuncture

Venipuncture is the technique that permits access to a vein, usually to withdraw a blood specimen, initiate an intravenous infusion, or instill a medication. The venipuncture must be a sterile procedure because the integrity of the skin is broken during the procedure. This skill is performed in the relative comfort and quiet of the garrison.

The veins used for drawing blood include:

- **Median cubital vein:** First choice, well supported, least apt to roll
- **Cephalic vein:** Second choice
- **Basilic vein:** Third choice; often the most prominent vein, but it tends to roll easily and makes venipuncture difficult

Perform a Venipuncture

This is a complex and detailed skill that we will cover both in-depth over the next few pages and in Skill Drill 23-1. To perform a venipuncture, first verify the request to obtain a blood specimen and check the physician's orders. Select the proper blood specimen tube for the test to be performed. Check the local laboratory standard operating procedures (SOPs).

The type of blood tube needed will depend on the specific test to be performed. For some tests, an anticoagulant or other additives are present in the tube **FIGURE 23-1 ▼**. The tubes' rubber stoppers are color-coded for different tests. Use the following mnemonic to help remember the order for filling the tubes: Red Blood Gives Life. The *red*-topped tube contains no additives and is intended to clot if blood typing is needed. The *blue*-topped tube contains the preservative

EDTA and is used to help determine a patient's prothrombin time and partial thromboplastin time (values that are used to calculate the patient's blood clotting time). The *green*-topped tube is filled with heparin to prevent clotting and is used to evaluate the patient's electrolyte and glucose levels. *Lavender*-topped tubes are filled with sodium citrate and are often used for a complete blood count, including hematocrit and hemoglobin values.

Stamp the label with the patient's addressograph plate. If there is no plate, write the patient's name, organization, social security number, prefix code, ward or clinic, facility, and date. Apply the label to the specimen tube.

Perform a patient care handwash and don sterile gloves. Identify the patient. Explain the procedure and purpose for collecting the blood specimen to the patient. Ask the patient about any allergies (ie, iodine or alcohol). Position the patient, either sitting or lying down. Never attempt to draw blood from a standing patient.

Position a protective pad underneath the patient's extended elbow and forearm. Expose the area for venipuncture. Roll the patient's garment above the elbow. Extend the patient's arm with the palm up. Select the vein for venipuncture. Palpate and select one of the most prominent veins in the antecubital fossa **FIGURE 23-2 ▼**. You may need to apply the constricting band at this point for venipuncture site selection.

Prepare the sponges for use by opening the Betadine or alcohol 2″ × 2″ gauze sponge packages. Place them within easy reach, while still keeping the sponges in the package. Apply a constricting band around the patient's limb with enough pressure to stop the venous return without stopping the arterial flow. A radial pulse should still be felt. Wrap the latex tubing around the limb about 2″ above the venipuncture site. Stretch the tubing slightly and hold it with one end longer than the other. Loop the longer end and draw it under the shorter end so that the tails are away from site **FIGURE 23-3 ▶**. If a commercial band is used, wrap it around the patient's limb and secure it by overlapping the Velcro ends.

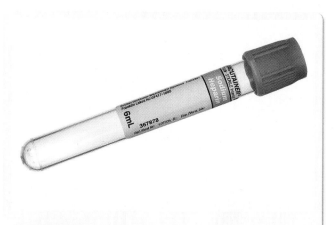

FIGURE 23-1 An anticoagulant or other additives may be present in the blood tube.

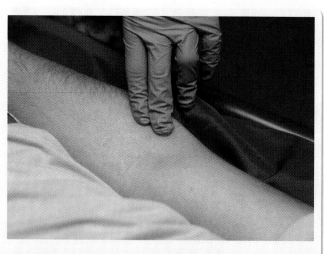

FIGURE 23-2 Find the prominent veins in the antecubital fossa.

Instruct the patient to clench and unclench his or her fist several times and then hold the clenched fist to trap the blood in the veins and distend them. Avoid veins that are infected, injured, irritated, or have an IV running distally. Palpate the selected vein along the length of the vein. To do this, trace your index finger up and down 1″ or 2″ from the selected site in both directions to determine the size and the direction of the vein. The vein should feel like a spongy tube.

Clean the patient's skin by moving the alcohol or Betadine wipe in a circular motion away from the selected venipuncture site. Do not palpate the vein after cleansing the skin.

Prepare to puncture the vein. Remove the protective cover from the needle. Position the needle in line with the vein and grasp the patient's arm below the entry point with your free hand. With your free hand, place your thumb 1″ below the entry site and pull the skin taut toward the patient's hand.

Align the needle, bevel up, with the vein and pierce the skin at a 15° to 30° angle. Decrease the angle until almost parallel to the skin's surface, then pierce the vein wall. A faint "give" will be felt when the needle enters the vein, and blood will appear in the needle.

If the venipuncture is unsuccessful, pull the needle back slightly (not above the skin's surface), and redirect the needle toward the vein and try again. If the needle is withdrawn above the skin's surface, do not attempt a venipuncture again with this same needle. If you are still unsuccessful, release the constricting band and place a 2″ × 2″ gauze sponge over the site. Quickly withdraw the needle and instruct the patient to elevate his or her arm slightly. The patient must keep his or her arm fully extended, applying pressure to the site for 2 to 3 minutes. Notify your supervisor before attempting another venipuncture.

Collect a Specimen

If the venipuncture is successful, you can now collect a blood specimen. To collect a single specimen, hold the **Vacutainer** sleeve and needle steady with your dominant hand. The collection tube is positioned against, but not through, the needle. With your other hand, place your index and middle fingers behind the flange of the Vacutainer FIGURE 23-4 ▾ . Push the tube as far forward as possible with your nondominant thumb without causing excessive movement. Instruct the patient to relax and unclench his or her fist after the blood has started flowing. Release the constricting band by pulling on the long end of the looped tubing or by releasing the Velcro fastener with your nondominant hand. When the tube is about two thirds full of blood or the blood stops, grasp the tube firmly and remove the tube. Prepare to withdraw the needle from the patient's vein.

To collect multiple specimens, follow the same steps for collecting a single specimen. Remove the first tube from the Vacutainer sleeve without dislodging the needle position. Insert the second tube into the Vacutainer sleeve. Push the tube as far forward as possible without causing excessive movement. Repeat these procedures until the desired number of tubes are filled or the blood stops flowing. Release the constricting band by pulling on the long end of the looped tubing or by releasing the Velcro fastener with your nondominant hand. Never withdraw the needle before the constricting band is released because of the potential for heavy blood loss and/or hematoma formation. Place a 2″ × 2″ sponge lightly over the venipuncture site. Withdraw the needle smoothly and quickly. Immediately apply pressure to the site with the 2″ × 2″ sponge, keeping the patient's arm fully extended.

Instruct the patient to elevate his or her arm slightly and keep it fully extended, applying firm manual pressure for 2 to 3 minutes. If the patient is unable to do this for him- or herself, you must do it for him or her. If the specimen tube contains an anticoagulant or other additive, gently invert the tube several times to mix with the patient's blood.

Apply an adhesive bandage to the venipuncture site after the bleeding has stopped. Dispose of the needle into a sharps container as soon as possible or in accordance with (IAW)

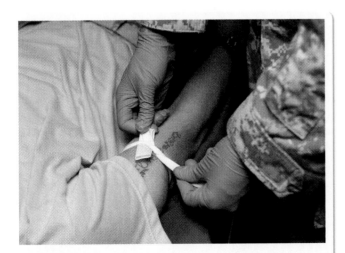

FIGURE 23-3 Applying the constricting band to the patient's limb makes it easier for you to locate a vein.

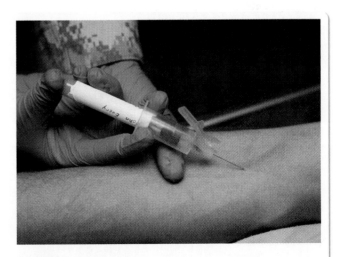

FIGURE 23-4 With your nondominant hand, place your index and middle fingers behind the flange of the Vacutainer.

local protocol. Never unscrew the needle from the Vacutainer sleeve with your hands. Never recap the needle.

Provide for the patient's comfort and safety. Remove the protective pad from underneath the patient's limb and roll down the patient's sleeve. Reposition the patient and raise the side rails if the patient is in a bed.

Remove all the equipment from the area. Dispose of all used supplies properly. Store reusable equipment and dispose of the needle IAW local SOPs. Remove your gloves and wash your hands. Check and complete the laboratory form IAW local SOPs. Apply prepared label(s) to specimen tube(s). Document the procedure IAW local SOPs.

Obtain a Blood Specimen Using a Vacutainer

To obtain a blood specimen using a Vacutainer, follow the steps in **SKILL DRILL 23-1 ▶**:

1. Verify the request to obtain a blood specimen.
2. Select the proper blood specimen tube for the test to be performed.
3. Prepare the label(s) and apply to the specimen tube.
4. Perform a patient care handwash.
5. Gather equipment (**Step ①**).
6. Don sterile gloves.
7. Assemble a Vacutainer and needle (**Step ②**).
8. Identify the patient. Question the patient about medication allergies.
9. Explain the procedure and purpose for collecting the blood specimen.
10. Position the patient comfortably either sitting or lying down.
11. Position a protective pad under the patient's extended elbow and forearm (**Step ③**).
12. Expose the area for venipuncture.
13. Select a vein for venipuncture in the antecubital fossa (**Step ④**).
14. Open Betadine and alcohol sponge packages and place them within easy reach (**Step ⑤**).
15. Apply the constricting band with enough pressure to stop venous return without stopping the arterial flow. A radial pulse should be felt (**Step ⑥**).
16. Wrap latex tubing around the limb about 2″ above the venipuncture site.
17. Stretch the tubing slightly and hold with one end longer than the other.
18. Loop the longer end and draw it under the shorter end so that the ends of the tubing are away from the site (**Step ⑦**).
19. Instruct the patient to clench and unclench his or her fist several times and then hold the clenched fist to trap blood in the veins and distend them.
20. Palpate along the length of the vein with your index finger up and down 1″ or 2″ from the selected site in both directions so that the size and direction of the vein can be determined (**Step ⑧**).
21. Cleanse the skin using Betadine, and then the alcohol pad, wiping in a circular motion away from the selected venipuncture site (**Step ⑨**).
22. Prepare to puncture the vein. Remove the protective cover from the needle. Position the needle in line with the vein and grasp the patient's arm below the entry point with your free hand (**Step ⑩**).
23. Place your thumb 1″ below the entry site and pull the skin taut toward the patient's hand (**Step ⑪**).
24. Puncture the vein. Align the needle, bevel up, with the vein and pierce the skin at a 15° to 30° angle (**Step ⑫**).
25. Attach the Vacutainer to the needle. Decrease the angle until almost parallel to the skin's surface, then pierce the vein wall.
26. A faint give will be felt when the needle enters the vein, and blood will appear in the needle.
27. If venipuncture is unsuccessful, pull the needle back slightly (not above the skin surface), and redirect the needle toward the vein and try again.
28. If still unsuccessful, release the constricting band.
29. Place a 2″ × 2″ sponge over the site.
30. Quickly withdraw the needle and instruct the patient to elevate the arm slightly, keeping the arm fully extended and applying pressure to the site for 2 to 3 minutes.
31. Notify your supervisor before attempting again (**Step ⑬**).
32. Collect a single specimen by holding the Vacutainer unit and needle steady with your dominant hand; place the collection tube against, but not through, the needle (**Step ⑭**).
33. Place your index and middle fingers of your nondominant hand behind the flange of the Vacutainer.

34. Push the tube as far forward as possible with the thumb of your nondominant hand without causing excessive movement (**Step** ⑮).

35. Instruct the patient to relax and unclench his or her fist after the blood has started flowing.

36. When the tube is two thirds full of blood, prepare to withdraw the needle.

37. Release the constricting band by pulling on the long end of the looped tubing with your nondominant hand (**Step** ⑯).

38. Place a 2″ × 2″ pad lightly over the venipuncture site.

39. Withdraw the needle smoothly and quickly. Immediately apply pressure to the site with the 2″ × 2″ pad, keeping the patient's arm fully extended (**Step** ⑰).

40. Instruct the patient to elevate his or her arm slightly, keeping the arm fully extended, and to apply firm manual pressure for 2 to 3 minutes (**Step** ⑱).

41. Remove the specimen tube from the Vacutainer (**Step** ⑲).

42. Apply an adhesive dressing to the venipuncture site after bleeding has stopped (**Step** ⑳).

■ Summary

If venipuncture is done smoothly and properly, there should be little pain for the patient and little risk to you. The procedural steps are designed to ensure a properly drawn specimen. With practice, obtaining a blood specimen can become a smooth routine.

SKILL DRILL 23-1

Obtain a Blood Specimen Using a Vacutainer

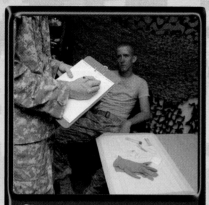

1 Verify the request to obtain a blood specimen. Select the proper blood specimen tube for the test to be performed. Prepare the label(s) and apply to the specimen tube. Perform a patient care handwash. Gather equipment.

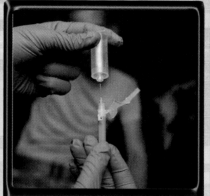

2 Put sterile gloves on. Assemble a Vacutainer and needle.

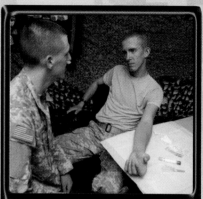

3 Identify the patient. Question the patient about medication allergies. Explain the procedure and purpose for collecting the blood specimen. Position the patient comfortably either sitting or lying down. Position a protective pad under the patient's extended elbow and forearm.

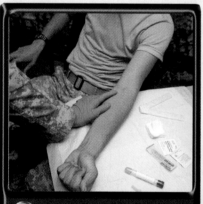

4 Expose the area for venipuncture. Select a vein for venipuncture in the antecubital fossa.

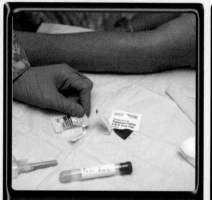

5 Open the Betadine and alcohol sponge packages and place them within easy reach.

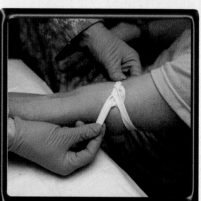

6 Apply the constricting band with enough pressure to stop venous return without stopping the arterial flow. A radial pulse should be felt.

SKILL DRILL 23-1

Obtain a Blood Specimen Using a Vacutainer (*continued*)

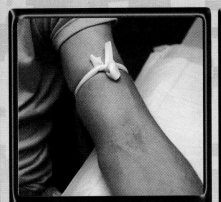

7 Wrap latex tubing around the limb about 2″ above the venipuncture site. Stretch the tubing slightly and hold with one end longer than the other. Loop the longer end and draw it under the shorter end so that the ends of the tubing are away from the site.

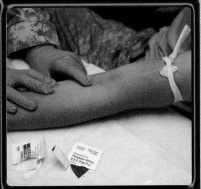

8 Instruct the patient to clench and unclench his or her fist several times and then hold the clenched fist to trap blood in the veins and distend them. Palpate along the length of the vein with your index finger up and down 1″ or 2″ from the selected site in both directions so that the size and direction of the vein can be determined.

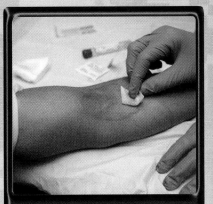

9 Cleanse the skin using Betadine, and then the alcohol pad, wiping in a circular motion away from the selected venipuncture site.

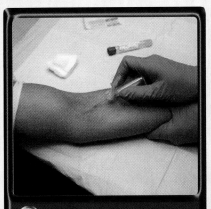

10 Prepare to puncture the vein. Remove the protective cover from the needle. Position the needle in line with the vein and grasp the patient's arm below the entry point with your free hand.

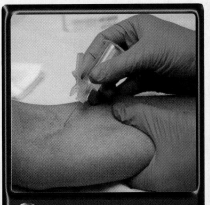

11 Place your thumb 1″ below the entry site and pull the skin taut toward the patient's hand.

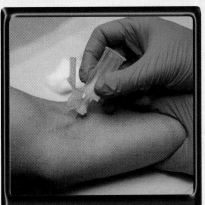

12 Puncture the vein. Align the needle, bevel up, with the vein and pierce the skin at a 15° to 30° angle.

(continues)

Obtain a Blood Specimen Using a Vacutainer (*continued*)

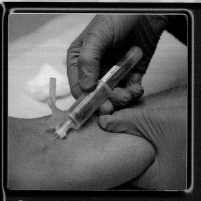

13 Attach the Vacutainer to the needle. Decrease the angle until almost parallel to the skin's surface, then pierce the vein wall. A faint give will be felt when the needle enters the vein, and blood will appear in the needle. If venipuncture is unsuccessful, pull the needle back slightly (not above the skin's surface), and redirect the needle toward the vein and try again. If still unsuccessful, release the constricting band. Place a 2″ × 2″ sponge over the site. Quickly withdraw the needle and instruct the patient to elevate the arm slightly, keeping the arm fully extended and applying pressure to the site for 2 to 3 minutes. Notify your supervisor before attempting again.

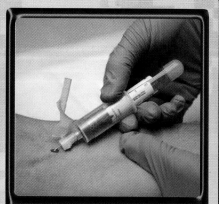

14 Collect a single specimen by holding the Vacutainer unit and needle steady with your dominant hand; place the collection tube against, but not through, the needle.

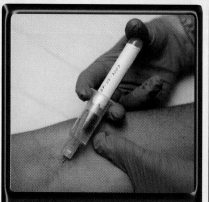

15 Place your index and middle fingers of your nondominant hand behind the flange of the Vacutainer. Push the tube as far forward as possible with the thumb of your nondominant hand without causing excessive movement.

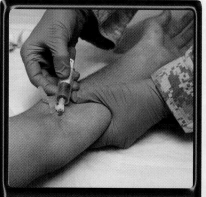

16 Instruct the patient to relax and unclench his or her fist after the blood has started flowing. When the tube is two thirds full of blood, prepare to withdraw the needle. Release the constricting band by pulling on the long end of the looped tubing with your nondominant hand.

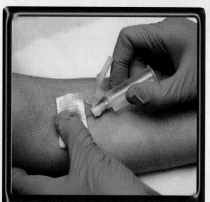

17 Place a 2″ × 2″ pad lightly over the venipuncture site. Withdraw the needle smoothly and quickly. Immediately apply pressure to the site with the 2″ × 2″ pad, keeping the patient's arm fully extended.

SKILL DRILL 23-1

Obtain a Blood Specimen Using a Vacutainer (*continued*)

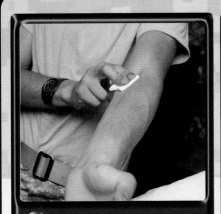

18 Instruct the patient to elevate his or her arm slightly, keeping the arm fully extended, and to apply firm manual pressure for 2 to 3 minutes.

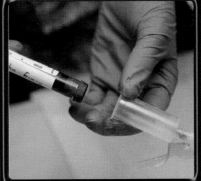

19 Remove the specimen tube from the Vacutainer.

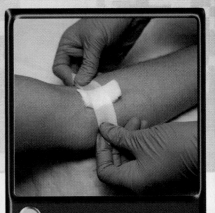

20 Apply an adhesive dressing to the venipuncture site after bleeding has stopped.

YOU ARE THE
COMBAT MEDIC

You are the combat medic on duty during sick call at the Battalion Aid Station. A soldier comes in and presents his documentation.

Assessment

He is trembling, sweating, and complaining of palpitations—classic symptoms of hypoglycemia (low blood glucose). After performing a complete patient assessment on this soldier, you report your findings to the medical officer (MO). The MO also suspects hypoglycemia and wants to test the patient's blood glucose levels. He requests that you draw the patient's blood.

Procedure

You verify his request and begin to collect the proper equipment for the venipuncture procedure. To evaluate the patient's blood glucose level, you select a green-topped specimen tube. The tube contains heparin to prevent clotting of the specimen. You stamp the labels with the patient's addressograph plate and apply them to the specimen tube.

Now you perform a patient care handwash and don sterile gloves. You verify the patient's identity by having him show you his ID card. You explain to the patient that you are going to draw a sample of his blood to test his blood glucose level. You advise him to look at a poster on the opposite wall if he has any needle phobias. The patient smiles and relaxes.

"Are you allergic to iodine or alcohol?" you ask as you position the patient in a sitting position. He shakes his head no and you continue with your preparations for the procedure. You place a protective pad underneath his extended elbow and forearm. He rolls his shirt sleeve up past his elbow for you, exposing the antecubital fossa. You palpate the arm, find the median cubital vein, and apply the constricting band.

After the patient clenches and unclenches his fist, you run your finger up and down the selected vein to assess its quality. It is a good vein, so you clean the patient's skin with an alcohol wipe. Once the skin is clean, you swiftly puncture the skin. You feel the faint give as the needle enters the vein—the venipuncture is a success.

Now you can continue and collect a blood specimen. You hold the Vacutainer sleeve and needle steady in your right hand and with your left hand, you place your index and middle fingers behind the flange of the Vacutainer. With your left thumb, you push the tube as far forward as possible.

"Relax and unclench your fist now," you instruct the patient. You release the constricting band and the specimen tube fills up with blood. When the tube is two thirds full, you grasp it firmly and remove it. Then you withdraw the needle from the patient's arm and apply a gauze pad over the puncture site.

"Are you all right?" you ask your patient as you elevate his arm and keep direct pressure on the puncture site. He gives you a wan smile and nods.

Ready for Review

- Venipuncture is the technique that permits access to a vein, usually to withdraw a blood specimen, initiate an intravenous infusion, or instill a medication.
- This skill is performed in the relative comfort and quiet of the garrison.

Vital Vocabulary

Vacutainer A device that connects to a catheter to assist with blood collection.

venipuncture The technique that permits access to a vein, usually to withdraw a blood specimen, initiate an intravenous infusion, or instill a medication.

COMBAT MEDIC *in Action*

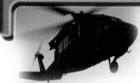

You are the combat medic on duty during sick call at the Battalion Aid Station. A soldier comes in and presents with signs of fatigue. After performing a thorough patient assessment, the exact cause of his fatigue is still unclear. You bring your findings to the MO. After listening to your report and reviewing the documentation, the MO wants to do a complete blood count on the patient.

1. What is the color of the top of the blood specimen tube you will use?
   - A. Red
   - B. Blue
   - C. Green
   - D. Lavender

2. Which vein could you use to draw the blood?
   - A. Median cubital vein
   - B. Cephalic vein
   - C. Basilic vein
   - D. All of the above

3. To pierce the skin, you hold the needle at a _____ angle to the skin.
   - A. 15º to 20º
   - B. 10º to 30º
   - C. 15º to 30º
   - D. 20º to 30º

4. You must notify your supervisor after _____ unsuccessful venipuncture attempts.
   - A. Two
   - B. Three
   - C. One
   - D. Four

5. After withdrawing the needle, the patient should keep his or her arm:
   - A. lowered.
   - B. elevated.
   - C. immobilized.
   - D. in traction.

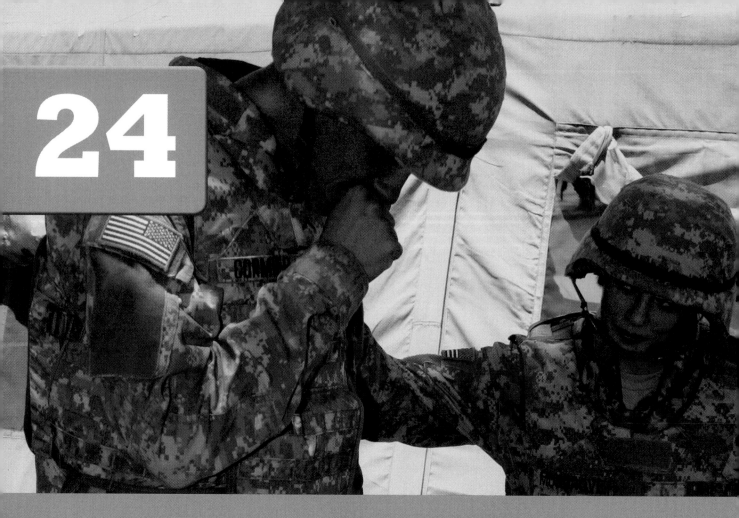

24

Respiratory Disorders

Objectives

Knowledge Objectives

- [ ] Describe the function of the respiratory system.
- [ ] Describe the anatomy of the respiratory system.

- [ ] Describe the physiology of respiration.
- [ ] Discuss pneumonia.
- [ ] Discuss asthma.
- [ ] Discuss upper respiratory infection.

Introduction

Coughing, shortness of breath, and difficulty breathing are all common symptoms seen in respiratory disorders. You must be able to recognize the signs and symptoms suggesting a respiratory disorder and possess the physical examination skills to identify the underlying condition. As a combat medic, you will treat common respiratory disorders within your scope of practice and you must know when to refer these soldiers to the medical officer for further evaluation.

Function of the Respiratory System

The respiratory system supplies oxygen to the individual tissue cells and removes their gaseous waste product (ie, carbon dioxide). Respiration has two components: external respiration and internal respiration. External respiration takes place only in the lungs, where oxygen from outside air enters the blood and carbon dioxide leaves the blood to be exhaled into the outside air. With internal respiration, gas exchange takes place between the blood and the body's cells, with oxygen leaving the blood and entering the cells at the same time that carbon dioxide is leaving the cells and entering the blood.

The primary components of the respiratory system are often compared to an inverted tree, with the trachea representing the tree's trunk and the **alveoli** resembling the tree's leaves. That is a nice analogy to get things started, but in reality a respiratory tree would have to branch 24 times and have nearly a billion leaves FIGURE 24-1 ▾. Imagine attempting to pull fluid from the ground into those leaves by exerting a negative pressure at the leaf ends, and you may begin to appreciate the complexities of breathing.

Respiratory System Anatomy Review

The Upper Airway

Air enters the upper airway primarily through the nares (nostrils) of the nose. The nares are lined with nasal hairs, which serve as filters that catch particulate matter in the air we breathe. The external nares are separated by the nasal septum. The nasal cavities are the two spaces located between the roof of the mouth and the cranium. They are covered with mucous membranes and contain many blood vessels. They also secrete a large amount of fluid (1 quart/day). Anyone with hay fever also can attest to the severe swelling that can occur in the nasal cavities.

The **sinuses** are small cavities lined with mucous membrane in the bones of the skull. They are open and drain into the nasal cavities. The sinuses are highly susceptible to infection.

At any given time, one nostril is usually more open than the other and would be the better choice for the insertion of a nasopharyngeal airway.

After passing through the nares, air is pulled over the **turbinates**. These ridges of tissue are covered with a mucous membrane and contain many blood vessels. Because of the many blood vessels, the turbinates easily swell (causing a stuffy nose) or bleed (**epistaxis**). The mucous membrane traps more particulate matter, and the large surface area of the turbinates warms and humidifies the air we breathe as the air passes over it. Processes such as intubation or a tracheotomy allow inhaled air to skip this trip through the nose, bypassing the humidification and filtering.

Quiet breathing typically allows air to flow through the nose FIGURE 24-2 ▸. Even people who breathe through their mouth usually have some nasal airflow. It is typically not necessary to tell patients that they must breathe through their nose when you apply a nasal cannula. Unless the nasal passages are actually swollen shut from edema or trauma, the cannula will function well.

The **pharynx** is divided into three parts: the nasopharynx, oropharynx, and laryngopharynx. The **nasopharynx** is the upper portion located immediately behind the nasal cavity and above the palate. The oropharynx is the middle section located between the palate and hyoid bone. The laryngopharynx is the lower section located below the hyoid bone, and is the transition point to the lower airway. The pharynx carries air into the respiratory system and carries food and liquids into the digestive system.

The **larynx** is an elastic membrane made of cartilage, moved by muscles, and lined with mucous membrane. It is located between the pharynx and the trachea, and is larger in males than in females. The vocal cords are located at the upper end of the larynx. They are set into motion by airflow from the lungs; the difference in size of the larynx makes the voice higher or lower.

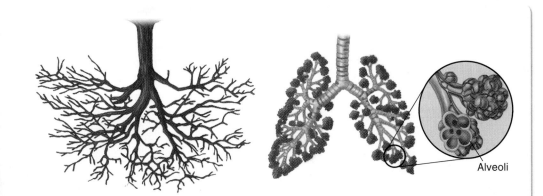

Alveoli

FIGURE 24-1 The tracheobronchial tree branches in much the same way as a tree, except that even the most branched tree has only half as many branchings as those inside the lung.

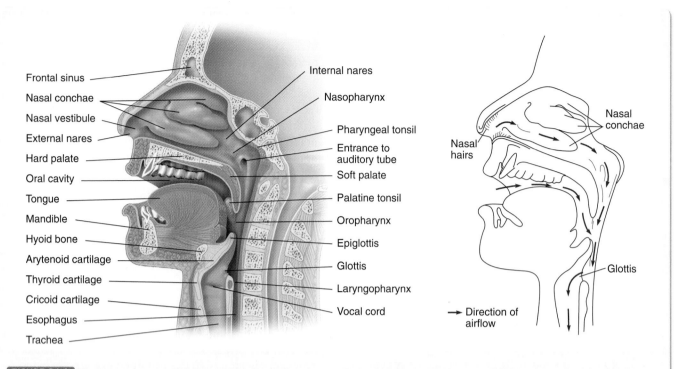

FIGURE 24-2 The upper airway contains many blood vessels and serves to heat and humidify the air we breathe. Note that an important filter is lost when we bypass the upper airway via intubation.

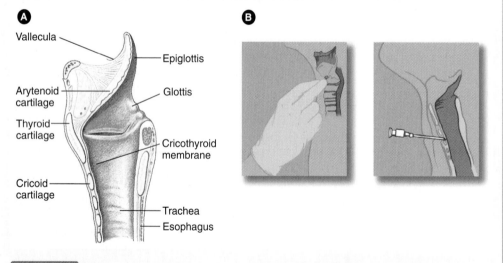

FIGURE 24-3 It is imperative that you completely understand the anatomy of the larynx in order to perform the most basic to the most advanced airway management skills. **A.** Anatomy of the larynx. **B.** Applying pressure to the cricoid cartilage, which compresses the esophagus while keeping the trachea open.

The **glottis** is the space between the vocal cords **FIGURE 24-3 ▲**. The glottis (hole) is covered by the epiglottis (leaf-shaped flap over the hole). Most of us were taught that the epiglottis covers the glottis like a trap door when we swallow, keeping food and liquid from entering the trachea. In reality, many people aspirate around their epiglottis, but others seem to swallow just fine even after their epiglottis has

been surgically removed. The glottis is lined with ciliated mucous membrane (thread-like projections that propel or sweep dust or mucus). The cilia trap dust and other particles, moving them upward to the larynx to be expelled by coughing.

The trachea is a tube that extends from the lower edge of the larynx to the upper part of the chest above the heart. It conducts air between the larynx and the lungs. A framework of C-shaped cartilage keeps it open. All of the open sections of the cartilage are posterior so the esophagus can bulge into this region while swallowing.

The **cricoid cartilage** can be palpated just below the thyroid cartilage in the neck. It forms a complete ring and maintains the trachea in an open position. Pressing on the anterior portion of this ring compresses the esophagus while keeping the trachea open. Applying pressure to the cricoid cartilage (Sellick maneuver) may be helpful in airway maintenance.

The small space between the thyroid and cricoid cartilages is the **cricothyroid membrane**. The membrane does not contain many blood vessels and is covered by only skin and minimal subcutaneous tissue. It is a potential site for performing a cricothyrotomy (an incision through the skin and cricothyroid membrane to relieve difficulty breathing caused by an obstruction in the airway). The rest of the neck contains large blood vessels, important nerves, and other critical anatomic structures that you must avoid cutting when performing a cricothyrotomy. Cricothyrotomies look easy when performed by skilled clinicians, but this procedure can turn into a bloody disaster if you are not absolutely certain of anatomic landmarks.

Trauma or swelling of any of the laryngeal structures can create a life-threatening airway obstruction. In the worst-case scenario, this entire anatomic region may be bypassed by a tracheotomy (a surgical opening into the trachea). By their very nature, traumatic injuries may alter the typical anatomy of the upper airway. Procedures such as a cricothyrotomy can prove highly challenging when the airway is filled with blood and vomit, and the anatomic landmarks are obscured by swelling or subcutaneous air.

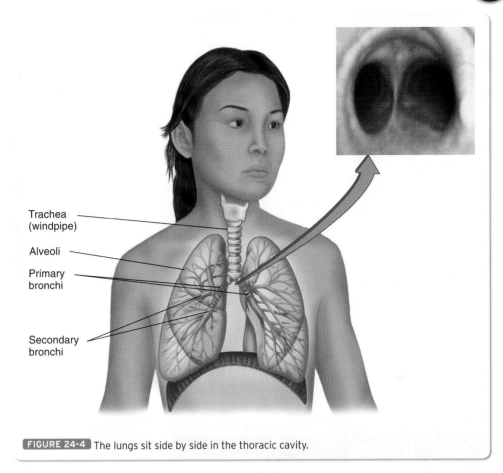

Trachea (windpipe)

Alveoli

Primary bronchi

Secondary bronchi

FIGURE 24-4 The lungs sit side by side in the thoracic cavity.

The Lower Airway

The trachea branches off into two bronchi that enter the lungs. These passageways bring air to the alveoli. The right bronchus is considerably larger in diameter than the left, and also extends downward in a more vertical direction than the left. The right bronchus is larger and straighter than the left, which increases the likelihood of inhaling foreign material or intubating the right bronchus. The notch or depression where the bronchus enters the lung is called the long hilus.

The lungs are extremely thin and delicate tissues. This is where external respiration takes place. Two lungs sit side by side in the thoracic cavity **FIGURE 24-4 ▲**. They are two cone-shaped structures with the bases lying on the diaphragm. The right lung is divided by fissures (clefts) into three lobes: superior, middle, and inferior. The left lung is subdivided into two lobes: superior and inferior.

The bronchial tree is the subdivision of the bronchus. Bronchioles are the smallest division of the bronchi. The terminal bronchioles are attached to the alveoli, which are clusters of air sacs resembling a bunch of grapes. **Surfactant** is a substance that prevents the alveoli from collapsing by reducing the surface tension of the fluids that line them. Gas exchange takes place as blood passes through the capillaries

Garrison Care TIPS

The lungs contain about three times more lung tissue than is necessary for life.

around the alveoli. Due to its number of air spaces, a lung is very lightweight, and if removed would float in water.

Lungs occupy a considerable portion of the thoracic cavity and are separated from the abdominal cavity by the diaphragm. The pleura is a double sac of serous membrane enveloping each lung. The **parietal pleura** is the portion of the pleura that lines the thoracic cavity. The **visceral pleura** is the portion that encloses the surface of the lung.

The **mediastinum** is the region between the lungs. It contains the heart, great blood vessels, esophagus, trachea, and lymph nodes. The pleural space is the space between the two membranes of the parietal and visceral pleura.

■ Physiology of Respiration

The physiology of respiration is accomplished through pressure changes in the lungs. It occurs in two phases: inhalation and exhalation **FIGURE 24-5 ▶**. **Inhalation** is an active process. Inspiration is the contraction of the respiratory system muscles. The diaphragm flattens and drops down. The intercostal muscles contract, causing the ribs and sternum to move

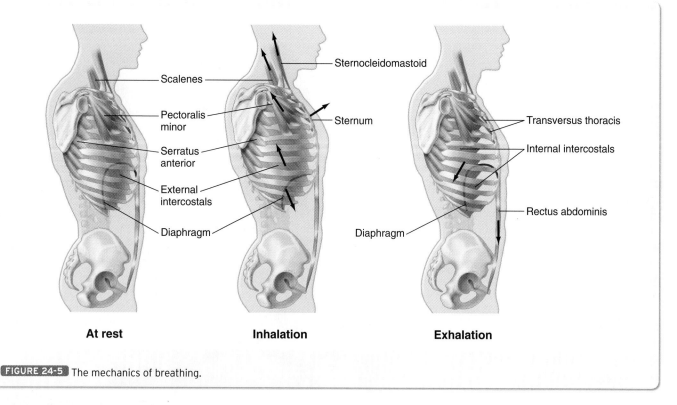

At rest **Inhalation** **Exhalation**

FIGURE 24-5 The mechanics of breathing.

up and out. The enlargement of the thorax causes pressure in the lungs to fall and pulls air into the lungs. In contrast, **exhalation** is a passive process. The respiratory muscles relax and the diaphragm moves upward. The chest wall relaxes; the intrathoracic pressure rises; and air is pushed out of the lungs.

Alveoli supply oxygen to the blood and remove carbon dioxide from the blood. This exchange is made by **diffusion** across the cell wall of the alveoli and capillaries. As you may recall from earlier chapters, diffusion is the natural migration of molecules from an area of greater concentration to an area of lesser concentration.

Normal respiratory drive depends on the level of carbon dioxide in the blood. When blood circulates through active tissue, it receives carbon dioxide. The blood circulated through the respiratory center in the brain stem (medulla oblongata and pons) senses increased carbon dioxide in the blood and increases the respiratory rate. A person performing vigorous exercise breathes more deeply and quickly to cope with the need for more oxygen. The larger the volume of air that moves into and out of the lungs, the more carbon dioxide is eliminated.

The amount of oxygen in the blood is directly proportional to the amount of oxygen delivered to the alveoli. Fluid in the alveoli, such as occurs with pneumonia or a pulmonary contusion, may prevent adequate oxygen exchange. Fluid accumulation in the lungs may be due to such pulmonary problems as pulmonary edema from heart failure, toxic inhalations, or drowning. The alveoli may be collapsed (atelectasis), thereby preventing adequate oxygenation of blood. Alveoli may also collapse from external forces such as pneumothorax or a flail chest, or from internal causes such as secretions plugging the airways or an ineffective cough.

■ Respiratory Disorders

Pneumonia

Pneumonia is inflammation of the lung caused by a reaction to an invading microorganism or noxious substance. It usually results in consolidation, which is the accumulation of fluid in a lung lobe. It is the sixth leading medical cause of death in the United States. When trying to determine the likely causes of pneumonia, you must consider where and how patients acquired it and what other medical problems, if any, they may have. These considerations are important because of the different types of infectious agents that cause pneumonia. Bacterial causes are common in young adults whereas viruses are the common cause in infants and young children.

During the focused history and physical exam, obtain a patient history. Symptoms of pneumonia include:

- A frequent productive cough with purulent sputum (green, brown, rusty colored)
- Chest pain, pleuritic (worse with a cough or a deep breath)

- Shortness of breath (SOB) at rest
- Malaise, lethargy
- Poor appetite

Perform a physical exam and look for the following signs:

- Fever, occasionally with shaking chills
- Tachycardia
- Tachypnea (may or may not be present)
- Respiratory distress, which may consist of any or all of the following:
  - Abnormal breath sounds: rhonchi, rales, wheezing
  - Abnormal pulse oximetry (< 95% oxygen saturation)
  - Use of accessory muscles
  - Patient experiences the sensation of SOB

The red flags of pneumonia include shortness of breath and a fever over 101°F. Treatment of pneumonia begins with administering aspirin or acetaminophen for the fever. Administer a decongestant like pseudoephedrine; do not give antihistamines because they can solidify secretions. Administer cough suppressants if the patient has trouble sleeping at night. Have the patient increase his or her fluid intake. Antibiotics are the mainstay of treatment, which requires the consult of a medical officer. Bronchodilators, such as the albuterol inhaler, may be administered to assist in breathing. Consider bed rest and evacuate the patient if you are in the field environment. Record all treatments in the patient's medical record. Seek the advice and assistance of a higher medical authority whenever possible.

Asthma

Asthma is a disorder of the tracheobronchial tree characterized by mild to severe obstruction of airflow. Symptoms vary in each patient. Symptoms may be episodic, paroxysmal, or persistent. The clinical hallmark is wheezing, but a chronic cough may be the predominant symptom. Acute symptoms result from narrowing of large and small airways due to spasm of bronchial smooth muscle, edema, inflammation of the bronchial mucosa, and the production of excessive mucus.

The trigger of the obstructive elements of asthma is the hyper-reactivity or hyper-responsiveness of the airway. This manifests as an exaggerated bronchoconstrictor response to many different stimuli. The degree of hyper-responsiveness is closely linked to the extent of inflammation and the severity of the disease. Precipitating factors may be the following:

- Emotional upsets
- Physical exertion (usually begins within 3 minutes after the end of exercise)
- Cold weather
- Upper respiratory infection (URI)
- Allergens such as pollen, mold, house dust, animal dander, smoke, etc.

During the focused history and physical exam, obtain a patient history, which may vary widely from mild to life-threatening asthma attacks. Symptoms may include:

- Shortness of breath after exercise or upon awakening
- History of wheezing

- Chronic cough (usually nonproductive)
- May be exacerbated by certain triggers
- Nocturnal attacks
- Chest tightness

Perform a physical exam, looking for the following signs:

- Wheezing is the hallmark of asthma, which may be mild or severe.
- The expiratory phase is prolonged.
- There is accessory muscle use with retractions.
- Tachycardia is present.
- Blood oxygenation is decreased (check with pulse oximeter).

The red flags of asthma include SOB, severe wheezing, and accessory muscle use. Treatment for an acute asthma attack begins with administering an inhaled bronchial dilator such as albuterol (either metered-dose inhaler or nebulizer). Administer intravenous fluids and supplemental oxygen. Refer this patient to the medical officer. Evacuate immediately if you and the patient are in the field environment. Record all treatment in the patient's medical record. Seek the advice and assistance of a higher medical authority whenever possible.

Upper Respiratory Infection

An upper respiratory infection is an acute, usually afebrile, viral infection of the respiratory tract, with inflammation in any or all airways, including the nose, paranasal sinuses, throat, larynx, and often the trachea and bronchi. During the focused history and physical exam, obtain a patient history. Look for the following symptoms:

- Nasal congestion
- Sore throat
- Cough (productive or nonproductive)
- Hoarseness
- Malaise
- Fatigue
- Headache
- Sinus pressure

Perform a physical examination. Look for the following signs:

- **Eyes:** Conjunctiva infected, increased lacrimation.
- **Ears:** Tympanic membrane (TM) may be infected; moves poorly with the Valsalva maneuver. The Valsalva maneuver is performed by having the patient close his or her mouth, pinch the nostrils closed, and gently attempt to blow air out of his or her closed nostrils. If the Eustachian tubes are not blocked with the middle ear fluid/congestion, you will see the TM move while observing through an otoscope.
- **Nose:** Mucoid or purulent nasal discharge, swollen mucous membranes, or decreased air movement.
- **Throat:** Oropharynx infected; tonsillar pillars may be swollen with or without exudate.
- **Neck:** Supple, tender to palpation, lymph nodes usually in the anterior chain.

- **Chest:** Lungs may be clear or have scattered rhonchi or mild wheezing; usually no retractions or accessory muscle use.
- **Vital signs:** Temperature, normal to low-grade (100°F to 101°F) fever

The red flags of something potentially more serious than an upper respiratory infection include:

- Fever > 101°F
- SOB
- Productive cough with chest pain
- Tonsillar swelling with exudates
- Pain when touching chin to chest
- Difficulty swallowing saliva

Treatment is symptomatic. Administer decongestants, throat lozenges, cough syrup, acetaminophen, increased fluids, and rest. Record all treatment in the patient's medical record. Seek the advice and assistance of a higher medical authority whenever possible.

■ Summary

Respiratory disorders are common, and your ability to recognize and accurately assess, treat, and/or refer for treatment is crucial. Early diagnosis and treatment will reduce the amount of time that soldiers are unable to perform their duties due to illnesses.

YOU ARE THE
COMBAT MEDIC

Insurgents have been targeting oil pipelines in your area. While the majority of their attacks have been prevented, one attack tore a hole in a pipeline and started a massive fire. The fire sent large, black, toxic clouds into the air. Although your garrison is miles away from the fires, the air around you does feel heavier and less clean.

Assessment

You are on duty during sick call at the Battalion Aid Station (BAS). A soldier comes into the BAS complaining of shortness of breath. You take him aside to perform a thorough patient assessment.

After taking the patient's information, you take the patient's vital signs. His temperature is 98.5°F, his pulse rate is 110 beats/min, his respiration rate is 28 breaths/min, his blood pressure is 108/54 mm Hg, and his oxygen saturation is 75%.

The patient states that his chief complaint is shortness of breath. Using the OPQRST mnemonic, you learn more about the history of the patient's chief complaint. The night before, he was kept awake by an annoying chronic cough. When he woke up this morning, the patient found that he couldn't quite catch his breath. While he has never experienced an asthma attack, his brother frequently has attacks during the winter.

While he is answering your questions, you notice that the patient is wheezing and his exhalations are prolonged. Combined with his tachycardia and decreased blood oxygenation, you suspect that this patient is experiencing an asthma attack due to the increased pollution in the air. You refer this patient to the medical officer for further assessment and care.

Aid Kit

Ready for Review

- As a combat medic, you will treat common respiratory disorders within your scope of practice, and you must know when to refer these soldiers to the medical officer for further evaluation.
- The respiratory system supplies oxygen to individual tissue cells and removes their gaseous waste product (ie, carbon dioxide).
- The physiology of respiration is accomplished through pressure changes in the lungs. It occurs in two phases: inhalation and exhalation.
- Pneumonia is inflammation of the lung caused by a reaction to an invading microorganism or noxious substance.
- Asthma is a disorder of the tracheobronchial tree characterized by mild to severe obstruction of airflow.
- An upper respiratory infection is an acute, usually afebrile, viral infection of the respiratory tract, with inflammation in any or all airways, including the nose, paranasal sinuses, throat, larynx, and often the trachea and bronchi.

Vital Vocabulary

alveoli Balloon-like clusters of single-layer air sacs that are the functional site for the exchange of oxygen and carbon dioxide in the lungs.

cricoid cartilage Forms the lowest portion of the larynx; also referred to as the cricoid ring. It is the first ring of the trachea and is the only upper airway structure that forms a complete ring.

cricothyroid membrane A thin, superficial membrane located between the thyroid and cricoid cartilages that is relatively avascular and contains few nerves; the site for emergency surgical and nonsurgical access to the airway.

diffusion Movement of a gas from an area of higher concentration to an area of lower concentration.

epistaxis Nosebleed.

exhalation Passive movement of air out of the lungs.

glottis The space between the vocal cords that is the narrowest portion of the adult's airway; also called the glottic opening.

inhalation The active process of moving air into the lungs.

larynx A complex structure formed by many independent cartilaginous structures that all work together; where the upper airway ends and the lower airway begins.

mediastinum The region between the lungs that contains the heart, great blood vessels, esophagus, trachea, and lymph nodes.

nasopharynx The nasal cavity; formed by the union of the facial bones.

parietal pleura Thin membrane that lines the chest cavity.

pharynx Throat.

sinuses Cavities formed by the cranial bones that trap contaminants and keep them from entering the respiratory tract and act as tributaries for fluid to and from the eustachian tubes and tear ducts.

surfactant A proteinaceous substance that lines the alveoli; decreases alveolar surface tension and keeps the alveoli expanded.

turbinates Three bony shelves that protrude from the lateral walls of the nasal cavity and extend into the nasal passageway, parallel to the nasal floor; serve to increase the surface area of the nasal mucosa, thereby improving the processes of warming, filtering, and humidifying inhaled air.

visceral pleura Thin membrane that lines the lungs.

COMBAT MEDIC *in Action*

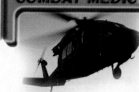

You are the combat medic on duty during sick call at the Battalion Aid Station. A soldier comes in with a cough that will not go away. During the focused history and physical exam, you learn that the soldier is coughing up green sputum. When he tries to take a breath, his chest hurts. "I just don't have any energy," he complains.

1. Physical signs of pneumonia include:
   - A. fever, occasionally with shaking chills.
   - B. tachycardia.
   - C. tachypnea.
   - D. all of the above.

2. Treatment of pneumonia begins with:
   - A. administering IV fluids.
   - B. administering ephedrine.
   - C. placing the patient in the shock position.
   - D. administering aspirin or acetaminophen for fever.

3. True or false? A patient with pneumonia may return immediately to duty.
   - A. True, after a dose of aspirin, the fever will disappear.
   - B. False, the patient needs bed rest to recover.
   - C. True, the patient needs lots of physical exercise to recover.
   - D. False, the patient needs to be isolated.

4. In adults, pneumonia is most often caused by:
   - A. bacteria.
   - B. viruses.
   - C. smoke.
   - D. dander.

5. Additional medications to be given to the patient include:
   - A. pseudoephedrine.
   - B. antihistamines.
   - C. albuterol.
   - D. both A and C.

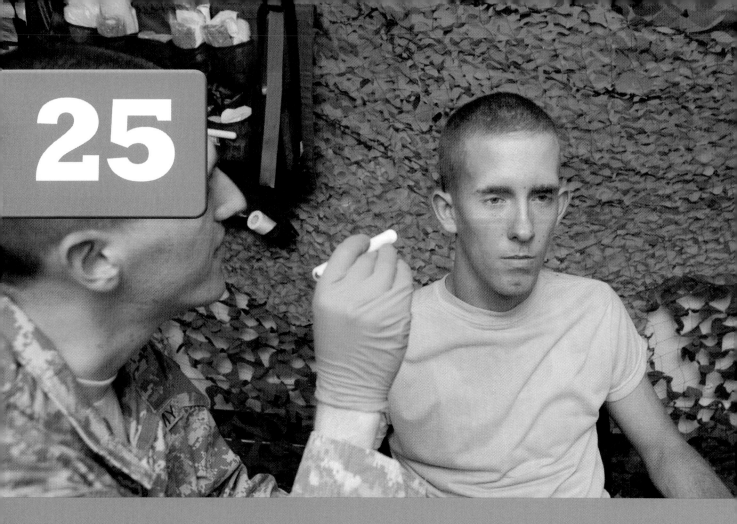

25

Eye, Ear, Nose, and Throat Care

Objectives

Knowledge Objectives

- Describe the anatomy of the eyes, ears, nose, sinuses, mouth, and throat.

- Describe the physical examination of the eye.

- Describe the physical examination of the ear.

- Describe the physical examination of the nose and sinuses.

- Describe the physical examination of the mouth and throat.

- Describe common eye, ear, nose, and throat complaints.

Skills Objectives

- Perform a visual acuity test.

■ Introduction

As a combat medic, you will need to attend to patients with eye, ear, nose, and throat (EENT) complaints. Although these complaints are commonplace, it's important to be able to recognize the red flags of more serious conditions as they present themselves. This chapter is designed to provide an overview of a basic EENT physical examination and to present some of the most common EENT conditions routinely seen by physicians and physician assistants in clinics, Battalion Aid Stations (BAS), and troop medical clinics (TMC) today.

■ Anatomy Review

The Eye

The **sclera** is the tough layer, or the white of the eye, that protects the inner structure of the eye and helps to maintain its shape **FIGURE 25-1 ▶**. It is connected to six muscles that allow the eye to look up, down, and side to side. The **conjunctiva** is the mucous membrane that lines the eyelid and extends from the eyelid to the front of the eyeball. It covers the anterior portion of the sclera. The **retina** is the inner layer of the eye. It contains the rods and cones, the receptors of vision that allow us to see images. The retina is a continuation of the optic nerve. The **cornea** is tough, transparent, and colorless. It covers the pupil and iris. Injuries may cause opacity in the cornea and stop light rays from entering the eye.

The **lens** is a circular structure filled with a jelly-like substance that adjusts to focus on both near and far away objects. The **iris** is the colored part of the eye. It is located between the cornea and lens and controls the amount of light entering the eye. The **pupil** is the circular opening in the iris. It is the window of the eye through which light passes to the lens and the retina. **Lacrimal glands** are the tear glands located in the upper-outer aspect of each upper eyelid **FIGURE 25-2 ▶**. They prevent infections, moisten the eye, and drain through ducts located in the eyelids.

The Ear

The external ear is made of the **auricle** or pinna **FIGURE 25-3 ▶**. The auricle is shaped to collect sound waves and direct them toward the external auditory meatus (opening to the ear canal).

The middle ear is an air-filled cavity within the temporal bone of the skull containing three **ossicles** (small bones): the malleus (hammer), incus (anvil), and stapes. The tympanic membrane (TM), or eardrum, is a thin, translucent (see-through) membrane. Sound vibrations from the environment travel through the external auditory canal (EAC), causing movement of the TM, which in turn causes movement of the ossicles to continue transference of the sound. The TM separates the external and middle ear.

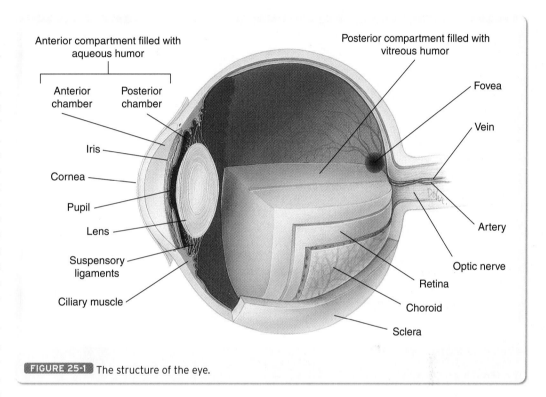

FIGURE 25-1 The structure of the eye.

Anterior compartment filled with aqueous humor
Anterior chamber
Posterior chamber
Iris
Cornea
Pupil
Lens
Suspensory ligaments
Ciliary muscle
Posterior compartment filled with vitreous humor
Fovea
Vein
Artery
Optic nerve
Retina
Choroid
Sclera

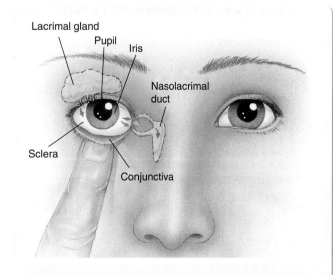

FIGURE 25-2 The lacrimal system consists of tear glands and ducts. Tears act as lubricants and keep the anterior part of the eye from drying.

Lacrimal gland
Pupil
Iris
Nasolacrimal duct
Sclera
Conjunctiva

The eustachian tube (auditory tube) drains the middle ear to the nasopharynx. Upper respiratory infections (URIs) or head colds commonly result in mucus build-up in the eustachian tube, possibly causing some hearing loss during the course of the infection.

The inner ear is a membranous curved cavity inside a bony labyrinth consisting of the cochlea (involved in hearing), the semicircular canals (involved in balance), and the vestibule (also involved in balance). Movement of the head stimulates the balance receptors in the inner ear.

The Nose and Sinuses

The nose is formed of bone and cartilage and is covered with skin. The nares are the bilateral anterior openings of the nose. The frontal and maxillary bones form the nasal bridge. The nose is covered by a vascular mucous membrane thickly lined with small hairs and mucous secretions. **Paranasal sinuses** are air-filled, paired extensions of the nasal cavity within the bones of the skull FIGURE 25-4 ▸ . Other sinuses include the maxillary sinus, frontal sinus, ethmoid sinus, and sphenoid sinus.

The Mouth and Throat

The functions of the mouth and throat include:

- Emission of air for vocalization and non-nasal inspiration
- Passageway for food, liquid, and saliva
- Initiation of digestion by masticating (chewing) foods and by salivary secretions
- Identification of taste

The tongue, teeth, mouth, and gums are located in the anterior portion of the oropharynx. The vestibule is the space between the buccal mucosa and the outer surface of the teeth and gums.

■ Assessment

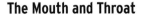

Ocular Complaints

Ocular injuries are classified as penetrating or nonpenetrating. A penetrating injury would include debris embedded in the eye. A nonpenetrating injury would include a chemical burn to the eye (see Chapter 7: *Head Injuries*). Trauma can lead to serious damage and the possible loss of vision for the soldier. Eye injuries are common in spite of protection of the eye by the bony orbit.

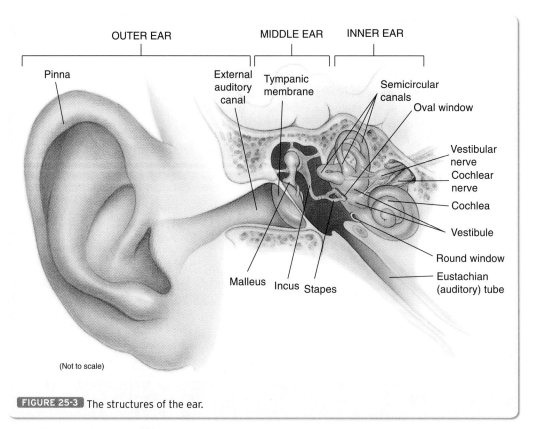

FIGURE 25-3 The structures of the ear.

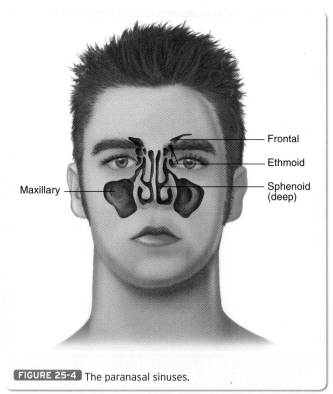

FIGURE 25-4 The paranasal sinuses.

During the focused history and physical exam, obtain the patient's history. An accurate history assists you in establishing a possible cause for the eye problem. Determine the mechanism of injury. If there is a patient history of injury, determine whether it was blunt trauma or penetrating injury. Was there a projectile or missile injury? Was the eye injured by glass from a motor vehicle accident, or was it a thermal, chemical, or laser burn? Does the patient wear glasses or contact lenses? Is there a history of eye disease or previous eye trauma or surgery? Is there eye pain or loss of vision? If there is vision loss, is it in one eye or both?

Perform a physical examination on the patient. Ensure that you have adequate lighting and avoid putting pressure on the globe while performing the physical examination. Determining the soldier's visual acuity is the most important step in evaluating ocular problems. For chemical burns to the eyes, immediately perform DCAP-BTLS and not the visual acuity test (see Chapter 7: *Head Injuries*). Screen visual acuity with any available printed material if you are in the field. If the patient is unable to read print, have the patient count your raised fingers or distinguish between light and dark. In the garrison, screen the patient utilizing a standard Snellen chart (eye chart).

The Snellen visual acuity test measures the smallest letters that a soldier can read from a standardized chart at a distance of 20′. This test measures distance vision and is performed initially on all patients presenting with an eye complaint, except for ocular burns. In children and the elderly, this test may be performed routinely to screen for any visual problems. To perform the Snellen visual acuity test, follow the steps in SKILL DRILL 25-1 ▶:

1. Position the patient 20′ away from the Snellen chart, making certain the area is well lit (**Step ①**).

2. Test each eye individually by covering one eye with an opaque card or gauze, being careful to avoid applying pressure to the eye.

3. Ask the patient to identify all of the letters beginning at the 20/20 vision level. If the patient can read this line, then no further distance vision testing is required for this eye. If the patient cannot read the 20/20 line, determine the smallest line on which the patient can identify more than half of the letters. Record the visual acuity designated by that line. One technique is to ask the patient to cover one eye and then read the smallest line that he or she can from left to right. Then have the patient cover the other eye and read the smallest line that he or she can from right to left. This reduces the chance the patient is merely memorizing the letters with a good eye and reciting them as you attempt to assess an injured eye. The abbreviation for the left eye is OS; for the right eye it is OD; for example, "V/A 20/20 OS, 20/40 OD uncorrected" (**Step ②**).

4. After testing the eyes individually, have the patient uncover both eyes and test both eyes at the same time. The abbreviation for both eyes is OU; for example, "V/A 20/20 OU uncorrected."

5. If a patient has corrective lenses, test him or her without glasses initially and then with the patient's glasses on. Do not forget to consider whether the patient may be wearing contact lenses. If he or she is wearing lenses, either have the patient remove the

TABLE 25-1	Levels of Vision
Acuity Level	**Description**
20/20	Normal vision. The fighter pilot minimum; the vision required to read numbers in a telephone book.
20/40	Able to pass a driver's license test in most states; most printed material is at this level.
20/80	Able to read an alarm clock at 10′; news headlines are this size.
20/200	Legal blindness; able to see stop sign letters.

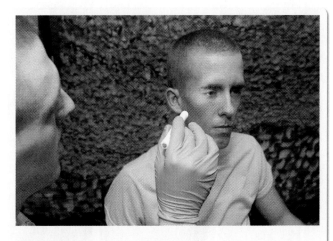

FIGURE 25-5 Hold a penlight at an oblique angle to the eye and move the light slowly across the cornea.

contact lenses or document that the patient's obtained visual acuity is corrected (**Step ③**).

Distance vision acuity is recorded as a fraction. The numerator indicates the distance from the chart (20′); the denominator indicates the distance from which the normal eye can read the line. Thus, 20/200 means that the patient can read at 20′ what the average person can read at 200′. TABLE 25-1 ▲ lists the common levels of vision.

After performing the visual acuity test, note any drainage or bleeding from the eye. Inspect the eyelid's ability to open wide and close completely. Inspect the eyelids for edema, discoloration, and foreign bodies. Inspect the position of the eyelids in relationship to the eyeballs. Ask the patient to look upward as you pull down the lower lid. Observe the patient's conjunctiva (pink to dark pink is normal) for erythema or **exudates** (pus). Note the color of the sclera; white is normal. Patients who have darker pigmented skin may have scattered areas of brown pigment as a normal finding in the sclera, and this observation should be noted.

The cornea should be clear and avascular (not bloodshot). Ask the patient to look straight ahead. Hold a penlight at an oblique angle to the eye and move the light slowly across the cornea FIGURE 25-5 ▲. Inspect the cornea for

Perform a Visual Acuity Test

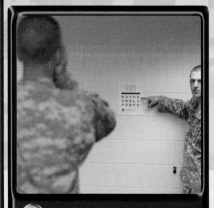

1 Position the patient 20′ away from the Snellen chart, making certain the area is well lit.

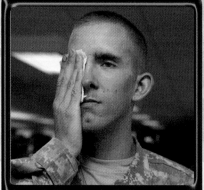

2 Test each eye individually by covering one eye with an opaque card or gauze, being careful to avoid applying pressure to the eye. Ask the patient to identify all of the letters beginning at the 20/20 vision level. If the patient can read this line, no further far vision testing is required for this eye. If the patient cannot read the 20/20 line, determine the smallest line on which the patient can identify more than half of the letters. Record the visual acuity designated by that line.

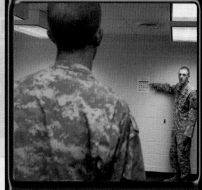

3 After testing each eye individually, have the patient uncover both eyes and test both eyes at the same time. If a patient has corrective lenses, test them without glasses initially and then with the patient's glasses on.

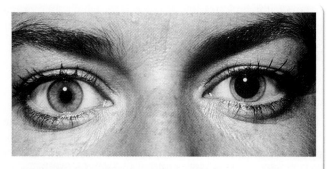

FIGURE 25-6 Assess the pupil size. Unequal pupil size may signal a serious problem.

clarity—it should be transparent, shiny, and smooth. Note any opacity (cloudy areas) in the lenses that may be visible through the pupil.

Note any irregularity in the shape of the pupils **FIGURE 25-6 ▲**. The pupils should be equal, round, regular,

and reactive to light (PERRL). Unequal size of the pupils (anisocoria) may be congenital. Approximately 20% of normal people have minor or noticeable differences in pupil size, but their reflexes should remain normal. Differences in pupil size also can be caused by eye medication.

Test the patient's pupillary reaction to light both directly and consensually. Dim the lights in the room so that the patient's pupils dilate. Do not shine the light into both eyes simultaneously. Shine a penlight directly into one eye and observe the pupil's constriction. Note the consensual reaction of the opposite pupil constricting simultaneously with the tested pupil.

Ear Examination

The physical examination of the ear consists of inspection, palpation, and an otoscopic examination of the ear. Inspect the ear size, shape, symmetry, landmarks, and color. Palpate the auricle for tenderness and swelling. Inspect the external auditory canal (EAC) for discharge.

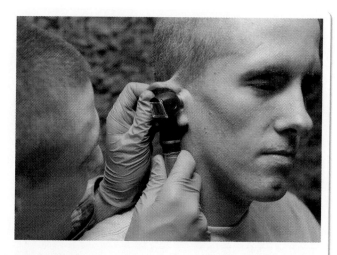

FIGURE 25-7 The otoscope is used to inspect the EAC and the middle ear.

The otoscope is used to inspect the EAC and the middle ear **FIGURE 25-7 ▲**. Use the largest speculum the ear canal will accommodate. Visualize the ear canal as you insert the speculum. Pull the auricle back and out and slowly insert the speculum, noting discharge, lesions, narrowing of the EAC, foreign bodies, or presence of cerumen (wax). Stabilize your examining hand against the patient's head to prevent injury. If the TM is obscured by cerumen, the canal can be cleaned by warm water irrigation. If you suspect perforation of the TM or if the auditory canal is filled with blood or discharge, it should never be irrigated. Consult with the medical officer prior to ear irrigation.

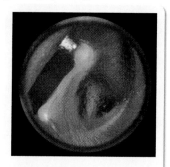

FIGURE 25-8 A healthy TM may be pearly gray to amber in color.

The TM should have no perforations. Look for air bubbles, air/fluid levels, or scarring. A healthy TM may be pearly gray to amber in color; redness indicates an infectious process **FIGURE 25-8 ◄**.

The inner ear is tested by evaluating the patient's hearing. Gross hearing testing begins when the patient responds or fails to respond to your questions. Complete hearing evaluations are performed through audiology services.

Nose and Sinus Examination

Inspect the external structure of the nose for shape, size, symmetry, color, and presence of deformities or lesions. The skin should be smooth without swelling and conform to the skin color of the patient's face. Palpate the external nose for tenderness, swelling, or masses. Inspect the frontal and maxillary sinus area for swelling. Palpate the frontal and maxillary sinuses for tenderness.

Mouth Examination

Inspect and palpate the lips for symmetry, color, edema, and surface abnormalities. The color of the patient's lips should be pink and have vertical and horizontal symmetry. Have the patient remove any dental appliances and open his or her mouth partially. Use a tongue blade and bright light to inspect the buccal mucosa, teeth, and gums. The mucous membrane should look pinkish-red, smooth, and moist. The gums should have a pink appearance with a clearly defined, tight margin at each tooth. The gum surface beneath the dentures should be free of inflammation, swelling, or bleeding.

Inspect and count the patient's teeth, noting cavities, ulcerations, lesions, or missing teeth. The tongue should appear dull red, moist, and glistening and should be smooth with increasing roughness. Ask the patient to tilt his or her head back for you to inspect the pinker soft palate and uvula. The whitish hard palate should be dome-shaped.

■ Eye, Ear, Nose, and Throat (EENT) Assessment

To perform an eye, ear, nose, and throat (EENT) assessment, follow these steps:

1. Identify the patient and explain the procedure to the patient.
2. Perform a patient care handwash.
3. Have the patient sit in a chair or on an examination table.
4. Inspect the patient's external ear anatomy.
5. Palpate the patient's outer ear for tenderness. Gently pull on the ear lobe and the outer ear to evaluate for tenderness in the patient's ear.
6. Insert an otoscope with a speculum a few millimeters into the external auditory canal (EAC) while gently pulling on the outer ear in a posterior direction. Inspect for abnormalities of the EAC or tympanic membrane (TM).
7. Have patient perform the Valsalva maneuver. While still observing the TM with the otoscope, have the patient pinch his or her nose closed and close his or her mouth. Then instruct the patient to gently blow air into the nose. Observe the TM for subtle movement, which is a normal finding.
8. Assess the visual acuity of the patient by performing Skill Drill 25-1.
9. Inspect the patient's eyelids for any abnormalities (swelling, drainage, etc.).
10. With clean hands, gently pull the patient's lower eyelid downward and inspect the conjunctiva and sclera for redness, drainage, or a foreign body. Use your free hand to shine light from an ophthalmoscope into the eye being examined.
11. With clean hands, gently pull the patient's upper eyelid upward and inspect the conjunctiva and sclera

for redness, drainage, or a foreign body. Use your free hand to shine a light from an ophthalmoscope into the patient's eye.

12. Inspect the pupil of each eye for size and shape.

13. Shine a light into each eye, one at a time, and note the reactivity of the patient's pupils to light.

14. Inspect the patient's exterior nose for obvious deformity, such as bleeding.

15. Using the same speculum that was used on the patient's ears, gently insert the otoscope 2 to 3 millimeters into each nostril. Note any congestion, swelling, discharge, bleeding, or discoloration in the patient's nostril.

16. Have the patient protrude his or her tongue as he or she says, "Ahh." Inspect the oropharynx with the otoscope light. Use the tongue depressor to move the patient's tongue out of your way if necessary. Note any discoloration, swelling, lesions, or discharge in the patient's throat. Note the midline movement of the uvula.

17. Inspect the patient's neck for obvious masses or lumps.

18. Palpate under the patient's jaw line and over the patient's neck muscles for any tenderness or enlarged lymph nodes.

19. Record your findings in the appropriate area of the SF-600.

■ Common EENT Disease Complaints

Eye

A red eye can be a sign and symptom of a variety of abnormalities of the eye. Infection, allergies, drugs, chemical exposure, trauma, or systemic disease may cause a red, painful eye. Eye discharge is mainly associated with viral or bacterial conjunctivitis. Loss of vision should *always* be considered a medical emergency.

With a foreign body (FB) in the eye, the patient usually presents with a history of injury and the sensation that something is in the eye. **Conjunctivitis** simply refers to inflammation of the conjunctiva. It can be due to chemical irritation, infections, or allergies. Vision is generally not affected except in cases of chemical irritation. The treatment will depend on the cause.

With chemical conjunctivitis, there is usually a history of a chemical splash in the eye(s). Treatment requires immediate irrigation. Allergic conjunctivitis usually affects both eyes (OU), with the patient commonly complaining of watery, itchy eyes. Patients may have associated sneezing and watery nasal discharge. The patient usually has a history of similar episodes. Bacterial conjunctivitis usually starts in one eye and may spread to the other eye. The sclera and conjunctivae are commonly reddened with a purulent (pus-like) discharge **FIGURE 25-9 ▶**. Viral conjunctivitis usually starts in one eye and may spread to both eyes. The sclera and conjunctivae are commonly reddened with a clear, watery discharge **FIGURE 25-10 ▶**.

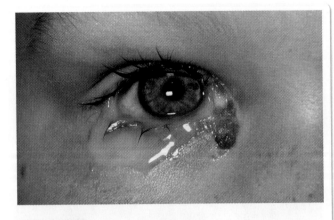

FIGURE 25-9 Bacterial conjunctivitis.

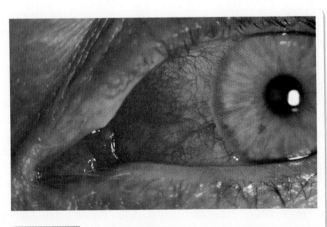

FIGURE 25-10 Viral conjunctivitis.

Garrison Care TIPS

In adults, up to 50% of all earaches are actually dental problems.

Eye pain with decreased visual acuity should be considered an emergency and should be evaluated on an urgent basis. A medical officer consultation is required in *all* ocular complaints.

Ear

Ear pain may be caused by an infection of the external canal or middle ear, or by eustachian tube dysfunction. It may be caused by a build-up of fluid in the middle ear tube, commonly seen in cases of the common cold or upper respiratory infections. Ear pain may be accompanied by **tinnitus** (ringing in the ears) or decreased hearing. **Otitis externa** (swimmer's ear) usually includes aggravation of pain when pressing on the tragus or tugging on the auricle, and requires antibiotic treatment.

With **otitis media** (middle ear infection), the patient usually complains of ear pain and decreased hearing in the affected ear. The TM will look red and/or bulging. The cone of light will commonly be absent during an otoscopic examination. This condition is typically unilateral (occurs in one ear). Treatment requires the administration of antibiotics and decongestants, so medical officer consultation is required.

The Valsalva maneuver can help raise or lower the suspicion of fluid behind the TM. It is performed by having the patient close his or her mouth, pinch the nose closed, and gently blow air out the nose. This maneuver forces air into the eustachian tube. Through the otoscope, you should see the ear drum move when the Valsalva maneuver is performed. Lack of movement could indicate otitis media or an eustachian tube dysfunction.

With cerumen impaction (wax in the ears), the patient usually presents with hearing loss and no pain. The TM cannot be seen during the otoscopic examination because it is obscured by the cerumen. Treatment requires irrigation of the ear. Curetting (scraping) should be done only by the medical officer. Prior to irrigation, triethanolamine polypeptide oleate-condensate (Cerumenex) or carbamide peroxide (Debrox) should be placed in the affected ear and allowed to soften the cerumen for approximately 15 minutes. Prior to irrigation, make sure there is no perforation in the TM.

With eustachian tube dysfunction, the patient usually presents with hearing loss, no pain, and commonly has associated symptoms of an upper respiratory infection (URI) or a head cold. Treatment requires administering a decongestant.

Nose and Throat

Nosebleeds

The most common type of nasal bleeding is in the front nasal passages. Bleeding is usually caused by external trauma, nose picking, nasal infection from plucking nose hairs, vigorous nose blowing, or the drying of the nasal mucosa. However, epistaxis (nasal bleeding) may be an early sign of a more significant illness such as hypertension (high blood pressure) or a blood clotting disorder. Most cases can be treated easily by having the patient sit up and lean forward. Tip the patient's head downward and pinch the patient's entire nose firmly for 10 to 15 minutes. If this does not control the bleeding, then a vasoconstrictive nasal spray such as Afrin or NeoSynephrine may be used. A cold pack applied to the area may also slow the bleeding.

If the patient has a history of multiple nosebleeds, he or she should be asked about family history of bleeding problems. Ask about medications such as aspirin or nonsteroidal anti-inflammatory drugs (NSAIDs) and any history of chronic illnesses that predispose the patient to nosebleeds, such as hypertension. If the patient does have a chronic illness, a referral to the medical officer is necessary.

As always, first stop the bleeding. Check the patient's blood pressure after treatment has been initiated. To prevent a recurrence when the cause is a dry nasal mucosa, the patient may be given bacitracin ointment or a nasal spray to use as a protective coating for the nasal mucosa.

Medical officer consultation is required for the following cases:

- Significant trauma
- Pain

- Blood pressure with systolic greater than 140 mm Hg and diastolic greater than 90 mm Hg
- Pulse greater than 100 beats/min
- Temperature greater than 100°F
- When pressure does not control bleeding
- Recurrent bleeding episodes
- When you are in doubt or uncomfortable with the case

Upper Respiratory Infection

A URI is an acute infection of the upper airway generally characterized by a cough, which may be either productive or nonproductive; sputum may be clear or purulent. There may be a low-grade fever. The lungs are typically clear to auscultation. Patients commonly complain of a sore throat, nasal congestion/discharge, low-grade fever, and sinus pressure. URIs are usually a result of a common cold virus. The physical examination is usually unremarkable except for nasal congestion and the appearance of a slightly reddened pharynx with mucus streaking. Vital signs are usually normal with the possible exception of a low-grade (slight) fever. Treatment is symptomatic in nature, such as administering cough suppressants, decongestants, throat lozenges, and analgesics such as acetaminophen for fever and body aches. Antibiotics are *not* indicated for URIs.

Medical officer consultation is indicated in the following cases:

- Temperature greater than 100°F
- Pain when touching the chin to the chest
- Purulent or dark sputum
- Hoarseness for 1 week
- Eardrum bulging
- Tonsils grossly swollen, necrotic, or heavily exudative
- Difficulty in swallowing
- Symptoms present for more than 1 week
- If you are in doubt or uncomfortable with the case

Sore Throat

A patient with the chief complaint of a sore throat without common cold symptoms is generally suffering from a nonspecific viral infection, streptococcal (strep) bacterial infection, mononucleosis viral infection, or, rarely, a peri-tonsillar abscess. Nonspecific viral or irritative pharyngitis is common in patients who smoke, and usually presents with few, if any, abnormal examination findings. These patients usually have associated symptoms consistent with a URI. Diagnostic tests such as blood work and throat cultures are rarely needed because the focused history and physical examination will lead to the correct diagnosis. Treatment is symptomatic in nature with the administration of throat lozenges.

Streptococcal (strep) pharyngitis is a bacterial infection that usually presents with a sudden onset of severe sore throat, fever, tender/swollen neck glands, nausea, and malaise. Exudate is commonly seen on very reddened tonsils and the pharynx. Diagnosis is confirmed with a throat culture but, depending on the situation, the health care provider may treat

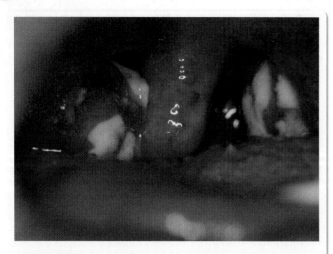

FIGURE 25-11 Infectious mononucleosis may present with a shaggy, white-purple tonsillar exudate.

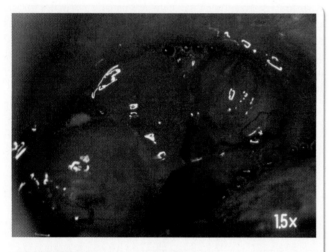

FIGURE 25-12 A peri-tonsillar abscess.

sports (football) for at least 30 days after diagnosis due to the increased risk of splenic rupture (rupture of spleen).

With a peri-tonsillar abscess, a patient complains of severe sore throat, has pain with swallowing, is usually febrile, and is very sick appearing. The peri-tonsillar abscess usually affects one side, resulting in a tonsil deviating toward the midline FIGURE 25-12 ◂ . It may result as a complication of strep pharyngitis. It commonly requires urgent surgical drainage and/or intravenous antibiotic therapy.

The red flags of sore throat are:

- Fever of 101°F or greater
- Difficulty or pain with swallowing
- Tonsillar exudates
- Swollen tonsils
- Tender or swollen lymph glands of the neck

Rhinitis

Rhinitis is the inflammation of the nasal membranes resulting in sneezing, itching, rhinorrhea, and nasal congestion. Patients with allergies often have family histories of multiple allergic disorders including hay fever, asthma, and eczema. People with fair skin such as those with red hair tend to be at the greatest risk. Allergic rhinitis is nonpurulent nasal discharge with associated sneezing. Hay fever symptoms include eye and nasal signs plus occasional wheezing. The patient's history may include symptoms that are seasonal in nature.

Treatment is aimed at identification and avoidance of the offending allergen, but the itching and sneezing can be treated symptomatically with an antihistamine. Decongestants should be used to treat the nasal congestion. If eye irritation is significant, add an antihistamine eye drop such as Visine. If nasal congestion is severe, a nasal decongestant spray may also be used for short periods, not to exceed 3 days. Sedating antihistamines should be used cautiously in the active duty soldier because they increase the risk of heat injury. Also, soldiers who are operating heavy equipment or driving need to be on profile during antihistamine use.

Hoarseness

Hoarseness or laryngitis is defined as a change in normal voice quality, with the most common cause being a viral infection. Other causes include bacterial infections, excessive use of the voice, allergic reactions, and inhalation of irritating substances. Viral laryngitis is self-limiting, with no specific treatment indicated. Some symptomatic relief may be gained with warm normal saline or hydrogen peroxide gargles or throat lozenges. Cepacol lozenges or a Chloraseptic gargle may be of some benefit. Bacterial laryngitis is more frequently seen in children and is treated with appropriate antibiotics.

Avoidance of irritating substances (such as tobacco smoke) should be stressed in cases where this is the cause of the laryngitis. All patients with laryngitis should rest their voice and should be advised to stop smoking, if applicable. Chronic hoarseness (> 2 weeks) may be due to dysfunction of

for this condition based on clinical suspicion alone. Strep requires antibiotic treatment.

Infectious mononucleosis is a viral infection that commonly presents in similar fashion as a streptococcal infection, but patients will also commonly complain of severe fatigue. These patients commonly have significant lymph node (gland) enlargement of the neck and may exhibit a shaggy, white-purple tonsillar exudate FIGURE 25-11 ▴ . Abdominal pain may indicate inflammation of the spleen. A blood test (Monospot) may be ordered along with a throat culture to rule out strep and confirm mononucleosis. When the diagnosis of mononucleosis is confirmed, the treatment is purely symptomatic with the administration of throat lozenges, acetaminophen, decongestants, and sometimes short courses of oral steroids. Antibiotics are not indicated. Patients are advised to avoid contact

the vocal cords from tumor growth or neurologic deficit and needs specialized care.

Sinuses

Patients who present with the complaint of sinusitis may or may not have true sinusitis. Most, in fact, do not. **Sinusitis** is a bacterial infection of one of the paranasal sinuses. Acute sinusitis may follow a URI, dental abscess, or a nasal allergy. As the term *acute* implies, in acute sinusitis, the symptoms are of recent, abrupt onset. The patient usually complains of sinus pressure or pain, commonly unilateral (one side or the other) and a productive cough that is very often worse when lying down compared to when standing or sitting. The affected sinus is commonly tender when palpated or percussed. The patient may have a sore throat that is worse at night and early in the morning due to the draining of mucus down the throat from the sinuses as a result of lying down. Rarely is the patient febrile. Antibiotics and symptomatic treatment are required because this is commonly due to bacterial infection.

As the term *chronic* implies, with chronic sinusitis the symptoms are of several weeks or even months in duration. The patient usually has minimal examination findings but reports a diffuse pressure sensation involving the affected sinuses and may complain of nasal congestion and discharge.

The patient may require antibiotics depending on clinical suspicion and diagnostic studies such as a CT (computed tomography) scan. Some cases are due to seasonal or environmental allergies.

Medical officer consultation is required for the following cases:

- Temperature greater than 100°F
- Retro-orbital headache
- Purulent nasal discharge
- Pain when touching chin to the chest
- Tenderness to percussion over the maxillary and/or frontal sinuses
- When you are in doubt or uncomfortable with the case

■ Summary

Primary care of the eyes, ears, nose, and throat begins with knowledge of their structure and function. To recognize and accurately assess, treat, and/or refer these patients for treatment, clinical observation, accurate vital signs, and appropriate history taking are essential. Early assessment and treatment will reduce the amount of time soldiers are unable to perform their duties due to debilitating illness.

YOU ARE THE
COMBAT MEDIC

You are the combat medic during sick call at the Battalion Aid Station (BAS). Two soldiers walk into the BAS. One soldier is leaning against his buddy and holding a bloody towel to his nose.

"I accidently hit him with my elbow during PE," the supporting soldier says sheepishly.

"I keep telling you, man, it's okay!" the patient says. "My mom is always saying that it's always getting in people's way."

Assessment

Clearly, the patient's nose is bleeding due to the trauma of an elbow to the face. You need to assess this patient to discover if this is simply a mild nosebleed or a fractured bone in the nose, but your first priority is to stop the bleeding. You have the patient sit down in a chair and lean forward. You tip the patient's head downward and pinch the patient's entire nose firmly. The patient winces, but allows you to apply pressure for 10 minutes. The bleeding does not stop, so you obtain a cold pack and have the patient apply it gently to his nose.

While the patient keeps the cold pack against his nose, you take his blood pressure using his free arm. It is 148/88 mm Hg. Because of the trauma to his nose, his high blood pressure, and the fact that his nose is still bleeding, you need to call in the medical officer for a consultation. The medical officer determines that the patient's nose is indeed fractured and transfers the patient on to a higher echelon of care.

Ready for Review

- As a combat medic, you will need to attend to patients with eye, ear, nose, and throat (EENT) complaints.
- Ocular injuries are classified as penetrating or nonpenetrating.
- A red eye can be a sign and symptom of a variety of abnormalities of the eye.
  - Infection, allergies, drugs, chemical exposure, trauma, or systemic disease may cause a red, painful eye.
- Eye discharge is mainly associated with viral or bacterial conjunctivitis.
- Loss of vision should always be considered a medical emergency.

Vital Vocabulary

auricle Part of the external ear that is shaped to collect sound waves and direct them toward the external auditory meatus.

conjunctiva A thin, transparent membrane that covers the sclera and internal surfaces of the eyelids.

conjunctivitis Inflammation of the conjunctiva.

cornea The transparent anterior portion of the eye that overlies the iris and pupil.

exudate Pus.

iris The colored portion of the eye.

lacrimal glands The structures in which tears are secreted and drained from the eye.

lens A transparent body within the globe of the eye that focuses light rays.

ossicles Three small bones in the middle ear.

otitis externa Swimmer's ear.

otitis media Middle ear infection.

paranasal sinuses Air-filled, paired extensions of the nasal cavity within the bones of the skull.

pupil The circular opening in the center of the eye through which light passes to the lens.

retina A delicate, 10-layered structure of nervous tissue located in the rear of the interior of the eye globe that receives light and generates nerve signals that are transmitted to the brain through the optic nerve.

rhinitis Inflammation of the nasal membranes resulting in sneezing, itching, rhinorrhea, and nasal congestion.

sclera The white part of the eye.

sinusitis A bacterial infection of one of the paranasal sinuses.

streptococcal (strep) pharyngitis A bacterial infection that usually presents with a sudden onset of severe sore throat, fever, tender neck glands, nausea, and malaise.

tinnitus Ringing in the ears.

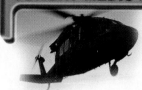

COMBAT MEDIC in Action

You are the combat medic during sick call at the Battalion Aid Station. A soldier comes into the BAS and presents with a headache and sore throat. During the assessment, he complains of pain in his left sinus and a cough that is keeping him awake at night. When you palpate his sinuses, they feel tender. He does not have a fever.

1. In acute sinusitis, the symptoms are:
   - A. of recent, abrupt onset.
   - B. very mild.
   - C. of several weeks.
   - D. of several months.

2. Acute sinusitis may follow:
   - A. an URI.
   - B. a dental abscess.
   - C. a nasal allergy.
   - D. all of the above.

3. In chronic sinusitis, the symptoms are:
   - A. of recent, abrupt onset.
   - B. very mild.
   - C. of several weeks or months.
   - D. very severe.

4. Red flags that require a medical officer consultation include:
   - A. pain when touching the chin to the chest.
   - B. nasal congestion.
   - C. a temperature over 98°F.
   - D. a productive cough.

5. Sinusitis is:
   - A. a virus in the sinuses.
   - B. a bacterial infection of one of the paranasal sinuses.
   - C. a reaction to allergies.
   - D. a bacterial infection of the throat.

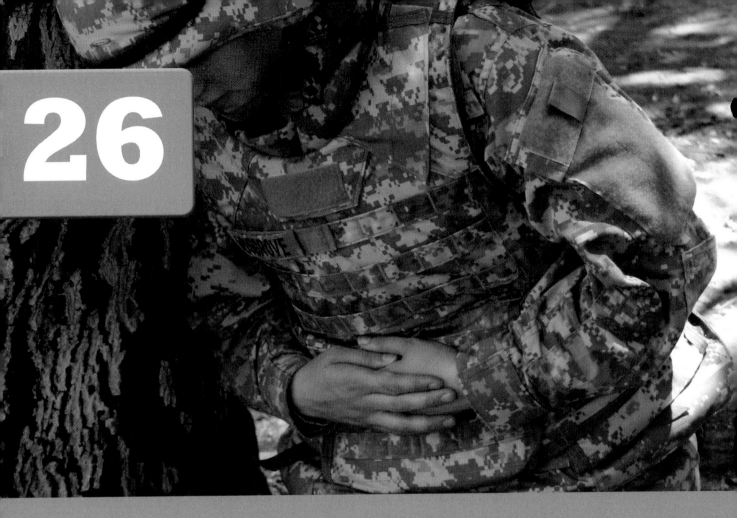

26

Abdominal Disorders

Objectives

Knowledge Objectives

☐ Discuss the anatomy and physiology of the abdomen.

☐ Discuss taking a focused history in a patient with gastrointestinal disorders.

☐ Describe how to give a physical examination of the abdomen.

☐ Describe the system-based approach to abdominal disorders.

Introduction

As a combat medic engaged in combat or peacekeeping operations, you will find that abdominal symptoms in soldiers are a common presentation during sick-call procedures. You must have a basic knowledge of the anatomy and function of the gastrointestinal system and an understanding of the common disorders you may encounter.

Nausea, vomiting, diarrhea, constipation, and abdominal pain are all common signs and symptoms that could potentially indicate a significant underlying problem. It is important to understand that some causes of abdominal distress may require surgical intervention. The failure to look for and find these causes may result in the death of a fellow soldier. As always, obtaining a good medical history and accurate vital signs, and performing an appropriate physical examination will greatly reduce the likelihood of overlooking such a problem.

Anatomy and Physiology of the Abdominal Organs

The abdominal cavity is below (inferior to) the diaphragm. Its boundaries include:

- Anterior abdominal wall
- Pelvic bones
- Spinal column
- Muscles of the abdomen and flank

The abdominal cavity is divided into four quadrants FIGURE 26-1 ▾. The right upper quadrant (RUQ) includes:

- Liver
- Gallbladder
- Head of the pancreas (retroperitoneal)
- Part of the colon (hepatic flexure and part of the transverse colon)

- A portion of the small intestine
- Abdominal aorta (along the line separating the RUQ from the left upper quadrant) (retroperitoneal)
- Right kidney (retroperitoneal)
- Right renal artery
- Inferior vena cava (retroperitoneal)

The left upper quadrant (LUQ) includes:

- Stomach
- Spleen
- Tail of the pancreas (retroperitoneal)
- Part of the colon (splenic flexure and portion of the transverse colon)
- A portion of the small intestine
- Abdominal aorta (along the line separating the RUQ from the LUQ)
- Left kidney (retroperitoneal)
- Left renal artery

The right lower quadrant (RLQ) includes:

- Part of the colon (ascending colon including cecum)
- Appendix (attached to cecum)
- A portion of the small intestine
- Part of the uterus (in women) and bladder
- Right fallopian tube and right ovary (in women)
- Right iliac artery and vein

The left lower quadrant (LLQ) includes:

- A portion of the small intestine
- Part of the colon (sigmoid/descending colon)
- Part of the uterus (in women) and bladder
- Left fallopian tube and left ovary (in women)
- Left iliac artery and vein

The **liver** stores about 10% of the human body's total blood volume (TBV) FIGURE 26-2 ▸. The liver filters bacteria from the blood and metabolizes carbohydrates (sugars), fat,

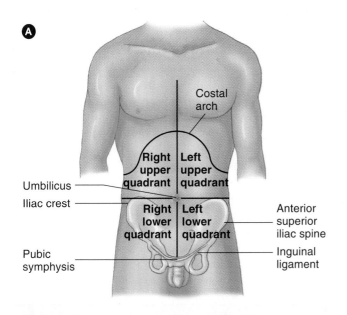

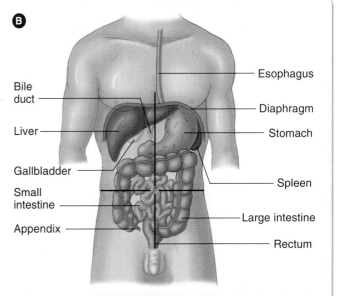

FIGURE 26-1 The anatomy of the abdomen. **A.** The four quadrants of the abdomen. **B.** Abdominal organs can lie in more than one quadrant.

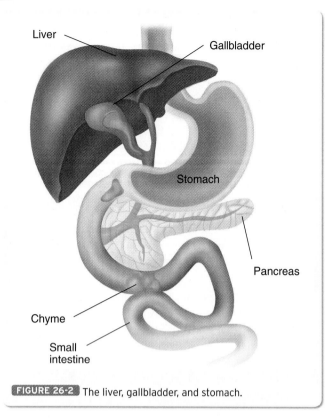

FIGURE 26-2 The liver, gallbladder, and stomach.

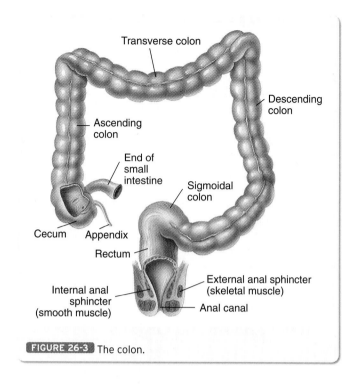

FIGURE 26-3 The colon.

and protein. In addition, it stores vitamins and iron and forms various blood clotting factors. It detoxifies and excretes and metabolizes many different drugs. It forms bile, which breaks down fat for digestion, and serves as a means for excreting certain waste products from the blood.

The **gallbladder** stores the bile formed by the liver. It empties the bile into the first part of the small intestine (duodenum) when there is high fat content in a meal. If stones form in the gallbladder, they may obstruct the drainage system (bile duct) to the small intestine.

The stomach stores large quantities of food until it can be accommodated by the duodenum (first portion of the small intestine). It secretes digestive juices. It is poor at absorption except for highly lipid-soluble substances like alcohol and some medications such as aspirin.

The **pancreas** produces and secretes digestive juices into the first part of the small intestine (duodenum) via the pancreatic duct. It produces and secretes hormones into the blood that regulate blood sugar (glucose) levels. The pancreas produces insulin, which promotes sugar (glucose) entry into most cells of the body. It also produces glucagon, which stimulates the release of glucose from the liver into the circulating body fluids.

The **small intestine** absorbs carbohydrates (sugars) and ions such as sodium, chloride, bicarbonate, calcium, iron, and potassium. The small intestine also absorbs the water that accompanies the ions being absorbed, as well as proteins and fat. The colon (large intestine) absorbs the majority of water and electrolytes (up to 5 to 7 liters per day) FIGURE 26-3 ▶. It stores fecal matter until it can be expelled.

The **spleen** stores red blood cells (RBCs). It filters bacteria from the blood, similar to the liver. It forms some of the lymphocytes and monocytes (white blood cells involved in fighting infections). It is a highly vascular organ that, if injured, may result in massive hemorrhaging. It may be inflamed and enlarged in patients with infectious mononucleosis (mono). As a result, these patients should be advised to avoid contact sports for up to 4 weeks after diagnosis due to the remote possibility of splenic rupture.

The **kidneys** excrete most of the end products of metabolism through filtration of blood and formation of urine. They regulate the water, electrolyte, and acid-base content of the blood.

■ Focused History and Physical Exam

Obtaining a detailed focused history and physical examination is critical to the proper diagnosis of a patient with abdominal disorders. You will need to obtain subjective data (history) and objective data (physical examination) from the patient.

Subjective Data

The subjective data includes:

- Age, sex, race, and in females, the first day of the last menstrual period (FDLMP)
- Chief complaint (usually stated in the patient's own words)
- History of present illness (HPI), using OPQRST:
  - **Onset:** Sudden? Gradual? Specific cause?
  - **Provoking/palliative:** What makes it worse or better?
  - **Quality:** What does the pain feel like? Sharp? Dull?
  - **Radiation/region:** Where is the pain? Is it localized to one area?

- **Severity:** How would you score the pain on a scale of 1 to 10? Does it limit your activity?
- **Timing:** Duration? Is the pain intermittent? Constant?
- **Associated symptoms and complaints:** Are there other complaints? Are they related?

The past history includes taking the SAMPLE history:

- Signs/symptoms
- Allergies
- Medications
- Past medical and surgical history including social history
  - Past medical history (PMH)
  - Past surgical history (PSH)
  - Social history (Soc. Hx)
- Last oral intake
- Events leading up to illness (especially recent foreign travel)

Objective Data

Obtain a complete set of vital signs, including postural blood pressure and pulse. What is the general appearance of the patient? Is the patient in distress or pain? Begin looking at the uppermost part of the gastrointestinal tract, the oral structures, such as the mouth and throat. Then, move down the patient's body for a full physical examination. The order of the examination of the abdomen is inspection, auscultation, and palpation.

Inspection

Expose the patient from his or her xiphoid process to the symphysis pubis. Ensure that the patient is warm and comfortable. Have the patient lie supine with his or her arms down at their side. Have the patient bend his or her knees or support him or her with a pillow to help relax the abdominal muscles. Begin inspecting from the patient's right; this view enhances shadows and contouring.

Inspect the skin. Look at the color of the skin and look for the following signs:

- **Jaundice:** Yellowing of the skin, eyes, and nails
- **Pale skin:** Pallor
- **Bruising:** Bluish discoloration of the umbilicus (Cullen's sign) suggests intra-abdominal bleeding
- **Redness:** May indicate inflammation

Look for scars and describe their location, shape, size, and color. Look for striae (stretch marks) and describe their location, size, and color **FIGURE 26-4**. Describe any rashes.

Inspect the skin's contour and symmetry. Flat skin is common in thin patients with good muscle tone. **Scaphoid** is a sunken appearance of the skin. It may be normal in thin patients or may denote a diseased state. Observe for distension or bulging. Have the patient take in a deep breath and hold it; the contour changes will be more obvious. Asymmetrical distension or protrusion may result from a hernia, tumor, cysts, bowel obstruction, or enlargement of abdominal organs.

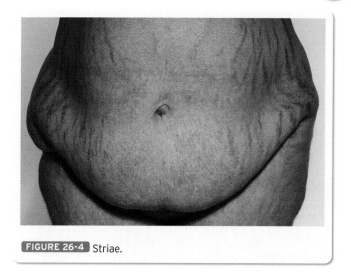

FIGURE 26-4 Striae.

Auscultation

Remember to do this prior to palpation. Never touch the abdomen until auscultation is completed because palpation can alter bowel sounds. Listen in all four quadrants of the abdomen. Warm the diaphragm of the stethoscope against your hand prior to touching the patient.

Listen to the bowel sounds in all four quadrants to ensure that no sounds are missed. The stage of digestion affects the sound characteristics. Note the frequency and character of the sounds:

- Hypoactive sounds indicate slow, sluggish sounds.
- Active bowel sounds usually sound like clicks and gurgles occurring irregularly, 5 to 35 times per minute.
- Hyperactive sounds indicate loud prolonged gurgles (borborygmi or stomach growling) associated with hunger.
- Increased bowel sounds may occur with gastroenteritis.
- Absent bowel sounds are established only after 5 minutes of continuous listening. Absent bowel sounds can be associated with an acute abdomen.
- Bruit (pronounced "broo-ee") is a harsh, blowing sound heard with auscultation that results from turbulent flow of blood through an artery. This could be caused by narrowing of an artery or weakening of the wall of an artery such as found with an aneurysm.

Palpation

The standard order of the examination is altered because palpation may cause altered bowel motility and heighten bowel sounds, resulting in a false interpretation of bowel sounds

Garrison Care **TIPS**

Anything other than normal, active bowel sounds should alert you to a problem.

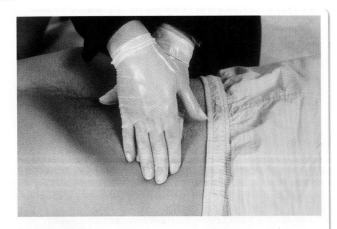

FIGURE 26-5 Check tenderness by gently palpating each of the four quadrants.

Field Medical Care TIPS

An extensive physical examination is not warranted in the field because the urgency to move the patient to a treatment facility may be great and the examination will have to be repeated at the garrison.

during auscultation. If the patient is in pain, have him or her point to the pain site. Palpate this area last.

When palpating the abdomen, you are assessing for muscle spasm, tenderness, and fluid. This assessment helps to substantiate findings and allows you to evaluate the shape, size, position, mobility, consistency, and tension of major abdominal organs.

To perform palpation, first wash and warm your hands. Keep your fingernails short. Position the patient's arms at the side, knees flexed to relax the abdominal muscles. Palpation techniques include light palpation, deep palpation, and bi-manual palpation (one hand on top of the other).

Begin with light palpation **FIGURE 26-5 ▲**. Slowly palpate all quadrants, first lightly and then deeply. With the patient supine, place your palm lightly on his or her abdomen and gently depress the abdominal wall about 1 cm with your fingers. This will allow you to detect guarding and tenderness, which may be caused by peritonitis.

Next, perform deep palpation to assess deeper abdominal structures. Indent the patient's abdomen by pressing into the abdominal wall with the distal half of your fingers. Check for rebound tenderness, which is sharp pain at the site of peritoneal inflammation when abdominal pressure is released. This should be done at the end of the examination, because a positive response produces pain and muscle spasm that can interfere with any subsequent examination.

Bi-manual palpation should be used if deep palpation is difficult due to obesity or muscular resistance; it is performed by placing one hand on top of the other. Some combat medics prefer this method with all patients. When evaluating specific

structures or organs, a bi-manual method of placing one hand on each side of the structure (or mass) is helpful in determining size and feeling for nodules and tenderness. Assess for abdominal masses. Note abdominal consistency, mobility, and movement with respiration.

Red Flags

The red flags that warrant urgent referral to a medical officer include:

- Progressive, severe pain that persists without improvement over 6 hours
- Severe abdominal pain with guarding or rebound tenderness
- Recent medical history (< 6 months) of abdominal surgery
- Abdominal pain with associated fever
- Abdominal pain with associated tachycardia
- Patient reporting blood in the stool or emesis (vomitus)
- Abdominal pain with dehydration
- Abdominal pain in a pregnant patient
- Abdominal pain in a female who is late having her menstrual period

Do not confuse normal abdominal structures for abdominal masses.

■ Symptom-Based Approach to Abdominal Disorders

Abdominal pain is a common presenting symptom. As with most other patient symptoms, the causes of abdominal pain can usually be identified if you first obtain an accurate set of vital signs and a good history of the complaint (OPQRST). For instance, a patient with a recent onset of RLQ abdominal pain with associated fever probably has appendicitis, at least until proven otherwise.

The physical examination you perform will be guided by the vital signs and patient history. Associating the patient history with vital signs and the anatomy in the region in which the patient is complaining of pain will help narrow the list of possible causes. If you failed to note a patient's temperature, you might attribute his or her pain to a pulled abdominal muscle. If you failed to consider appendicitis as the cause, the patient could have been discharged only to suffer from a ruptured appendix followed by a serious and diffuse abdominal infection (peritonitis) that could lead to death. Given the complexity of abdominal anatomy, you can see there are many problems that could cause abdominal pain, and if overlooked some of these could result in serious complications or even death.

The retroperitoneum is a space behind (posterior to) the peritoneum. Retroperitoneal organs include the pancreas and kidneys. This is significant because the location of these organs commonly means that problems associated with these organs will result in back or flank pain instead of abdominal pain. As a matter of routine, all patients complaining of abdominal or flank pain should also have their lungs examined. Examination of the heart and chest may also be necessary, especially in patients with upper abdominal symptoms.

You must always consider the possibility of pregnancy in any female complaining of abdominal pain, regardless of whether she denies the possibility of being pregnant.

Retroperitoneal Causes of Pain

The possible causes of retroperitoneal pain include:

- **Pyelonephritis:** Kidney infection
- **Nephrolithiasis:** Kidney stones
- **Pancreatitis:** Inflammation or infection of the pancreas

Pyelonephritis

Pyelonephritis is a kidney infection. It usually occurs in females as a progression of a bladder infection (cystitis). It may occur in males, though it is uncommon. Patients usually present with fever, pain with urination (dysuria), frequent urination, and back pain in the region of the affected kidney (flank pain), and may report bloody-appearing urine (hematuria). The patient may exhibit shaking, chills, nausea, vomiting, fever with tachycardia, and costovertebral angle tenderness (CVAT) that is elicited by tapping your fist on the patient's back over the kidney. Treatment always involves referral to a medical officer because antibiotics and possibly hospitalization are required.

Nephrolithiasis

Nephrolithiasis is also called kidney stones. They occur more commonly in men than women and tend to occur more often during the hot summer months. As a result, kidney stones are a common finding when operating in an environment such as the desert. Pain usually develops suddenly and may awaken the patient from sleep. The onset of pain is usually in the flank, is typically severe and colicky (comes and goes or varies in intensity in a rhythmic nature), and will migrate as the stone makes its way through the urinary tract. The patient may report bloody-appearing urine (hematuria).

The physical examination will reveal a patient who appears to be in significant pain. The patient is commonly restless and constantly moving. Fever is common, as is tenderness to palpation (TTP) in the vicinity of the stone.

Treatment must always involve referral to the medical officer because narcotic pain medication and close observation are required. Most kidney stones will pass through the urinary tract on their own time. Increase the fluid intake (sometimes intravenously) and give appropriate pain control medications. Prevention is centered on ensuring adequate fluid intake, especially in hot climates.

Diffuse Abdominal Pain

The possible causes of diffuse abdominal pain include:

- **Early appendicitis:** Inflammation or obstruction of the appendix
- **Colitis:** Inflammation of the colon
- **Mesenteric thrombosis:** A blood clot in the intestinal artery
- **Gastroenteritis:** Stomach and intestinal infection

- **Peritonitis:** Inflammation of the abdominal wall
- **Pancreatitis:** Inflammation or infection of the pancreas

Early Appendicitis

Early appendicitis is initiated by the obstruction of the appendix by a **fecalith** (hardened feces), inflammation, foreign body, or **neoplasm** (cancerous process). Obstruction leads to increased pressure within the appendix, congestion of venous blood, infection, and thrombosis (clotting) of blood within the wall of the appendix. If untreated, gangrene and perforation can develop within 36 hours. Treatment is an appendectomy (surgical removal of the appendix). The signs and symptoms include:

- Pain, early in the course, in the peri-umbilical region (around the navel)
- Pain, later in the course, localized to the RLQ
- Loss of appetite, nausea, vomiting, and extreme constipation
- Low-grade fever, elevated white blood cell (WBC) count

Gastroenteritis

Gastroenteritis is stomach and intestinal inflammation. It is commonly manifested by a cramping abdominal pain, nausea, vomiting, and/or diarrhea. It is usually caused by infection, commonly viral. Gastroenteritis is rapid in onset, self-limited to a few days' duration, and occasionally complicated by dehydration. Treatment is limited to symptomatic treatment such as Pepto-Bismol or Kaopectate to help bind up and remove bowel contaminants. Antibiotics are not given. Antispasmodic medications such as Imodium can alleviate cramping pain. Have the patient avoid foods and beverages likely to upset the GI tract (such as fried, fatty, greasy, or spicy foods and alcoholic beverages) and increase the patient's daily liquid intake. Patients with fever, bloody diarrhea or vomitus, tachycardia at rest, hypotension, or an inability to drink liquids without vomiting require prompt referral to the medical officer.

Peritonitis

Peritonitis is the inflammation of the wall of the abdominal cavity. It commonly results from perforation of a viscus (organ) such as the appendix, stomach, or bowel. Pain is usually abrupt in onset, but may be localized to the region of origin, such as RLQ in appendicitis, or may be diffuse and involve the entire abdomen. Peritonitis is usually associated with vomiting. The physical examination usually reveals a high fever, decreased or absent bowel sounds on auscultation, and abdominal distension. These patients look ill. Treatment begins with prompt referral to the medical officer because this is almost always a surgical emergency.

Right Upper Quadrant Pain

The possible causes of right upper quadrant (RUQ) pain include:

- Dissecting aneurysm (rupturing artery wall)
- Gallbladder disease (cholecystitis)
- Hepatitis

- Pneumonia
- Appendicitis (if retro-cecal [behind the cecum])
- Pyelonephritis
- Nephrolithiasis
- Pancreatitis
- Peptic ulcer disease

Hepatitis

Hepatitis is the inflammation of the liver. It can be caused by a variety of agents including viral infections, bacterial infections, and physical or chemical agents (drugs and alcohol). Among soldiers, viral and alcoholic hepatitis are most common. These conditions rarely result in abdominal pain except when palpating the liver. The typical presentation includes anorexia (loss of appetite), nausea, vomiting, malaise, fever, enlarged and tender liver, and jaundice (yellowing of skin, nails, and sclera). Treatment always involves referral to a medical officer because serious complications can result from this condition.

Peptic Ulcer Disease

Peptic ulcer disease (PUD) results from a break in the mucosa (lining) of the stomach or the first part of the small intestine (duodenum). It is usually manifested by pain in the middle upper abdomen (dyspepsia). It more commonly occurs in smokers and patients taking anti-inflammatory medications such as ibuprofen or aspirin for prolonged periods of time. Pain may or may not be associated with eating or drinking. PUD may be caused by the bacteria *Helicobacter pylori* (*H pylori*). The patient may report black, tarry looking stools (melena), a result of bleeding from the ulcer site.

Patients have usually had dyspepsia for an extended period of time before an actual ulcer develops. Physical examination findings are usually unremarkable with the possible exception of tenderness to palpation (TTP) in the middle upper abdomen (midepigastric area). Rectal examination may reveal blood in the stool. Patients who smoke should be advised to quit and to avoid foods, beverages, and medications that aggravate symptoms. Treatment always involves referral to a medical officer because serious complications can result from this condition.

Left Upper Quadrant Pain

The causes of left upper quadrant (LUQ) pain can include:

- Dissecting aneurysm (rupturing artery wall)
- Gastroesophageal reflux disease (GERD)
- Pancreatitis
- Peptic ulcer (that progresses to a perforated stomach)
- Acute myocardial infarction (AMI)
- Pneumonia
- Pyelonephritis
- Nephrolithiasis
- Cholecystitis (that progresses to perforated/ruptured gallbladder)
- Ectopic pregnancy (pregnancy in a fallopian tube)
- Pelvic inflammatory disease (PID) (infection in uterus/fallopian tubes)

Gastroesophageal Reflux Disease (GERD)

The lower esophageal sphincter (LES) is a band of smooth muscle tissue where the esophagus meets the stomach. The muscle tone of this sphincter controls the gradient of air pressure in the lower esophagus relative to the air pressure in the stomach. Normally air pressure in the lower esophagus is greater than the pressure in the stomach. This creates the tendency for stomach contents to remain in the stomach. Various factors can influence this normal air pressure gradient, resulting in the reverse situation—air pressure being greater in the stomach than in the lower esophagus. The esophagus was not designed to tolerate the destructive power of gastric juices. Given the proximity of the esophagus to the heart and the burning sensation experienced by the patient, patients who suffer from gastroesophageal reflux disease (GERD) frequently complain of heartburn.

GERD affects 20% of adults, who report at least weekly episodes of heartburn; up to 10% complain of daily symptoms. Though most patients have mild disease, up to 50% develop esophageal mucosal damage (reflux esophagitis) and a few develop more serious complications. Patients commonly complain of heartburn that may be aggravated by meals, bending, or lying down. Patients usually get relief from taking antacids. It is important to remember that these symptoms could also be the result of a stomach ulcer, gallstones (stones in the gallbladder), or angina pectoris (chest pain due to coronary artery disease).

Physical examination is usually normal in uncomplicated cases. The heart and lungs should be examined as with any other patient with GI symptoms. The diagnosis is usually made based on symptoms and the absence of findings that would suggest other causes. Special diagnostic tests may be necessary.

Treatment always involves referral to the medical officer, with the possible exception of patients who have already been diagnosed with this condition who require symptomatic treatment. GERD is a lifelong disease that requires lifestyle modification and medical intervention. The best advice is to avoid lying down within 3 hours after meals, weight loss if indicated, cessation of smoking, and avoidance of foods, beverages, and activities known to precipitate symptoms. Over-the-counter (OTC) liquid antacids such as Maalox, Mylanta, or milk of magnesia usually provide rapid, though short-term, symptomatic relief. Prescription acid-blocking medications to be taken on a daily basis are typically required to minimize the severity and reduce the frequency of GERD symptoms.

Gastritis

Gastritis is the inflammation of the stomach, and is most commonly seen in alcoholics, critically ill patients, or patients taking anti-inflammatory medications such as ibuprofen or aspirin. *H pylori* may also be a cause. These patients usually present with pain in the middle upper abdomen and/or nausea and vomiting. Bloody vomitus (hematemesis) that looks like coffee grounds may be reported. The patient may also report black, tarry-looking stools (melena). The patient may also be anorexic (presenting with weight loss due to loss of appetite).

Physical examination may reveal tachycardia at rest and/or hypotension if there has been significant blood loss. There is commonly tenderness to palpation (TTP) in the middle upper abdomen (midepigastric area). Rectal examination often reveals evidence of blood in the stool.

Treatment always involves referral to the medical officer because invasive testing and hospitalization may be required. Maintenance therapy involves smoking cessation, avoidance of alcohol, and avoidance of all medications that can cause stomach inflammation, such as anti-inflammatory medications like ibuprofen and aspirin. Acid-blocking medications are usually necessary.

Left Lower Quadrant Pain

The possible causes of left lower quadrant (LLQ) pain include:

- Gastroenteritis
- Cystitis
- Nephrolithiasis
- Testicular torsion
- Ovarian torsion
- Pelvic inflammatory disease
- Ectopic pregnancy

Cystitis

Cystitis (also known as a bladder infection or a urinary tract infection [UTI]) is an infection of the urinary bladder. It is more common in women then men and often occurs after sexual intercourse. The patient usually presents with painful urination (dysuria), frequent urination, and discomfort in the suprapubic area. The patient may report gross blood in the urine (hematuria). If treatment is delayed, the infection can migrate up the ureter to the kidneys resulting in pyelonephritis. Physical examination is usually unremarkable, with the possible exception of tenderness to palpation of the suprapubic area. Urine testing (urinalysis) commonly reveals the presence of blood and bacteria.

Treatment always involves referral to the medical officer because antibiotics are indicated. The patient can benefit from increasing oral fluid intake. Recurrences can be prevented by encouraging the patient to urinate after sexual intercourse and advising females to wipe only from front to back after urinating.

Testicular Torsion

Testicular torsion is a condition whereby a testicle essentially twists upon itself. This may occur spontaneously or after strenuous activity. The result of the twisting (torsion) is that the testicle is deprived of blood flow causing ischemic pain. It commonly occurs in patients between the ages of 10 and 20 years. Immediate symptoms of torsion are sudden onset of severe local pain, nausea, and vomiting followed by scrotal edema and fever. Pain is also commonly felt in either lower abdominal quadrant. The affected testicle is commonly elevated in the scrotum as compared to the unaffected testicle.

If this condition is suspected, urgent surgical referral is essential. If surgery is not performed within 2 to 4 hours of the onset of pain, it is possible that the testicle will have to be removed. Your medical officer may need to attempt a manual detorsion whereby the testicle is twisted in the opposite direction of the torsion for temporary relief. This is usually performed from a medial to lateral direction to reduce the torsion (counterclockwise for the right testicle, clockwise for the left testicle).

Ovarian Torsion

Ovarian torsion is similar to testicular torsion in the male except that it involves the ovary in the female. It also has an abrupt onset with severe, unilateral pain but in the lower abdomen or pelvis. The ovary involved will dictate which side is painful. Nausea and vomiting are common and the patient may have a low-grade fever. If the torsion occurs on the right side, it may be difficult to distinguish from appendicitis.

If this condition is suspected, urgent surgical referral is essential. If surgery is not performed within 2 to 4 hours of the onset of pain, it is possible that the ovary will have to be removed.

Constipation

The normal frequency of bowel movements varies from one person to another. Normal may be defined as 3 per week by some and 12 per week by others. Patients usually complain of **constipation** when they cannot have a bowel movement (BM) when they feel the urge to do so or when they have painful or straining bowel movements with firm, hard stools. Inadequate fluid and dietary fiber intake are the most common causes in soldiers. It is uncommon for patients to report abdominal pain as a result of constipation unless the constipation is severe. Physical examination of the abdomen is usually unremarkable unless there is severe constipation, in which case you may palpate a firm mass in the LLQ.

Treatment is focused on prevention by increasing fluid intake and dietary fiber intake, like eating whole grain cereals. Fiber supplements such as Metamucil, Citrucel, or Fibercon taken on a daily basis will help the patient to maintain regular bowel habits. Stool softeners such as docusate sodium (Colace) taken by mouth for several days and short-term use of a stimulant laxative like bisacodyl (Dulcolax) are beneficial. Persistent cases of constipation or significant abdominal pain or discomfort warrant referral to the medical officer.

Diarrhea

Diarrhea is the frequent passage of unformed watery bowel movements. Diarrhea can range in severity from an acute self-limiting episode to a life-threatening illness. It is helpful to distinguish acute from chronic diarrheas because treatment may differ. With acute diarrhea, the symptoms are acute in onset and persist for less than 3 weeks. Acute diarrhea is most commonly caused by viral, bacterial, or parasitic infections, frequently resulting from consumption of unpurified water or improperly stored or prepared food. Noninfectious causes include medications (such as antibiotics) and food allergies.

Chronic diarrhea persists for longer than 3 weeks, and also may be bacterial, viral, or parasitic in nature. Diarrhea not caused by infections could be attributed to a number of malabsorptive, secretory, inflammatory, or motility disorders. Sometimes the cause of chronic diarrhea remains unknown. All cases of chronic diarrhea should be referred to the medical officer.

The subjective signs include frequent loose or watery stools, which may contain blood, mucus, or pus; fever; abdominal pain/tenderness; cramping; and a history of travel (outside contiguous United States [OCONUS]). The objective signs include orthostatic hypotension (tilts). This is a drop in blood pressure when the patient changes position from lying to sitting or from sitting to standing. A patient feeling dizzy or lightheaded upon standing may indicate a fluid volume deficit.

If symptoms are chronic, document the patient's weight. Other objective signs include signs of viral URI on ear, eye, nose, and throat (EENT) examination. Note the abdomen's appearance—is it flat, protuberant, or distended? Listen to the bowel sounds—are they normal, increased, decreased, or absent?

Note any tenderness on abdominal palpation; if there is tenderness, note whether it is guarding or rebound. With guarding tenderness, a patient with abdominal pain may experience abdominal wall muscle spasm during palpation of the abdomen in an effort to guard against aggravation of pain. The patient may also attempt to block you from examining a painful area. During deep palpation of the abdomen, if the patient experiences greater pain upon quick release of your hands than during the actual palpation, this is rebound tenderness. This finding suggests inflammation of the peritoneum (parietal). Potential causes include perforated viscera such as a ruptured appendix or bowel.

Treatment begins with fluid resuscitation—IV or oral fluid and electrolyte replacement (Gatorade). Antidiarrheal medications include loperamide (Imodium), Pepto-Bismol, or Kaopectate for simple or minimal diarrhea. Do not give if fever or blood in stool are present. Antibiotic therapy is recommended for moderate to severe bacterial diarrhea with fever or with bloody stools, so consult with the medical officer. The patient should be on a liquid diet and then progress to a bland diet. He or she should avoid caffeine, dairy products, and raw fruits and vegetables. They should consume food and water only from approved sources. Use only the IV route for resuscitation and medication administration if any signs of inflammation such as guarding are present.

Hemorrhoids

Hemorrhoids are varicose (blood engorged) veins in the lower rectum or anus caused by straining at stool, constipation, prolonged sitting, and a diet poor in fiber. The subjective signs are:

- Itching
- Irritation and pain with bowel movements
- Bleeding either in the toilet or on the toilet paper, typically bright red

The objective signs are obvious external hemorrhoids or internal hemorrhoids found on inspection of the rectum. If no obvious source of bleeding is found, refer the patient to the medical officer for further examination.

Treatment includes giving the patient a diet high in fiber (vegetables, fruits, grains) and increased water intake. This helps promote soft, formed regular movements. A sitz bath (sitting in warm water) for 15 minutes three times a day reduces pain and swelling. A stool softener like docusate sodium (Colace) may be administered by mouth daily. Give the patient a bulk-forming laxative like Metamucil, Citrucel, or Fibercon. Pain control includes NSAIDs (nonsteroidal anti-inflammatory drugs like ibuprofen, acetaminophen, and topical anesthetics [Dibucaine]). The patient should avoid straining (such as with sit-ups or heavy lifting). If bleeding is excessive or no source is found for the bleeding, the medical officer must be notified immediately.

■ Summary

Abdominal disorders are common, and your ability to recognize and accurately assess, treat, and/or refer the patient for treatment is crucial. Early diagnosis and treatment will reduce the amount of time that soldiers are unable to perform their duties due to illness.

YOU ARE THE
COMBAT MEDIC

You are the combat medic at sick call in the Battalion Aid Station (BAS). A soldier shuffles into the BAS, holding his abdomen. "I am in some serious pain, sir," he says. The soldier appears pale and diaphoretic, so you take him aside to a quiet room to perform a patient assessment.

Assessment

You begin the focused history and physical exam. The patient is 26, male, and Caucasian. His chief complaint is that his stomach "really hurts." The pain began in the middle of the night and has been getting progressively worse. Nothing makes the pain dissipate. The pain feels sharp and it is focused around the navel. On a scale of 1 to 10, he rates his pain as an 8.

You begin to take his SAMPLE history. The patient complains of nausea and a complete loss of appetite. He is allergic to mold and he is not currently taking any medications. He's been healthy all his life, has never had a surgery, and does not drink alcohol. His last meal was lunch yesterday, when he managed to have a bowl of soup and some water. He has been stationed at this garrison for about 4 months.

Next, you obtain a complete set of vital signs, including the patient's postural blood pressure and pulse. You have the patient lie down on an examination table and expose him from the xiphoid process to the symphysis pubis. You place a pillow underneath the patient's knees to help relax his abdominal muscles. His skin is pale and free of any striae or rashes.

You warm your stethoscope against your hand, and then place it on his stomach to listen to his bowel sounds. After listening, you palpate the patient's abdomen. You begin with light palpation and find nothing usual. When you perform the deep palpation, you discover rebound tenderness. Rebound tenderness is a red flag and warrants an urgent referral to a medical officer. The patient is evacuated to a higher echelon facility where his appendix is surgically removed.

Aid Kit

Ready for Review

- As a combat medic engaged in combat or peacekeeping operations, you will find that abdominal symptoms in soldiers are a common presentation during sick-call procedures.
- Obtaining a detailed focused history and physical examination is critical in the proper diagnosis of a patient with abdominal disorders.
- You will need to obtain subjective data (history) and objective data (physical examination) from the patient.
- Abdominal pain is a common presenting symptom.
- As with most other patient symptoms, the causes of abdominal pain can usually be identified if you first obtain an accurate set of vital signs and a good history of the complaint (OPQRST).

Vital Vocabulary

constipation Inability to have a bowel movement, or a painful straining bowel movement with firm, hard stools.

cystitis Also known as urinary tract infection (UTI); an infection of the urinary bladder.

diarrhea Liquid stool.

fecalith Hardened feces.

gallbladder A sac on the undersurface of the liver that collects bile from the liver and discharges it into the duodenum through the common bile duct.

gastritis Inflammation of the stomach.

gastroenteritis Stomach and intestinal inflammation.

hemorrhoids Varicose veins in the lower rectum or anus.

hepatitis Inflammation of the liver.

kidneys Two retroperitoneal organs that excrete the end products of metabolism as urine and regulate the body's salt and water content.

liver A large solid organ that lies in the right upper quadrant immediately below the diaphragm; it produces bile, stores sugar for immediate use by the body, and produces many substances that help regulate immune responses.

neoplasm Cancerous process.

nephrolithiasis Kidney stones.

ovarian torsion A condition whereby an ovary twists upon itself.

pancreas A flat, solid organ that lies below the liver and the stomach; it is a major source of digestive enzymes and produces the hormone insulin.

peptic ulcer disease (PUD) Abrasion of the stomach or small intestine.

peritonitis Inflammation of the wall of the abdominal cavity.

pyelonephritis Kidney infection.

scaphoid Sunken appearance of the skin.

small intestine The portion of the digestive tube between the stomach and the cecum, consisting of the duodenum, jejunum, and ileum.

spleen An organ of the lymphatic system that is located in the left upper quadrant of the abdomen and consists of two types of lymph tissue that are associated with drainage of the spleen.

testicular torsion A condition whereby a testicle essentially twists upon itself.

COMBAT MEDIC in Action

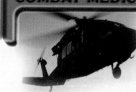

You are the combat medic during sick call at the Battalion Aid Station. On a hot summer night, a soldier presents with severe pain in his right flank. The pain is so severe that it actually woke the soldier up out of a sound sleep. As he was walking to the BAS, the pain lessened a bit, but now it is more severe than when he first woke up. The patient also reports that there was blood in his urine when he woke up.

1. The possible causes of retroperitoneal pain include:
   A. pyelonephritis.
   B. nephrolithiasis.
   C. pancreatitis.
   D. all of the above.

2. Another common term for nephrolithiasis is:
   A. kidney infection.
   B. gall stones.
   C. kidney stones.
   D. gall bladder infection.

3. Prevention of nephrolithiasis is centered on:
   A. increasing fiber in the diet.
   B. avoiding alcohol.
   C. ensuring adequate fluid intake.
   D. surgery.

4. The possible causes of diffuse abdominal pain include:
   A. colitis.
   B. mesenteric thrombosis.
   C. peritonitis.
   D. all of the above.

5. The red flags that warrant urgent referral to a medical officer include:
   A. abdominal pain with dehydration.
   B. abdominal pain in a pregnant patient.
   C. abdominal pain with associated fever.
   D. all of the above.

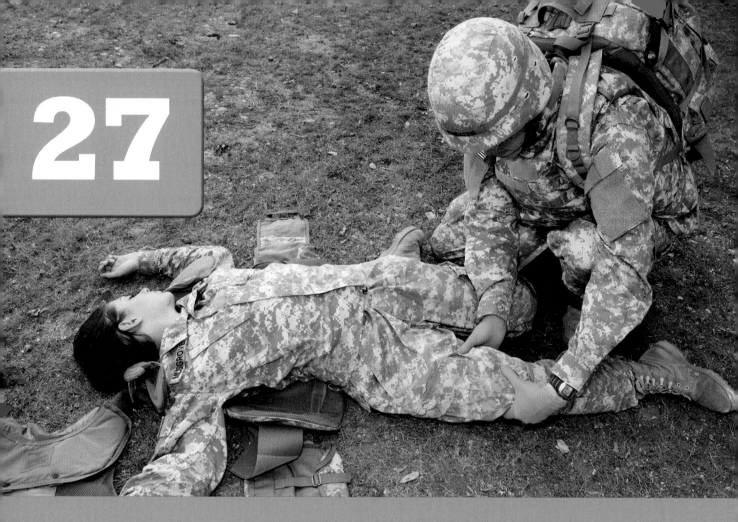

27

Orthopaedics

Objectives

Knowledge Objectives

- Describe the approach to evaluating an orthopaedic complaint.
- Describe the shoulder examination.
- Describe the lower back examination.
- Describe the knee examination.
- Describe the ankle examination.

Introduction

Musculoskeletal injuries and disorders rank second only to upper respiratory infections (URIs) for the numbers encountered by combat medics. These injuries are frequently encountered in the field; however, many times there will not be any obvious findings on the physical examination. Appropriate assessment and management techniques can prevent further painful injury and even prevent permanent disability or death of your fellow soldiers.

The ability to accurately recognize and treat musculoskeletal injuries is one of the many skills that, as a combat medic, you will need to perform in both clinical and field environments. These skills will enable you to successfully manage patients with musculoskeletal complaints. If these tenets are consistently applied in the performance of your daily clinical duties, you will be doing your part in preserving the fighting strength of our Army.

Musculoskeletal System Anatomy Review

The musculoskeletal system gives the body its shape and allows for its movement. It is essential that you understand its basic anatomy and physiology.

Functions of the Musculoskeletal System

The musculoskeletal system performs many important functions within the body. Bones help support the soft tissues of the body and form a framework that gives the human body its shape and allows it to maintain an erect posture. Movement is generated because muscles are attached to bones by **tendons**. (Reminder: Muscles-to-bones [MTB] means muscles–tendons–

bones.) When a muscle contracts, the force generated by the muscle is transferred to a bone on the opposite side of the **joint** from the muscle, leading to motion. Bones also offer protection to the more fragile organs and structures beneath them—for example, the skull protects the brain, the rib cage protects the heart and lungs, and the spinal column protects the spinal cord.

The Body's Scaffolding: The Skeleton

The integrated structure formed by the 206 bones of the body is called the skeleton. It can be divided into two distinct portions: the **axial skeleton** and the **appendicular skeleton**. The axial skeleton is composed of the bones of the central part, or axis, of the body; its divisions include the vertebral column, skull, ribs, and sternum. The skull is composed of the cranium, basilar skull, face, and inner ear FIGURE 27-1 ▾ .

The spine is composed of 33 spinal vertebrae: 7 cervical, 12 thoracic, 5 lumbar, 5 sacral, and 4 coccygeal. Moving anteriorly, the thorax is formed by the sternum and 12 pairs of ribs.

The appendicular skeleton is divided into the **pectoral girdle**, the **pelvic girdle**, and the bones of the upper and lower extremities.

Shoulder and Upper Extremities

The pectoral girdle FIGURE 27-2 ▸ , also referred to as the shoulder girdle, consists of two scapulae and two clavicles. The **scapula** (shoulder blade) is a flat, triangular bone held to the rib cage posteriorly by powerful muscles that buffer it against injury. The **clavicle** (collarbone) is a slender, S-shaped bone attached by ligaments at the medial end to the sternum and at the lateral end to the raised tip of the scapula, called the **acromion**. The clavicle acts as a strut to keep the shoulder

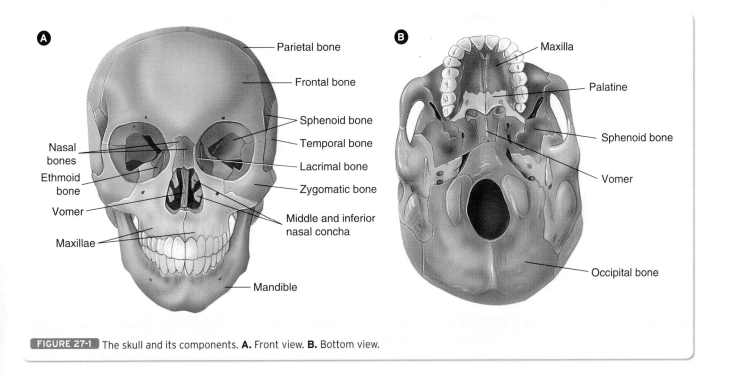

FIGURE 27-1 The skull and its components. **A.** Front view. **B.** Bottom view.

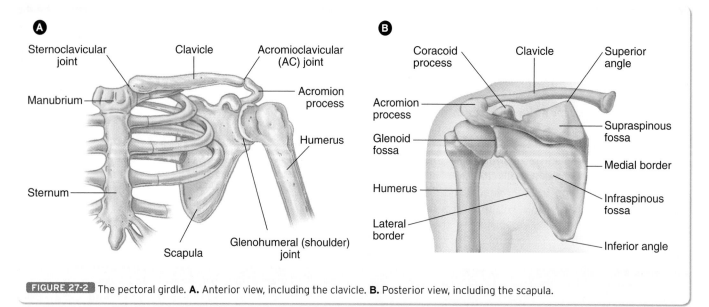

A Sternoclavicular joint · Clavicle · Acromioclavicular (AC) joint · Manubrium · Acromion process · Humerus · Sternum · Scapula · Glenohumeral (shoulder) joint

B Coracoid process · Clavicle · Superior angle · Acromion process · Glenoid fossa · Supraspinous fossa · Medial border · Humerus · Infraspinous fossa · Lateral border · Inferior angle

FIGURE 27-2 The pectoral girdle. **A.** Anterior view, including the clavicle. **B.** Posterior view, including the scapula.

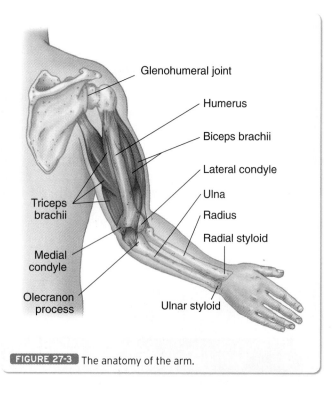

Glenohumeral joint · Humerus · Biceps brachii · Lateral condyle · Ulna · Radius · Radial styloid · Triceps brachii · Medial condyle · Olecranon process · Ulnar styloid

FIGURE 27-3 The anatomy of the arm.

propped up; however, because it is slender and very exposed, this bone is vulnerable to injury.

The upper extremity **FIGURE 27-3 ▲** joins the shoulder girdle at the glenohumeral joint. The proximal portion contains the **humerus**, a bone that articulates proximally with the scapula and distally with the bones of the forearm—the radius and ulna—to form the hinged elbow joint.

The **radius** and **ulna** make up the forearm. The radius, the larger of the two forearm bones, lies on the thumb side of the forearm. Distally, the ulna is narrow and is on the small finger side of the forearm. It serves as the pivot around

Garrison Care TIPS

To remember the difference between supination and pronation, think of soup. The *SUP*-inated hand can hold a cup of *soup*.

which the radius turns at the wrist to rotate the palm upward (**supination**) or downward (**pronation**). Because the radius and the ulna are arranged in parallel, when one is broken, the other is often broken as well.

The hand **FIGURE 27-4 ▶** contains three sets of bones: wrist bones (**carpals**), hand bones (**metacarpals**), and finger bones (**phalanges**). The carpals, especially the scaphoid, are vulnerable to fracture when a person falls on an outstretched hand. Phalanges are more apt to be injured by a crushing injury, such as being slammed in a car door.

Pelvis and Lower Extremities

The pelvic girdle **FIGURE 27-5 ▶** is actually three separate bones—the **ischium**, **ilium**, and **pubis**—fused together to form the innominate bone. The two iliac bones are joined posteriorly by tough ligaments to the sacrum at the **sacroiliac joints**; the two pubic bones are connected anteriorly to one another by equally tough ligaments at the symphysis pubis. These joints allow very little motion, so the pelvic ring is strong and stable.

The lower extremity consists of the bones of the thigh, leg, and foot **FIGURE 27-6 ▶**. The **femur** (thigh bone) is a long, powerful bone that articulates proximally in the ball-and-socket joint of the pelvis and distally in the hinge joint of the knee. The head of the femur is the ball-shaped part that fits into the **acetabulum**. It is connected to the shaft, or long tubular portion of the femur, by the femoral neck. The femoral neck is a common site for fractures, generally referred to as hip fractures, especially in the older population.

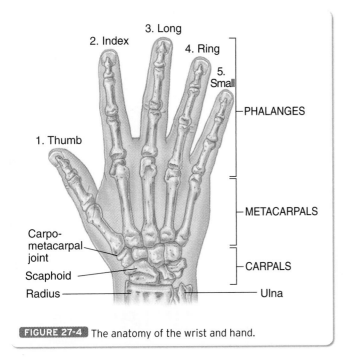

FIGURE 27-4 The anatomy of the wrist and hand.

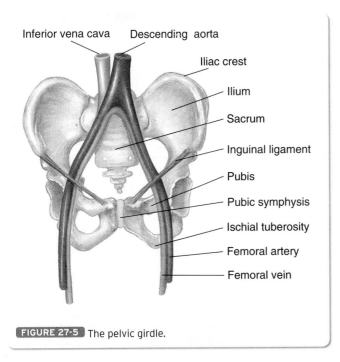

FIGURE 27-5 The pelvic girdle.

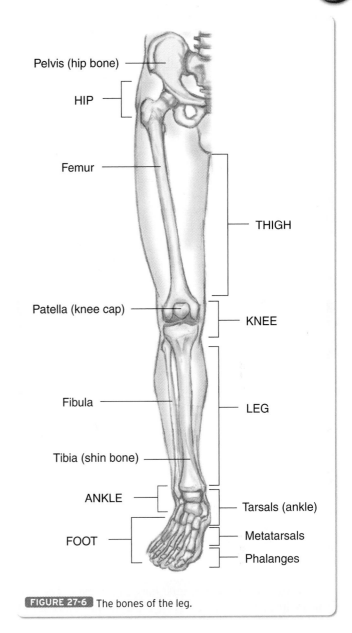

FIGURE 27-6 The bones of the leg.

The foot **FIGURE 27-7 ▶** consists of three classes of bones: ankle bones (**tarsals**), foot bones (**metatarsals**), and toe bones (phalanges). The largest of the tarsal bones is the heel bone, or **calcaneus**, which is subject to injury when a person jumps from a height and lands on his or her feet.

Characteristics and Composition of Bone

Bone Shapes

Bones may be classified based on their shape. **Long bones** are longer than they are wide; examples include the femur, humerus, tibia, fibula, radius, and ulna. **Short bones** are nearly as wide as they are long; they include the phalanges, metacarpals, and metatarsals. **Flat bones** are thin, broad bones; they include the sternum, ribs, scapulae, and skull. **Irregular bones** do not fit into one of the other categories but rather have a shape that is designed to perform a specific function, such as the bones of the vertebral column and the

The lower leg consists of two bones, the **tibia** and the **fibula**. The tibia (shin bone) forms the inferior component of the knee joint. Anterior to this joint is the **patella** (knee-cap), a bone that is important for knee extension. The tibia runs down the front of the lower leg, where it is vulnerable to direct blows, and can be felt just beneath the skin. The much smaller fibula runs posteriorly and laterally to the tibia. The fibula is not a component of the knee joint, but it does make up the lateral knob of the ankle joint (lateral **malleolus**) at its distal articulation.

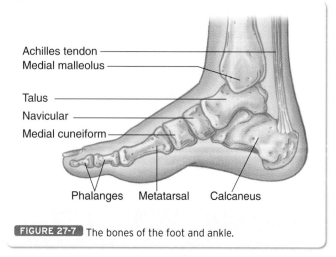

FIGURE 27-7 The bones of the foot and ankle.

mandible. <u>**Round bones**</u> are generally found in proximity to a joint and help with movement. They are often referred to as sesamoid bones because of their location within a tendon. The patella is the largest of these bones.

Typical Long Bone Architecture

Long bones have several distinct regions and anatomic features **FIGURE 27-8 ▶**. These bones can grow to such long lengths because of the presence of the growth plate, or <u>**physis**</u>, in children. Once a person reaches adulthood, the growth plate closes and the mature adult bone is complete. The long bone is divided into three regions: the diaphysis, the epiphysis, and the metaphysis.

The articular surfaces of a long bone come in contact with other bones to form <u>**articulations**</u> (joints). These regions of the bone are covered by articular <u>**cartilage**</u>, a substance that acts as a cushion to protect the bone from damage and wear. The portion of bone that is not covered by articular cartilage is, instead, covered by the <u>**periosteum**</u>. This dense, fibrous membrane contains capillaries and cells that are important for bone repair and maintenance. In the inner portion of the long bone, blood enters through a nutrient artery. Once it penetrates the bone's outer cortex, the artery enters the <u>**medullary canal**</u>, the hollow inner portion of the shaft that is lined by the <u>**endosteum**</u> (similar to the periosteum, but on the inside) and contains yellow (fatty) marrow in adults.

Joints

When two bones come together, they articulate with one another to form a joint. Some joints are fused and allow for no motion, such as the joints of the skull. Other joints allow

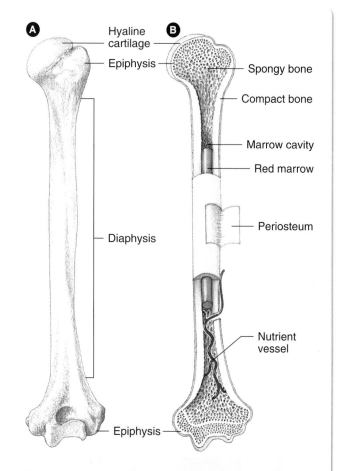

FIGURE 27-8 Anatomy of the long bone. **A.** The humerus. Notice the long shaft and dilated ends. **B.** Longitudinal section of the humerus showing compact bone, spongy bone, and marrow.

for motion by permitting movement between the two bones, typically within a certain plane of motion that is defined by the structure of the bones that form it. The various motions that a joint may allow include flexion, extension, <u>**abduction**</u>, <u>**adduction**</u>, rotation, circumduction, pronation, and supination **FIGURE 27-9 ▶**.

Types of Joints

The three general types of joints are fibrous, cartilaginous, and synovial **FIGURE 27-10 ▶**. <u>**Fibrous joints**</u>, also referred to as synarthroses or fused joints, contain dense fibrous tissue that does not allow for movement. Examples include the bones of the skull and the distal tibiofibular joint.

<u>**Cartilaginous joints,**</u> also called amphiarthroses, allow for very minimal movement between the bones. The pubic symphysis and the joints connecting the ribs to the sternum are examples of this type of joint.

<u>**Synovial joints**</u>, or diarthroses, are the most mobile joints of the body. They are surrounded by an extension of the periosteum called the <u>**joint capsule**</u>, with the bones that form them being held in place by very strong <u>**ligaments**</u>. Within the joint are the articular cartilage and the

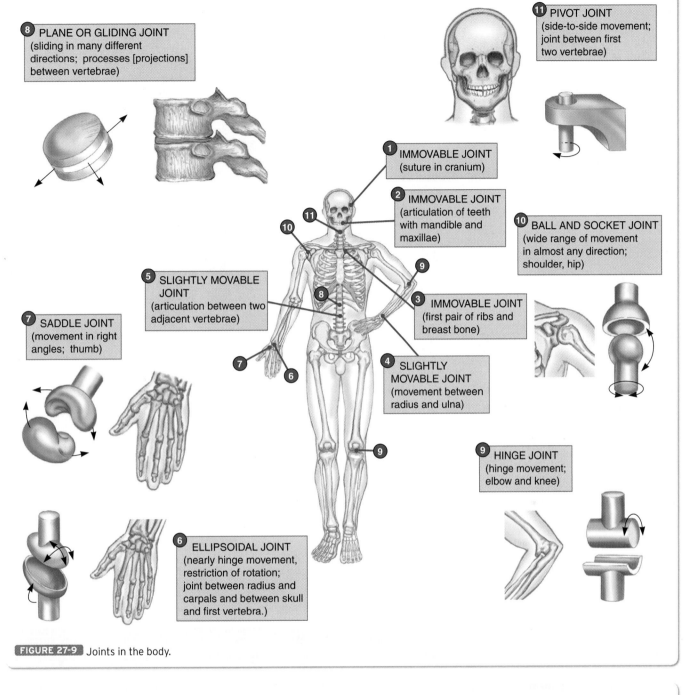

8 PLANE OR GLIDING JOINT
(sliding in many different directions; processes [projections] between vertebrae)

11 PIVOT JOINT
(side-to-side movement; joint between first two vertebrae)

1 IMMOVABLE JOINT
(suture in cranium)

2 IMMOVABLE JOINT
(articulation of teeth with mandible and maxillae)

10 BALL AND SOCKET JOINT
(wide range of movement in almost any direction; shoulder, hip)

5 SLIGHTLY MOVABLE JOINT
(articulation between two adjacent vertebrae)

3 IMMOVABLE JOINT
(first pair of ribs and breast bone)

7 SADDLE JOINT
(movement in right angles; thumb)

4 SLIGHTLY MOVABLE JOINT
(movement between radius and ulna)

9 HINGE JOINT
(hinge movement; elbow and knee)

6 ELLIPSOIDAL JOINT
(nearly hinge movement, restriction of rotation; joint between radius and carpals and between skull and first vertebra.)

FIGURE 27-9 Joints in the body.

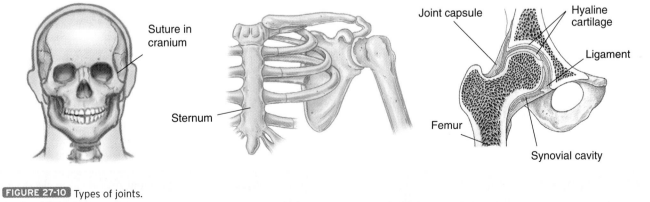

Suture in cranium

Sternum

Joint capsule

Hyaline cartilage

Ligament

Femur

Synovial cavity

FIGURE 27-10 Types of joints.

synovial membrane, which secretes synovial fluid into the joint cavity to lubricate it.

Bursa

A **bursa** is a padlike sac or cavity located within the connective tissue, usually in proximity to a joint. It may be lined with a synovial membrane and typically contains fluid that helps reduce the amount of friction between a tendon and a bone or between a tendon and a ligament. Examples include the olecranon bursa of the elbow and the prepatellar bursa of the knee. **Bursitis** is inflammation of a bursa.

Skeletal Connecting and Supporting Structures

Tendons connect muscle to bone. These flat or cordlike bands of connective tissue are white and have a glistening appearance.

Ligaments connect bone to bone and help maintain the stability of joints and determine the degree of joint motion. These inelastic bands of connective tissue have a structure similar to that of tendons.

Cartilage consists of fibers of collagen embedded in a gelatinous substance. This flexible connective tissue forms the smooth surface over bone ends where they articulate, provides cushioning between vertebrae, gives structure to the nose and external ear, forms the framework of the larynx and trachea, and serves as the model for the formation of the skeleton in children. Cartilage has a very limited neurovascular supply—it receives nutrients through diffusion from the outer covering of the cartilage or from the synovial fluid—so it does not heal well if it is injured.

The Moving Forces: Muscles

Muscles are composed of specialized cells that contract (shorten) when stimulated to exert a force on a part of the body. Three types of muscle are found in the body: smooth muscle, cardiac muscle, and skeletal muscle **FIGURE 27-11** .

Skeletal Muscle

Skeletal muscle **FIGURE 27-12** is also called **voluntary muscle**, because its contractions are largely under voluntary control, or **striated muscle**, because striations can be seen in it during microscopic examination. Skeletal muscle includes all of the muscles attached to the skeleton and forms the bulk of the tissue of the arms and legs. It is also found along the spine and buttocks. By maintaining a state of partial contraction, this type of muscle allows the body to maintain its posture and to sit or stand. It varies greatly in size and shape, from thin strands to the large muscles of the thigh and back. It also constitutes the muscles of the tongue, soft palate, scalp, pharynx, upper esophagus, and eye. About 40% to 50% of normal body weight is skeletal muscle, because it has a high water content. In addition, because of its high metabolic rate and demand for energy and oxygen, skeletal muscle has a very rich blood supply, which causes it to bleed significantly when injured.

Skeletal muscles are profoundly affected by the amount of training and work to which they are subjected. Unused

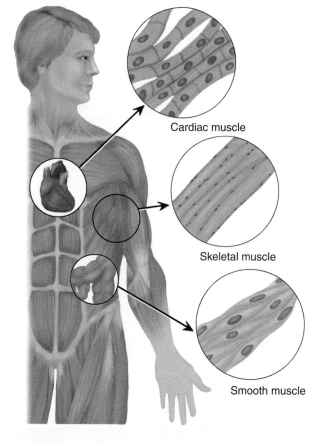

FIGURE 27-11 The three types of muscle are skeletal, smooth, and cardiac.

muscles tend to **atrophy** (shrink or waste away), whereas physical training promotes **hypertrophy** (increase in size).

Skeletal muscles are attached to bones by tendons. Tendons cross joints to create a pulling force between two bones when a muscle contracts. The biceps muscle, for example, has its origin on the scapula; the biceps tendon passes over the head of the humerus, where it fuses with the body of the biceps muscle. At the distal end of the biceps, a tendon passes over the anterior surface of the elbow and inserts on the radius. Thus, when the biceps muscle contracts, the force causes the elbow to bend (flex).

Muscle contraction requires energy. This energy is derived from the metabolism of glucose and results in the production of **lactic acid** (lactate). Lactic acid, in turn, must be converted into carbon dioxide and water, a process that requires oxygen. For that reason, vigorous muscular activity is often followed by an increased respiratory rate, which increases oxygen delivery to and carbon dioxide removal from the tissues.

The sensation of **muscle fatigue** occurs when the energy supply to the muscle is inadequate to meet the energy demands. If muscle fatigue occurs as a result of excessive muscular activity, rest produces quick recovery. If it occurs from a lack of oxygen or essential nutrients or electrolytes

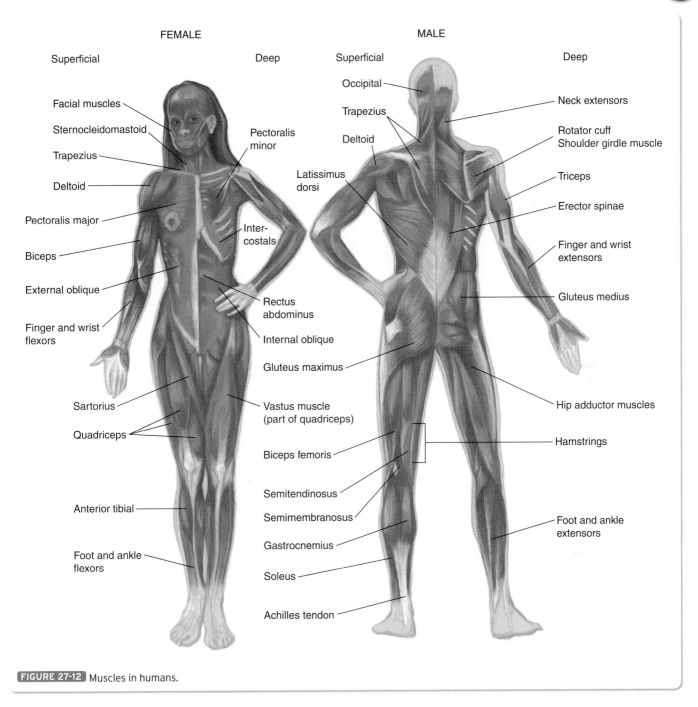

FEMALE

Superficial   Deep

Facial muscles

Sternocleidomastoid

Trapezius   Pectoralis
                                                minor
Deltoid

Pectoralis major

Biceps   Inter-
                                                costals
External oblique

Finger and wrist   Rectus
flexors   abdominus

                                                Internal oblique

Sartorius   Gluteus maximus

Quadriceps   Vastus muscle
                                                (part of quadriceps)

                                                Biceps femoris

Anterior tibial   Semitendinosus

                                                Semimembranosus

Foot and ankle   Gastrocnemius
flexors
                                                Soleus

                                                Achilles tendon

MALE

Superficial   Deep

Occipital   Neck extensors

Trapezius   Rotator cuff
                                                Shoulder girdle muscle
Deltoid

Latissimus   Triceps
dorsi
                                                Erector spinae

                                                Finger and wrist
                                                extensors

                                                Gluteus medius

                                                Hip adductor muscles

                                                Hamstrings

                                                Foot and ankle
                                                extensors

FIGURE 27-12 Muscles in humans.

Musculoskeletal Blood Supply

When a person has a musculoskeletal injury, the arteries that supply the injured region may also be damaged. Therefore, it is important to realize which arteries are present in each part of the extremity **FIGURE 27-13 ▶**.

The upper extremity's blood supply originates from the **subclavian artery**. When the subclavian artery reaches the axilla, it is referred to as the **axillary artery**. After giving off several branches that supply the shoulder region with blood,

(such as sodium or calcium), however, rest will not lead to such a quick recovery.

the artery leaves the axilla and becomes the **brachial artery**. After the brachial artery passes through the elbow, it divides into the **radial artery** and **ulnar artery**. In the hand, the radial and ulnar arteries form superficial and deep arcades of blood vessels that branch to form the arteries of each finger, the **digital arteries**.

In the lower extremity, the blood supply originates from the external iliac artery. When the external iliac artery reaches the leg, it becomes the **femoral artery**. When it reaches the knee, the femoral artery turns posteriorly and laterally and is referred to as the **popliteal artery**. The popliteal artery divides into the **anterior tibial artery** and the **posterior tibial artery**.

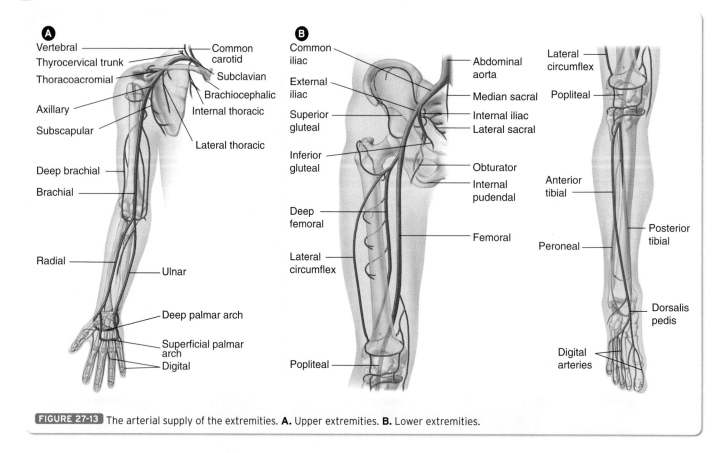

FIGURE 27-13 The arterial supply of the extremities. **A.** Upper extremities. **B.** Lower extremities.

The anterior tibial artery travels along the anterior and lateral surface of the tibia until it reaches the ankle, where it proceeds along the **dorsal** surface of the foot toward the great toe and becomes the dorsalis pedis artery. The posterior tibial artery travels along the posterior aspect of the tibia until it reaches the ankle, where it follows a path just behind the medial malleolus until it reaches the **plantar** aspect of the foot. Within the foot, arcades of arteries supply the various structures with blood and give off branches that form the digital arteries of the toes.

■ Using the SOAP Method

Use the SOAP method to evaluate a musculoskeletal complaint. The SOAP method is the standard for documentation in medical treatment records and is designed to allow for easy reference for follow-up care. The method follows the standard and natural flow of a patient interview, beginning with the *Subjective* data, proceeding to the *Objective* findings, arriving at an *Assessment*, and formulating a treatment *Plan*. Chapter 17, *Sick Call Procedures and Medical Documentation*, covers the SOAP method in detail.

Subjective Data

Obtain a relevant history of the patient's presenting symptoms or complaints. Note the patient's age, sex, race, and if the patient is female, first day of the last menstrual period (FDLMP). Note the patient's chief complaint by having the patient state in one sentence the reason for the visit; for example, "I twisted my ankle while running this morning."

Garrison Care **TIPS**

Maintain a high index of suspicion. Paying close attention to the degree of pain and disability reported by the patient will ensure you give appropriate consideration to the possibilities that could account for the symptoms. Consider the mechanism of injury. Any injury reported by the patient should raise or lower your index of suspicion for the potential severity of the injury. A patient complaining of knee pain after twisting it while running probably has less potential for a significant injury compared to a patient who twisted his or her knee when landing following a parachute jump.

Obtain the patient's history of present illness (HPI) using the OPQRST method. The HPI contains all of the information relevant to the patient's chief complaint:

- **Onset:** Sudden? Gradual? Specific injury?
- **Provoking/palliative factors:** What makes it worse/better?
- **Quality:** What does the pain feel like? Sharp? Dull?
- **Radiation/region:** Where is the pain? Is it localized to one area?
- **Severity:** How would you score the pain on a scale of 1 to 10? Does it limit your activity?
- **Timing:** Duration? Is the pain intermittent? Constant?
- **Associated symptoms and complaints:** Are there other complaints? Are they related?

Obtain the patient's past history using the SAMPLE method. This contains information that may contribute to the HPI. This information may be helpful in determining possible causes of the chief complaint or ruling out other possible causes. This information may also impact your treatment decisions. Its principle components are:

- **Signs/symptoms:** Mostly unnecessary if you obtained a thorough HPI.
- **Allergies:** List any allergies and reactions to medications.
- **Medications:** List all medications and dosages, including over-the-counter (OTC) medications that the patient is presently taking.
- Past medical and surgical history including social history:
  - **Past medical history (PMH):** List any significant medical diagnosis or disease condition the patient has; for example, hypertension, diabetes, etc.
  - **Past surgical history (PSH):** List any significant surgical procedures that have been performed; for example, appendectomy, tonsillectomy, C-section.
  - **Social history (Soc. Hx):** Document the patient's use of tobacco, alcohol, and/or illegal substances. Occupational and leisure activities may be relevant and would be entered in this section.
- **Last oral intake:** The last thing the patient had to eat and drink and when it was consumed.
- **Events leading up to illness or injury:** The situation that led to the illness or injury, if known.

Objective Data

The objective information includes vital signs, general impression, and the physical examination findings by body area. At a minimum, the vital signs should include blood pressure, temperature, pulse, and respiratory rate. The general impression is a statement of your initial impression of the current state of the patient's general health; for example:

GEN—patient in no acute distress (NAD) or
GEN—patient appears to be in severe pain.

Examine the body areas that are potentially related to the history you obtained under the subjective section. In the case of orthopaedic complaints it is common to abbreviate this as "MUSC" for musculoskeletal. If a patient is complaining of joint symptoms, it is advisable to also evaluate the joint above and below the area of complaint; for example:

MUSC—full range of motion (FROM) left knee. Positive tenderness to palpation (TTP) of patellar tendon. No joint instability appreciated.

During the physical examination, perform an inspection. Is there a gross or obvious deformity, soft-tissue swelling (STS), erythema (redness of skin), or ecchymosis (bruising)? Can the patient bear weight on the extremity? Compare the injured extremity to the uninjured extremity. Determine the patient's range of motion (ROM)—is it full or limited? Compare the ROM to the uninjured extremity.

Next, palpate the injured extremity. Is there tenderness to palpation (TTP)? Can it be localized to one point or is it diffuse? Consider the anatomy you are palpating to help determine what may potentially be injured. If a joint is involved, is it stable or is there laxity of the ligaments?

Perform special maneuvers as indicated by the location of the complaint and compare to the uninjured extremity. Determine the patient's muscle strength—is it full or limited? Compare the patient's muscle strength to the uninjured extremity.

Assessment

The assessment is your suspected diagnosis. If you suspect a particular injury, but are not 100% certain, then your assessment might read as follows:

A. R/O MMT. Translation: Assessment = rule out medial meniscus tear.

If would also be appropriate to simply restate the patient's chief complaint; for example:

A. Knee pain.

Plan

Your treatment plan should be noted. It could be as simple as:

P. Refer to medical officer.

At a minimum, this plan should include:

- Medication and dosage, if prescribed.
- Duty and activity restrictions, if any.
- When the patient should return for follow-up evaluation. Every SOAP note should conclude with the circumstances under which the patient should return (eg, Return to clinic [RTC] if symptoms persist, worsen, or other symptoms develop).

■ Shoulder Examination

The shoulder region and upper arm are susceptible to a wide variety of both traumatic and nontraumatic disorders. Most complaints in the military are a result of overuse and repetitive motions. As a result, conservative treatment measures and

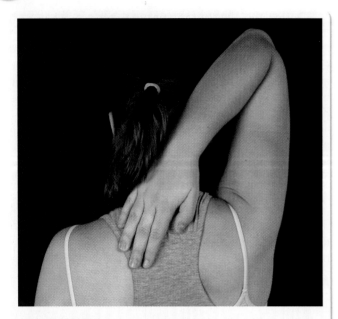

FIGURE 27-14 Test the shoulder for external rotation and abduction by having the patient attempt to reach his or her hand over the shoulder and behind the head to touch his or her fingertips to the top of the opposite shoulder blade.

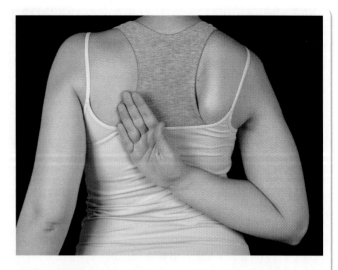

FIGURE 27-15 Test the shoulder for internal rotation and abduction by having the patient attempt to reach his or her hand behind the back to touch his or her fingertips to the bottom of the opposite shoulder blade.

a reasonable period of time avoiding aggravating activity are commonly all that is necessary. The first step in evaluating a patient with any symptom is to obtain a good focused history (subjective data). The second step is the physical examination (objective data).

Inspection of the shoulder begins by comparing the painful shoulder to the unaffected side. Note whether the patient has difficulty moving his or her shoulder. Observe for abnormalities of the neck and elbow (the joint above and the joint below). Inspect for obvious deformities, soft-tissue swelling (STS), erythema (redness), and ecchymosis (bruising).

Test the patient's range of motion (ROM). Test the shoulder for external rotation and abduction by having the patient attempt to reach his or her hand over the shoulder and behind the head to touch his or her fingertips to the top of the opposite scapula (shoulder blade) **FIGURE 27-14 ▲**. Test the shoulder for internal rotation and abduction by having the patient attempt to reach his or her hand behind the back to touch his or her fingertips to the bottom of the opposite scapula **FIGURE 27-1 5 ▶**. The patient is said to have full range of motion (FROM) if he or she can successfully perform each of the above maneuvers. Make certain to compare the range of motion to the unaffected shoulder.

Next, perform palpation on the anterior, posterior, lateral, and superior aspects of the shoulder girdle, noting any tenderness to palpation (TTP) or deformities. Compare your findings to the unaffected shoulder.

Test the patient's muscle strength. Assess flexion by having the patient pull his or her arm anteriorly while you pull the arm in the opposite direction, resisting his or her effort. Note any weakness compared to the unaffected extremity.

Assess extension by having the patient pull his or her arm posteriorly while you pull the arm in the opposite direction, resisting his or her effort. Note any weakness as compared to the unaffected extremity.

Assess abduction by having the patient push his or her arm laterally away from the body while you push in the opposite direction, resisting the patient's effort. Note any weakness as compared to the unaffected extremity.

Assess adduction by having the patient pull his or her arm medially toward the body while you pull in the opposite direction, resisting the patient's effort. Note any weakness compared to the unaffected extremity.

Assess external rotation by having the patient keep his or her elbow tucked against his or her side and rotate the forearm laterally and away from the body as you resist the patient's effort. Note any weakness as compared to the unaffected extremity.

Assess internal rotation by having the patient keep his or her elbow tucked against his or her side and rotate the forearm medially and toward the midline as you resist the patient's effort. Note any weakness as compared to the unaffected extremity.

Assessment

Document your presumptive diagnosis based on the focused history and the physical examination findings. Common causes of shoulder pain in the soldier population include **tendinitis**, bursitis, muscle strains, and contusions. If you are unsure of the diagnosis, simply restate the chief complaint of the patient, such as "A. shoulder pain."

Plan

Document what your plan is to treat the patient based on the assessment you have made. Any numbness, muscle weakness, decreased range of motion, or radiating pain requires a prompt referral to the medical officer. Minor sprains, strains, tendinitis, and contusions are commonly treated with rest, ice compresses, short-term use of a sling, and the administration of oral anti-inflammatory medications.

Red Flags

The red flags of shoulder pain are the signs and symptoms that warrant urgent referral to a medical officer:

- Muscle weakness in either upper extremity
- Severe pain or decreased ROM
- Numbness or diminished sensation in either upper extremity
- A significant mechanism of injury (MOI)
- Chronic or long-standing pain or disability
- Pain that radiates to other areas or pain radiating from other areas to the shoulder, such as from the neck to the shoulder
- Associated chest pain, shortness of breath, or fever

■ Lower Back Examination

Lower back pain is a common symptom among soldiers. The most common cause of lower back pain in soldiers is a strain of the lower back musculature. Muscle spasms are common as well. The focused history will commonly lead you to a correct diagnosis or assessment.

A patient with no history of injury is worrisome because the possible causes include malignancy (cancer) of the pelvis or spine or an abdominal organ disorder. Pain that radiates into the buttock and/or lower extremity may indicate nerve root involvement such as a herniated intervertebral disk. More concerning than pain that radiates from the lower back would be weakness of either lower extremity because this could indicate significant nerve root involvement that may require urgent surgery to correct.

Objective Data

Inspect the following items:

- Observe the patient's walk and posture.
- Inspect for loss or absence of the usual lumbar lordosis (curvature).
- Inspect for skin changes, visible muscle spasm, obvious deformities, soft-tissue swelling (STS), erythema (redness), or ecchymosis (bruising).

Inspect the patient's ROM. Test for lumbar flexion by having the patient attempt to bend over and touch his or her toes while keeping the legs straight. Note how close the fingertips come to the toes. Test for lumbar extension by having the patient arch his or her back in a posterior direction as far

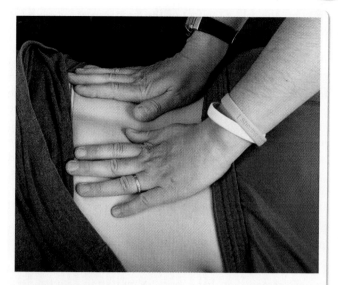

FIGURE 27-16 Palpate the muscles that parallel the middle lumbar spine.

as possible. Test for lateral bending at the waist by having the patient bend to the left and to the right. The patient should be able to bend the same distance on each side. Test for rotation at the waist by having the patient pivot to the left and right while his or her hips remain in a fixed position. The patient should be able to rotate to the same degree on each side.

Palpate the spinous processes that run up the middle of the lumbar spine and note any depressions. Palpate the paraspinal muscles (the muscles that parallel the middle lumbar spine) **FIGURE 27-16 ▲**. Note any TTP or palpable muscle spasm.

Test the patient's muscle strength by performing the hamstring muscle test. With the patient lying in a prone position, have him or her attempt to flex the hamstring muscles by pulling his or her foot toward the buttock. At the same time, grasp his or her ankle and resist the patient's effort. Repeat this with the opposite extremity and note any difference in strength.

Perform the quadriceps muscle test. With the patient sitting on the edge of an examination table, have the patient attempt to flex his or her quadriceps muscles by extending the lower leg against your hand as you resist the effort. Repeat this with the opposite extremity and note any difference in strength.

Perform the calf muscle strength test. With the patient sitting on the edge of the examination table or chair, have the patient attempt to plantar flex his or her foot (press the foot down) against the resistance of your hand. Alternately you could have the patient attempt to stand on his or her tiptoes. Repeat this with the opposite extremity and note any difference in strength.

Test the patient's anterior leg muscle strength. With the patient sitting on the edge of the examination table or chair, have the patient attempt to dorsiflex his or her foot (pull the foot up) against the resistance of your hand. Alternately, you could have the patient attempt to stand on his or her heels and raise the ball of the foot off the floor. Repeat this with the opposite extremity and note any difference in strength.

Assessment

Document your presumptive assessment based on the focused history and physical examination findings. Consider that the presence of lower back pain without a precipitating injury could be more significant than back pain with a precipitating injury. Common causes of lower back pain in soldiers include muscle strains and muscle spasms that will typically respond to a brief period of rest, application of moist-hot compresses, and the administration of oral anti-inflammatory medications. If you are unsure of the diagnosis, simply restate the chief complaint of the patient; for example, "A. back pain."

Plan

Document what your plan is to treat the patient based on the assessment you have made. Minor strains and muscle spasms can be treated with short periods of rest, moist-hot compresses, and the administration of oral anti-inflammatory medication as needed. Oral muscle relaxants are sometimes necessary for the relief of a muscle spasm. Any muscle weakness, numbness, loss of control of bowel or bladder function, or decrease in range of motion requires prompt referral to a medical officer.

Red Flags

The signs and symptoms that warrant urgent referral to a medical officer include:

- Patient with loss of bowel or bladder control (incontinence)
- Muscle weakness in either lower extremity
- Severe pain or decreased ROM
- Numbness or loss of sensation in buttocks, groin, or lower extremity
- Significant MOI
- Chronic or long-standing pain or disability
- Pain that radiates to other areas
- Associated abdominal pain, fever, or bloody urine

■ Knee Examination

Most unilateral knee pain is traumatic in origin. Acute trauma usually causes ligament sprains or meniscal damage. Repeated mild trauma over long periods of time can lead to chondromalacia (softening of cartilage), tendinitis, bursitis, chronic arthritis, or other problems. The focused history that you obtain will lead you to the most likely cause. The physical examination will help confirm your suspicions.

Objective Data

Compare the problem knee to the unaffected knee. Determine whether the patient can walk more than a few steps on the affected extremity. The inability to bear weight should raise concern. Determine whether the patient is also having problems with the hip or ankle. Inspect for an obvious deformity, erythema, ecchymosis, or STS.

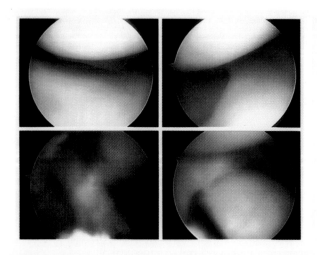

FIGURE 27-17 A meniscal injury may need to be repaired with surgery.

Test the patient's ROM. Have the patient perform a deep knee bend by flexing his or her knees until the buttocks touch the heels and then rise again to a standing position. This indicates that the patient has FROM. If the patient is unable to perform the deep knee bend, then assess his or her ROM while he or she is seated on the edge of an examination table. A popping sensation or sound during ROM could indicate torn knee cartilage or meniscus.

Palpate the lateral aspect of the knee including the lateral collateral ligament (also known as the fibular collateral ligament). TTP could indicate a tear or sprain of the ligament. Palpate the medial aspect of the knee including the medial collateral ligament (also known as the tibial collateral ligament). TTP could indicate a tear or sprain of the ligament.

With the patient's knee flexed to about 90°, palpate the anterior joint line. This is the superior aspect of the tibia where a portion of the medial and lateral meniscus can be palpated. TTP here could indicate a meniscal injury **FIGURE 27-17 ▲**. Medial meniscus injuries are more common than lateral meniscus injuries. Palpate the patella and along the patellar tendon down to its insertion into the tibia. TTP of the patella, patellar tendon, or its insertion could indicate bursitis or tendinitis.

Apply stress to the lateral collateral (fibular collateral) ligament (LCL). Use one hand to brace the patient's knee on its medial side. With your other hand, apply pressure to the patient's extended lower leg in a medial direction. This is known as varus stress. Repeat the procedure on the unaffected extremity. A normal, intact ligament should prevent the lower leg from deviating toward the midline.

Apply stress to the medial collateral (tibial collateral) ligament (MCL). Use one hand to brace the patient's knee on its lateral side. With your other hand, apply pressure to the patient's extended lower leg in a lateral direction; this is known as valgus stress. Repeat the procedure on the unaffected extremity. A normal, intact ligament should prevent the lower leg from deviating away from the midline. **FIGURE 27-18 ▶** demonstrates the valgus stress while

FIGURE 27-19 ▾ demonstrates the varus stress.

Apply stress to the anterior cruciate ligament (ACL). With the patient's knee flexed to about 90° and his or her foot stabilized, apply anterior stress to the lower leg. Repeat the procedure on the unaffected extremity. A normal, intact ACL should result in no movement of the tibia in relation to the femur. Movement of the tibia anteriorly would be called a positive anterior drawer sign.

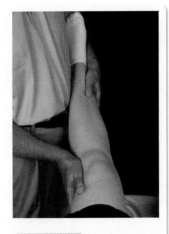

FIGURE 27-18 Apply valgus stress to assess the patient's knee.

Apply stress to the posterior cruciate ligament (PCL). With the patient's knee flexed to about 90° and his or her foot stabilized, apply posterior stress to the lower leg. Repeat the procedure on the unaffected extremity. A normal, intact PCL should result in no movement of the tibia in relation to the femur. Movement of the tibia posteriorly would be called a positive posterior drawer sign.

Perform the quadriceps muscle test. Have the patient sit on the edge of the examination table with his or her knee flexed to about 90°. Then have him or her attempt to extend the lower leg against the resistance of your hand. Compare to the unaffected extremity and note any weakness.

Perform the second hamstring muscle test. Have the patient lie in the prone position on the examination table with his or her lower extremity fully extended. Then have the patient attempt to flex his or her knee as the lower leg pulls against the resistance of your hand. Compare the unaffected extremity and note any weakness.

Assessment

Document your presumptive assessment based on the focused history and the physical examination findings. In soldiers, anterior knee pain in the absence of trauma is often due to overuse injuries such as patellar tendinitis. Twisting injuries of the knee, especially when the foot was planted firmly on the ground, can result in meniscal or ligamentous injuries. If you are unsure of the possible diagnosis, simply restate the chief complaint, for example, "A. knee pain."

Plan

Document what your plan is to treat the patient based on the assessment you have made. Minor sprains and tendinitis can be treated with short periods of rest, ice compresses, and the administration of oral anti-inflammatory medication as needed. Any muscle weakness, numbness, laxity of ligaments, decrease in range of motion, or difficulty walking requires prompt referral to a medical officer.

Red Flags

The signs and symptoms that warrant referral to a medical officer are:

- A joint that is red (erythematous) or warm to the touch (urgent referral)
- A joint with signs of instability such as a positive drawer sign
- Any condition significantly limiting the activity or duties of the patient
- Any condition where the patient has difficulty bearing weight
- When a tear of a tendon, muscle, or ligament is suspected
- Any chronic or long-standing condition
- Any situation where there is a suspected compromise of circulation (urgent referral)
- Any swelling of the knee (effusion)

■ Ankle Examination

Ankle sprains are common in the active duty population due to the high level of physical activity. Most ankle sprains are a result of ankle inversion and therefore result in pain of the lateral aspect of the ankle. Ankle sprains can be grouped as grade I (simple sprains), or as grade II or grade III sprains, which are significant. A grade I sprain is confined to the anterior talofibular ligament (ATFL) and demonstrates no instability. A grade II sprain involves injury to both the ATFL and calcaneofibular ligament (CFL), with mild laxity of one or both ligaments. A grade III sprain involves injury and significant laxity of both the ATFL and CFL. Fractures are frequently associated with significant sprains.

Objective Data

Compare the problem ankle to the unaffected ankle. Determine whether the patient can bear weight on the affected extremity. Inspect for apparent pain with the knee or lower leg and for obvious deformity, erythema, ecchymosis, or STS.

Test the patient's plantar flexion by having the patient stand on his or her tiptoes. If the patient is unable to do so, have the patient sit down in a chair or on the edge of an examination table. Then see if the patient can flex his or her

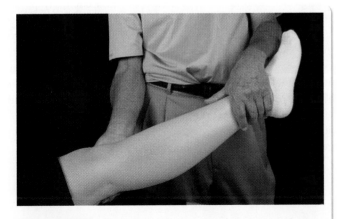

FIGURE 27-19 Apply varus stress to assess the patient's knee.

foot downward. Note the location of any area the patient says is painful with this motion. Compare to the unaffected side.

Test the patient's dorsiflexion by having the patient stand on his or her heels and raise the ball of the foot off of the floor. If the patient is unable to do so, have the patient sit down in a chair or on the edge of an examination table. Then see if the patient can flex his or her foot upward. Note the location of any area the patient says is painful with this motion. Compare to the unaffected side.

Test inversion by having the patient stand on the lateral borders of his or her feet, raising the medial borders up off of the floor. If the patient is unable to do so, have the patient sit down in a chair or on the edge of an examination table. Grasp the patient's midfoot and rotate the sole toward the midline, noting any pain produced and its location. Compare to the unaffected side.

Test eversion by having the patient stand on the medial borders of his or her feet, raising the lateral borders up off the floor. If the patient is unable to do so, have the patient sit down in a chair or on the edge of an examination table. Grasp the patient's midfoot and rotate the sole away from the mid-line, noting any pain produced and its location. Compare to the unaffected side.

Palpate the medial malleolus (distal tibia) and lateral malleolus (distal fibula). TTP over the malleoli could indicate a fracture or a site where a ligament has pulled away from its bony attachment. Compare to the unaffected side.

Palpate the area inferior to each malleolus. TTP here could indicate a sprained or torn ligament. Compare to the unaffected side.

Palpate the base of the fifth metatarsal. TTP here could indicate a fracture where a tendon has pulled away from its insertion. This is not unusual in the case of ankle inversion injuries. Compare to the unaffected side.

Stress the lateral ankle ligaments by grasping the patient's lower leg with one hand and the heel with the other. While stabilizing the leg, apply an inversion force to the heel. Compare with the unaffected ankle and note any laxity of the lateral ligaments.

Stress the medial ankle ligaments. Grasp the patient's lower leg with one hand and the heel with the other. While stabilizing the leg, apply an eversion force to the heel. Compare with the unaffected ankle and note any laxity of the medial ligaments.

Stress the ligaments, providing anterior and posterior ankle stability. Grasp the patient's lower leg with one hand and the heel with the other. While stabilizing the leg apply an anterior drawer force to the heel. Compare with the unaffected ankle and note any laxity of the ATFL and CFL. Laxity with this maneuver is abnormal and known as a positive anterior drawer test.

Assess the Achilles tendon for integrity. Have the patient flex the knee of the injured extremity (while standing on the other leg) and rest his or her shin on the seat of a chair. With your hand, squeeze the calf muscles. If the Achilles tendon is not ruptured you should see the foot plantar flex as the calf muscles are squeezed. Compare to the unaffected extremity.

Assess the calf muscles for weakness. Have the patient hop up and land on the ball of his or her foot. It is normal if the patient can do this. It is abnormal if the patient lands flat-footed. Compare to the unaffected extremity.

An alternate method for assessing the calf muscles for weakness is having the patient stand on his or her tiptoes. If he or she is unable to do so, have the patient sit down in a chair or on the edge of an examination table. Then see if the patient can flex the foot downward against the resistance of your hand. Note any weakness as compared to the unaffected side.

Assess the anterior leg muscles for weakness. Have the patient stand on his or her heels and raise the ball of the foot off of the floor (dorsiflexion). If the patient is unable to do so, have him or her sit down in a chair or on the edge of an examination table. Then see if the patient can flex the foot upward against the resistance of your hand. Note any weakness as compared to the unaffected side.

Assessment

Document your presumptive assessment based on the history and your physical examination findings. Most ankle sprains are due to inversion injury. With rare exception, patients with a minor (grade I) sprain are able to walk on the injured extremity shortly after the injury, although it may be painful to do so. More significant injuries usually present with significant difficulty bearing weight on the extremity shortly after the injury. Tendon ruptures are not common, but weakness on examination should clue you in to this possibility. If unsure of the possible diagnosis, simply restate the chief complaint; for example, "A. ankle pain."

Plan

Document what your plan is to treat the patient based on the assessment you have made. Minor sprains and tendinitis can be treated with short periods of rest, ice compresses, and administering oral anti-inflammatory medication as needed. Wrapping the injured ankle with an elastic bandage such as an ACE wrap can minimize STS, provide stability for walking, and minimize pain. Elevation of the injured ankle above the level of the heart is also beneficial to minimize pain and STS. More significant injuries will also require the avoidance of bearing weight on the injured extremity until the patient can be evaluated by the medical officer. Any muscle weakness, numbness, laxity of ligaments, decrease in range of motion, or difficulty walking requires prompt referral to the medical officer.

Red Flags

The signs and symptoms that warrant urgent referral to a medical officer include:

- Any pain that makes it difficult for the patient to walk
- A joint with signs of instability such as a positive drawer sign
- Any condition significantly limiting the activity or duties of the patient
- Any ankle or other joint that is hot or warm to the touch compared to the opposite or unaffected joint
- When a tear of a tendon, muscle, or ligament is suspected
- Any chronic or long-standing condition
- Any situation where there is a suspected compromise of circulation

■ Summary

Musculoskeletal injuries are a frequently encountered complaint with few obvious findings on the physical examination. The ability of the combat medic to apply appropriate principles and techniques of assessment and management may mean the difference in preventing further painful injury and permanent disability or even death for the patient.

YOU ARE THE
COMBAT MEDIC

You are the combat medic during sick call in the Battalion Aid Station (BAS). Three soldiers come into the BAS. Two soldiers are supporting the third soldier, who is hopping on his left leg. While dismounting a vehicle, the soldier twisted his knee. The surface on the running board was unexpectedly slick, and the soldier's right leg slipped out and twisted in front of him. When he stood up and placed his full weight on his right leg, he felt unsteady and experienced a burning pain in his knee, thus the expletive.

Assessment

You take the patient into an examination area. First, you have the patient sit at the end of the examination table, where you compare his knees. His right knee appears to be swollen compared to his left knee. You ask him to try and bear weight on his right leg, but when he attempts this, he winces in pain and immediately balances on his left foot.

You have the patient sit back on the table and begin to test his range of motion. The patient bends his knee at almost a 90º angle and you gently place your hand beneath his right foot. You slowly push the foot and the leg up. The patient winces. "It feels like it's popping," he says. You also hear some noise from the knee joint. You begin to suspect that the patient has torn his meniscus.

After completing the remainder of the physical assessment, it appears that only the meniscus in his right knee is injured. This type of injury requires a prompt referral to a medical officer. The medical officer confirms your diagnosis and the patient to evacuated to a higher echelon facility where he undergoes surgery.

While the mechanism of injury (MOI) seems relatively harmless compared to the potential MOI of the battlefield, a simple twist of the knee can cause major physical damage to a soldier.

Ready for Review

- Musculoskeletal injuries and disorders rank second only to upper respiratory infections (URIs) for the numbers encountered by combat medics.
- These injuries are frequently encountered in the field; however, many times there will not be any obvious findings on the physical examination.
- The musculoskeletal system gives the body its shape and allows for its movement.
- Use the SOAP method to evaluate an orthopaedic complaint. The method follows the standard and natural flow of a patient interview, beginning with the Subjective data, proceeding to the Objective findings, arriving at an Assessment, and formulating a treatment Plan.
- The shoulder region and upper arm are susceptible to a wide variety of both traumatic and nontraumatic disorders.
  - Most shoulder complaints in the military are a result of overuse and repetitive motions.
- Lower back pain is a common symptom among soldiers.
  - The most common cause of lower back pain in soldiers is a strain of the lower back musculature.
- Most unilateral knee pain is traumatic in origin.
  - Acute trauma usually causes ligament sprains or meniscal damage.
  - Repeated mild trauma over long periods of time can lead to chondromalacia (softening of cartilage), tendinitis, bursitis, chronic arthritis, or other problems.
- Ankle sprains are common in the active duty population due to the high level of physical activity.
  - Most ankle sprains are a result of ankle inversion and therefore result in pain of the lateral aspect of the ankle.

Vital Vocabulary

abduction Movement away from the midline of the body.

acetabulum The cup-shaped cavity in which the rounded head of the femur rotates.

acromion Lateral extension of the scapula that forms the highest point of the shoulder.

adduction Movement toward the midline of the body.

anterior tibial artery The artery that travels through the anterior muscles of the leg and continues to the foot as the dorsalis pedis.

appendicular skeleton The part of the skeleton comprising the upper and lower extremities.

articulations The locations where two or more bones meet; joints.

atrophy Wasting away of a tissue.

axial skeleton The part of the skeleton comprising the skull, spinal column, and rib cage.

axillary artery The artery that runs through the axilla, connecting the subclavian artery to the brachial artery.

brachial artery The artery that runs through the arm and branches into the radial and ulnar arteries.

bursa A fluid-filled sac located adjacent to joints that reduces the amount of friction between moving structures.

bursitis Inflammation of a bursa.

calcaneous The heel bone; the largest of the tarsal bones.

carpals The eight small bones of the wrist.

cartilage Tough, elastic substance that covers opposable surfaces of moveable joints and forms part of the skeleton.

cartilaginous joints Joints that are spanned completely by cartilage and allow for minimal motion.

clavicle The collar bone.

digital arteries The arteries that supply blood to the fingers and toes.

dorsal Referring to the back or posterior side of the body or an organ.

endosteum The inner lining of a hollow bone.

femoral artery The main artery supplying the thigh and leg.

femur The proximal bone of the leg that extends from the pelvis to the knee.

fibrous joints Joints that contain dense fibrous tissue and allow for no motion.

fibula The smaller of the two bones of the lower leg.

flat bones Bones that are thin and broad, such as the scapula.

humerus The bone of the upper arm.

hypertrophy An increase in size.

ilium The broad, uppermost bone of the pelvis.

irregular bones Bones with unique shapes that allow them to perform a specific function and that do not fit into the other categories based on shape.

ischium The lowermost dorsal bone of the pelvis.

joint The point at which two or more bones articulate, or come together.

joint capsule A saclike envelope that encloses the cavity of a synovial joint.

lactic acid A metabolic end product of the breakdown of glucose that accumulates when metabolism proceeds in the absence of oxygen.

ligaments Tough bands of tissue that connect bone to bone around a joint or support internal organs within the body.

long bones Bones that are longer than they are wide.

malleolus The large, rounded bony protuberance on either side of the ankle joint.

medullary canal The hollow center portion of a long bone.

metacarpals The five bones that form the palm and back of the hand.

metatarsals The five long bones extending from the tarsus to the phalanges of the foot.

muscle fatigue The condition that arises when a muscle depletes its supply of energy.

patella The kneecap.

pectoral girdle The shoulder girdle.

pelvic girdle The large bone that arises in the area of the last nine vertebrae and sweeps around to form a complete ring.

periosteum The fibrous tissue that covers bone.

phalanges The bones of the fingers or toes.

physis The growth plate in long bones.

plantar Referring to the sole of the foot.

popliteal artery The artery in the area or space behind the knee joint.

posterior tibial artery The artery that travels through the calf muscles to the plantar aspect of the foot.

pronation The act of turning the palm of the hand backward or downward, performed by internal rotation of the forearm.

pubis One of two bones that form the anterior portion of the pelvic ring.

radial artery The artery pertaining to the wrist.

radius The bone on the thumb side of the forearm.

round bones The small bones that are found adjacent to joints that assist with motion.

sacroiliac joints The points of attachment of the ilium to the sacrum.

scapula The shoulder blade.

short bones The bones that are nearly as wide as they are long.

skeletal muscle Muscle that is attached to bones and usually crosses at least one joint; striated or voluntary muscle.

striated muscle Skeletal muscle that is under voluntary control.

subclavian artery The artery that travels from the aorta to each upper extremity.

supination To turn the forearm laterally so that the palm faces forward (if standing) or upward (if lying supine).

synovial joints Joints that permit movement of the component bones.

synovial membrane The lining of a joint that secretes synovial fluid into the joint space.

tarsals The ankle bones.

tendinitis Inflammation of a tendon that most commonly results from overuse.

tendons The fibrous portions of muscle that attach to bone.

tibia The shin bone.

ulna The larger bone of the forearm, on the side opposite the thumb.

ulnar artery The artery of the forearm that travels along its medial aspect.

voluntary muscle Muscle that can be controlled by a person.

COMBAT MEDIC in Action

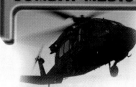

During sick call at the Battalion Aid Station, your battle buddy shuffles into the facility. He is grimacing and holding his lower back. "Too much basketball again, Martin?" you ask. Your buddy doesn't even crack a smile, so you know he is in serious pain. "Let's take a look at you," you say as you lead him into an examination room.

1. The red flags of back pain include:
   A. loss of bowel or bladder control.
   B. pain that radiates to other areas.
   C. bloody urine.
   D. all of the above.

2. While assessing the lower back, you will inspect the following items:
   A. visible muscle spasm.
   B. soft-tissue swelling.
   C. erythema.
   D. all of the above.

3. To test the patient's muscle strength, you will perform the:
   A. hamstring test.
   B. scapula test.
   C. flexion test.
   D. girdle test.

4. The most common cause of lower back muscle pain is:
   A. falls.
   B. tripping.
   C. strain.
   D. muscle spasms.

5. Pain that radiates could indicate a problem with the:
   A. nerve roots.
   B. spinal cord.
   C. hamstrings.
   D. spinal column.

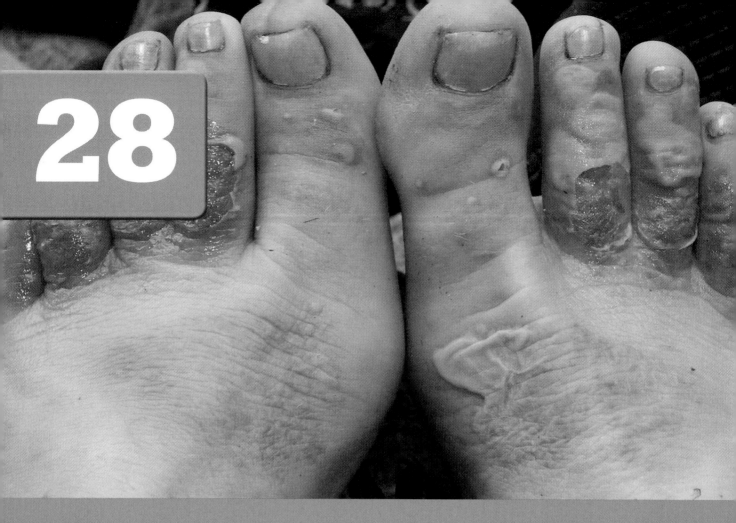

28

Skin Diseases

Objectives

Knowledge Objectives

- ☐ Describe the anatomy and physiology of the skin.
- ☐ Describe the physical examination of the skin.
- ☐ List viral skin diseases.
- ☐ List bacterial skin diseases.
- ☐ Describe contact dermatitis.
- ☐ Describe fungal skin diseases.
- ☐ Describe blisters, corns, and calluses.

Introduction

The skin is an effective barrier against ordinary environmental intrusions. In time of war, however, when the soldier is deployed to environments quite foreign to ordinary peacetime conditions, minor skin problems and irritation can progress quickly to significant illness. When the skin is compromised by blisters and cuts and is attacked by insects and bacteria, its protective barrier is breached and soldiers may become incapacitated. The role you play in educating, implementing preventive measures, and treating common skin disorders is vital to the well-being of the soldiers in your unit.

Skin diseases are of major importance in military operations. Although they cause few fatalities, they are a significant source of combat ineffectiveness, troop morbidity, and poor morale. The loss of soldiers, whether due to missile injury, accident, systemic infection, or skin disease, has the same effect: fewer soldiers are available to accomplish the mission. Certain skin diseases, such as immersion foot and frostbite, often require extended recovery periods or evacuation, compounding the problem and delaying the soldier's return to duty.

Anatomy Review

The skin is the largest organ of the human body, making up 15% of our total body weight (TBW). It provides a water-tight barrier to keep body fluids in and environmental fluids out. It also provides sensory perception through nerve endings and specialized receptors.

The skin consists of two principal layers: the epidermis and the dermis **FIGURE 28-1 ▾**. The **epidermis** (outer layer) is composed mostly of dying and dead cells that shed constantly and are replaced from beneath by new cells. The epidermis has no blood vessels, so the dermis must supply its nutrition.

The **dermis** is a thick layer of connective tissue below the thin epidermis. The dermis is rich in blood supply and nerve endings. It contains hair follicles and sebaceous glands that secrete oil to lubricate the epidermis. The ridges and grooves caused by elevations and depressions in the epidermis and dermis are determined by heredity. These ridges and grooves form fingerprints, which are unique to each individual.

The subcutaneous tissue (hypodermis) underneath the dermis contains fat and hair follicles. The subcutaneous tissue provides insulation, cushioning, and a reserve energy source.

Functions of the Skin

The skin is a covering for the underlying deeper tissues, protecting them from dehydration and injury. The skin helps to regulate body temperature. In cold weather, blood vessels constrict to help conserve heat; in hot weather, the blood vessels in the skin dilate to allow more blood to be brought to the skin's surface to allow for the release of heat into the air. The skin is the site of many nerve endings and temporarily stores fat, glucose, water, and salts. It also has properties that allow it to absorb certain medications and other chemicals.

Physical Examination of the Skin

Physical examination of the skin is performed by inspection and palpation. The most important tools are your own eyes and your powers of observation. Adequate exposure of the skin is necessary. If the skin condition is on an extremity, inspect the skin on both extremities for symmetry or differences. Begin by inspecting the skin for color and uniform appearance, thickness, symmetry, and the presence of any skin lesions. A **skin lesion** is a catch-all term that describes any change in skin appearance.

As you inspect the skin, palpate for moisture, temperature, and turgor. **Turgor** checks the hydration status of the patient. To check turgor, pinch the skin on the patient's arm, abdomen, or sternum. Release the skin and note how long it takes to return to normal position **FIGURE 28-2 ▸**. The skin should feel and move easily when pinched and should immediately return to its original position when released. Turgor will be altered when the patient is dehydrated or if edema or swelling is present. Turgor should not be tested on the back of a patient's hand (a common mistake). The looseness and thinness of the skin in that area makes it an unreliable location for testing turgor and mobility.

When describing skin lesions, note the lesion's size, shape, color, and location, and the presence of drainage (if any). A **macule** is flat and small (< 1 cm) **FIGURE 28-3 ▸**. The color varies from white to brown to red to purple. A **patch** is a large macule (> 1 cm). Examples of

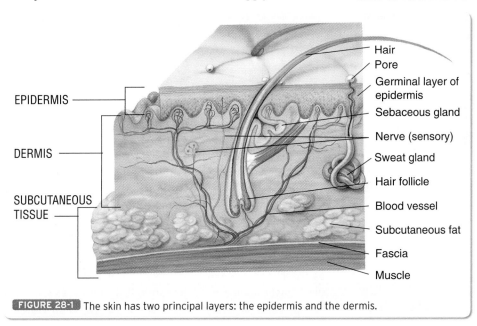

EPIDERMIS

DERMIS

SUBCUTANEOUS TISSUE

Hair
Pore
Germinal layer of epidermis
Sebaceous gland
Nerve (sensory)
Sweat gland
Hair follicle
Blood vessel
Subcutaneous fat
Fascia
Muscle

FIGURE 28-1 The skin has two principal layers: the epidermis and the dermis.

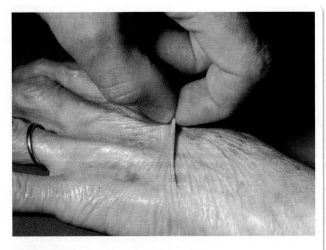

FIGURE 28-2 Tenting is evident with extreme dehydration.

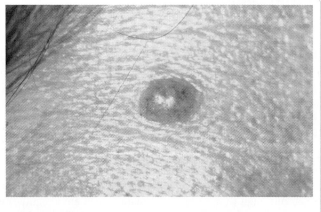

FIGURE 28-5 A papule is a solid, raised skin lesion.

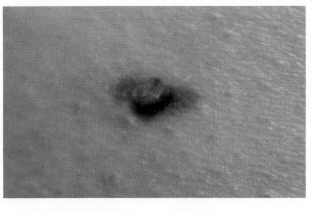

FIGURE 28-3 A macule is a small, flat skin lesion.

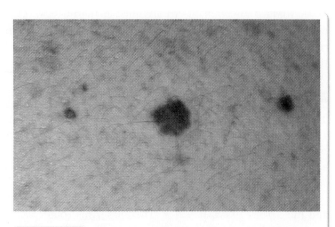

FIGURE 28-6 A plaque is a large papule or a group of papules.

FIGURE 28-4 A patch is a large macule, and can include freckles, flat moles, and tattoos.

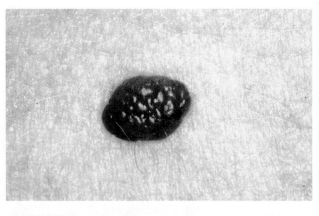

FIGURE 28-7 A nodule is a palpable, solid, elevated skin lesion.

patches include freckles, flat moles, and tattoos FIGURE 28-4. A **papule** is a solid, raised lesion < 1 cm FIGURE 28-5. A **plaque** is a papule > 1 cm or a group of papules. Examples of

plaque include warts, some moles (nevi), and some types of skin cancer FIGURE 28-6.

A **nodule** is a palpable, solid lesion, 1–2 cm and elevated FIGURE 28-7. Nodules are deeper in the dermis than papules. Larger nodules (> 2 cm) are called tumors. Examples of nodules include cysts or lipomas. A **vesicle** is an elevated lesion containing serous fluid that is < 1 cm; if > 1 cm, it is

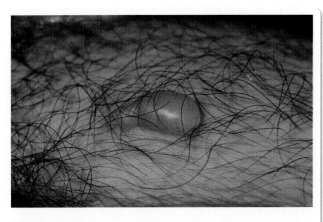

FIGURE 28-8 A vesicle is an elevated lesion containing serous fluid.

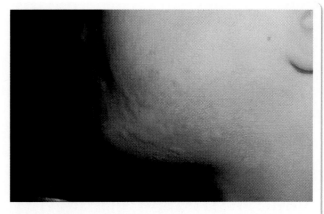

FIGURE 28-10 Wheals (hives) are transient, elevated lesions caused by localized edema.

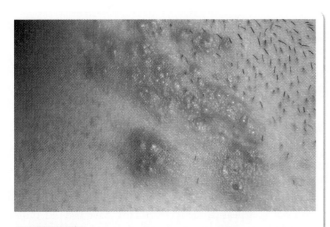

FIGURE 28-9 Pustules are superficial and elevated lesions containing pus.

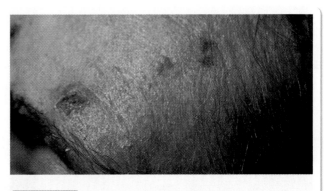

FIGURE 28-11 Crusts (scabs) consist of dried serum, blood, or pus.

called a **bulla** **FIGURE 28-8 ▲**. Vesicles or bullae are commonly caused by contact dermatitis, physical trauma, or sunburn. **Pustules** are superficial and elevated lesions < 1 cm, containing pus, that result from infection **FIGURE 28-9 ▲**. Some causes are impetigo, acne, and folliculitis.

Wheals (hives) are transient, elevated lesions caused by localized edema. Wheals are a common allergic reaction (eg, from drug reactions, insect stings or bites, or sensitivity to cold, heat, pressure, or sunlight) **FIGURE 28-10 ▶**. Crusts (scabs) consist of dried serum, blood, or pus. **Crusting** occurs in many inflammatory and infectious diseases **FIGURE 28-11 ▶**.

■ Viral Skin Diseases

Herpes Simplex

Herpes simplex is an infection from the herpes simplex virus (HSV). It is characterized by one or many clusters of small vesicles filled with clear fluid on slightly raised inflammatory bases. The fluid inside the vesicle is extremely contagious. Herpes simplex infections are caused by two different viral types: HSV 1 and HSV 2. Both types produce identical pat-

terns of infection. Asymptomatic carriers can still shed the virus and spread the disease.

The signs and symptoms of herpes simplex include lesions that may appear anywhere on the skin or mucosa but are most frequent around the mouth, on the lips (fever blisters), and in the genital area, accompanied by tingling, discomfort, and itching. Single clusters vary in size. The lesions persist for a few days and then begin to dry, forming a thin yellowish crust or ulcer.

The primary (initial) infection is generally the most severe, with fever, lymphadenopathy (swollen lymph nodes), and urinary symptoms (if the outbreak is genital). Recurrent infection is common. Local skin trauma or systemic stressors (fatigue, illness) may reactivate the virus. It is common to see HSV recurrences in a field or combat environment.

A **herpetic whitlow** is an HSV infection of the fingers, resulting from the inoculation of HSV through a skin break **FIGURE 28-12 ▶**. These are more common in health care workers. Symptoms of a herpetic whitlow include swelling and pain over the lesions on the finger.

Healing generally occurs in 8 to 12 days following onset. Individual herpetic lesions usually heal completely, but recurrent lesions at the same site may cause atrophy and scarring.

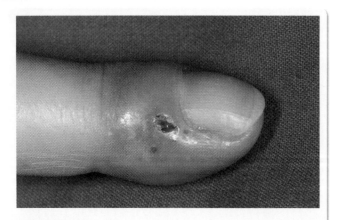

FIGURE 28-12 A herpetic whitlow is an HSV infection of the fingers.

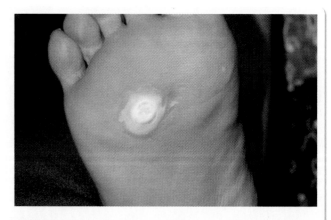

FIGURE 28-14 Warts are transmitted by touch and commonly appear on the hands, around the fingernails, and on the bottom of the feet.

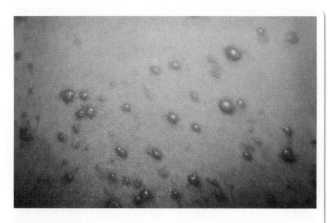

FIGURE 28-13 Herpes zoster.

Antiviral medications (eg, acyclovir) are used for initial out-breaks, recurrent infections, and suppressive therapy. Second-ary bacterial infections are treated with systemic antibiotics.

Advise the patient to avoid sexual intercourse while genital lesions are present; however, viral shedding may occur even if the patient is symptom free. Discuss condom usage with all genital herpes patients. Treatment with medications reduces the symptoms of the infection, but does not destroy the virus. HSV is a recurrent illness without a cure at this time. Refer the patient to a doctor or physician assistant for treatment of herpes infections.

Herpes Zoster

Herpes zoster (shingles) is an infection caused by the chicken-pox virus FIGURE 28-13 ▲. The signs and symptoms include pain, tenderness, and itching occurring along the site of the future rash. This usually precedes the rash by 2 to 3 days. Characteristic crops of vesicles on an erythematous base then appear. Headache, fever, and chills occur occasion-ally. The pain may be severe and narcotic analgesics may be required. The rash occurs most often in the thoracic or lum-bar region and is unilateral (usually only on one side). Lesions

usually continue to form for about 3 to 5 days. Crusting occurs by 7 to 10 days and resolves by 14 to 21 days.

Treatment begins with applying wet compresses to soothe the skin. Antiviral medications are used to treat herpes zoster. Refer the patient to a doctor or physician assistant for treatment.

Warts

Different types of viruses cause different types of warts. Warts commonly occur in children and young adults. Most warts resolve spontaneously; others may last a lifetime. At least 55 human papilloma viruses (HPVs) have been identified that cause warts. At least three types of HPV have been identified as a cause of cervical cancer and venereal warts.

Warts are transmitted by touch and commonly appear at the site of minor trauma, on the hands, around the fingernails from nail biting, and on the bottom of the feet FIGURE 28-14 ▲. The wart virus also may penetrate normal intact skin.

Some types of warts respond to a single treatment, whereas others may be resistant. Explain to patients that most warts require several treatments. Topical wart medications and liquid nitrogen "freezing" are the best methods for initial treatment.

■ Bacterial Skin Diseases

Bacterial skin infections are among the most common dis-abling skin infections that occur during wartime and field exercises. There are several reasons for this: irregular bathing habits, irritation of the skin from rough clothing and equip-ment, and minor trauma from abrasions, insect bites, and crowded living conditions. Bacterial skin infections need to be treated aggressively because of their rapid spread, particularly in a field or combat environment.

Cellulitis

Cellulitis is an acute bacterial infection of the dermis and subcutaneous tissues FIGURE 28-15 ▶. It may arise from an entry of bacteria through the skin, for example through a lac-

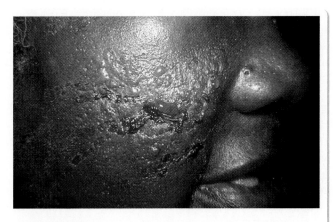

FIGURE 28-15 Cellulitis is an acute bacterial infection of the dermis and subcutaneous tissues.

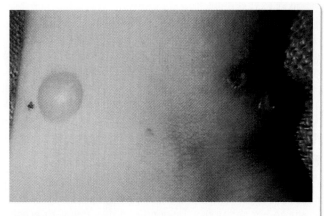

FIGURE 28-16 Impetigo is a superficial bacterial skin infection.

eration or a puncture wound, or through an extension from an abscess. Cellulitis is a serious disease process because of the possibility of the infection spreading to the lymphatic and blood systems, resulting in **bacteremia** (blood infection) and sepsis.

Cellulitis is more common in the lower extremities. The major findings are local redness, tenderness, and enlarged regional lymphadenopathy. The skin is hot, red, and edematous (marked by edema). The presence of cellulitis with chills or fever suggests that bacteremia is present. Local abscesses form occasionally, requiring incision and drainage (I&D).

For treatment, refer the patient to a doctor or physician assistant. If a medical officer is not present, evacuate the patient on a priority basis to a medical officer. Oral antibiotic therapy to cover streptococci and staphylococci is required as first line outpatient therapy. For severe infections that require hospitalization, such as head and neck cellulitis with fever or chills or large areas of infection, IV antibiotics are used. Immobilization and elevation of the affected area help reduce edema. A good way to make sure that the infection is getting better is to circle the red area. When the patient returns on a follow-up visit, ensure that the redness is inside the lines. Make sure to document your findings on each follow-up visit.

Impetigo

Impetigo is a superficial bacterial skin infection, occurring most frequently on exposed parts of the body, especially on the face, hands, neck, and extremities **FIGURE 28-16**. Risk factors include crowded living conditions, neglected minor wounds, and poor hygiene. Lesions are initially pea-sized papules, becoming vesicular and rupturing, leaving the classic honey-colored crusts. Regional lymphadenopathy is seen in the majority of cases. Constitutional symptoms such as fever and chills are absent.

Refer the patient to a doctor or physician assistant for antibiotic treatment. Impetigo is extremely contagious, so avoidance of the patient's towels, clothing, or linen is crucial to prevent the spread of infection.

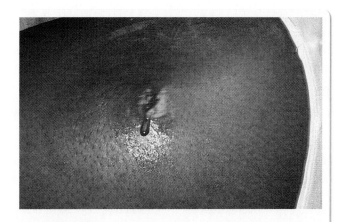

FIGURE 28-17 A cutaneous abscess begins as a deep, tender, red papule that becomes pus filled.

Cutaneous Abscesses

Everyone has normal, non-disease-producing bacteria on their skin. The number and type of bacteria vary in relation to the anatomic site, environmental factors (heat, humidity), general hygiene, and the underlying health of the person. Because the skin provides a strong barrier against pathogenic (illness-producing) bacteria, abscesses often occur in an area of the skin that has been injured. Most patients first complain of a localized area of pain and swelling. The **cutaneous abscess** begins as a deep, tender, red papule that becomes fluctuant (pus-filled) **FIGURE 28-17**. Fever is usually not present. Cellulitis may or may not be present.

Refer the patient to a doctor or a physician assistant for incision and drainage (I&D) of all abscesses. Antibiotics may be given following I&D. An abscess is not ready for drainage until the overlying skin has thinned and the mass is fluctuant. Warm compresses will help localize the infection. Incision of the fluctuant area is performed by a medical officer under sterile conditions. The abscess cavity is then packed loosely with a gauze wick that is removed 24 to 48 hours later. Follow-up wound care on the drained abscess cavity will continue until the wound has closed.

Wet-to-dry dressings require moist packing that dries between dressing changes. When the packing is removed, it debrides the wound by removing the dead cells that stick to it. The packing should never dry completely. If it does, dressing changes should be performed more often. During dressing changes, the packing is removed, the wound is irrigated, and the packing is replaced until the wound closes (usually 1 to 3 weeks). Localized heat also helps to resolve tissue inflammation.

Folliculitis

Folliculitis is an inflammation of a hair follicle caused by infection, chemical irritation, or minor physical injury such as shaving or abrasions. The condition may follow or accompany other skin infections. Chronic low-grade irritation or inflammation without significant infection may occur when stiff hairs in the bearded area emerge from the follicle, curve, and re-enter the skin. This is called pseudofolliculitis barbae (PFB) or razor bumps. Topical or oral antibiotics are used to treat folliculitis. Refer the patient to the doctor or the physician assistant for treatment.

Bites

One to three million animal bites to humans occur annually in the United States. Dog bites represent 70% to 90% of all bites. Cat bites represent 7% to 20%, but have a higher incidence of infection. Humans and rodents make up the remainder of bites. Dog bites cause a crushing type of injury due to their rounded teeth and strong jaws. The pressure may cause damage to deeper structures such as bones, vessels, muscles, and nerves. Cats, due to their sharp, pointed teeth, usually cause a puncture wound with the bacteria going into deeper tissues. Commonly, a cat tooth will be a foreign body within the wound.

The extremities are involved in 75% of cases when victims handle or attempt to avoid the animal. Head and neck injuries are the next most common injury sites. Bites on the hands have a higher risk of infection due to poor blood supply, and the hand anatomy makes adequate cleansing of the wound more difficult.

Wounds should be described as to size, location, and type. Include diagrams of the wound in the patient's chart for follow-up visits. If infected, describe any lymph node enlargement and diagram the extent of the cellulitis, if present. These organisms are resistant to many antibiotics but are generally sensitive to penicillin. All bite injuries are potentially dangerous and can cause significant infection.

Wash the skin with warm soapy water. Irrigate wounds with soapy water using a needle catheter and syringe (prefera-

bly a large syringe to provide adequate pressure). Flush puncture wounds with a minimum of 200 mL of soapy water. All animal bites are tetanus prone. Provide tetanus prophylaxis, as indicated. Systemic antibiotics are also given. The type of antibiotic given is dependent on the type of animal involved.

Review rabies postexposure prophylaxis guidelines. Exposure is defined as an open bite or wound in contact with the body fluids of a rabid animal. Rabies is a rare, but potentially fatal viral disease transmitted by the bite of a rabid animal. Among wild animals, skunks, raccoons, foxes, and bats are common suspects for rabies transmission. Rabbits and rodents (rats and mice) are rarely infected with rabies. Unprovoked attacks by any animal, however, should raise suspicion for rabies exposure.

With human bites, review for the possibility of HIV, hepatitis B, or hepatitis C transmission and provide treatment, if necessary. Refer all bite wounds to a doctor or physician assistant for assessment and treatment. Close follow-up is needed for all bite wounds.

■ Contact Dermatitis

Contact dermatitis is a skin inflammation caused by exposure to irritants (eg, poison oak) or allergens (eg, medications). One of the most frequent disorders requiring both inpatient and outpatient therapy that arises during military conflicts is dermatitis caused by contact with environmental or work-related materials. Under wartime conditions, inadequate facilities may limit personal hygiene and increase exposure to common chemical irritants and allergens.

Examples of agents that may cause contact dermatitis include:

- Topical medications
- Plants: poison oak, ivy, or sumac
- Chemicals used in the manufacture of shoes and clothing, metal compounds, dyes, and cosmetics
- Industrial agents, dyes
- Rubber and latex in gloves or condoms
- Perfumes, personal hygiene products
- Jewelry metals (copper, silver, nickel)

Photo dermatitis occurs when a patient wearing photo sensitizers is exposed to sunlight. Aftershave lotions, sunscreens, and antibiotics all can exaggerate the sun's effects.

Signs and symptoms of contact dermatitis include transient redness to severe swelling with bullae. With poison oak, ivy, or sumac, linear streaks are characteristic. The fluid inside the vesicle or bulla is not infectious. Pruritus and vesiculation are common. Typically the dermatitis is limited to the site of contact but may later spread. Vesicles and bullae may rupture, ooze, and crust. Secondary bacterial infections may occur. As inflammation subsides, scaling and some temporary thickening of the skin can occur. Continued exposure to the causative agent may perpetuate the dermatitis.

Take the patient's history. The patient's occupation, hobbies, duties, vacations, clothing, topical drug use, current medications, cosmetics, hygiene products, and activities must be considered. The site of the initial lesion is often an impor-

---

Garrison Care TIPS

In general, the better the blood supply, the easier the wound is to clean, thus lowering the risk of infection. This is why lacerations are easier to clean than puncture wounds.

tant clue in making a correct diagnosis. For example, hand dermatitis may result from lotions, jewelry, soaps, detergents, rubber, or latex gloves.

Unless the causative agent is identified and removed, treatment will be ineffective. Patients with photo dermatitis should also avoid the photo-sensitizing chemical or exposure to light. An oral corticosteroid may be given for 7 to 14 days in extensive cases, or even in limited cases when facial inflammation is present or the mission dictates.

Topical corticosteroids are not helpful in the blistering phase, but once the dermatitis is less acute, a topical corticosteroid cream, ointment, or spray can be used. Antihistamines are ineffective in suppressing allergic contact dermatitis but help the itch. Careful thought must be given to issuing antihistamines to soldiers in the field. Antihistamines make most people drowsy, so you don't want soldiers operating heavy equipment or driving. Antihistamines also make people at higher risk for heat injury.

Counsel the patient not to scratch the rash because of the risk of spreading the rash. Refer patients with contact dermatitis to a medical officer for treatment.

■ Fungal Skin Diseases

Fungal infections are common on the feet and the body. Fungal infections may be pruritic (itchy) or asymptomatic. Occasionally there is tenderness and inflammation. Although most superficial skin infections merely produce discomfort and large numbers of outpatient visits, significant numbers of soldiers have been hospitalized for complications from secondary bacterial infections. In a 1-year period in Vietnam, 7% of all hospital admissions were for skin conditions. Superficial fungal infections are most commonly acquired from humans, but may also be acquired from the soil and animals. This point is important to remember because soldiers in combat are more likely to be exposed to and become infected with fungi that inhabit the soil and infest local wild animals.

Superficial skin infections are named according to their anatomic location:

- Body (tinea corporis), also known as ringworm
- Feet (tinea pedis), also known as athlete's foot
- Scalp (tinea capitis)
- Groin (tinea cruris), also known as jock itch

Tinea Corporis

Tinea corporis (ringworm) is an erythematous plaque with central clearing and well-defined and usually raised margins **FIGURE 28-18 ▶**. These usually appear in a ring shape that looks as though a worm is under the skin. Remember, ring-

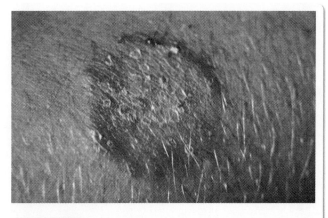

FIGURE 28-18 Tinea corporis.

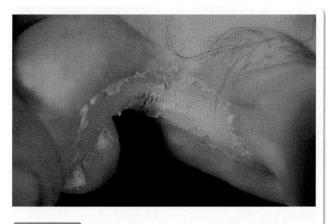

FIGURE 28-19 Tinea pedis.

worm is not due to an actual worm. Intense inflammation with or without pustules may be present.

Most skin infections respond very well to topical antifungal preparations. Cases not clearing with topical therapy or those with widespread involvement require oral antifungal therapy. Affected areas should be kept clean and dry. Two weeks of antifungal treatment is usually required.

Tinea Pedis

Tinea pedis (athlete's foot) is the most common superficial fungal infection **FIGURE 28-19 ▲**. Infections typically begin in the web spaces of the toes and may later involve the bottom surface of the foot. Toe web lesions often are macerated (softened) and have scaling borders. These lesions may be vesicular or they may become dry, scaly, cracking, and bleeding. Acute flare-ups, with many vesicles and bullae, are common during warm weather. Tinea pedis may be complicated by secondary bacterial infection, cellulitis, or lymphangitis, which may recur.

Minor foot infections can be treated with topical agents. Good foot hygiene is essential. Toes and feet must be dried after bathing, macerated skin is gently debrided, and a bland,

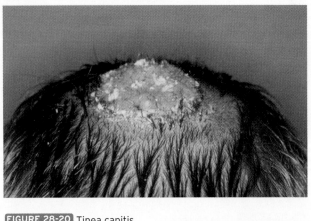

FIGURE 28-20 Tinea capitis.

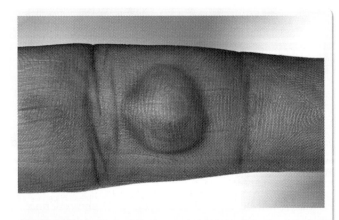

FIGURE 28-22 Blisters form as a result of heat, moisture, and friction.

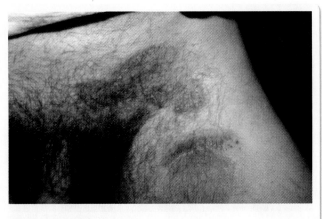

FIGURE 28-21 Tinea cruris.

drying antifungal powder (miconazole) applied. Taking boots off and letting feet dry out several times a day is helpful. If possible, soldiers should frequently change into dry socks.

Tinea Capitis

Tinea capitis (scalp infection) mainly affects children FIGURE 28-20 ▲ . It is contagious and may become epidemic. The signs and symptoms include inflammation that is low-grade and persistent. Alopecia (hair loss) may occur with characteristic black dots on the scalp which result from broken hairs. Topical treatment is not advised; oral antifungal therapy is indicated. Refer the patient with alopecia or scalp infections to a medical officer for treatment.

Tinea Cruris

Tinea cruris (jock itch) is a type of fungal infection that occurs almost exclusively in men FIGURE 28-21 ▲ . Typically, a ringed lesion extends from the skin fold between the scrotum and upper thigh. One or both sides may be affected. It may be extremely itchy and may produce pain (due to friction) on walking or running. Recurrence is common because fungi may repeatedly infect susceptible persons. Flare-ups occur more often during the summer, due to heat and humidity of

the skin area. Tight clothing or obesity tends to favor growth of the organisms. Cotton briefs tend to stay wet, also contributing to their growth.

Topical therapy with a cream or lotion is often effective. Instruct the patient to keep the area as clean and dry as possible. Instruct the patient to switch to boxers or to stop wearing underwear until the infection is under control.

■ Blisters, Corns, and Calluses

Blisters form as a result of heat, moisture, and friction FIGURE 28-22 ▲ . First, a tear occurs within the upper layers of the skin (epidermis) forming a space between the layers while leaving the surface intact. Then fluid seeps into the space. The soles of the feet and palms of the hands are the most common areas because the hands and feet rub up against boots and other equipment. Blister formation requires thick and immobile epidermis, as found in these areas. Additionally, blisters form more easily on moist skin than dry or soaked skin, and warm conditions favor blister formation.

Blisters on the feet may be a short-lived medical problem, but for soldiers, blisters are not a trivial condition. Blister treatment occupies a great deal of sick call time for the combat medic and the soldier engaged in self-aid. One complication associated with friction blisters is cellulitis. One study found that 84% of cellulitis treated in a recruit population was caused by friction blisters, with an average loss of 8 days per patient.

To prevent blisters, you need to minimize friction for the feet. This begins with the proper boot selection. Socks can decrease friction between the feet and boots. Choosing socks made of a material that helps move moisture away from the foot, such as Gore-Tex, will help. Layering of socks can minimize friction forces. Counsel patients on changing socks frequently and allowing the feet, socks, and boots to dry.

Small intact blisters that don't cause discomfort do not need treatment. To protect the blister roof, cover with a small bandage. Larger or painful blisters that are intact should be drained without removing the roof. First, clean the blistered area with soap and water. Then lance the bottom of the blister with a sterile needle or scalpel and allow the blister to drain. For added protection, surround the unroofed blister with donut-shaped moleskin and a bandage. Do not remove the skin from the blister if at all possible. The skin is the body's natural dressing to protect underlying tissue. Blisters with small tears are treated the same as those that you punctured. Blisters with larger tears should be unroofed carefully with fine scissors and the base cleaned with soap and water. Apply antibiotic ointment and a bandage.

Corns and calluses differ in where they occur. Corns appear on the bony areas on top of the toes, or on skin between the toes. Corns feel hard to the touch, are tender, and have a roundish appearance. Calluses commonly appear on the ball or the heel of the foot or the big toe, but can appear anywhere on the body that experiences continued pressure or irritation.

To prevent corns and calluses, make certain that the soldiers' boots and shoes fit properly. Small corns may be treated with extra padding. Shaving off the upper layers of corns and calluses may be performed by a medical officer.

■ Summary

When the skin is compromised by blisters and cuts and is attacked by insects and bacteria, its protective barrier is breached and soldiers may become incapacitated. The role you play in educating, implementing preventive measures, and treating common skin disorders is vital to the well-being of the soldiers in your unit.

YOU ARE THE
COMBAT MEDIC

While on patrol, a soldier comes across an orange tabby cat cornered by two neighborhood dogs. The soldier yells at the dogs and they quickly scatter. The soldier approaches the cat and reaches out to give the tabby a reassuring pat. In thanks, the cat bites him on the hand on the soft spot between the thumb and the first finger.

Assessment

Now the soldier is sitting in front of you, the combat medic, during sick call in the Battalion Aid Station. Because of your knowledge of animal bites, you know that the soldier's puncture wound is probably filled with bacteria. You also won't be surprised to find a small tooth inside the wound.

Treatment

You note and diagram the size, location, and the type of wound. Then you wash the skin with warm soapy water. Next you irrigate the puncture wound with soapy water using a needle catheter and a syringe. You flush the wound out with 400 mL of soapy water. The treatment of the patient continues with the administration of a tetanus booster and an antibiotic to prevent infection.

Aid Kit

Ready for Review

- The skin is an effective barrier against ordinary environmental intrusions.
  - In time of war, when the soldier is deployed to environments quite foreign to ordinary peacetime conditions, minor skin problems and irritation can progress quickly to significant illness.
- The skin is the largest organ of the human body, making up 15% of our total body weight (TBW).
  - It provides a water-tight barrier to keep body fluids in and environmental fluids out.
  - It provides sensory perception through nerve endings and specialized receptors.
- Physical examination of the skin is performed by inspection and palpation.
  - The most important tools are your own eyes and your powers of observation.
- Bacterial skin infections are among the most common disabling skin infections that occur during wartime and field exercises.
- Contact dermatitis is a skin inflammation caused by exposure to irritants (eg, poison oak) or allergens (eg, medications).
- Fungal infections are common on the feet and the body.
  - Fungal infections may be pruritic (itchy) or asymptomatic.

Vital Vocabulary

bacteremia Blood infection.

bulla An elevated lesion (> 1 cm) containing serous fluid.

cellulitis An acute bacterial infection of the dermis and subcutaneous tissues.

contact dermatitis Skin inflammation caused by exposure to irritants or allergens.

crusting Also called scabs; skin lesions that consist of dried serum, blood, or pus.

cutaneous abscess A deep, tender, red papule that becomes pus-filled.

dermis The inner layer of skin containing hair follicle roots, glands, blood vessels, and nerves.

epidermis The outermost layer of the skin.

folliculitis Inflammation of a hair follicle caused by infection, chemical irritation, or minor physical injury.

herpes simplex An infection from the herpes simplex virus (HSV).

herpes zoster Also called shingles; an infection caused by the chicken-pox virus.

herpetic whitlow An HSV infection of the fingers, resulting from the inoculation of HSV through a skin break.

impetigo A superficial bacterial skin infection.

macule A flat, small (< 1 cm) skin lesion colored white to brown to red to purple.

nodule A palpable, solid lesion, 1-2 cm, and elevated.

papule A solid, raised lesion (< 1 cm).

patch A large macule (> 1 cm), such as freckles, flat moles, and tattoos.

plaque A papule > 1 cm or a group of papules.

pustules Superficial and elevated lesions < 1 cm containing pus that result from infection.

skin lesion A term that describes any change in skin appearance.

tinea capitis Fungal infection on the scalp.

tinea corporis Also called ringworm; an erythematous plaque with central clearing and well-defined and usually raised margins.

tinea cruris Also called jock itch; a ringed lesion that extends from the skin fold between the scrotum and upper thigh.

tinea pedis Also called athlete's foot; a common superficial fungal infection.

turgor Loss of elasticity in the skin.

vesicle An elevated lesion containing serous fluid that is < 1 cm.

wheals Also called hives; transient, elevated lesions caused by localized edema.

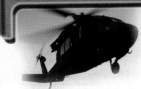

COMBAT MEDIC *in Action*

During sick call at the Battalion Aid Station, a soldier presents with itchy feet. It's difficult for him to sleep because the skin between his toes is so itchy. You have the soldier take off his socks and find dry, cracking lesions in between his toes. You've seen this type of infection before in the high school locker room. This soldier has athlete's foot.

1. The medical term for athlete's foot is:
   A. tinea corporis.
   B. tinea pedis.
   C. tinea capitis.
   D. tinea cruris.

2. Athlete's foot is caused by a(n):
   A. bacteria.
   B. infection.
   C. fungus.
   D. virus.

3. Athlete's foot can be prevented by:
   A. keeping the feet moist.
   B. soaking the feet after a shower.
   C. walking barefoot.
   D. changing the socks often.

4. Athlete's foot can be treated with:
   A. topical agents.
   B. antibiotics.
   C. aspirin.
   D. fluids.

5. Acute flare-ups are complicated by:
   A. stress.
   B. walking.
   C. cold weather.
   D. warm weather.

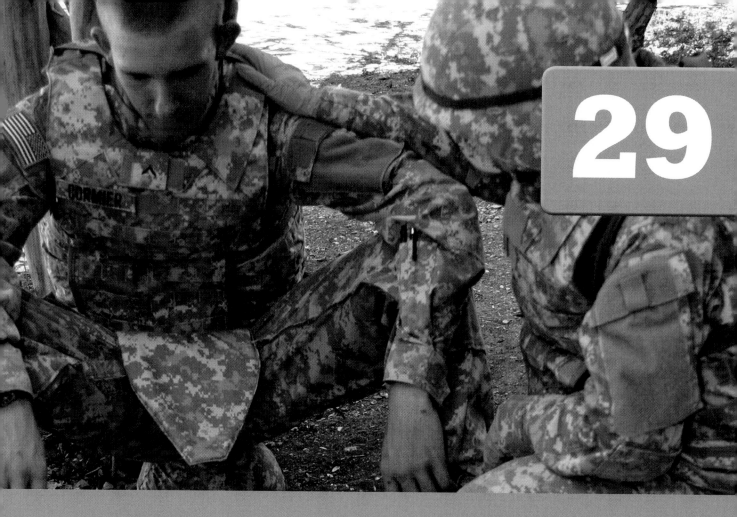

29

Mental Health

Objectives

Knowledge Objectives

- [ ] List the types of stress and stressors.
- [ ] Discuss the effects of stress.
- [ ] Discuss stress behaviors in combat.
- [ ] Define battle fatigue.
- [ ] Describe battle fatigue reactions.
- [ ] List the triage categories of battle fatigue.
- [ ] List the principles of battle fatigue treatment.
- [ ] Discuss noncombat arms battle fatigue casualties.

- [ ] Discuss the signs and symptoms of depression.
- [ ] Discuss the suicide prevention responsibilities of the combat medic.
- [ ] Discuss the myths versus facts on suicide.
- [ ] Identify the historic risk factors associated with suicide.
- [ ] List the immediate danger signals related to suicide.
- [ ] Discuss what to do when confronted with a suicidal soldier.

■ Introduction

As a combat medic, you may assist the commander in assessing the impact of sustained operations on his or her soldiers. You may recommend which, if any, soldiers need help dealing with stress and/or battle fatigue due to the extreme situations they encounter. This block of instruction applies to every type of military unit regardless of mission or level of combat intensity. History shows that most battle-fatigued soldiers can be restored to duty quickly if they are rapidly identified and properly treated. However, history also shows us that soldiers not treated effectively can become permanently disabled.

In the United States every 16.6 minutes, someone dies by suicide. In addition, for every completed suicide it is estimated that there are more than 100 suicide attempts. Following a 27% increase in the number of reported suicides within the Army between 1997 and 1999, in 2000 the Chief of Staff identified suicide as a serious problem and called for a refinement of the Army Suicide Prevention Program (ASPP). Suicide prevention, although at one time recognized as a leadership responsibility, is now the business of everyone, including leaders, supervisors, soldiers, and civilian employees. As a combat medic, you must be able to identify soldiers who may be at risk for suicide and encourage soldiers to seek help by defining help-seeking behavior as a sign of strength, courage, and maturity.

■ Combat/Operational Stress Control

Combat/Operational Stress Control (COSC) encompasses programs developed and actions taken by military leadership to prevent, identify, and manage adverse combat stress reactions (CSR) in units to:

- Optimize mission performance
- Conserve fighting strength
- Prevent or minimize adverse affects of combat stress on soldiers' physical, psychological, intellectual, and social health
- Return the unit or service member to duty expeditiously

Given the many and varied circumstances of our current operations and combat operational tempo (OPTEMPO), each of us, in our own way, experience stress. In each combat operation, be it high- or mid-intensity conflict or operations other than war (OOTW), we can expect individuals to demonstrate the effects of stress. Most of these stress reactions, however unpleasant, do not cause long-term problems. However, in some cases, stress from an operational environment can cause problems that are difficult to overcome without

> **Garrison Care TIPS**
>
> FM 22-51, Leader's Manual for Combat Stress Control, and FM 8-51, Combat Stress Control in a Theater of Operations, Tactics, Techniques, and Procedures, are both excellent references.

help. Effectively addressing the psychological effects of such stress, both before and after it occurs, can greatly improve a unit's readiness status.

■ Definitions

Fatigue is the weariness or decreased performance capability due to hard or prolonged work. **Battle fatigue** is a broad group of physical, mental, and emotional signs that naturally result from the heavy mental and emotional work of facing danger under difficult conditions. Battle fatigue is the Army's doctrinal term for combat stress behaviors.

Stress is a general concept describing a "load" on the system. It is one of the body's processes for dealing with uncertain changes and danger. It involves physical, mental, automatic perceptual, and cognitive processes and an accompanying emotional response for evaluating uncertainty or threat. **Combat stress** is an individual soldier's internal psychological and physiological processes of reacting to and dealing with combat stressors. Combat stress is the cause of battle fatigue.

A **stressor** is an event or situation that creates personal conflict or poses a threat that requires the body to adapt or change. **Combat stressors** are any stressors that occur in the context of performing one's combat mission (whether under fire or not). **Stress behaviors** are stress related actions that can be observed by others. For example, moving or keeping still and speaking or not speaking. These behaviors may be intended to overcome and turn off a stressor, to escape it, or to adapt to it. A **combat stress casualty** is a soldier who is rendered combat ineffective due to battle fatigue.

■ Types of Stress and Stressors

There are four deployment-related stress problems:

- **Posttraumatic stress disorder (PTSD):** Occurs after battle
- **Acute stress disorder:** Occurs due to constant stress on the mind and body
- **Adjustment disorder:** Occurs when the soldier returns home and has to readjust to daily life
- **Combat stress reactions (COSRs):** Also called battle fatigue

Combat or operational stress can be the result of direct exposure or indirect exposure. **Direct exposure** is the effect of being exposed to situations or circumstances that directly cause a stressful or emotional reaction. **Indirect exposure** is the effect of being exposed to situations or circumstances that others may experience that indirectly cause a stressful or emotional reaction. Stressful reactions can be caused by either direct or indirect exposure to:

- **Cultural issues:** Having to deal with morals and ethics different from your own may cause stressful feelings or reactions.
- **Combatant casualties:** Dealing with or helping the enemy when they may be wounded may cause a stressful reaction due to feelings of hostility or loss.
- **Civilian casualties:** Having to deal with possible injuries to noncombatants may cause anxiety or stressful feelings.

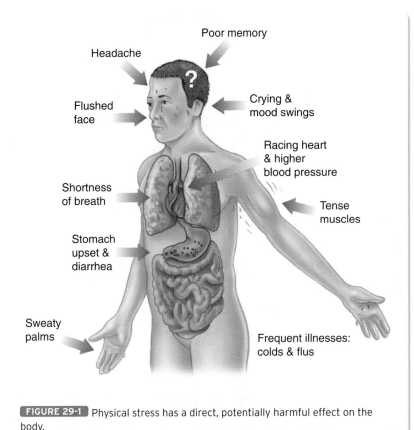

Poor memory

Headache

Flushed face

Crying & mood swings

Racing heart & higher blood pressure

Shortness of breath

Tense muscles

Stomach upset & diarrhea

Sweaty palms

Frequent illnesses: colds & flus

FIGURE 29-1 Physical stress has a direct, potentially harmful effect on the body.

be overwhelmed. Physical stressors can result in mental stress because they cause discomfort and impair performance. They can interfere directly with brain functioning and perceptual and cognitive mental abilities, thus increasing stress. Noise, light, and physical discomfort may interfere with sleep. Examples of physical stressors include:

- Environmental
  - Heat and cold
  - Vibration or noise
  - Hypoxia (may come from fumes or poisons)
  - Physical work
  - Difficult terrain
  - Bright lights, darkness, haze (can cause eye strain)
- Physiologic
  - Sleep debt
  - Dehydration
  - Malnutrition
  - Poor hygiene
  - Muscle fatigue
  - Overuse or underuse of muscles
  - Illness or injury

- **Body recovery:** Having to deal directly with death may cause stress due to the feeling of loss.
- **Humanitarian aid:** Having to deal with populations of people who may need food, water, shelter, and other basic necessities of life can cause significant stressful effects.
- **Separation issues:** Being away from your normal environment and loved ones can take its emotional toll.
- **Communication:** The loss of information about your home while serving in a combat zone may be very stressful.
- **Loss:** The effect of losing a fellow soldier, spouse, child, or someone else you have feelings and emotions for can have a stressful impact.
- **Cumulative loss:** Dealing with multiple losses of persons to whom you are emotionally tied can have a significant stressful effect.

Physical Stress

Physical stress has a direct, potentially harmful effect on the body **FIGURE 29-1 ▲**. It may come from external environmental conditions or internal physiologic demands required by or placed upon the human body.

Physical stressors evoke specific stress reflexes such as shivering when cold or sweating when hot. A soldier's stress reflexes can counteract the damaging impact of the stressors up to a point, but these reflexes and coping mechanisms can

Sleep

Sleep is essential to maintain brain efficiency and mental performance. Because of the body's natural rhythms, the best quality and longest duration of sleep is obtained during the night, from 2300 to 0600. These rhythms also make daytime sleep more difficult and less restorative, even in sleep-deprived soldiers. Forcing the body to go to sleep earlier in the evening impairs the soldier's ability to fall and remain asleep. This is why eastward travel across time zones initially produces greater deficits in alertness and performance than westward travel.

The ideal amount of sleep is 7 to 8 hours of continuous, uninterrupted night-time sleep each and every night. There is no minimum sleep requirement, though anything less than 7 to 8 hours per 24 hours will result in some level of performance degradation.

Although it is not ideal, sleep can be divided into two or more shorter periods to help soldiers obtain 7 to 8 hours per 24 hours. For example, sleep from 0100–0600, plus a nap from 1300–1500. Good nap zones, times when sleep onset and maintenance are the easiest, occur in the early morning, early afternoon, and night-time hours. Poor nap zones occur in the later morning and early evening hours, when the body's rhythms most strongly promote alertness. Sleep and rest are not the same. Resting does not restore performance, although it may briefly improve the way the soldier feels.

Sleep inertia is the degraded alertness/performance that lasts 10 to 20 minutes immediately upon waking. The long-term benefits of sleep generally far outweigh the short-term deficits resulting from sleep inertia, however. There is no such thing as too much sleep. Mental performance and alertness always benefit from sleep. Napping and sleep are not signs of laziness or weakness. They are signs of foresight, planning, and effective human resource management.

Mental Stress

Information is sent to the brain with only indirect physical impact on the body. The information may place demands on and cause reactions from the perceptual/cognitive system, the emotional system, or both. The perceptual/cognitive system refers to the process by which human beings interpret and organize sensation to produce a meaningful experience of the world. Perception typically involves the processing of sensory input (see, touch/feel, hear, taste, smell), and cognition is the mental activity used to interpret the sensory input. Cognition includes thinking, knowing, and remembering.

Mental stress can also produce some physical stress reflexes such as vasoconstriction, sweating, and adrenaline release. The distinction between mental and physical stress is rarely obvious. Because of the overlapping of mental and physical stress, no great effort needs to be made to distinguish between them, unless physical stressors have reached the point where they require protective measures or treatment. Both physical and mental stressors may be present in a soldier. Examples of mental stressors include:

- Perceptual/cognitive
  - Too much or too little information
  - Sensory overload or deprivation
  - Ambiguity, uncertainty, isolation
  - Time pressure or waiting
  - Unpredictability
  - Rules of engagement, difficult judgment
  - Hard choice or no choice
- Emotional
  - Fear- and anxiety-producing threats (of death, injury, failure, loss)
  - Grief-producing losses
  - Resentment, anger- and rage-producing frustration, threat, loss, and guilt
  - Boredom-producing inactivity
  - Conflicting motives (worries about home, divided loyalties)
  - Spiritual confrontation or temptation causing loss of faith

Positive Stress (Eustress)

Eustress is the degree of stress that is necessary to sustain and improve tolerance to stress without overstraining and disrupting the human system. Some level of stress is helpful and necessary for health. Insufficient stress leads to physical and/or mental weakness. Progressively greater exposure to a physical stressor is often required to achieve greater tolerance

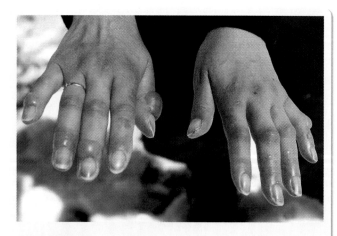

FIGURE 29-2 This frostbite injury will permanently reduce the soldier's tolerance to cold.

(acclimatization) to that stressor. Examples of progression include:

- Cardiovascular and muscle fitness
- Heat and cold acclimatization

Stressors that overstrain the adaptive capability of the body do not hasten acclimatization or increase tolerance to the stressor, but clearly impede acclimatization and can cause permanent impairment. Examples of stressors that can lead to impairment include:

- Extreme cold exposure that leads to frostbite, which permanently reduces the soldier's tolerance to cold **FIGURE 29-2** ▲
- Extreme heat exposure that leads to heat stroke, which permanently reduces the soldier's tolerance to heat

It is important to remember that once acclimatization is achieved, it must be maintained through continued exposure. Remember the "use it or lose it" rule. Up to a point, mental stress, even painful mental stress, may increase tolerance to future stress without causing impairment. Severe overstrain, however, can significantly weaken a soldier's tolerance to future stress. It is believed that immediate treatment can greatly reduce the potential for chronic disability, even for impairing emotional overstrain.

Successfully facing and mastering stressors increases tolerance to mental stress. Airborne and air assault training are good examples of confronting and mastering stressors. They require the soldier to master his or her instinctive fear of heights under controlled circumstances that are deliberately stressful.

■ Effects of Stress

Stress is an internal process that helps the soldier to function better, stay alive, and cope successfully. There is an optimal range of stress for any given task. Too little stress results in a job done haphazardly or not at all because the soldier is easily distracted, makes errors of omission, or falls asleep. If stress is too intense, the soldier may be too distracted or too focused on one aspect of the task to complete the mission. If the soldier is not familiar with his or her own stress reflexes and perceives the stress reflex as dangerous, the stress itself can become a stressor and magnify itself. Extreme stress may cause the soldier to freeze or become agitated and flee in panic.

■ Stress Behaviors in Combat

Adaptive Behaviors

Positive combat stress behaviors include heightened alertness, strength, endurance, and tolerance to discomfort. Ultimate positive combat stress behaviors are acts of extreme courage and almost unbelievable strength. They may even involve deliberate self-sacrifice. Positive adaptive behaviors include:

- Strong personal bonding between combat soldiers
- Sense of pride and shared identity with unit history and mission (esprit de corps)
- Unit cohesion

Dysfunctional Behaviors

Misconduct stress behaviors (MCSBs) range from minor breaches of unit orders or regulations to serious violations of the Uniform Code of Military Justice (UCMJ). This is more likely to occur in poorly trained, undisciplined soldiers. MCSBs predominate in military OOTW and ambiguous conflict scenarios with light combat operations. Dysfunctional behaviors can be prevented by enacting stress control measures. Once serious misconduct has occurred, it must be punished to prevent further erosion of discipline. Examples of misconduct stress behaviors include:

- Mutilating enemy dead
- Not taking prisoners
- Killing enemy prisoners, noncombatants, or animals
- Fighting with allies
- Alcohol or drug abuse
- Recklessness or lack of discipline
- Looting, pillage, or rape
- Fraternization
- Excessive use of sick call, malingering, or shirking duties
- Negligent disease or injury
- Self-inflicted wounds (SIW)
- Combat refusal
- Threatening/killing own leaders (fragging)
- AWOL or desertion

Battle Fatigue

Battle fatigue may also be called combat stress reaction (CSR). It feels unpleasant and interferes with the mission. It is best treated with reassurance, rest, replenishment, and restored confidence. The term *battle fatigue* is applied to any combat stress reaction that is treated.

Warning signs of battle fatigue deserve immediate attention from a leader, combat medic, or battle buddy. Early intervention can prevent potential harm to the soldier, others

---

> ## Garrison Care **TIPS**
>
> The distinction among positive combat stress behaviors, misconduct stress behaviors, and battle fatigue is not always clear.

in the unit, and the mission. The warning signs, in order from least serious to most serious, are:

- Hyperalertness
- Fear, anxiety
- Irritability, anger, or rage
- Grief, self-doubt, or guilt
- Physical stress complaints
- Inattention or carelessness
- Loss of confidence
- Loss of hope or faith
- Depression or insomnia
- Impaired duty performance
- Erratic actions or outbursts
- Freeze-up (unable to respond to danger) or immobility
- Terror or panic running
- Total exhaustion or apathy
- Loss of skills and memories
- Impaired senses (speech, vision, touch, hearing)
- Weakness or paralysis
- Hallucinations or delusions

Posttraumatic Stress Disorder

Posttraumatic stress disorder (PTSD) symptoms are normal responses after extremely abnormal and distressing events. It is normal for the survivor of one or more horrible events to have painful memories, anxiety, guilt, and/or unpleasant dreams. This behavior only becomes PTSD when either the pain of the memories or the actions the soldier takes to escape these memories interfere with occupational or personal life goals. PTSD and battle fatigue symptoms have much in common, but the behavior does not become PTSD until the trauma is over.

The warning signs of PTSD are:

- Intrusive, painful memories
- Trouble sleeping or nightmares
- Social isolation or withdrawal
- Jumpiness or acute startle response
- Guilt
- Alcohol or drug misuse or misconduct

> ## Garrison Care **TIPS**
>
> Studies show that immediate, far-forward treatment and rapid return to duty protect battle fatigue casualties against subsequent PTSD, whereas premature evacuation of battle fatigue casualties often results in chronic PTSD.

■ Battle Fatigue

Battle fatigue is the Army term for combat stress symptoms and reactions that feel unpleasant, interfere with mission performance, and are best treated with reassurance, rest, replenishment of physical needs, and activities to restore confidence. Battle fatigue can be present in soldiers who are physically wounded or ill. It may co-exist with misconduct stress behaviors. There are four major contributing factors that cause battle fatigue:

- Sudden exposure to intense fear, shocking stimuli, and the life or death consequences of battle
- Cumulative exposure to the dangers, responsibilities, and horrible consequences of battle
- Physical stressors and stress symptoms that reduce the soldier's coping ability
- Homefront and preexisting domestic problems

Battle-fatigued soldiers have often lost confidence in themselves, their equipment, their buddies, support units, or leaders. The signs and symptoms of battle fatigue are listed in TABLE 29-1 ▾ . Leaders and combat medics must ensure that battle fatigue casualties are given positive expectations. Never refer to these soldiers as psychiatric casualties, because this

Garrison Care TIPS

Individual personality does not predict susceptibility to battle fatigue.

TABLE 29-1 Signs and Symptoms of Battle Fatigue

Simple fatigue	• Tiredness • Loss of initiative • Indecisiveness • Inattention • General apathy
Anxiety	• Verbal expression of fear • Pronounced startle responses • Tremors • Sweating • Rapid heart rate • Insomnia with terror dreams
Depression	• Slow speech and movement • Restless and easily startled • Elements of self-doubt and self-blame • Hopelessness • Symptoms of grief or bereavement • Pessimistic attitude
Memory loss	• Inability to remember recent orders and instructions (mild) to loss of memory for well-learned skills • Inability to remember a traumatic event or period of time • Total amnesia (serious)

Garrison Care TIPS

Physical causes for memory loss must be ruled out before diagnosing a soldier with battle fatigue. The physical causes for memory loss include: traumatic brain injury (TBI), hypothermia, hyperthermia, drug intoxication or withdrawal, toxic illnesses, lasers, radiation, and chemical agents.

projects a negative attitude. Encourage these solders to feel empowered and in control of their emotions and feelings.

Physical Function Disturbance

Battle fatigue can cause a variety of physical disturbances TABLE 29-2 ▾ . You must be alert to the physical reactions of battle fatigue that mimic physical injury, particularly those injuries that can be attributed to lasers, radiation, or chemical agents, such as muscle weakness. In other words, be careful not to label what is actually a laser injury as battle fatigue.

Psychosomatic Disturbance

Psychosomatic refers to the interaction of the mind and the body. A **psychosomatic disturbance** is an expression of an emotional conflict through physical symptoms. TABLE 29-3 ▸ lists the types of psychosomatic disturbances.

Triage Categories of Battle Fatigue

The categorizing or sublabeling of battle fatigue cases is based solely on where they can be treated. Hence, sublabels depend as much on the situation of the unit as on the symptoms shown by the soldier. The labels *light* and *heavy*, *duty* and *rest*, *hold* and *refer*, when added to the label *battle fatigue*, are nothing more than a short hand or brevity code for saying where

TABLE 29-2 Types of Physical Disturbances

Motor disturbances	• Weakness/paralysis • Muscle contractions making it impossible to straighten a limb • Gross tremors • Pseudoconvulsive seizures
Visual disturbance	• Blurred vision • Double vision • Tunnel vision • Total blindness
Auditory (hearing) disturbance	• Tinnitus (ringing in the ears) • Deafness • Dizziness
Tactile (skin) sensory disturbances	• Anesthesia (loss of sensation) • Paresthesia (abnormal sensation such as pins and needles)
Speech disturbances	• Stuttering • Hoarseness • Muteness

TABLE 29-3 Types of Psychosomatic Disturbances

Cardiorespiratory psychosomatic disturbances	• Rapid irregular heartbeat • Shortness of breath • Lightheadedness • Tingling/cramping of toes, fingers, and lips
Gastrointestinal psychosomatic disturbances	• Stomach pain • Indigestion • Nausea • Vomiting • Diarrhea
Musculoskeletal psychosomatic disturbances	• Back or joint pain • Excessive pain • Disability from minor or healed wounds • Headache
Disruptive disturbances	• Disorganized, bizarre, impulsive, or violent behavior • Total withdrawal • Persistent hallucinations

the soldier is being treated or sent. These labels have no other meaning and have only a transient significance. The sublabel should be updated as the soldier improves or arrives at a new level of care.

The first triage categories of battle fatigue are light and heavy. Light battle fatigue is managed by self- or buddy aid or the unit combat medic, or through leader action. Most soldiers in combat will experience light battle fatigue at some time. If symptoms persist after rest, the soldier should be sent to sick call as suffering from heavy battle fatigue, which requires medical attention at a medical treatment facility (MTF). Symptoms of heavy battle fatigue may be temporarily too disruptive to the unit mission. These soldiers are triaged based on where they can be treated.

The battle fatigue categories are further classified as duty, rest, hold, and refer. Light battle fatigue cases can be treated immediately and returned to duty at their unit. Rest battle fatigue cases are sent to the unit's nonmedical combat service support element for brief rest, placed on light duty for 1 to 2 days, and no medical observation is required. Hold battle fatigue cases are held for treatment at the MTF because of the tactical situation and because the soldier's symptoms persist.

Refer battle fatigue casualties must be referred and transported to the next higher echelon for evaluation and treatment **FIGURE 29-3 ▶**. The refer category becomes hold when the soldier reaches an MTF where he or she can be held and treated.

■ Principles of Treatment

Prevention is the first principle of treatment for any medical condition. The primary goal of prevention is to control and/or reduce the stressors that are known to increase battle fatigue and misconduct stress behaviors. These stressors include:

- Being a new soldier
- Homefront worries
- Intense battle that incurs many soldiers killed in action (KIAs) and wounded in action (WIAs)
- Insufficient tough, realistic training
- Lack of unit cohesion
- Lack of trust in leaders
- Sleep deprivation
- Poor physical conditioning
- Debilitating environmental exposure
- Inadequate information
- High degree of uncertainty
- Absence of achievable end to the mission in sight
- Inadequate sense of purpose

The primary prevention is a leader's responsibility. Most of these stressors can be overcome through tough, realistic training that builds confidence and by looking out for each other. The secondary goal is to minimize acute disability by training leaders, chaplains, and medical personnel to:

- Identify the early warning signs and symptoms of battle fatigue
- Intervene immediately by treating warning symptoms and controlling relevant stressors
- Prevent contagion by rapidly segregating and treating dramatic battle fatigue casualties and disciplining minor misconduct stress behaviors
- Re-integrate recovered battle fatigue casualties back into the unit
- Take and publicize appropriate disciplinary actions for criminal misconduct stress behaviors

The tertiary goal is to minimize the potential for chronic disability, such as PTSD, in both soldiers who show battle fatigue and those who do not. You need to have an active prevention program in place during and immediately after combat and/or a traumatic incident. Conduct end of tour debriefings for units and their families. Remain sensitive and provide positive intervention to delayed or covert posttraumatic stress signs and symptoms.

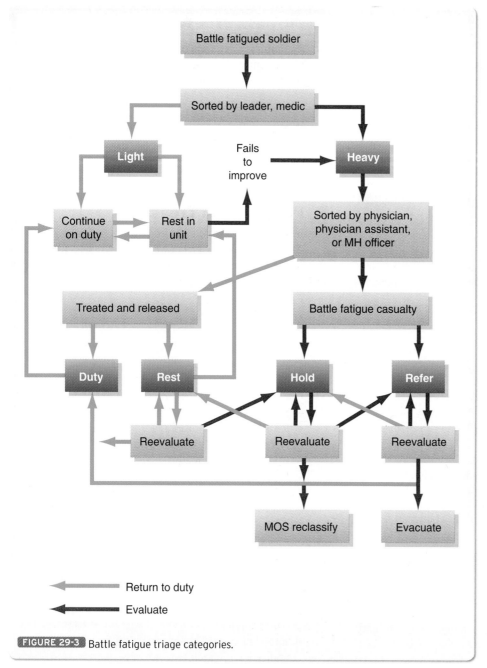

Return to duty
Evaluate

FIGURE 29-3 Battle fatigue triage categories.

PIES

All treatment plans should be based on certain principles characterized by the mnemonic *PIES*. These principles help to prevent permanent disability. PIES stands for:

- **Proximity:** Treat soldiers as close to their unit and the battle as possible.
- **Immediacy:** Battle fatigue requires immediate treatment.
- **Expectancy:** The battle fatigue casualty is provided a positive expectation for full recovery and early return to duty.
- **Simplicity:** Use simple, brief, straightforward methods to restore physical well-being and self-confidence by using nonmedical terminology and techniques.

Physical Assessment and Treatment

All casualties require an initial assessment and physical exam. A brief physical exam, including mental status assessment, must be performed to rule out illness or injury. Observe for conditions that mimic battle fatigue.

Conditions That Mimic Battle Fatigue

Many physical conditions and complaints can mimic, contribute to, or co-exist with battle fatigue, including:

- Dehydration causes altered mentation (the process of thinking).
- Chronic diarrhea or fever from a virus contributes to battle fatigue.
- Hyperthermia leads to irritability, disorientation, and confusion.
- Hypothermia causes a soldier to move or speak slowly.
- Head trauma causes amnesia, confusion, and impulsive behavior.
- Apparent loss of spinal cord function (sensory or motor) can occur as a result of trauma or can be a sign of battle fatigue.
- Postconcussion syndrome shows symptoms of a concussion (dizziness, poor concentration, headache, and anxiety) that may persist for weeks after the initial injury.
- Abdominal trauma causes shock, making the soldier unresponsive except for guarding because of pain from peritonitis.
- Air emboli/focal brain ischemia from a blast injury may cause stroke-like symptoms such as speech disturbances, loss of motor/sensory functions.
- Laser eye injury may cause loss of vision.
- Soldiers may experience vision loss for psychological reasons also, such as fear of losing their vision.
- Middle ear injury can cause hearing loss, tinnitus, and perceiving noises in the ear.
- Peripheral neuropathies are functional disturbances in the extremities that might be due to compression

(such as numbness and tingling in the arms/hands when carrying a rucksack).

- Nerve agent exposure can cause mild personality changes, insomnia with bad dreams, chronic and persistent depressive symptoms, and seizures.

Begin treatment for battle fatigue while covertly watching for more serious psychiatric conditions. First, give the soldier a reprieve from extreme stress. The soldier should remain in the combat zone, away from immediate danger, but still within sound of artillery to remind the soldier that his or her unit is still in battle. Other distant noises such as helicopters and aircraft are acceptable but should not be so noisy as to disrupt sleep.

Reassure the soldier by telling him or her that he or she has battle fatigue, a temporary condition that will improve quickly. Reassure the soldier that this is a normal reaction to terribly severe conditions. Also reassure the soldier that he or she will be able to return to duty after a brief period of rest and physical replenishment.

Separate soldiers with battle fatigue from patients with serious medical, surgical, or psychiatric conditions because association with patients often causes worsening symptoms and delays recovery. Soldiers with overly dramatic symptoms of panic or anxiety may need to be separated from other soldiers with battle fatigue. It is not necessary to separate soldiers with battle fatigue from soldiers who are convalescing, or who have minor illnesses or minor injuries because they often also have some degree of battle fatigue.

Provide simple treatment that includes rehydration, sleep, hygiene, and relative relief from danger. Maintain a tactical atmosphere. Restore confidence with structured military work details, physical exercise, and recreation. Reinforce the soldier's identity as a soldier and a member of his or her unit, not as a patient. Provide the soldier with battle fatigue an opportunity to express his or her feelings and regain perspective.

Avoid sedatives and tranquilizers unless these medications are absolutely essential to manage sleep or agitated behavior. Soldiers need to maintain a normal state of alertness so that they can take care of themselves and respond to treatment. Evacuate and/or hospitalize a soldier only if absolutely necessary, because hospitalization delays recovery and sig-

nificantly increases the possibility of chronic psychiatric disability. If evacuation is necessary it is better to use a general-purpose vehicle and not an ambulance.

Unmanageable cases of battle fatigue should be evacuated only to the next higher echelon of care. Soldiers with manageable battle fatigue who do not improve sufficiently within the allotted time to return to duty may also be sent unobtrusively to the next higher echelon of care.

A soldier with battle fatigue should be hospitalized only if absolutely necessary for the casualty's or the unit's safety. Move the soldier back to the nonhospital setting as soon as possible. If a soldier arrives at the hospital as an inappropriate evacuee, he or she should be told that he or she is only experiencing battle fatigue and returned to his or her unit area or appropriate forward area as soon as possible to recover in a nonhospital facility.

Restoration and reconditioning are programs to treat soldiers with battle fatigue in the combat zone. The Forward Support Medical Company (FSMC) is the first line for restoration. Restoration lasts 1 to 3 days and is conducted in the division or corps area by the medical detachment or mental health section. Reconditioning lasts 7 to 14 days and requires hospital admission for accountability, but treatment is conducted in the nonhospital setting by the mental health section. Both the restoration and reconditioning programs assist soldiers with battle fatigue to regain the skills and abilities needed for combat duty, including concentration, work tolerance, psychological endurance, and physical fitness.

■ Physical Restraints

Physically restraining soldiers with presumed battle fatigue goes against the treatment message of normality and positive expectation. However, some conditions may require the use of physical restraints to ensure the safety of the soldier and personnel or for medical evacuation:

- Serious disorientation or confusion
- Paranoid
- Delusional
- Hallucinating
- Suicidal
- Agitated
- Reckless
- Manic
- Intrusive
- Threatening violence

The best way to subdue and restrain agitated or disruptive soldiers is verbally, through reassurance and reorientation.

If verbal intervention fails, then a show of strength and force may suffice. Use a five-person takedown team with one person as leader and one person for each extremity. Begin by gathering around the leader with an air of confidence. The leader states, "Come calmly, or you will go in restraints," and then state why restraints are needed. Give the soldier an opportunity to back down, but this should only last a few seconds.

If the soldier does not cooperate, the following takedown method is used to position for restraints. At the signal of the leader, each team member controls his or her designated extremity and the leader holds the soldier's head. The soldier is brought to the ground or floor in a backward motion and then rolled over onto his or her abdomen. Once the soldier is face down, mechanical restraints, such as a leather restraint system, may be applied.

The leather restraint system includes two adjustable wrist cuffs and two adjustable ankle cuffs with an adjustable, lockable securing strap for each cuff. If mechanical restraints are not available, an improvised litter restraint method may be used by securing the soldier between two litters using patient securing (litter) straps.

Once restrained, the soldier's extremities must be checked frequently for impaired circulation and sensation to prevent nerve injury, skin ulcer, or gangrene. Do not leave this soldier alone if at all possible because the restrained soldier is at risk for airway compromise. Place the soldier in the supine position once restraints have been applied to prevent positional asphyxia.

Noncombat Arms Battle Fatigue Casualties

Medical personnel may experience increased stress associated with supporting combat operations. Combat support and combat service support, especially supply, transport, maintenance, and medical troops, may be tasked with prolonged/sustained operations, with increased risk from enemy forces that were bypassed. They tend to have more battle fatigue casualties (per wounded in action) than combat arms when they do have casualties. Seeing and having to touch the maimed bodies left behind by an attack may produce battle fatigue and/or PTSD in inadequately prepared troops, even if they are not under fire themselves.

Stressors pertaining to medical personnel include providing 24-hour care for severely injured patients. There are also moral dilemmas, such as triaging casualties into the Expectant category; saving severely injured soldiers, even if they beg to be allowed to die; placing casualties into a "return to duty" category; sending a soldier back to the dangers of combat when you do not have to face that same danger; and caring for wounded soldiers who are related to them or someone whom they know.

It is also difficult and taxing to maintain appropriate interpersonal relationships when everyone is under stress. Knowing how to unwind during lulls in the action without slipping into misconduct stress behaviors is an additional challenge. The final challenging stressor is the boredom when patient activities come to a halt for long periods of time.

Methods to reduce stress for medical personnel include:

- Establishing a sleep plan and shift schedules
- Developing time management skills
- Building team and unit cohesion
- Providing leisure time and recreational activities
- Training on how to conduct routine and special after-action debriefings

Depression

Depression is a mood disorder. Moods affect how you act and how you feel about yourself and life in general. Depression is a sad or unhappy mood that you cannot control. Depression may be caused by a stressful change in life or by chemical changes in the body. There also appears to be a genetic link to depression.

Depression is often associated with suicide. In 75% to 80% of suicides, depression is a contributing factor. Sadness and an occasional "case of the blues" are normal emotions for everyone. As an abnormal state, depression is a profound sadness that is present nearly every day for at least 2 weeks.

Signs and Symptoms of Depression

Medical conditions that present with similar symptoms must be ruled out, prior to a diagnosis of depression being made. The signs and symptoms of depression include:

- Mood changes
  - Sadness
  - Crying spells or inability to cry
  - Discouragement
  - Inability to feel pleasure
- Negative perception of self, the environment, and the future leading to
  - Pessimism
  - Negativism
  - Helplessness and hopelessness
  - Heightened sense of guilt
- Alterations of biologic function
  - Insomnia or hypersomnia (oversleeping)
  - Significant weight loss when not dieting, or weight gain
  - Constipation
  - Fatigue or loss of energy
  - Agitation
  - Indecisiveness
  - Dwelling on things
  - Recurrent thoughts of death or suicide

Suicide Prevention Responsibilities

Each year in the United States, approximately 500,000 people require emergency room treatment as a result of attempted suicide. In October 2001, a national vital statistics report showed that suicide was the second leading cause of death for both sexes from age 35 to 44, and the third leading cause of death for men and women who were age 20 to 24.

The former Surgeon General Dr. David Satcher said, "Suicide is a serious public health problem." During the 1990s, the Army lost the equivalent of a battalion—a total of 802 soldiers—to suicide. General Shinseki, the former Army chief of staff, called suicide a "serious problem," and directed a revision of the old suicide prevention program that placed primary responsibility for minimizing suicide upon leaders.

Many incidents of suicide are preventable; however, leaders and soldiers must be trained to recognize and respond to symptoms so they can help troubled soldiers and family members to discover alternatives to suicide. You may think that suicide was covered fairly intensively during basic training and stress management classes; however, stress management is not the total answer to preventing suicide. Here's a bigger picture of what we're dealing with. In 1996, following Admiral Jeremy Boorda's suicide, the Assistant Secretary of Defense for Health Affairs called for an analysis of the Department of Defense Suicide Prevention Programs. This study showed that suicide within the military was not primarily associated with stress in an individual's life. Suicide appeared to be associated with a diagnosable psychiatric disorder such as depression and/or substance abuse. Researchers also discovered that the military discouraged soldiers from seeking help from mental health professionals.

Suicide is an equal opportunity destroyer that cuts across rank, race, and gender. You must be able to recognize soldiers and other members of the military community who display behavior that might make them at high risk for attempting suicide. The Army Suicide Prevention Program Model is based on prevention, intervention, and the integration of installation/community resources. You must be aware of your responsibilities when it comes to preventing suicide and ensuring that you properly respond to soldiers who may be in danger of suicide, and safeguarding soldiers who express suicidal thoughts.

Prevention is primary in the Army's efforts to reduce suicide. When it comes to prevention, combat medics must be able to:

- Identify high-risk soldiers
- Be proactive and care for soldiers
- Encourage help-seeking behavior
- Promote positive life-coping skills to deal with life crises
- Be aware of suicidal thoughts and behavior in soldiers
- Know the community-wide resources for referral of soldiers demonstrating self-destructive behavior
- Ensure that soldiers' problems are properly addressed

Many soldiers come into the Army after experiencing many adverse events as a child such as physical or sexual abuse, parental violence, family alcoholism, family incarceration, or parental divorce. As a result, many soldiers come from homes that have not adequately prepared them to cope with crises in a positive way. Research has shown that adverse childhood events increase the risk of attempting suicide two- to five-fold.

Myths Versus Facts on Suicide

Why do people try to kill themselves? There is no simple answer as to why this occurs. The majority of all suicides within the Army are secondary to some form of psychiatric disorder like depression in combination with substance abuse. Suicidal people tend to feel a tremendous sense of loneliness and isolation. They feel helpless, hopeless, and worthless. Often, they believe that it does not matter if they live or die and that no one would miss them.

How can you tell if a soldier is depressed? Indicators of depression include:

- Mood changes
- Sadness
- Crying spells or inability to cry
- Discouragement
- Inability to feel pleasure
- Negative perception of self, the environment, and the future leading to
  - Pessimism
  - Negativism
  - Helplessness and hopelessness
  - Heightened sense of guilt
- Changes in biologic function
  - Insomnia or hypersomnia (oversleeping)
  - Significant weight loss when not dieting, or weight gain
  - Constipation
  - Fatigue or loss of energy
  - Agitation
- Indecisiveness
- Dwelling on things
- Recurrent thoughts of death or suicide

Why would a soldier commit suicide? There are numerous reasons a soldier may choose suicide. There are three major psychological reasons:

- Death as retaliatory abandonment
- Death as a retroflexed murder
- Death as self-punishment

With death as retaliatory abandonment, the individual is angry with a significant other for rejection and wants the rejector to feel the pain he or she is feeling. For example, a soldier kills himself after finding out that his wife left him for another man. The soldier attempts to regain control over the situation and dictate the final outcome, which is to reject life.

With death as a retroflexed murder, the individual tries to kill others through his or her own death. For example, after a deployment a soldier finds out his wife is having an affair. Instead of murdering her, he turns his murderous rage into suicide.

With death as self-punishment, the individual feels guilty and unworthy of living. For example, a soldier has serious Uniform Code of Military Justice (UCMJ) actions pending. She feels like a failure, is embarrassed and humiliated, and feels she does not deserve to live.

What causes or triggers suicide? Is there a difference for younger and older soldiers? Younger soldiers tend to resort to suicide because of negative life-coping skills. Their negative life-coping skills, combined with relationship problems, financial problems, pending civilian legal action, or UCMJ disciplinary action, forces them over the edge. Older soldiers tend to resort to suicide as a result of facing major life transitions, such as a failed marriage or being passed over for promotion. Other soldiers may suffer from chronic substance abuse or a mood disorder. A common feeling among both the young and old is an overwhelming feeling of isolation and loneliness.

Army Suicide Triggers

A review of suicidal cases in the Army revealed that 75% of completed suicides were triggered by relationship problems, 50% occurred while soldiers were pending UCMJ action, 42% were experiencing financial problems, and 34% were having drug and alcohol problems. Additional reasons included:

- A bad evaluation for an enlisted soldier or officer
- The breakup of a close relationship
- The anniversary of a suicide of a close friend or family member
- Drug or alcohol abuse
- Leaving old friends
- Alone with concerns about self or family
- Financial stressors
- New military assignment
- Death of a loved one: spouse, child, parent, sibling, friend, or pet
- Loss of esteem/status
- Humiliation
- Rejection (job loss, failed promotion, discharged)
- Disciplinary or legal difficulty
- Suicide of a friend or family member
- Retirement

At times, beliefs about addressing soldiers who may be suicidal interfere with reaching out to soldiers who may be in danger. **TABLE 29-4 ▶** lists the myths and facts of suicide.

Identifying Historic Risk Factors Associated With Suicide

It is important to know your soldiers so you are able to recognize those soldiers who, because of adverse events, are at higher risk of resorting to suicide. Studies have shown that historic factors are a major contributor to suicidal behavior. What historic factors might make a person more prone to attempting or committing suicide?

- Made a previous suicide attempt
- A family or friend lost through suicide
- A victim of childhood abuse or witnessed family violence
- Previously abused drugs and/or alcohol
- Alcohol abuse or dependency by a significant family member

Life-coping skills are affected by some of the previously mentioned historic factors. Some of the factors are created by genetic vulnerabilities such as alcoholism and psychiatric illnesses like depression; developmental history such as childhood trauma, abuse, neglect, or parental abandonment; and the current environment such as work and home conditions.

TABLE 29-4 **Myths and Facts of Suicide**

Myth	Fact
People who talk about suicide rarely attempt or commit suicide.	Nearly 80% of those who attempt or commit suicide give some warning of their intentions. When people talk about committing suicide, they may be giving a warning that should not be ignored.
Talking to people about their suicidal feelings will cause them to commit suicide.	Talking to people about their suicidal feelings usually makes them feel relieved that someone finally recognizes their emotional pain, and they feel safer talking about it.
All suicidal people want to die, and there is nothing that can be done about it.	Most suicidal people are undecided about living or dying. They may gamble with death, leaving it to others to rescue them. Often, they call for help before and after a suicide attempt.
Suicide is an impulsive act with no prior planning.	Most suicides are carefully planned and thought about for weeks.
A person who attempts suicide will not try again.	Most people who commit suicide have made previous attempts.
Improvement in a suicidal person means the danger is over.	Most suicides occur within about 3 months following the beginning of improvement when the individual has the energy to act on suicidal thoughts and feelings.
Suicidal persons are crazy or psychotic.	Studies of hundreds of suicide notes indicate that, although suicidal persons are extremely unhappy and may abuse substances, they are not necessarily psychotic.
Because it includes the holiday season, December has a high suicide rate.	Nationally, December has the lowest suicide rate of any month. During the holiday season, depressed persons feel some sort of belonging and feel things may get better. Statistics have shown that the majority of suicides tend to occur in January, April, September, and October.

It is important to create a supportive environment that promotes positive coping skills for all soldiers.

Immediate Danger Signs Related to Suicide

When one or more of the following signs are observed in a soldier, suicidal behavior may be imminent, especially if the soldier has experienced some life stress events associated with suicide, appears to be depressed, and/or has a history known to cause an increased risk of suicide:

- Talking about death or hinting at suicide
- Giving away important possessions
- Making a will in connection with the disposal of personal property
- Obsession with death, sad music, or sad poetry
- Themes of death in letters or artwork
- Specific plans to commit suicide and access to lethal means
- Buying a gun

■ What to Do and What Not to Do When Confronted With a Suicidal Soldier

Asking About Suicide

Ask the soldier directly:

- Are you thinking about suicide or taking your life?
- What has happened to make you want to die?
- How will you do it?

If you suspect that a soldier is suicidal, begin asking questions and be direct. Take all suicide threats seriously. The warning signs given by many soldiers can be very subtle, so trust your suspicions. Do not be afraid of discussing suicide with the soldier. Getting the soldier to talk about it is a positive step. Be a good listener. Do not make moral judgments, act shocked, or make light of the situation. Confronting these feelings may lead the soldier away from actually attempting suicide by demonstrating that someone cares.

Express your concerns about the impact of the soldier's behavior on significant others such as family, friends, and battle buddies. Those who attempt suicide most often feel alone, worthless, and unloved. You can help by letting this soldier know that he or she is not alone and that you are there. By assuring the soldier that help is available, you are literally throwing a lifeline. Remember, although individuals may think that they want to die, human beings have an innate will to live and are more than likely hoping to be rescued.

Garrison Care TIPS

Offering advice such as, "Be grateful for what you have" or "You're so much better off than most people" may only deepen the sense of guilt the soldier may already feel.

TABLE 29-5 Do's and Don'ts of Working With a Suicidal Soldier

Do's	Don'ts
Go with the soldier or send an escort to get help.	Do not leave anyone alone if you believe the risk for suicide is imminent.
Realize that suicide is an equal opportunity destroyer.	Do not assume the soldier is not the suicidal "type."
Remain calm.	Do not act shocked when the person tells you he or she is contemplating suicide.
Tell a commander, mental health provider, or other members of the military support system what you suspect.	Do not keep deadly secrets.

Get Help

Help the soldier understand you are getting help because of your concerns. The most useful thing you can do is to get someone who is considering suicide professional help. Getting help for someone you believe may be suicidal involves respect and the safeguarding of his or her welfare. Every soldier deserves dignity, and you must be compassionate toward the needs of others. Go with the soldier or send an escort with the soldier. Do not send the soldier alone TABLE 29-5 ▲. The Army community offers many resources for help including the Community Mental Health Service, Social Work Services, Chaplain, Army Community Service (ACS), and the chain of command.

■ Summary

Battle fatigue occurs in units, often all at once. Stress levels remain high in almost all Army units due to continually changing missions and a potential for terrorist attacks anytime and anywhere in the world. As a combat medic, one of your jobs is to monitor the mental health of soldiers in your assigned unit and advise the unit command when stress levels are high. It is the responsibility of the command and the combat medic to take the necessary measures to prevent combat fatigue. You will treat battle fatigue as close to your unit as possible and evacuate only when necessary.

Remember that suicide is a traumatic event for the soldier and for all those people who have some connection with the soldier. A founding president of the American Association of Suicidology stated, "Human understanding is the most effective weapon against suicide. The greatest need is to deepen awareness and sensitivity of people to their fellow man."

YOU ARE THE
COMBAT MEDIC

You and your team are on a field mission in a remote, isolated area. Your unit is nearing the end of its tour of duty and you have experienced a great deal on the battlefield. Two days into the mission, you notice that your battle buddy's behavior is out of character. Team members have to repeat commands to him and you've seen him stare remotely out into the distance during marches.

You take the soldier aside for a talk. He admits that he's been having trouble sleeping for the past week. Lately, he feels so tired that he's beginning not to care about much anymore.

Assessment

You perform an initial assessment and a brief physical exam in order to rule out any illness or injury. After ruling out any illness or injury, you determine that this soldier is indeed experiencing a light case of battle fatigue.

You reassure the soldier that he is experiencing battle fatigue and that these feelings will pass with rest and physical replenishment. You tell him that his reactions are normal in a severely stressful situation.

Treatment

You meet with the unit leader and determine the best course of action to treat this soldier. You decide to allow the soldier to remain at the base camp. While his focus is on rest and recovery, he will be performing duties to assist in maintaining the base camp.

After 3 days away from the active combat zone, the soldier begins to sleep a solid 7 hours. He begins to ask you and the unit leader how his buddies are doing on their mission. By the fifth day, he is requesting to return to active duty. "I just want to complete the mission with my unit, sir," he explains.

Ready for Review

- As a combat medic, you may assist the commander in assessing the impact of sustained operations on his or her soldiers.
- There are four deployment-related stress problems:
  - Posttraumatic stress disorder (PTSD): Occurs after battle
  - Acute stress disorder: Occurs due to constant stress on the mind and body
  - Adjustment disorder: Occurs when the soldier returns home and has to readjust to daily life
  - Combat stress reactions (CSR): Also called battle fatigue
- Positive combat stress behaviors include heightened alertness, strength, endurance, and tolerance to discomfort.
  - Ultimate positive combat stress behaviors are acts of extreme courage and almost unbelievable strength.
- *Battle fatigue* is the Army term for combat stress symptoms and reactions that feel unpleasant, interfere with mission performance, and are best treated with reassurance, rest, replenishment of physical needs, and activities to restore confidence.
- The first triage categories of battle fatigue are light and heavy.
  - Light battle fatigue is managed by self- or buddy aid or the unit combat medic, or through leader action.
  - Heavy battle fatigue requires medical attention at a medical treatment facility (MTF).
- Prevention is the first principle of treatment for any medical condition.
- The primary goal of prevention is to control and/or reduce the stressors that are known to increase battle fatigue and misconduct stress behaviors.
- Physically restraining soldiers with presumed battle fatigue goes against the treatment message of normality and positive expectation.
  - Some conditions may require the use of physical restraints to ensure the safety of the soldier and personnel or for medical evacuation.
- Combat support and combat service support, especially supply, transport, maintenance, and medical troops, may be tasked with prolonged/sustained operations, with increased risk from enemy forces that were bypassed.
- Depression is a mood disorder.
  - Moods affect how you act and how you feel about yourself and life in general.
  - Depression is a sad or unhappy mood that you cannot control.
- Many incidents of suicide are preventable.
  - Leaders and soldiers must be trained to recognize suicidal tendencies and respond to help troubled soldiers and family members to discover alternatives to suicide.

Vital Vocabulary

battle fatigue A broad group of physical, mental, and emotional signs that naturally result from the heavy mental and emotional work of facing danger under difficult conditions.

Combat/Operational Stress Control (COSC) Encompasses programs developed and actions taken by military leadership to prevent, identify, and manage adverse combat stress reactions in units to optimize mission performance, conserve fighting strength, prevent or minimize adverse affects of combat stress on soldiers' physical, psychological, intellectual, and social health, and return the unit or service member to duty expeditiously.

combat stress The individual soldier's internal psychological and physiological processes of reacting to and dealing with combat stressors.

combat stress casualty A soldier who is rendered combat ineffective due to battle fatigue.

combat stressors Any stressors that occur in the context of performing one's combat mission.

depression A sad or unhappy mood that you cannot control.

direct exposure The effect of being exposed to situations or circumstances that directly cause a stressful or emotional reaction.

eustress The degree of stress necessary to sustain and improve tolerance to stress without overstraining and disrupting the human system.

fatigue The distress and impaired performance that come from doing something too hard or for too long.

indirect exposure The effect of being exposed to situations or circumstances that others may experience that indirectly cause a stressful or emotional reaction.

physical stressors Evoke specific stress reflexes such as shivering or sweating.

posttraumatic stress disorder (PTSD) Symptoms such as painful memories, anxiety, guilt, and unpleasant dreams that are normal responses after extremely abnormal and distressing events.

psychosomatic disturbance An expression of an emotional conflict through physical symptoms.

stress A load on the system; one of the body's processes for dealing with uncertain changes and danger.

stress behaviors Stress related actions that can be observed by others.

stressor An event or situation that creates personal conflict or poses a threat that requires the body to adapt or change.

COMBAT MEDIC *in Action*

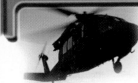

You are concerned about your battle buddy. His clothes are looking looser and looser on him and he's been getting less and less sleep. He has a lot on his mind, with his wife and two kids back home. Lately, his wife has been sounding strange over the phone and her e-mails are becoming shorter and fewer. His oldest is mentioning, "Uncle Steve," a close friend from high school, more and more often. One evening after reading his e-mail, your battle buddy appears, face ashen, his wife has admitted to having a relationship with his friend, Steve. "My life is over," he says.

1. Of all completed suicides, 75% were triggered by:
   A. relationship problems.
   B. pending UCMJ action.
   C. financial problems.
   D. drug and alcohol problems.

2. Indicators of depression include:
   A. mood changes.
   B. discouragement.
   C. inability to feel pleasure.
   D. all of the above.

3. Suicidal behavior may be imminent if:
   A. the soldier gives away important possessions.
   B. the soldier is obsessed with death, sad music, or sad poetry.
   C. the soldier refers to themes of death in letters or artwork.
   D. all of the above.

4. If you suspect that a soldier is suicidal, you should notify:
   A. a commander.
   B. a mental health provider.
   C. other members of the military support system.
   D. all of the above.

5. The historic factors that might make a person more prone to attempt or commit suicide include:
   A. a previous suicide attempt.
   B. the death of a family member or friend through suicide.
   C. previous abuse of drugs or alcohol.
   D. all of the above.

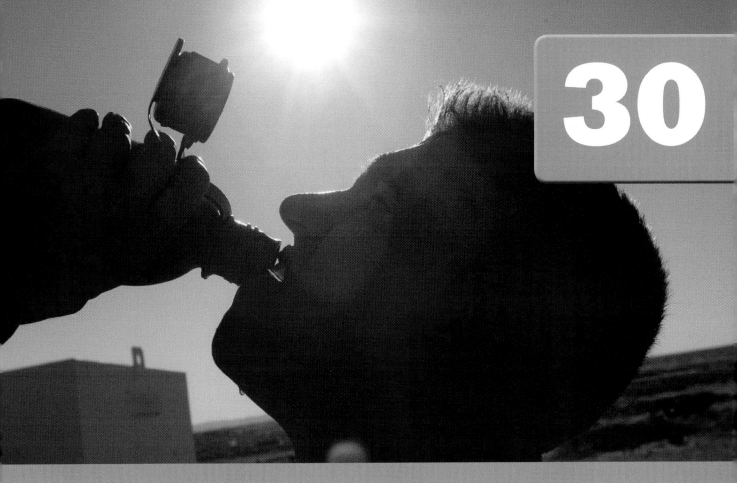

30

Environmental Emergencies

Objectives

Knowledge Objectives

- [ ] Describe an environmental emergency.
- [ ] Identify and manage a heat injury.
- [ ] Discuss how to prevent heat illness.
- [ ] Explain how to perform a general assessment of cold weather injuries.
- [ ] Discuss how to manage cold injuries.

- [ ] Describe how disease is spread by arthropods.
- [ ] Discuss the threats posed by arthropods.
- [ ] List the types of scorpions, spiders, and snakes that pose a threat to soldiers.
- [ ] Describe the types of altitude illness.
- [ ] Discuss how to manage altitude illness.

■ Introduction

During EMT-B training, you learned that heat injuries are a type of environmental injury resulting from exposure to extreme temperatures. However, when wearing protective equipment (MOPP), all soldiers are at risk for a heat injury regardless of the outdoor temperature. Wearing proper clothing and operating at appropriate activity levels are key methods for prevention, but may not always be possible. As a combat medic, one of your key duties is prevention. You need to identify high-risk personnel such as basic trainees, soldiers with a previous history of heat injury, and overweight soldiers. Acclimatization and protection from undue heat exposure can help both leaders and individuals prevent unnecessary injury.

Cold injuries are most likely to occur when an unprepared individual is exposed to winter temperatures. The cold weather and the type of combat operation in which the individual is involved impact on whether he or she is likely to be injured and to what extent. Clothing, physical condition, and mental makeup also are determining factors. However, cold injuries can usually be prevented. Well-disciplined and well-trained individuals can be protected even in the most adverse circumstances.

You must know the hazards of exposure to the cold and how to provide care for cold injuries. The extent of the cold injury depends on duration of exposure and adequacy of protection. Individuals with a history of cold injury are likely to be more easily affected for an indefinite period. The body parts most easily affected by cold are the cheeks, nose, ears, chin, forehead, wrists, hands, and feet. Proper treatment and management depend on accurate diagnosis.

Altitude illness can affect anyone exposed to altitudes over 4,921′ (1,500 m) in elevation. The military's capability to deploy worldwide in support of the National Command Authority strategic directives implies that we must be capable of mounting combat operations anywhere in the world—including high altitudes. Numerous combat operations conducted throughout Operation Enduring Freedom have seen combat forces airlifted to an area of operations several thousand feet higher than their staging base. These rapid changes in altitude can lead to a spectrum of medical problems known collectively as altitude illness. Altitude illness can significantly affect a soldier's performance and effectiveness during combat operations.

■ Recognize an Environmental Emergency

Heat

An <u>environmental emergency</u> is a medical condition caused or exacerbated by the weather, terrain, atmospheric pressure, or other local factors. Many military campaigns have been lost due to the lack of heat acclimatization and subsequent <u>heat illness</u>. King Edward and his metal-armored crusaders allegedly lost the final battle of the Holy Land against the well-adapted and well-ventilated Arab horsemen because of heat illnesses. Modern military organizations continue to encounter heat illness because of the requirement to train unacclimatized troops with forced heavy physical exercise.

The US Army reported at least 125 deaths from heat stroke during basic training during the years 1941–1944; mortality rates range from 10% to 75%. In the United States alone, more than 4,000 people die of heat stroke annually. Athletes also are prone to heat illness. Between 1961 and 1971, 46 American football players died of heat stroke, which is the second leading cause of death in young athletes. Recently, a professional baseball pitcher died of heat stroke.

The environmental factors that induce or exacerbate other medical or traumatic conditions include:

- **Climate:** High ambient temperature reduces the body's ability to lose heat by radiation. High relative humidity reduces the body's ability to lose heat through evaporation.
- **Seasons:** Winter can produce extremely low temperatures while summer can produce extremely high temperatures.
- **Weather:** Variables such as the wind can effect the temperature.
- **Atmospheric (barometric) pressure:** The pressure exerted by the weight of the air; an increase in altitude decreases pressure.
- **Terrain:** Altitude can effect the temperature.

The risk factors for heat injury include:

- **Age:** Persons at the extremes of age are at greater risk for environmental emergencies. Small children have a large body surface area, especially of the head, and a very limited ability to compensate for acute major changes in temperature. Older people lose their ability to internally regulate their temperature and are more susceptible to temperature extremes. They get colder or warmer quicker and with less awareness than younger individuals.
- **General health:** Anyone who has a serious underlying medical condition (eg, heart failure, cancer), especially if the person is undernourished, is more susceptible to environmental influences.
- **Fatigue:** When people are tired, they may not exercise appropriate judgment in potentially dangerous environmental situations (eg, staying outside in the heat for too long). In addition, fatigue may upset the body's normal regulatory mechanisms, making the person more likely to incur injury.
- **Predisposing medical conditions:** Particularly risky conditions include diabetes (decreased sensation in the extremities), congestive heart failure (alterations of autonomic nervous system function), and thyroid disease (excess or abnormally low sensitivity to heat or cold).
- **Medications:** Both prescription and over-the-counter (OTC) medications may predispose persons to environmental injury, especially heat injury. Many common medications such as antihistamines impair the body's ability to sweat and dissipate heat. Heat

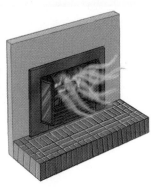
Radiation

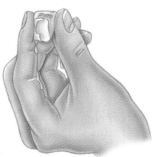
Conduction

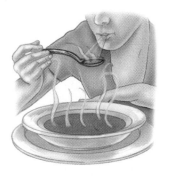
Convection

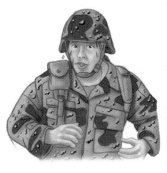
Evaporation

FIGURE 30-1   Heat is dissipated from the body through radiation, conduction, convection, and evaporation.

intolerance is a common side effect of these drugs, whether they are prescription or OTC drugs. In addition, diuretics can contribute to dehydration.

Thermolysis refers to the body's normal methods of heat loss and gain. Heat is generated by muscular activity and through metabolic reactions in the body. As body temperature increases, changes occur in each organ system. If an individual is gradually exposed to a hot environment, the body acclimates, or becomes used to the heat. Heat is dissipated from the body by four mechanisms FIGURE 30-1 ▲ :

- **Radiation:** Transmission of heat through space (eg, warmth from a radiant heater or fireplace)
- **Conduction:** Transmission of heat from warmer to cooler objects in direct contact (eg, touching a cold surface, lying on a cold floor)
- **Convection:** Transfer of heat by circulation of heated particles (eg, wind chill, cold water exposure, or cooling soup by blowing on it)
- **Evaporation:** Loss of heat at the surface from vaporization of liquid (eg, sweating, spraying water mist on the body to keep cool while sunbathing)

Cold

Hannibal lost half of his force of 46,000 crossing the Pyrenean Alps. Napoleon's retreat from Moscow in the dreadful winter of 1812 to 1813 was one of the most famous mass casualty incidents in military history. Cold weather injuries can significantly impact other injuries and illnesses and produce more casualties. The risk factors include:

- **Age:** The very young and very old are more susceptible to cold weather injuries.
- **General health:** Poor general health makes you more susceptible to cold weather injuries.
- **Fatigue:** Fatigue makes individuals more lax in taking proper precautions for cold weather.
- **Predisposing medical conditions:** Atherosclerosis, hypovolemia, diabetes, alcohol consumption, and

previous cold injury can make an individual more sensitive to cold injuries.

- **Medications:** Peripheral vasodilator medications cause vessels to dilate and the body to lose more heat. Diuretics along with the cold cause more fluid to be excreted, making dehydration more common. Nicotine causes peripheral vasoconstriction, which decreases circulation to the extremities.

The mechanisms of heat loss include:

- **Conduction:** Transfer of heat from one substance to another due to difference in temperature
- **Convection:** Transfer of heat through gas or liquid by circulated heat particles
- **Evaporation:** Loss of heat at the surface from vaporization of liquid (eg, sweating)
- **Radiation:** Energy in the form of heat radiates in waves through the air or other mediums (water)

The environmental risks for cold injury include:

- **Climate, season, weather:** All are factors that make you more susceptible to cold weather injuries (eg, fall and winter with their cool, damp climates cause more cold weather injuries than warm spring or summer).
- **Atmospheric (barometric) pressure:** The pressure exerted by the weight of the air. An increase in altitude decreases pressure. The higher the elevation, the colder the climate.
- **Terrain:** There are more environmental exposures on mountains and ridges than in valleys or depressions.

■ Identify and Manage a Heat Injury

Heat Cramps

A **heat cramp** is a muscle cramp or spasm of the voluntary muscles of the arm, leg, or abdomen caused by depletion in the body of water and salt. Painful spasms of skeletal muscles can occur including muscles of the extremities and the abdomen. Heat cramps often occur in individuals who are perspiring heavily and drinking large quantities of water or other hypotonic solutions.

The patient's skin may be moist or dry. The core temperature is normal or minimally elevated. In order to obtain an accurate core temperature, you must obtain a rectal temperature reading. Do not eliminate heat exhaustion as a possibility, because heat cramps and heat exhaustion may coexist. The treatment for heat cramps includes:

- Move the patient into the shade.
- Loosen clothing.
- Gently stretch cramped muscles.
- Provide oral hydration with an electrolyte solution. If the patient is nauseated, provide IV hydration with Ringer's lactate solution. See Chapter 13, *Intravenous Access*, for detailed information.
- Obtain further medical advice from the medical officer if the patient's symptoms continue.

Heat Exhaustion

Heat exhaustion is a systemic reaction to prolonged heat exposure and is due to sodium depletion and dehydration. The symptoms of heat exhaustion include:

- Profuse sweating with pale, moist, and cool skin
- Headache, often with weakness and fatigue
- Thirst
- Dizziness
- Loss of appetite
- Nausea (with or without vomiting)
- Confusion
- Core temperature varies from normal to 104°F

The treatment of heat exhaustion begins by moving the patient to a cool, shady area. Loosen or remove the patient's clothing and boots. Provide oral hydration with electrolyte solution, if tolerated by the patient. If the patient cannot tolerate oral hydration, provide IV hydration with Ringer's lactate solution. Keep the patient supine.

Monitor the patient and always evacuate. The patient may be treated at the Battalion Aid Station (BAS) and return to duty (RTD) after appropriate rest and rehydration if the combat situation dictates.

Heat Stroke

Heat stroke is caused by failure of the temperature-regulating system in the brain. Heat stroke usually involves excessive exposure to strenuous physical activity under hot conditions; however, elderly or chronically ill patients may develop heat stroke without strenuous physical activity. The hallmark of this condition is an altered mental status.

Heat stroke is a medical emergency that will result in death if treatment is delayed; it has an 80% fatality rate if left untreated. You must act without delay, because body temperature may exceed 105°F. The signs and symptoms of heat stroke include:

- Sweat may or may not be present
- Red (flushed), hot, usually dry skin
- Headache

> ### Garrison Care TIPS
>
> Heat stroke is a medical emergency that will result in death if treatment is delayed.

- Dizziness
- Nausea
- Confusion, bizarre, or combative behavior
- Weakness
- Seizures
- May progress to coma
- Rapid and weak respiration and pulse
- Core temperature above 104°F

To treat heat stroke, start cooling measures immediately and continue them while waiting for transportation and during evacuation. Act quickly to prevent further injury. Remove the patient from the environment and remove the patient's clothing. Perform active cooling by misting the patient with water and fanning, applying moist wraps, applying ice packs to the groin or axilla, or immersing the patient in cool water. Do not lower the patient's core temperature below 102°F. The patient's temperature will continue to drop after removal from the water. Provide fluid therapy via IV hydration with Ringer's lactate solution.

> ### Garrison Care TIPS
>
> Prompt evaporative cooling is the preferred method; however, be aware of potential complications such as shivering.

> ### Garrison Care TIPS
>
> IV fluids should be infused as close to normal body core temperature as possible.

Prevention of Heat Illness

The predisposing factors of heat injuries include:

- Previous heat injury
- Age (pediatric and geriatric patients are high risk; extremes of age)
- General health and medications
- Cardiac disease
- Diabetes (circulation impairments that may interfere with thermoregulatory input)
- Obesity
- Recent illness
- Fatigue
- Medications that inhibit sweating (atropine, antihistamines, tranquilizers, cold medications, and diuretics)

- Acclimatization, length of exposure, intensity of exposure
- Environment, including humidity, wind chill, and ambient air temperature
- Alcohol intake within the last 24 hours
- Food consumption
- Fever
- Clothing, interceptor ballistic armor (IBA) and especially chemical, biological, radiation, nuclear, explosion (CBRNE) gear

The wet bulb globe thermometer (WBGT) index is used to determine the heat condition. The use of MOPP or IBA gear increases the WBGT by about 10°F. Heat stress is an important factor to consider in an environment in which protective gear or MOPP gear is worn. In environments with moderate and relatively comfortable temperatures, MOPP gear can greatly increase temperatures to the most severe and debilitating level of heat stress. It is important that soldiers in MOPP gear maintain adequate water consumption, are frequently rotated to reduce occurrence of heat injuries, and establish appropriate rest and work periods to ensure adequate manpower is available.

Water consumption recommendations can be found on a heat category chart. When to drink is as important as how much—if you wait until you are thirsty to consume water, you have waited too long.

Additional heat injury prevention recommendations include:

- Follow work/rest guidelines on a heat category chart.
- Restrict or modify strenuous physical activities during high heat stress conditions, if the combat situation permits.
- Have soldiers take breaks in the shade and drink water.
- Hold formations in the shade or off blacktop and concrete surfaces whenever possible.
- Allow 2 weeks for soldiers to become acclimated to the heat. Progressively increase the workload during the second week. During periods of sudden temperature change, treat all soldiers as nonacclimated.
- Heat effects build up cumulatively during the day and over several days. Recovery is slow even after temperatures have decreased.
- Always stress prevention. Perform heavy work earlier in the day. Follow the highest heat category reached for the remainder of the day. Verify heat injury reporting procedures.

Salt tablets are not used in the prevention of heat injury. Usually, eating field rations or liberally salting the garrison diet will provide enough salt to replace what is lost through sweating in hot weather. Soldiers are more likely to keep hydrated if the fluids are cold. Some units buy electrolyte replacement solutions to supplement the flavor and to aid with self-hydration.

■ Identify and Manage a Cold Injury

Chilblains

Chilblains are caused by the repeated prolonged exposure of bare skin in damp, nonfreezing temperatures. It is often precipitated by acute repeated exposure to cold. Chilblains are more common in cold, damp climates. The signs and symptoms of chilblains include redness or cyanosis of the affected areas and blue-red patches, commonly on the lower extremities and the face, hands, and feet. Another symptom is hot, tender, and itching skin. Subcutaneous nodules may be present. The patient may have ulcerated or bleeding lesions with chronic repeated episodes.

Emergency care for chilblains includes warming the injured body part, elevating the affected body part, and placing the injured body part in contact with a warm object, such as your hands or the patient's body. Instruct the patient to cross his or her arms and place his or her hands underneath the armpits. Do not rub the injured tissue. Do not apply direct heat or ice to the injured tissue. Protect the rewarmed area from further cold exposure or trauma.

Immersion Syndrome

Immersion syndrome (immersion foot/trench foot/paddy foot) involves injuries that result from prolonged exposure of the feet to cool or cold water or mud FIGURE 30-2 ▾. Inactive feet in damp or wet socks and boots or tightly laced boots that impair circulation are even more susceptible to injury. Trench foot occurred frequently during World War I because soldiers stood in cold, wet, muddy trenches for extended periods of

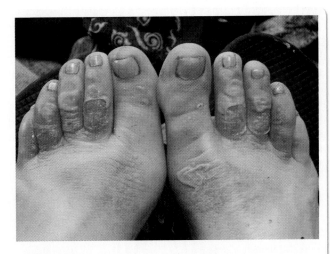

FIGURE 30-2 Immersion foot/trench foot/paddy foot involves injuries that result from prolonged exposure of the feet to cool or cold water or mud.

time awaiting orders. During Vietnam, soldiers were also faced with similar environmental conditions. Paddy foot was a condition that frequently occurred during this period due to wet feet, even though the temperatures were higher.

The early stages (first phase) develop slowly over hours or days. The affected area is cold and pale. There is numbness and tingling. The patient's pulses will be diminished or absent. In the later stages (advanced), the patient will complain of his or her limbs feeling hot and burning and he or she will experience shooting pains. The affected area is pale. Blisters, swelling, redness, and ulceration may occur. Complications include anesthesia (numbness), which may persist for weeks, along with hyperhydrosis (excessive sweating), and cold sensitivity. In very severe cases, infection and **gangrene** may occur.

The treatment for immersion syndrome consists of protecting the extremity from trauma and infection. Gradually rewarm the affected area by exposing it to warm air. Do not apply heat or ice, or massage it. Dry the patient's feet thoroughly and have him or her avoid walking. Elevate the affected part. Seek medical treatment and evacuate the patient.

To prevent immersion syndrome, make certain that soldiers in your unit keep their feet warm and dry and change out of wet socks several times daily. Ensure that all soldiers' boots fit well. Soldiers should never sleep in wet socks and boots.

Snow Blindness

Snow blindness is a burn to the eye from UV radiation. Damage is to the cornea and is similar to a welding flash burn to the eye. It is more likely to occur in hazy, cloudy weather than in sunny weather. The signs and symptoms of snow blindness include a scratchy feeling in the eyes as if from sand or dirt, watery eyes, and redness of the eyes.

The emergency treatment for snow blindness begins by testing the patient's visual acuity (see Chapter 18, *Preventive Medicine*). Cover the patient's eyes with a dark cloth. Patch both eyes and evacuate the patient for further medical care.

Hypothermia

Hypothermia is a systemic cold injury. Hypothermia is the decrease of body temperature below 95°F and generally occurs from prolonged exposure to low temperatures (often above freezing), especially from immersion in cold water. Hypothermia also occurs in wet, cold conditions or from the effects of wind. Physical exhaustion and insufficient food intake may also increase the risk of hypothermia. Hypothermia is a medical emergency. The elderly and very young are much more susceptible to hypothermia.

The signs and symptoms of hypothermia include:

- Mild hypothermia (core body temperature 90°F to 95°F)
  - Conscious, but usually apathetic or lethargic
  - Shivering
  - Pale, cold skin
  - Slurred speech
  - Poor muscle coordination
  - Faint pulse

- Severe hypothermia (core body temperature 90°F or lower)
  - Slow and shallow breathing
  - Irregular heart action
  - Weak or absent pulse
  - Stupor or unconsciousness
  - Ice cold skin
  - Rigid muscles
  - Glassy eyes

Emergency care for hypothermia includes:

- Mild hypothermia
  - Rewarm the body evenly. (Must provide a heat source, a campfire, or another soldier's body.)
  - Keep the patient dry and protected from the elements.
  - Give warm liquids.
  - Evacuate the patient to the nearest treatment facility immediately.
- Severe hypothermia
  - Gently handle the patient.
  - A cold heart is more prone to V-fib if handled roughly.
  - Avoid further heat loss, move the patient to a warm environment, cut to remove wet clothing, and avoid unnecessary movement.
  - Initiate an IV 250–500 mL bolus warmed to 104°F.
  - Place the patient on a cardiac monitor, if available. If V-fib is present, CPR should be initiated.
  - Evacuate the patient to the nearest medical treatment facility as soon as possible. Provide continuous monitoring of vital signs and level of consciousness while en route.
  - Rewarming should begin passively in a dry sleeping bag. If possible, heated humidified air should be given with any device available. Active rewarming should be confined to the trunk only. Rewarming the extremities before the core can result in acidosis and hyperkalemia (excessive potassium), and actually lower the core temperature.

Dehydration

Dehydration occurs when the body loses too much fluid, salt, and minerals. When soldiers engage in any strenuous exercises or activities, an excessive amount of fluid and salt is lost through sweat. The danger of dehydration is as prevalent in cold regions as it is in hot regions. In cold weather, it is extremely difficult to realize that this condition exists. Thirst is not as prevalent in the cold as it is in warm climates. The signs and symptoms of dehydration include:

- Parched and dry mouth, tongue, and throat
- Difficulty swallowing
- Nausea and dizziness
- Fainting
- Tired and weak
- Muscle cramps, especially in the legs
- Dark urine

Emergency care for dehydration in the cold begins by keeping the patient warm. Loosen the patient's clothes to improve circulation. Give oral and/or IV fluids for fluid and electrolyte replacement (not caffeine). Allow the patient to rest and seek medical assistance.

Frostbite

Frostbite is the freezing injury of tissue caused from exposure to cold, usually below 32°F depending on the wind-chill factor, duration of exposure, and adequacy of protection. The body parts most easily frostbitten are the cheeks, nose, ears, chin, forehead, wrists, hands, and feet FIGURE 30-3 ▾. The signs and symptoms in the following paragraphs are listed in the order in which they would appear with increased exposure and time.

The signs and symptoms of superficial frostbite include loss of sensation or numb feeling in any part of the body; sudden whitening of the skin in the affected area followed by a momentary tingling feeling; and redness of the skin in light-skinned soldiers, grayish coloring in dark-skinned soldiers FIGURE 30-4 ▾.

Deep frostbite is a very serious injury that requires immediate first aid and subsequent medical treatment to avoid or minimize loss of body parts. The signs and symp-

toms of deep frostbite include blisters. Blisters with clear fluid indicate a less severe injury whereas hemorrhagic blisters indicate a deeper, more severe injury. The patient will have swelling or tender areas. There may be a loss of previous feeling of pain in the affected area. The patient's skin may be pale, yellowish, and waxy-looking. The frozen area will feel solid or wooden to the touch.

Do not attempt to thaw the patient's feet or other seriously frozen areas if the patient will be required to walk or travel to receive further treatment. Thawing in the field increases the possibilities of infection, gangrene, or other injuries FIGURE 30-5 ▾. Warm the area at the first sign of frostbite using firm, steady pressure of the hand, underarm, or abdomen (the patient's or a buddy's), depending on the area affected. For the face, ears, or nose, cover the area with the patient's or a buddy's hands until sensation and color return. For the hands, place the patient's hands under his or her armpits inside the clothing against the body, and close the clothing. For the feet, loosen and remove all footgear. Place the patient's bare feet under clothing and against the body of another soldier.

Next, loosen or remove all tight clothing, watches, and jewelry. Cover the patient with a blanket or other dry material. The casualty should be prepared for pain when thawing occurs. Evacuate the patient to an appropriate facility. Pain medication may be required TABLE 30-1 ▸.

Prevention

The predisposing factors for cold injuries include:

- Previous cold injury
- Lack of discipline, training, experience
- Race/geographic origin

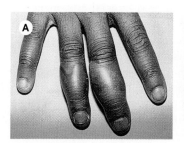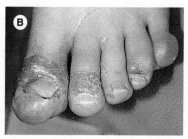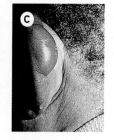

FIGURE 30-3 The extremities (**A** and **B**) and the ears (**C**) are particularly susceptible to frostbite.

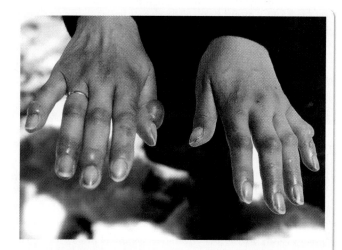

FIGURE 30-4 Frostbitten parts are hard and usually waxy to the touch.

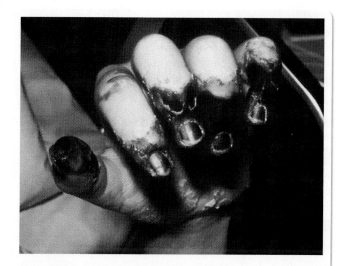

FIGURE 30-5 Gangrene can occur when the tissue is frozen.

TABLE 30-1	What Not to Do With Frostbite
DO NOT	soak the frostbitten part.
DO NOT	rub the affected area with snow.
DO NOT	expose the area to any extreme heat source.
DO NOT	rub or move the part in any way to increase circulation.
DO NOT	allow the casualty to smoke or drink alcohol. (Alcohol and tobacco can reduce blood flow to the extremities and worsen the condition.)
DO NOT	treat seriously frostbitten parts if the casualty must walk or travel to receive further treatment (avoid freeze-thaw-refreeze).

- Poor general health
  - Hypothyroidism
  - Malnutrition, dehydration
  - Hypoglycemia
  - Various medications
  - Fatigue and exhaustion
- Climate factors
  - Low temperature
  - Strong wind (wind chill)
  - Precipitation
  - High humidity
- Activity factors
  - Type of combat
  - Limited mobility
- Extended or intense exposure
- Tobacco usage (vasoconstriction)

To prevent cold injury, follow these precautions. Remember the mnemonic COLD (*Clean*, don't *Overdress*, *Loose* and in *Layers*, *Dry*) when dressing. Promote rest; soldiers should not overwork in order to prevent sweating. Provide more food than usual, because more calories are required in cold weather to continue to generate heat. Limit a soldier's exposure to the cold.

The injury control officer/NCO plans operations around the weather. Provide rewarming tents and warm liquids to soldiers in the field. Be sure to take carbon monoxide precautions—sleeping in tents and vehicles can be hazardous. Use frequent rotations for guards on outdoor posts. And finally, always use the buddy system.

■ Bites and Stings

How Disease Spreads

With all of the high-tech weapons systems, why does the Army concern itself with something as small as a mosquito or a spider? History is full of examples of armies that were demolished by arthropod-borne diseases. In fact, worldwide, 1 million deaths occur annually from malaria—a disease passed on by mosquitoes. An African child dies every 30 seconds from malaria. That means that if your unit deploys to a malaria-prone area, they will be at very high risk unless necessary precautions are taken. It's up to you to make sure the soldiers in your unit are aware of and realize the medical threat. Train your soldiers in the proper precautionary measures to protect themselves in both peacetime and wartime operations.

Overview

American soldiers are frequently deployed to regions of the world in which disease-carrying arthropods and animals flourish. The diseases involved are usually **endemic**—the disease exists at low levels among the natives at all times so the local population has had an opportunity to develop a degree of immunity. The American soldier, however, raised in a relatively sanitized environment, seldom develops this type of immunity and readily becomes ill when exposed to these diseases.

Arthropods are animals, including ticks, spiders, mites, and other insects as well as crustaceans such as shrimp, lobster, and crabs. A vector is a carrier and describes an arthropod that transports a disease-causing organism or pathogen from one host to another. **Venom** is a toxin produced by some animals, such as scorpions, spiders, and snakes. An **envenomation** is the process of injection of venom by the bites or stings of arthropods or snakes.

Passive transmission is also called mechanical transmission. This method of transmission occurs when an arthropod carries a pathogen from one host to another. During this transmission, the pathogen does nothing except go along for the ride. Filth flies carry bacteria or other disease-causing organisms on their mouthparts and feet from infected human feces. If soldiers eat food that has been contaminated by a fly landing on it and depositing these pathogens, then dysentery or other diarrheal disease may occur. Cockroaches provide a similar taxi service by carrying disease organisms on their legs, feet, and mouthparts. These pathogens can cause diarrheal diseases such as cholera.

Active transmission is also called biological transmission. In this method of transmission, the disease-causing agent undergoes some change in the body of the arthropod. The pathogen may multiply or simply develop into an infectious form.

There are four ways a pathogen can be passed to humans via active transmission. **Inoculation** is when a vector injects the pathogen into the host with its saliva while it feeds on the host. Mosquitoes transmit malaria by inoculation. **Regurgitation** is when the vector vomits the pathogen into the host while it feeds on the host. Fleas transmit bubonic plague by regurgitation. The bacteria that causes bubonic plague multiplies rapidly in the flea's gut and blocks it like stopping up a drain. When the flea attempts to eat, it cannot ingest the host's blood due to the blockage. The flea ends up regurgitating the bacteria into the host.

<u>Fecal contamination</u> is when the vector defecates into a wound on the host. As the wound itches, scratching and rubbing by the host causes the pathogen to enter the host's body. Chagas disease, also known as North American sleeping sickness, is transmitted in this way by the kissing bug. The kissing bug bites the host, causing a wound, then takes a few steps forward and defecates into the wound. <u>Crushing the vector</u> is when the vector is smashed onto the skin of the host. When the host wipes off the dead bug, the pathogen is rubbed into the skin. The body louse transmits epidemic typhus in this manner.

Mosquitoes

Mosquitoes are the most important arthropod to the military for a number of reasons FIGURE 30-6 ▾ . Mosquitoes are found

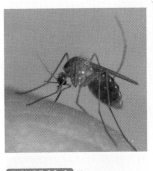

everywhere and in high numbers. They are capable of transmitting a large number of diseases, some of which have been war stoppers. During World War II, Korea, and Vietnam, entire units were rendered combat ineffective by malaria. Malaria was the most important health hazard encountered by American troops in the South Pacific during World War II, where about 100,000 men were infected and the success of the military campaign was jeopardized for a short time. In Southeast Asia, those US troops who did not practice effective preventive measures contracted malaria.

FIGURE 30-6 Know your enemy.

Mosquito larvae inhabit areas with standing water such as ponds, puddles, and ditches. Anything that can hold water provides a habitat for mosquito larvae. Adult mosquitoes continue to inhabit their larval habitats without venturing too far away.

Malaria

Malaria is a mosquito-borne disease of military importance. It is an ancient disease and is one of the most important preventable diseases in humans. Humans get malaria from the bite of a malaria-infected female mosquito. When the mosquito bites an infected person, it ingests microscopic malaria parasites found in the person's blood. When the mosquito then bites another person, the parasites go from the mosquito's mouth into the new person's blood. Malaria is a tremendous problem in tropical, developing countries where it causes 300 to 500 million cases each year.

The time between the infective bite and the appearance of symptoms is approximately 7 to 30 days, depending on the type of mosquito. Malaria must always be considered in a soldier deployed in a malaria-risk country with an unexplained febrile illness. Symptoms and signs of malaria include: fever alternating with chills, headache, muscle aches, sweats, and abdominal pain with diarrhea. A complication of malaria, called blackwater fever, is an acute and potentially fatal hemorrhagic state, which includes kidney failure. Mortality is from 20% to 30%. Soldiers with an acute febrile illness must be evaluated by a medical officer.

Measures for the prevention and control of malaria fall into two categories: preventing bites by mosquitoes and preventing development of the disease. The most effective means of malaria control is avoiding mosquito bites. Such prevention includes personal protective measures and the control of the mosquito and its environment. Prevention of disease development includes chemoprophylaxis and effective early treatment of cases. Malaria prophylaxis provides no protection against other mosquito-borne diseases. Due to multidrug resistance, malaria chemoprophylaxis should not be thought of as being 100% effective.

The most effective means of malaria prevention is avoiding mosquito bites. This can be done by using Insect Bar (bednets). Mosquitoes are night-biters and can bite more easily when a soldier is asleep. After the bednet is applied, the soldier then uses an aerosol on the inside of the net to kill any mosquitoes that may be under the net with him or her. Soldiers should wear long-sleeved, loose-fitting clothing because mosquitoes can only bite through clothing when it is worn tightly against the skin. Use chemical repellents. DEET should be applied to all exposed skin surfaces and reapplied every 4 to 6 hours. Permethrin is used to impregnate fabrics (battle dress uniform, bednets, tent screens, sleeping bags). Permethrin should not be applied to inner clothing, however. Soldiers should not wear flea collars to repel insects—flea collars are not labeled for human use. Contact with the skin may cause severe chemical burns and absorption of toxic levels of insecticide through the skin.

Dengue Fever

The *Aedes* mosquito transmits the viral disease dengue fever. The disease is endemic in most areas in the tropics. The military significance of dengue fever is its explosive nature,

> **Garrison Care TIPS**
>
> About 1,200 cases of malaria are diagnosed in the United States each year. Most of these cases are in immigrants and travelers returning from malaria-risk areas. Each year in the United States, a few cases of malaria result from blood transfusions, mother to fetus transmission during pregnancy, or from locally infected mosquitoes.

> **Garrison Care TIPS**
>
> Prevention also includes education on eliminating or destroying mosquito larval habitats. Remove all water-holding containers within human habitations.

resulting in a high percentage of casu-alties in a short time, and a prolonged convalescent period. There is no spe-cific therapy for dengue fever. Treatment is supportive. Vaccines are currently under development. The same preven-tion techniques used in malaria should be utilized for all mosquito-borne diseases.

Yellow Fever

The *Aedes* mosquito also transmits the viral disease yellow fever, which is uncommon in the United States but occurs in jungle environments in Africa and Central/South America. Treatment is supportive. Soldiers are immunized with yellow fever vaccine prior to deployment in endemic areas. Booster doses are recommended every 10 years. The same mosquito control measures used in malaria should be utilized for all mosquito-borne diseases.

Encephalitis

The mosquito-borne viral encephalitides are acute inflam-matory diseases that involve the central nervous system. The *Aedes* and *Culex* mosquitoes carry several forms of this viral disease. West Nile virus (WNV) is a strain of encephalitis. Other types of encephalitis include St. Louis encephalitis, Japanese B encephalitis, and California encephalitis. The WNV was first identified in 1937 in Africa. Epidemics have occurred in the Middle East and Europe.

WNV is spread when mosquitoes bite birds and infect them with the virus. The bird becomes ill and then the virus is spread to new mosquitoes when they bite the bird. Some-times the virus spreads to other species, such as horses.

WNV was first identified in the United States in 1999. It is not known how the WNV arrived in New York. Most people who are infected with WNV have no symptoms. It is estimated that 20% of the people infected will develop West Nile fever. Mild symptoms include fever, headache, and body aches. About 1 in 150 people infected will develop a more severe disease. The symptoms of severe infection include high fever, neck stiffness, coma, seizures, and paralysis. Death can occur in the elderly population. Treatment is supportive. A vaccine is currently being developed.

Filth Flies and Cockroaches

The habits of flies and cockroaches make them easy vectors for disease **FIGURE 30-7 ▸**. Cholera, dysentery, typhoid, and food-borne gastroenteritis outbreaks are associated with filth flies and cockroaches. These creatures pick up organisms from sewage, garbage, manure, and decaying animal bodies. The organisms are then passed on to humans and animals through the feces and vomit of the fly and the taxi ride of the cockroach.

Filth flies and cockroaches live in or near animal or human waste, garbage, decomposing plants and animals, or in mud with high organic content. A large population of flies

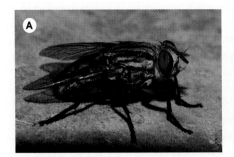
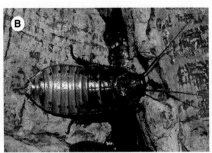

FIGURE 30-7 The habits of flies and cockroaches make them easy vectors for disease. **A.** Fly. **B.** Cockroach.

and/or cockroaches is usually a good indicator of unsanitary conditions.

Prevention and personal protective measures include locating and removing the food sources of the filth fly and cockroach. This is the key to eliminating them from any environment. Field latrines and soakage pits should be con-structed, used, maintained, and closed so as not to foster fly breeding. Sprays, fogs, and sticky traps are useful tools but are successful only when used with pest elimination measures.

Sandflies

Sandflies are small, blood-sucking gnats that look like small mosquitoes **FIGURE 30-8 ▸**. Sandflies attack the wrists, ankles, or any exposed part of the body. The diseases of mili-tary importance are sandfly fever and leishmaniasis. Sandfly fever is an acute, self-limiting viral disease transmitted through the bite of the sandfly. It occurs in tropical and subtropical areas of Europe, Africa, South America, and Asia.

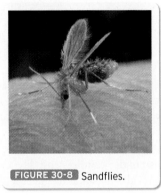

FIGURE 30-8 Sandflies.

Epidemics are seen in non-native persons such as US troops entering endemic areas. Sandfly fever may recur. The proper wearing of the uniform and application of repellents will prevent most infections. Dogs and other domesticated animals should be avoided.

Leishmaniasis, which is transmitted by the bite of an infected sandfly, is found in most third-world countries. There is no vaccine for leishmaniasis. Control measures are based on protection from and destruction of sandflies and the avoidance of domesticated animals.

Fleas

Adult fleas are not only persistent and painful biters, but also are efficient vectors of plague, typhus, and tularemia **FIGURE 30-9 ▸**. Plague and typhus have been identified as potential biowarfare agents. Fleas become infected feeding on rodents (chipmunks, rats, squirrels) and other mammals infected with the disease. Fleas then transmit the bacteria to

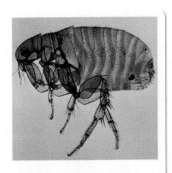

FIGURE 30-9 Fleas are efficient vectors of plague, typhus, and tularemia.

humans when they feed (bite). Large populations of fleas can usually be found around animal beds, burrows, and nests. Outdoors, fleas are abundant during rainy summers and in high humidity areas.

People usually get plague from being bitten by a flea that is carrying the plague bacterium or by handling an infected animal. Millions of people in Europe died of plague in the Middle Ages, when flea-infested rats inhabited human homes and places of work. Wild rodents in certain areas around the world are infected with plague. Outbreaks still occur in developing rural communities. They are usually associated with infected rats and rat fleas that live in the home. The World Health Organization (WHO) reports 1,000 to 3,000 cases of plague occur each year. Modern antibiotics are effective against plague. There is a plague vaccine, but it is currently not in use.

Locating and removing the rodents in the area is the key to eliminating the diseases they carry. Sprays, fogs, powders, and traps are useful tools but are successful only when used with pest elimination measures.

Ticks

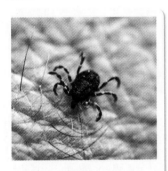

FIGURE 30-10 Ticks are the most efficient arthropod when it comes to disease transmission.

Ticks are the most efficient arthropod when it comes to disease transmission **FIGURE 30-10**. This is because the female tick can pass the pathogen to her eggs so that when the larvae hatch they are already able to pass on the disease upon eating their first meal. Ticks and mites are generally found in areas of tall grass or underbrush in close proximity to mammal resting places and watering holes. Ticks are important disease vectors in many regions of the United States, Europe, Asia, and Australia.

Diseases of military importance caused by ticks include Lyme disease, which was named in 1977 when arthritis was noticed in a cluster of children in and around Lyme, Connecticut. These bacteria are transmitted to humans by the bite of infected deer ticks and cause more than 16,000 infections in the United States each year. Lyme disease is the most common vector-borne infectious disease in the United States.

The signs and symptoms of Lyme disease include the development of a red, slowly expanding "bulls-eye" rash with tiredness, fever, headache, stiff neck, muscle, and joint aches.

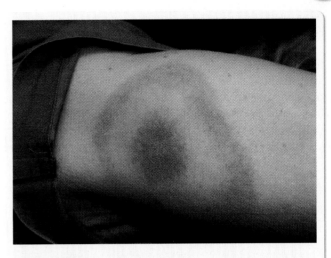

FIGURE 30-11 This distinctive skin lesion is called erythema migrans. This is a sign of Lyme disease.

These symptoms can occur in combinations over a period of months to years. If untreated with antibiotics, the patient may develop arthritis, or neurologic or cardiac problems. The illness typically presents in summer, and the first symptom in about 90% of patients appears as a red macule or papule that expands slowly in a circular manner, sometimes with a central clearing (bulls-eye). This distinctive skin lesion is called erythema migrans (EM) **FIGURE 30-11**. EM may be single or multiple.

The proper wearing of the uniform and application of repellents will prevent most infections. Search the total body area daily and remove ticks promptly. Remove any attached ticks by using gentle, steady traction with forceps or tweezers applied close to the skin to avoid leaving mouthparts in the skin. Use gloves when removing ticks. Following removal, cleanse the skin site with soap and water. A Lyme disease vaccine is currently not available.

Maintain a high index of suspicion for Lyme disease when deployed in areas that are endemic for Lyme disease. Many diseases are transmitted to humans by tick vectors. The incidence of tick-borne diseases, especially Lyme disease, has been increasing as a result of reforestation and military deployments. Ticks can also transmit infections with viruses, bacteria, rickettsia, and parasites. Other tick-borne diseases include Rocky Mountain spotted fever, tularemia, and tick paralysis.

Mites

Mites are tiny arthropods, barely visible to the naked eye **FIGURE 30-12**. Scabies is a highly contagious infestation of humans caused by the itch mite. Scabies may

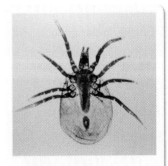

FIGURE 30-12 Mites are tiny arthropods, barely visible to the naked eye.

occur in all populations. Scabies are common in developing countries.

Mites are usually found in skin folds, such as finger and toe webs, axilla, or genital areas. Treatment includes ointment application and clothes laundering. Prevention rests in the practice of personnel cleanliness, with emphasis on frequent handwashing, bathing, and avoidance of potentially infested persons.

Chiggers

Chiggers are also known as redbugs, jiggers, or harvest mites. They are the immature stages of a tiny red mite and are found in most areas of the world. They inhabit areas of tall grass associated with low wet spots such as ponds and forest underbrush. They attach themselves to the clothing of people. Chiggers then move to an area of the body to feed.

Symptoms of chigger infestation include itching and small welts appearing over the bite area. Bites may continue to itch up to 2 to 3 weeks after the chigger has dislodged. The proper wearing of the uniform and application of repellents will prevent most infestations from occurring.

Lice

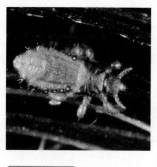

FIGURE 30-13 Lice.

Louse-borne diseases have always been a threat to fighting forces **FIGURE 30-13 ◄** . Three species are of military importance: the body louse, the head louse, and the crab louse. Anyone may become louse infested under suitable conditions of exposure. Lice are easily transmitted from person to person under direct contact. Head lice infestations are frequently found in schools and other institutions. Crab lice are spread through sexual contact. Body lice infestation can be found in people living in crowded, unsanitary conditions where clothing is infrequently changed or laundered. Soldiers who do not practice good personal hygiene can become infested with lice and pass them on to other soldiers when they come in contact with their hair, clothing, sleeping bags, or other linens.

If troops are deployed in areas where the civilian population is lousy, chances are high that the troops will become infested. Good personal hygiene, regular changing of clothes, and effective laundry procedures will control lice. Do not share clothing or bedding with other people.

Scorpions

Scorpions are part of the arachnid family, which includes mites, ticks, and spiders. Scorpions are about 3″ long and have eight legs and a small pair of claws **FIGURE 30-14 ►** . A scorpion's stinger is

at the end of its long tail. There are about 650 species of scorpions in the world and about 40 species in the southwestern United States. In the United States, only one type of scorpion can kill people. Most scorpions are relatively harmless, producing only localized sting reactions. The initial sting is very painful with little or no swelling or redness.

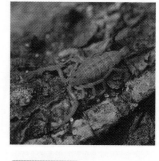

FIGURE 30-14 The bark scorpion.

Treatment includes evaluation by a medical officer to determine the risk of a potentially severe reaction to the sting. Ice application may relieve localized pain.

Spiders

The brown recluse spider has a dark, violin-shaped area on its back **FIGURE 30-15 ►** . It is found in woodpiles and other dark places. The venom causes local tissue destruction. The bite initially seems mild or goes unnoticed **FIGURE 30-16 ▼** . Pain at the site begins 1 to 4 hours later and a red area appears along with a central pustule or vesicle. The pustule may grow and form a crater over 3 to 4 days. Healing is slow.

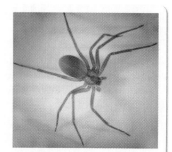

FIGURE 30-15 Brown recluse spiders are dull brown and have a dark, violin-shaped mark on the back.

The patient may have a low-grade fever, myalgias, nausea, and vomiting. Treatment is usually supportive. Ice and elevation may help with localized pain. Tetanus should be updated. Antibiotics are given when a secondary infection exists. Occasionally, surgical excision of the ulcerated area is needed. Treatment also includes evaluation by a medical officer.

The female black widow spider is shiny black, with a red hourglass marking on her abdomen **FIGURE 30-17 ►** . The black widow's bite is usually minor and often goes unnoticed at first. Symptoms of envenomation occur within 10 to

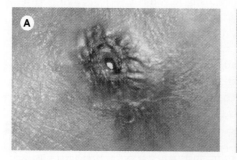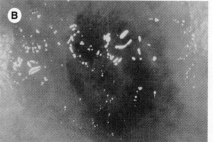

FIGURE 30-16 Brown recluse spider bite in early stage (**A**) and late stage (**B**).

60 minutes, including severe pain in the bitten extremity and muscle spasms of the abdomen and trunk. Headache, nausea, and vomiting may occur. Death is rare; at greatest risk are the very young and the very old. Symptoms may last 24 to 36 hours. Treatment includes evaluation by a medical officer and analgesics. All patients who have been bitten by a black widow spider should be evacuated to a treatment facility that can observe the patient for 12 to 24 hours. Antivenin is given in rare cases and is ordered by a medical officer.

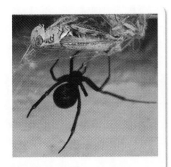

FIGURE 30-17 The female black widow spider is shiny black, with a red hourglass marking on her abdomen.

Snakes

Snake bites require special care, but are usually not life threatening. In the United States, there are two types of poisonous snakes—the pit vipers (including rattlesnakes, copperheads, and water moccasins) and coral snakes **FIGURE 30-18 ▼**. Every person reacts differently to a snake bite, so consider all snake bites to be from a poisonous snake. Symptoms are variable depending on the type of snake involved. Signs and symptoms may include a noticeable bite or scratch on the skin. There may be only one fang mark. Pain and swelling may

TABLE 30-2	**What Not to Do After a Snake Bite**
DO NOT	delay treatment by attempting to capture the snake.
DO NOT	suction or cut into the bite site.
DO NOT	place ice on the bite.
DO NOT	touch the head of the snake because dead snakes can still bite.
DO NOT	transfer a live snake with the patient.

occur in the bite area. The patient may experience rapid pulse, labored breathing, nausea, and vomiting. The patient may experience progressive weakness to unconsciousness or anaphylaxis and anaphylactic shock.

Field treatment of snakebites includes initial ABCs, looking for an allergic reaction or anaphylaxis. Apply oxygen, if available. Start an IV in all snakebite victims in the unaffected extremity. Remove watches and jewelry from the affected extremity.

Keep the patient as calm and inactive as possible; this will slow down the absorption of the venom. Place and tie a constricting band (cravat, Penrose drain, rope, or piece of clothing) 4″ to 6″ above the bite. The band should restrict superficial venous and lymphatic flow, but not arterial. The constricting band should be snug, but loose enough to easily slide a finger underneath. Always check pulses after applying the band; remember, this is not a tourniquet. This technique is the same technique as applying a restricting band to start an IV. Gently clean around the snakebite to remove any venom from the skin. Immobilize and splint the affected limb. Evacuate the patient to the nearest treatment facility. Tetanus prophylaxis must be assessed **TABLE 30-2 ▲**. If possible, the dead snake should be brought to the treatment facility with the patient for identification.

■ Altitude Illness

Altitude illnesses are caused by the effects of hypobaric (low atmospheric pressure) hypoxia on the central nervous system (CNS) and pulmonary system as a result of unacclimatized people ascending to a high altitude. They run the gamut from the common **acute mountain sickness (AMS)** to the rare deaths from **high-altitude cerebral edema (HACE)** and

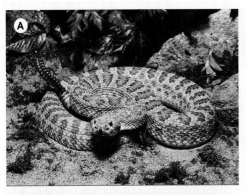
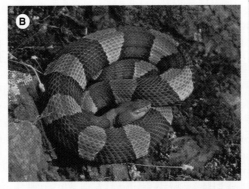
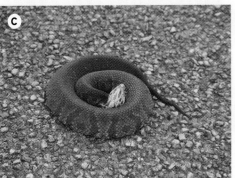
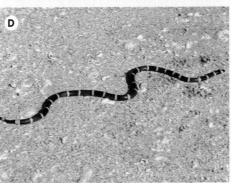

FIGURE 30-18 **A.** Rattlesnake. **B.** Copperhead. **C.** Cottonmouth. **D.** Coral snake.

high-altitude pulmonary edema (HAPE). Altitude illness typically occurs in people who rapidly ascend to heights above 8,000', but can occur at altitudes as low as 6,500'. Symptoms usually occur within 6 to 10 hours. Studies have shown that, among skiers who go from sea level to higher western US resorts but sleep at lower altitudes than climbers, there is a 25% chance of developing AMS. AMS is even more common among climbers of Mt. Rainier (who summit and descend in as quickly as 1 to 2 days), averaging 67% of all climbers.

Altitude illness is a problem of hypoxia caused by low atmospheric pressures. The partial pressure of oxygen in the atmosphere decreases with increasing altitude but remains a constant 21% of the earth's barometric pressure. For example, the partial pressure of alveolar oxygen (Pao_2) is 103 mm Hg at sea level but only 81 mm Hg in Denver (5,280'). Barometric pressure varies according to how far north you are located and is typically lower in the winter. Interestingly, local changes in barometric pressures can alter the "relative altitude" by 500' to 2,500'.

Risk Factors for Altitude Illness

Several factors predispose a person to altitude illnesses. The most important risk factor is a history of AMS, in which case slow ascents and use of prophylactic medicines are recommended. Normal residence below 3,000', physical exertion, presence of chronic obstructive pulmonary disease, and sleeping above 8,000' also increase the risk of developing altitude illness. Physical fitness is not a factor. Indeed, older people may be less likely to develop such an illness. Another individual factor is the hypoxic ventilatory drive. The brain stem normally responds to rising carbon dioxide levels. If you suddenly find yourself at a high altitude, the brain stem senses the lowered oxygen levels and responds by increasing ventilations.

The Clinical Picture of Altitude Illness

The following definitions have been established for altitude illness:

- **Acute mountain sickness (AMS):** Headache plus at least one of the following: fatigue or weakness, gastrointestinal symptoms (nausea, vomiting, or anorexia), dizziness or lightheadedness, or difficulty sleeping. The headache is often described as throbbing that is worse over the temporal or occipital areas and is exacerbated by the Valsalva maneuver.
- **High-altitude pulmonary edema (HAPE):** At least two of the following symptoms: dyspnea at rest, cough, weakness or decreased exercise performance, or chest tightness or congestion. Also, at least two of the following signs: central cyanosis, audible rales or wheezing in at least one lung field, tachypnea, or tachycardia.
- **High-altitude cerebral edema (HACE):** HACE requires the presence of a change in mental status and/or ataxia in a person with AMS or the presence of mental status changes and ataxia in a person without AMS.

Other conditions can mimic AMS, and the emergence of symptoms 3 or more days after being at higher elevations, a lack of a headache, or the failure of descent to improve signs or symptoms points to other causes.

Acute Mountain Sickness

Acute mountain sickness (AMS) is the most commonly experienced form of high-altitude illness. It is also the initial medical condition in the spectrum of altitude illness that can culminate with the development of high-altitude cerebral edema (HACE). AMS occurs shortly after arrival at an altitude typically over 7,500' and usually occurs 6 to 10 hours after ascent, with a peak at 24–72 hours.

The predominant symptom of AMS is headache, typically throbbing and global. It is often worse upon waking from sleep. AMS symptoms are usually nonspecific and if they occur after 72 hours or persist despite treatment, other diagnoses must be considered.

Although the development of AMS does not mandate descent, the patient should not progress higher. The patient should make an acclimatization stop and remain at the present elevation until the symptoms abate. However, descent of 500 to 1,000 meters usually relieves symptoms.

If descent is not possible or moderate to severe symptoms are present, medical care may be necessary. The majority of AMS can be treated symptomatically. Aspirin, ibuprofen, and acetaminophen have all been utilized effectively to treat headaches. Antiemetics are indicated for nausea and vomiting. Acetazolamide has the advantage of not only reducing symptoms but also facilitating acclimatization. Give acetazolamide (Diamox) 125 mg to 250 mg orally twice daily. In sulfa-allergic individuals who cannot take acetazolamide, dexamethasone may be used in a dose of 2 to 4 mg every 6 hours. Because dexamethasone does not facilitate acclimatization and has potential side effects, it should be reserved for moderate to severe symptoms. Although low-dose oxygen by nasal cannula and short duration treatment in a portable hyperbaric chamber can also rapidly improve symptoms, this equipment is not routinely available during standard tactical operations. Finally, symptoms may recur when therapy is stopped.

High-Altitude Cerebral Edema (HACE)

This neurologic syndrome represents the end stage of AMS and is potentially fatal. The diagnosis of HACE is clinical. HACE can run a rapid course with death from brain herniation occurring as early as 12 hours after onset. The typical onset for HACE is approximately 5 days after arrival at a new elevation.

HACE presents with typical symptoms and signs seen in patients with cerebral edema. Any person with AMS and ataxia and/or altered mental status should be considered to have HACE. Ataxia may begin as a swaying of the upper body, particularly when walking, which progresses to include an ataxic gait. The individual may appear to be intoxicated. Behavior and mental status changes may include extreme fatigue, confusion, disorientation, drowsiness, impaired thinking, reduced level of consciousness, and coma.

Symptoms and signs of cerebral edema include central cyanosis, audible rales or wheezing in at least one lung, tachypnea, and tachycardia. High-altitude pulmonary edema (HAPE) often coexists with HACE. Hypoxia and cyanosis may also be observed. Any rapid onset of neurologic symptoms, associated trauma or fever, or continued neurologic symptoms despite therapy or ascent arrest should raise concern for the possibility of another diagnosis. Carbon monoxide poisoning, cerebral vascular accident, metabolic disorder, toxic ingestion, migraine headache, and seizure disorder are some of the diseases that may mimic HACE.

Immediate descent is mandatory. Definitive treatment of HACE is immediate descent, and the greater the amount of descent the better the outcome for the individual. Descent of more than 1,000′ is recommended, and descents to altitudes of less than 8,000′ are optimal. Also, evaluation by an advanced provider is strongly recommended even if symptoms resolve.

Administer dexamethasone and oxygen. Dexamethasone should be administered as an initial 8 mg dose by any available route (eg, oral, rectal, intravenously, or intramuscularly) followed by 4 mg every 6 hours. Careful attention to blood pressure and cerebral perfusion pressure should be maintained, especially if the patient requires intubation and/or concomitant treatment for HAPE. Individuals who develop HACE should not re-ascend for at least several days after complete resolution of symptoms, and at a minimum ascend at a much slower rate than done so previously.

Although no definitive evidence for any type of HACE prophylaxis exists, preventative guidelines for AMS, as described in the previous section, should be followed. Early recognition of symptoms is critical. Prophylactic measures for HACE should be considered for individuals with a previous history. Prophylaxis includes use of staged or graded ascent, and use of oral acetazolamide.

High-Altitude Pulmonary Edema (HAPE)

HAPE is the most lethal high-altitude illness. Although HAPE has a high mortality if untreated, with appropriate descent and therapy it can be easily reversed. HAPE typically occurs 2 to 3 days and rarely 4 days after arrival at a new altitude. Occurrence is higher at night. HAPE is most typically seen at elevations over 8,000′ (2,440 m).

Initial symptoms of HAPE are a dry cough, chest tightness, decreased exercise tolerance, and dyspnea at rest. Consider anyone with dyspnea at rest and a cough to have the onset of HAPE and initiate treatment. You may note tachypnea, tachycardia, crackles, and a relative cyanosis or decreased oxygen saturation compared to other healthy team members. As HAPE progresses, dyspnea at rest worsens. The cough increases and may become frothy or blood tinged. Rales and wheezing may progress to being diffuse and audible without the use of a stethoscope. The patient becomes progressively more hypoxic and cyanotic. Mental status worsens with increasing hypoxemia, and ranges from initial anxiety to a reduced level of consciousness, and even coma.

The mainstay for treatment of HAPE is descent. This should be initiated once HAPE is suspected and before the patient becomes incapacitated and unable to assist in his or her descent. Descent of 1,000′ is recommended and can be lifesaving. Oxygen should always be administered if available. Nifedipine is a pulmonary vasodilator, which will reduce pulmonary arterial pressure. For HAPE treatment, nifedipine may be administered as 10 mg sublingually repeated in 10–15 minutes if required or as 20 mg orally followed by 30 mg orally three times daily. Salmeterol acts as a bronchodilator to open closed airways. Positive end-expiratory pressure may also be utilized to improve gas exchange. Because HAPE does not involve fluid overload, treatment with morphine is of minimal benefit and in some cases may be harmful. Finally, if for some reason descent is impossible, treatment in a portable hyperbaric chamber is recommended.

After descent to a level sufficient for resolution of symptoms, an individual should precede no higher until he or she remains asymptomatic for 72 hours. At that time, ascent can be attempted at a slower rate than what previously induced HAPE. In individuals who must ascend sooner or who must ascend at a rate that may likely induce HAPE, 10 mg of nifedipine orally three times daily may be utilized as a prophylactic agent. Salmeterol may also be given. Both medications should be administered 24 hours prior to ascent and continued for 72 hours after ascent to a higher elevation.

General Altitude Illness Prevention

Obviously, it is ideal to anticipate and prevent altitude illness rather than to treat it. Remember, a prior history of altitude illness is the strongest predictor. The primary method of preventing an altitude illness is through adequate acclimatization. Further ascent should halt immediately if signs or symptoms of illness develop. Those who must ascend faster than this rate or who become ill even when ascending at this rate should consider taking medications. The commonly used mantra for acclimatization is "climb high, sleep low," meaning hike or carry loads to a higher elevation but return to a lower point for a day before advancing to the level of the sleeping location. Unfortunately, the unpredictability of combat operations makes initiating routine medication therapy or climb-rest cycles impractical; therefore, you must be prepared to treat symptoms as they occur. You must also be prepared to advise the tactical commander on potential detrimental effects to the overall effective combat power of the unit.

The preferred method for altitude illness prevention always begins with staged ascent. However, despite careful planning and use of staged ascent, some individuals will still develop altitude illness easily and could benefit from medications.

The most well-known, studied, and utilized agent is acetazolamide. Acetazolamide reduces the production of cerebral spinal fluid (CSF), which may inhibit the development of cerebral edema. There are several downsides to acetazolamide. It is a sulfa-derived drug and thus cannot be used in those with sulfa allergies. Side effects of acetazolamide include drowsiness, anorexia, polyuria (excessive urination), and photosensitivity. Acetazolamide has been shown to decrease exercise ability by up to 30%. The prophylactic dose of acetazolamide is 125 to

250 mg orally twice daily. Acetazolamide is started 24 hours before ascent and continued for 24 to 72 hours after arrival at the new altitude, varying dose and length based on symptoms.

Dexamethasone is the second most commonly prescribed drug for use in AMS prevention. For rapid ascents, dexamethasone has been shown to be more effective than acetazolamide. It is unclear how dexamethasone works to prevent AMS, but it may be due to its suppression of cerebral edema as well as its potent anti-inflammatory effects. Dexamethasone does not aid the body in acclimatization to altitude like acetazolamide; it can only assist in prevention and treatment. The side effects of dexamethasone are hyperglycemia and depression. The typical dose used for prophylaxis is 4 mg orally two to four times a day, 12 to 24 hours prior to ascent and typically only utilized for 24 to 72 hours depending on side effects and altitude symptoms.

High-Altitude Pharyngitis and Bronchitis

These are common conditions that occur frequently in persons spending a prolonged time at altitude. They typically occur after 2–3 weeks at altitude and are due to prolonged environmental exposure to cold, dry air; dehydration; or rapid ventilation rather than to any actual effect of altitude. Symptoms consist of sore throat and chronic, predominantly dry cough. There is not typically an infectious component. These conditions are differentiated from HAPE by the historical feature of occurring after a prolonged time at altitude as well as by the lack of dyspnea at rest, which is present in HAPE.

Treatment is symptomatic with lozenges, decongestant nasal sprays, and if coughing spasms are severe, a cough suppressant. Albuterol may be helpful in selected cases. Breathing through a porous mask or balaclava (ski mask) can also be helpful.

Sleep Disorders

Insomnia and sleep disorders are common at altitude. Cheyne-Stokes respirations are seen in almost all individuals. The associated apneic periods both cause broken sleep and potentiate the development of AMS and pulmonary edema.

Sleeping agents should be utilized with extreme caution if used at all. Acetazolamide has been shown to improve sleep and decrease the length of apneic episodes during periodic breathing. If medication is required for sleep, zolpidem is the agent of choice, because it does not suppress respiration.

High-Altitude Peripheral Edema

This is altitude-related edema of the hands and face. It is not specifically related to the AMS-to-HACE spectrum of illnesses but can be seen with all forms of AMS. It tends to be recurrent on repeat altitude exposure and is more common in females. Although treatment is not typically required, diuretics may be used.

Altitude Descent Basics

All forms of altitude illness improve markedly with descent if it occurs expeditiously. Descent is the gold standard for treatment of all forms of altitude illness. If a patient is showing signs or experiencing symptoms of severe AMS, HAPE, or HACE it is best to have the person descend 500 to 1,000 meters even if the diagnosis is merely suspected. Minimal delays in descent often allow symptoms to rapidly develop, which may inhibit the patient from aiding in his or her own descent and rescue evacuation. In situations where descent is impossible due to weather or other constraints, the use of portable fabric hyperbaric chambers such as the Gamow, Chamber lite, or Certec SA bag can delay or often improve altitude symptoms of a patient until descent is possible. These devices create a hyperbaric environment around the patient and effectively give the effect of the patient having descended several hundred to several thousand feet. The higher in elevation one is when the bag is used, the higher the relative descent obtained by the use of the bag.

■ Summary

Always be prepared for extreme weather conditions. Once a heat or cold injury has occurred, a person is more susceptible to recurrence. Prevention is critical and may save someone's life. Don't let the weather become your worst enemy.

As you have learned, arthropods, spiders, scorpions, and snakes can affect a soldier's health in many ways. Many people have the tendency to overlook the impact these animals can have on military operations, even though history is full of examples of their devastating impact. An important part of your job is to inform your unit about the impact that these animals can have on military operations and the ways in which unnecessary exposure to them can be avoided.

High-altitude illness is a disease process that spans a spectrum from the discomfort of AMS to the life-threatening conditions of HAPE and HACE. In all cases, altitude illness results from ascending to an altitude too quickly for the human body to acclimatize. All forms of high-altitude illness improve with expeditious descent, but this is only mandatory for HAPE and HACE. In no case should a sick individual move his or her sleeping altitude higher until symptoms have resolved. It is important to be familiar with the pathophysiology, recognition, and treatment of altitude-related medical conditions. Furthermore, proper preventative measures and correct equipment will help minimize morbidity from altitude-related illnesses.

YOU ARE THE
COMBAT MEDIC

You and your unit are on a mission in a mountainous region. Having grown up in the mountains, your battle buddy seems to be a bit overconfident in the cold environment. "You call this a blizzard? Back home, we call these flurries."

Despite the frigid wind and temperatures, he keeps taking off his gloves for extended periods of time because his fingers, "just work better bare."

You just shake your head and keep your gloves on. You also keep on extra eye on his hands.

While tying another knot, your battle buddy pauses and starts to shake out his hand. "Man, my fingers hurt."

You immediately ask to see his fingers and find that the skin is yellowish. When you touch his fingers, they feel as if they were made of wood. "We have to get you warmed up," you say as you lead your battle buddy into a tent.

Now that you and your battle buddy are protected from the elements, you have him remove his BDU and place his fingers underneath his armpits. You zip up his coat as far as you can, then you wrap him up in a blanket to trap his remaining body heat. He says that his fingers still feel tender, so you give him a pain medication before you call for the MEDEVAC.

1. LAST NAME, FIRST NAME	RANK/GRADE	X	MALE
Lemming, Steven	PFC		FEMALE

SSN	SPECIALTY CODE	RELIGION
000-111-0000	00A	Methodist

2. UNIT

FORCE				NATIONALITY
A/T	AF/A	N/M	MC/M	

BC/BC		NBI/BNC		DISEASE		PSYCH

3. INJURY

	AIRWAY
	HEAD
FRONT BACK	WOUND
	NECK/BACK INJURY
	BURN
	AMPUTATION
	STRESS
	X OTHER (*Specify*)

Frostbite on

fingers

4. LEVEL OF CONSCIOUSNESS

X	ALERT		PAIN RESPONSE
	VERBAL RESPONSE		UNRESPONSIVE

5. PULSE	TIME	6. TOURNIQUET		TIME
60 bpm	1430	X NO ☐ YES		

7. MORPHINE	DOSE	TIME	8. IV	TIME
X NO ☐ YES				

9. TREATMENT/OBSERVATIONS/CURRENT MEDICATION/ALLERGIES/NBC (ANTIDOTE)

Deep frostbite on the fingers. Skin yellow and hard to touch. Warmed skin in the field.

10. DISPOSITION	RETURNED TO DUTY		TIME
	X EVACUATED		1500
	DECEASED		

11. PROVIDER/UNIT	DATE (YYMMDD)
Deforge, Mike	

Aid Kit

Ready for Review

- As a combat medic, one of your key duties is prevention.
- An environmental emergency is a medical condition caused or exacerbated by the weather, terrain, atmospheric pressure, or other local factors.
- The major heat injuries are heat cramps, heat exhaustion, and heat stroke.
- The major cold injuries are chilblains, immersion syndrome, hypothermia, dehydration, and frostbite.
- American soldiers are frequently deployed to regions of the world in which disease-carrying arthropods and animals flourish. The diseases involved are usually endemic.
- Altitude illnesses are caused by the effects of hypobaric (low atmospheric pressure) hypoxia on the CNS and pulmonary system as a result of unacclimatized people ascending to altitude.
  - It runs the gamut from the common acute mountain sickness (AMS) to the rare deaths from high-altitude cerebral edema (HACE) and high-altitude pulmonary edema (HAPE).

Vital Vocabulary

active transmission A disease-causing agent undergoes some change in the body of an arthropod before being transmitted.

acute mountain sickness (AMS) An altitude illness characterized by headache plus at least one of the following: fatigue or weakness, gastrointestinal symptoms (nausea, vomiting, or anorexia), dizziness or lightheadedness, or difficulty sleeping.

altitude illnesses Conditions caused by the effects from hypobaric (low atmospheric pressure) hypoxia on the CNS and pulmonary systems as a result of unacclimatized people ascending to altitude; they range from acute mountain sickness (AMS) to high-altitude cerebral edema (HACE) and high-altitude pulmonary edema (HAPE).

conduction Transfer of heat to a solid object or a liquid by direct contact.

convection Mechanism by which body heat is picked up and carried away by moving air currents.

crushing the vector When the vector is smashed into the skin of the host and the host wipes off the dead bug, the pathogen is rubbed into the skin.

deep frostbite A type of frostbite in which the affected part looks white, yellow-white, or mottled blue-white and is hard, cold, and without sensation.

dehydration Condition where the body loses too much fluid, salt, and minerals.

endemic When a disease exists at low levels among the local population who have a degree of immunity.

envenomation The poisonous effects of the bites or stings of arthropods or snakes.

environmental emergencies Medical conditions caused or exacerbated by the weather, terrain, or unique atmospheric conditions such as high altitude or underwater.

evaporation The conversion of a liquid to a gas.

fecal contamination When the vector defecates into a wound on the host.

frostbite Localized damage to tissues resulting from prolonged exposure to extreme cold.

gangrene Permanent cell death.

heat cramps Acute and involuntary muscle pains, usually in the lower extremities, the abdomen, or both, that occur because of profuse sweating and subsequent sodium losses in sweat.

heat exhaustion A clinical syndrome characterized by volume depletion and heat stress that is thought to be a milder form of heat illness and on a continuum leading to heat stroke.

heat illness The increase in core body temperature due to inadequate thermolysis.

heat stroke The least common and most deadly heat illness, caused by a severe disturbance in thermoregulation, usually characterized by a core temperature of more than 104°F (40°C) and altered mental status.

high-altitude cerebral edema (HACE) An altitude illness in which there is a change in mental status and/or ataxia in a person with AMS or the presence of mental status changes and ataxia in a person without AMS.

high-altitude pulmonary edema (HAPE) An altitude illness characterized by dyspnea at rest, cough, severe weakness, and drowsiness that may eventually lead to central cyanosis, audible rales or wheezing, tachypnea, and tachycardia.

hypothermia Condition in which the core body temperature is significantly below normal.

immersion syndrome A process similar to frostbite but caused by prolonged exposure to cool, wet conditions.

inoculation When a vector injects the pathogen into the host with its saliva while it feeds on the host.

passive transmission When an arthropod carries a pathogen from one host to another.

radiation Emission of heat from an object into surrounding, colder air.

regurgitation When a vector vomits a pathogen into a host while it feeds on the host.

snow blindness A burn to the eye from UV radiation.

superficial frostbite A type of frostbite characterized by altered sensation (numbness, tingling, or burning) and white, waxy skin that is firm to palpation, but the underlying tissues remain soft.

thermolysis The liberation of heat from the body.

venom A toxin produced by some animals.

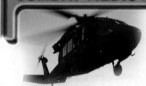

COMBAT MEDIC *in Action*

Your unit is on a field mission high in the mountains. Over the past two nights, a member of your unit has been having trouble sleeping. At dawn this morning, he mentioned that he had a headache. You gave him some oral pain medication and he said that he was ready to continue his duties. While taking a short break for a midday meal, he suddenly vomits.

1. Acute mountain sickness (AMS) can occur in altitudes over:
   A. 8,000'.
   B. 7,500'.
   C. 6,500'.
   D. 8,500'.

2. Additional symptoms of AMS include:
   A. fatigue.
   B. weakness.
   C. dizziness.
   D. all of the above.

3. Treatment for AMS begins with:
   A. evacuation by helicopter.
   B. climbing to a higher elevation.
   C. remaining in place and not climbing any higher.
   D. rappelling down the mountain rapidly.

4. A swaying of the upper body is a sign of:
   A. successful treatment.
   B. fatigue.
   C. HACE.
   D. intoxication.

5. Treatment of HACE begins with:
   A. immediate decent by at least 1000'.
   B. BVM ventilation.
   C. IV therapy.
   D. remaining in place and not climbing any higher.

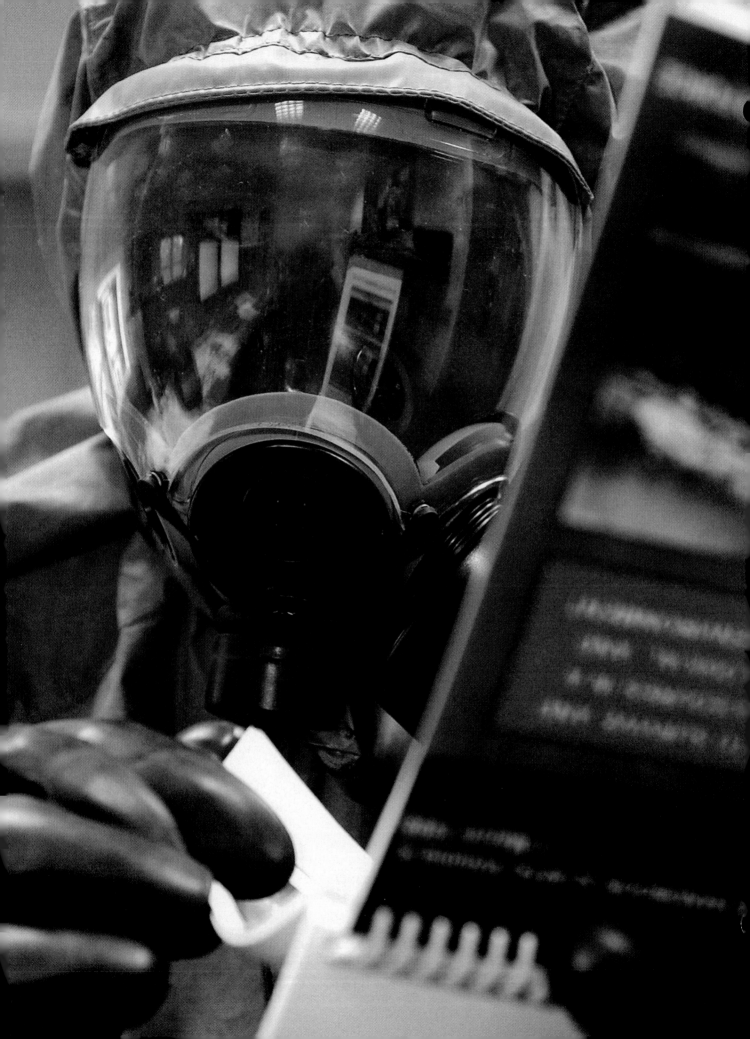

Nonconventional Incidents

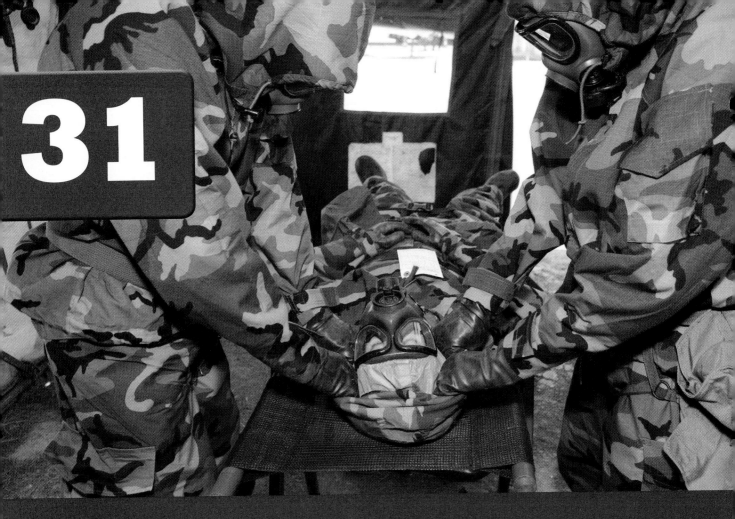

31

Introduction to CBRNE

Objectives

Knowledge Objectives
- [ ] Define CBRNE.
- [ ] Describe the CBRNE dissemination methods.
- [ ] Define chemical agents.
- [ ] Define biologic agents.
- [ ] Define radiologic devices.
- [ ] Define nuclear devices.
- [ ] Define high explosives.
- [ ] Discuss the roles of national, state, and local agencies in response to a CBRNE event.

■ Introduction

Today, the potential for a CBRNE attack by an enemy is real. This chapter identifies your role, as a combat medic, in support of CBRNE defense operations. It also describes the threats, methods of dissemination, and collective defensive agencies that may support and react to a CBRNE attack in accordance with FM 3-4: *Multiservice Tactics, Techniques, and Procedures for Nuclear, Biological, and Chemical (NBC) Protection*, FM 3-5: *NBC Decontamination*, FM 3-9: *Potential Military Chemical/Biological Agents and Compounds*, domestic preparedness programs, and the Technician EMS course.

CBRNE is defined as chemical, biologic, radiologic, nuclear, and high yield explosive devices. CBRNE actually stands for:

- Chemical agents
- Biologic agents
- Radiologic agents
- Nuclear devices
- Explosive devices

■ CBRNE Threats

The lone individual, such as Theodore Kaczynski, also known as the Unabomber, is by far the most difficult threat to detect. For almost 20 years, Kaczynski remained at large and planted mail bombs, killing 3 people and wounding 22. The lone individual is a wildcard, striking without a predictable motive or pattern, copying a previous event for the publicity, or just acting on a whim. Fortunately, individual terrorists have been the least successful in their attacks. Lacking the funding, organization, and sophistication of larger groups, they account for many of the recently failed attempts and hoaxes.

Local terrorist groups and nonaligned groups form the larger threat of domestic CBRNE terrorism because they may have the funding, organization, and ability to build or purchase CBRNE agents. The primary differences between these groups are the cause, the home base, and the source of their funding. Local terrorist groups have one distinct advantage over foreign organizations: the members fit into the local society and are often unnoticed until they strike.

Availability of Agents

CBRNE agents are available and relatively easy to acquire or manufacture. Crude chemical and biologic agents can be made from readily available components by individuals with the knowledge presented in college-level science courses. More sophisticated CBRNE weapons require advanced technical knowledge and materials that are much more difficult to acquire.

Radiologic materials are found in many facilities, such as research labs, hospitals, and in industry. In fact, almost every home has a small amount of radioactive material in the home's smoke detectors. Toxic industrial chemicals and the materials to make chemical warfare agents are readily available in school laboratories, are legitimately used in industry, and are employed in various research facilities. Biologic pathogens may be obtained from nature, hospital labs, and university research facilities, among other places. Instructions for making crude CBRNE weapons have been described in various handbooks, terrorist guides, and on the Internet.

Lethal Amounts

Advanced CBRNE weapons developed for use in warfare were designed for open-air delivery to inflict multiple casualties or deny terrain. Use of CBRNE agents by terrorists are likely to be of smaller quantities and use less sophisticated delivery systems. Release of CBRNE agents in enclosed spaces may maximize their effects. Large amounts of CBRNE are not needed in enclosed spaces. CBRNE agents are extremely toxic at very low doses. If these agents were released into an enclosed space, their lethal effects would be magnified. For comparison purposes, a fragmentation hand grenade has an effective casualty radius of 50′. The same quantity of chemical agent, about 1.7 lb, could fill a 600′-long subway platform with a concentration that would injure or kill every person who remained on the platform for 2 minutes. In addition, the facility might have to be shut down until it could be thoroughly decontaminated. A radiologic agent, spread in the same location, would likely not cause immediate injury, but would have the potential to shut down the facility until it could be thoroughly decontaminated. One study indicates that the same quantity of the most toxic biologic material, disseminated under ideal conditions, could cause deaths or injuries over an area of more than 3.25 square miles.

CBRNE Incidents

Although knowledge of the capabilities and characteristics of chemical, biologic, and radiologic agents is useful in the remediation effort after an incident, the ability to recognize both the potential for an event and the tools of a CBRNE terrorist may enable responders to anticipate and prevent or mitigate the effects of the attack. In many cases, security is often an issue regarding such activities as spray insecticide and crop dusting.

Since the 1970s, there has been an increase of actual terrorist activity involving CBRNE agents. There have also been hoaxes, such as the letter, sent in April 1997 to the B'nai B'rith headquarters in Washington, DC, that was alleged to contain anthrax, as well as the numerous hoaxes seen around the country in which letters, claiming to contain anthrax, have been sent to institutions such as clinics and media organizations. In the months following September 11, 2001, however, letters actually containing anthrax were mailed in the United States. Twenty-two citizens developed either the skin form or the pulmonary form of anthrax and five citizens died. The concern over the hoaxes is that they require the same initial response as an actual terrorist attack.

There was one reported CBRNE event in the 1970s, three more in the 1980s, and an exponential increase of events in the 1990s. Some significant incidents include:

- In 1972, members of a US fascist group called Order of the Rising Sun were found in possession of 30 to 40 kg of typhoid bacteria cultures, with which they planned to contaminate water supplies in Chicago, St. Louis, and other large midwestern cities.

- In 1984, two members of an Oregon cult cultivated *Salmonella* bacteria (which causes food poisoning) and used it to contaminate restaurant salad bars in an attempt to affect the outcome of a local election. Although some 751 people became ill and 45 were hospitalized, there were no fatalities.

Terrorist weapons may include nuclear devices, radiologic material, chemical agents, and biologic agents. The conventional wisdom is that a nuclear weapon is very difficult for a terrorist group to acquire; in contrast, radioactive material, chemical agents, and biologic agents are relatively easy to obtain and thus pose a greater threat.

Note that both the availability and the impact of chemical and biologic threat materials are high, with potentially devastating consequences FIGURE 31-1 ▶. This chapter will focus on the most likely terrorist weapons—radioactive material, chemical agents, and biologic agents—and also will touch on the potential result of terrorist use of nuclear devices.

CBRNE Dissemination Methods

There are many methods by which CBRNE can be disseminated. Breaking devices such as light bulbs and vacuum bottles pose a minimal hazard and are used for chemical dissemination. Bursting devices pose a moderate hazard and are used to disseminate all CBRNE agents. Exploding devices pose a moderate hazard and are used for radiologic dissemination. Exploding devices can also disseminate chemical and biologic agents although the heat and explosive forces are likely to significantly degrade the biologic agent to be delivered.

Spraying devices are used to disseminate chemical or biologic agents FIGURE 31-2 ▶. Line sources (such as moving vehicles and airplanes) release the agent along a moving line and pose significant downward hazards. Point sources (such as aerosol cans and garden hoses) are

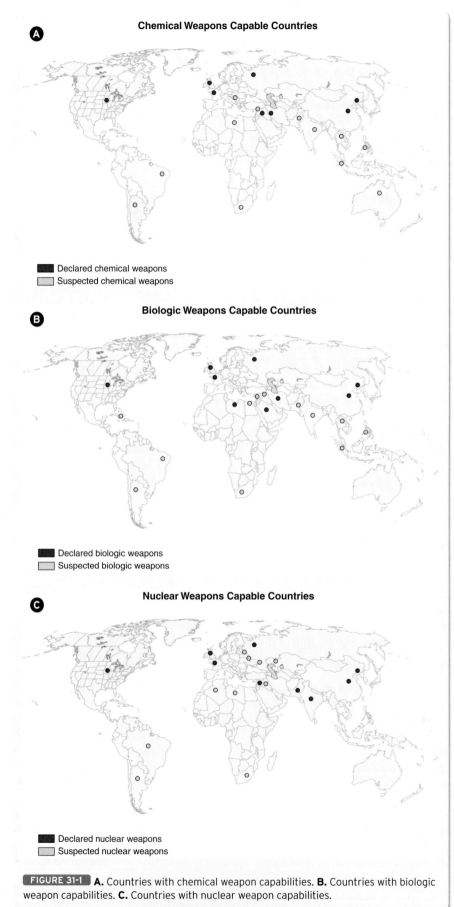

FIGURE 31-1 **A.** Countries with chemical weapon capabilities. **B.** Countries with biologic weapon capabilities. **C.** Countries with nuclear weapon capabilities.

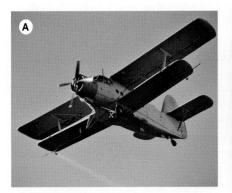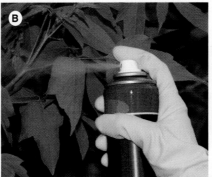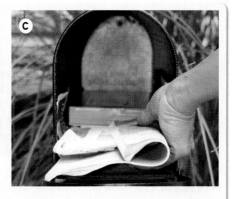

FIGURE 31-2 **A.** Line sources include moving vehicles and airplanes. **B.** Point sources include aerosol cans and garden hoses. **C.** Vectors include letters and packages, insects and animals, contaminated clothing, contaminated food, and contaminated water.

static and pose moderate to significant downward hazards. **Vectors** are objects that carry the agent from point of release to the target. They are unpredictable and can spread biologic or chemical agents. Vectors include letters and packages, insects and animals, contaminated clothing, contaminated food, and contaminated water.

■ Chemical Agents

The most common chemical agents are:

- **Nerve agents:** Sarin and VX
- **Blood agents:** Cyanide and chloride
- **Blister agents:** Mustard and Lewisite
- **Choking agents:** Phosgene and chlorine

Some of the chemical warfare agents are said to have characteristic odors, such as a horseradish or mustard smell for mustard agent, Lewisite's aroma of geraniums, or the freshly mown hay smell of phosgene. However, these are not adequate warning properties for the purpose of protecting yourself against adverse health effects associated with exposure.

Nerve Agents

Nerve Agents are among the most deadly chemicals ever developed. Nerve agents are designed to kill large numbers of people with small quantities. They can also cause cardiac arrest within seconds to minutes of exposure. Nerve agents, which were discovered while in search of a superior pesticide, are a class of chemical called *organophosphates*, which are found in household bug sprays, agricultural pesticides, and some industrial chemicals, at far lower strengths.

There are almost 900 different pesticides available for use in the United States. Approximately 37 of these belong to the organophosphate class of insecticides. The chemicals in this class kill insects by disrupting their brains and nervous systems. Unfortunately, at greater strengths, these chemicals or nerve agents also can harm the brains and nervous systems

of animals and humans. These chemicals block the essential enzyme cholinesterase in the nervous system from working, causing the body's organs to become overstimulated and burn out.

Types of Agents

G agents came from the early nerve agents, the G series, which were developed by German scientists (hence the G) in the period after WWI and into WWII. There are three G-series agents; all contain the same basic chemical structure with slight variations to produce different properties. The two variations of these agents are lethality and volatility. The following G agents are listed from high volatility to low volatility:

- **Sarin (GB):** Highly volatile colorless and odorless liquid. It turns from liquid to gas within seconds to minutes at room temperature. It is highly lethal, with an LD_{50} of 1,700 mg/70 kg (about 1 drop, depending on the purity). The **LD_{50}** is the amount that will kill 50% of people who are exposed to this level. Sarin is primarily a vapor hazard, with the respiratory tract as the main route of entry. This agent is especially dangerous in enclosed environments such as office buildings, shopping malls, or subway cars. When it comes into contact with skin, it is quickly absorbed and evaporates. When sarin is on clothing, it has the effect of **off-gassing**, which means that the vapors are continuously released over a period of time (like perfume). This renders the casualty as well as the casualty's clothing contaminated.
- **Soman (GD):** Twice as persistent as sarin and five times as lethal. It has a fruity odor as a result of the type of alcohol used in the agent, and generally has no color. Soman is both a contact and an inhalation hazard that can enter the body through skin absorption and through the respiratory tract. A unique additive in GD causes it to bind to the cells that it attacks faster than any other agent. This irreversible binding is called

aging, which makes it more difficult to treat casualties who have been exposed.

- **Tabun (GA):** Approximately half as lethal as sarin and 36 times more persistent; under the proper conditions it will remain for several days. It also has a fruity smell and an appearance similar to sarin. The components used to manufacture tabun are easy to acquire and the agent is easy to manufacture, which makes it unique. GA is both a contact and an inhalation hazard that can enter the body through skin absorption as well as through the respiratory tract.

V agent (VX) was developed by the British after World War II and has similar chemical properties to the G-series agents. It is a clear oily agent that has no odor and looks like baby oil. The difference is that VX is over 100 times more lethal than sarin and is extremely persistent **FIGURE 31-3 ◄**. In fact, VX is so persistent that given the proper conditions it will remain relatively unchanged for weeks to months. These properties make VX primarily a contact hazard, because it lets off very little vapor. It is easily absorbed into the skin, and the oily residue that remains on the skin's surface is extremely difficult to decontaminate. **TABLE 31-1 ▼** provides a quick reference and comparison of the nerve agents.

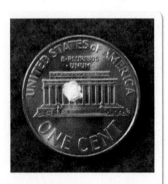

FIGURE 31-3 VX is the most toxic chemical ever produced. The dot on the penny demonstrates the amount needed to achieve a lethal dose.

Volatile nerve agents, such as sarin, are nonpersistent chemicals that pose primarily an inhalation hazard. Symptoms of exposure develop within seconds, but tend not to worsen if the casualty can be evacuated from the area. Casualties who either inhale a toxic dose or are unable to be evacuated from the release site will experience the highest mortality rates. Casualties who are able to leave the release area quickly or who are exposed to low levels of the agent will experience the least amount of symptoms and will require minimal medical intervention (the "walking wounded"). Because these agents are highly volatile, combat medics are at risk of becoming secondarily contaminated from agent off-gassing. This occurs if the casualty's clothing is not properly handled and you fail to wear appropriate respiratory protection. Symptomatic casualties require immediate treatment, including airway management and antidote therapy.

Nerve agents such as VX are very persistent agents, do not readily vaporize, and pose primarily a liquid threat. The symptoms from such a contamination may be delayed for minutes to hours depending on the concentration, dose, and location of the contaminant on the skin. Absorption occurs more readily on moist areas of the skin. Symptoms may even develop slowly in cases where liquid exposure is high. Because casualties of a VX attack are contaminated with a liquid, decontamination takes on a higher priority to limit the amount of agent absorption and to minimize the risk of spreading the contamination. Decontamination should ideally be provided simultaneously with antidote administration and airway management, when necessary.

Nerve Agent Symptoms

Nerve agents all produce similar symptoms, but have varying routes of entry. Nerve agents differ slightly in lethal concentration or dose and also differ in their volatility. Some agents are designed to become a gas quickly (nonpersistent or highly volatile), whereas others remain liquid for a period of time (persistent or nonvolatile). These agents have been used successfully in warfare and to date represent the only type of chemical agent that has been used successfully in a terrorist act.

Once the agent has entered the body through skin contact or through the respiratory system, the casualty will begin

TABLE 31-1 Nerve Agents

Name	Code Name	Odor	Special Features	Onset of Symptoms	Volatility	Route of Exposure
Tabun	GA	Fruity	Easy to manufacture	Immediate	Low	Both contact and vapor hazard
Sarin	GB	None (if pure) or strong	Will off-gas while on victim's clothing	Immediate	High	Primarily respiratory vapor hazard; extremely lethal if skin contact is made
Soman	GD	Fruity	Ages rapidly, making if difficult to treat	Immediate	Moderate	Contact with skin; minimal vapor hazard
V agent	VX	None	Most lethal chemical agent; difficult to decontaminate	Immediate	Very low	Contact with skin; no vapor hazard (unless aerosolized)

to exhibit a pattern of predictable symptoms. Like all chemical agents, the severity of the symptoms will depend on the route of exposure and the amount of agent to which the casualty was exposed. The resulting symptoms are described using the mnemonic SLUDGEM:

S Salivation
L Lacrimation (tears)
U Urination
D Defecation
G GI distress
E Emesis (vomiting)
M Miosis (pupil constriction)

Miosis is the most common symptom of nerve agent exposure and can remain for days to weeks. Only a handful of medical conditions are associated with the bilaterally pinpoint-constricted pupils (miosis) that are seen with nerve agent exposure. Conditions such as a suspected stroke, direct light to both eyes, and a drug overdose all can cause bilateral constricted pupils. You should therefore assess the casualty for all of the SLUDGEM signs and symptoms to determine whether the casualty has been exposed to a nerve agent.

Treatment

Fatalities from severe exposure occur as a result of respiratory complications, which lead to respiratory arrest. Once the casualty has been decontaminated, you should be prepared to treat aggressively, if the casualty is to be saved. You can greatly increase the casualty's chances of survival simply by providing airway and ventilatory support. As with all emergencies, managing the ABCs is the best and most important treatment that you can provide.

Often casualties exposed to these agents will begin seizing and will not stop. These casualties will require administration of **nerve agent antidote kits (NAAKs)** in addition to the support of the ABCs. NAAKs contain two auto-injector medications: atropine and 2-PAM chloride (pralidoxime chloride). These medications are delivered using the same technique as the EpiPen auto-injector; however, multiple doses may need to be administered.

Atropine is used to block the nerve agent's overstimulation of the body; however, because the nerve agent may remain in the body for a long period of time, 2-PAM chloride is used to eliminate the agent from the body. The 2-PAM chloride antidote is effective at relieving the respiratory muscle paralysis and twitching caused by the nerve agent. Many of the symptoms will be reversed with the use of atropine; however, many doses may need to be administered to see these results.

Blood Agents

Hydrogen cyanide (AC) and cyanogen chloride (CK) are both agents that affect the body's ability to use oxygen. **Cyanide** is a colorless gas that has an odor similar to almonds. The effects of the cyanides begin on the cellular level and are very rapidly seen at the organ system level. Besides the nerve agents, metabolic agents are the only chemical weapons known to kill within seconds to minutes. Unlike nerve agents, however, these deadly gases are commonly found in many indus-

trial settings. Cyanides are produced in massive quantities throughout the United States every year for industrial uses such as gold and silver mining, photography, lethal injections, and plastics processing. They are often present in fires associated with textile or plastic factories. In fact, cyanide is naturally found in the pits of many fruits in very small quantities. There is very little difference between the symptoms found in AC and CK. In low doses, these chemicals are associated with dizziness, lightheadedness, headache, and vomiting. Higher doses will produce symptoms that include:

- Shortness of breath and gasping respirations
- Tachypnea
- Flushed skin color
- Tachycardia
- Altered mental status
- Seizures
- Coma
- Apnea
- Cardiac arrest

The symptoms associated with the inhalation of a large amount of cyanide will all appear within several minutes. Death is likely unless the casualty is treated promptly. Cyanide binds with the body's cells, preventing oxygen from being used. Several medications act as antidotes. Once the combat medic in the proper personal protective equipment (PPE) has removed the casualty from the source of exposure, even if there is no liquid contamination, all of the casualty's clothes must be removed to prevent off-gassing. Trained and protected personnel must decontaminate any casualties who may have been exposed to liquid contamination before initiating treatment. Then you should support the ABCs and gain IV access.

Mild effects of cyanide exposure will generally resolve by simply removing the casualty from the source of contamination and administering supplementary oxygen. Severe exposure, however, will require aggressive oxygenation and perhaps ventilation with supplementary oxygen. Always use a bag-mask device to ventilate a casualty exposed to a metabolic agent. The agent can easily be passed on from the casualty to the combat medic through mouth-to-mouth or mouth-to-mask ventilations. If no antidote is available, initiate evacuation immediately.

Blister Agents

The primary route of exposure of blister agents, or **vesicants**, is the skin (contact); however, if vesicants are left on the skin or clothing long enough, they produce vapors that can enter the respiratory tract. Vesicants cause burn-like blisters to form on the casualty's skin as well as in the respiratory tract. The vesicant agents consist of sulfur mustard (H), Lewisite (L), and phosgene oxime (CX). (The symbols H, L, and CX are military designations for these chemicals.) The vesicants usually cause the most damage to damp or moist areas of the body, such as the armpits, groin, and respiratory tract. Signs of vesicant exposure on the skin include:

- Skin irritation, burning, and reddening
- Immediate intense skin pain (with L and CX)
- Formation of large blisters

- Gray discoloration of skin (a sign of permanent damage seen with L and CX)
- Swollen and closed or irritated eyes
- Permanent eye injury (including blindness)

If vapors were inhaled, the casualty may experience the following:

- Hoarseness and stridor
- Severe cough
- Hemoptysis (coughing up of blood)
- Severe dyspnea

Sulfur Mustard

Sulfur mustard (H) is a brownish, yellowish oily substance that is generally considered very persistent. It is both a vapor inhalation and a liquid contact hazard. When released, mustard has the distinct smell of garlic or mustard and is quickly absorbed into the skin and/or mucous membranes. As the agent is absorbed into the skin, it begins an irreversible process of damage to the cells. Absorption through the skin or mucous membranes usually occurs within seconds, and damage to the underlying cells takes place within 1 to 2 minutes. The clinical effects do not begin for hours.

Mustard is considered a **mutagen**, which means that it mutates, damages, and changes the structures of cells. Eventually, cellular death will occur. On the surface, the casualty will generally not produce any signs or symptoms until 4 to 6 hours after exposure (depending on concentration and amount of exposure) **FIGURE 31-4 ▾**. There is no pain, skin discoloration, or eye irritation immediately after exposure.

Mustard causes injury to the eyes, skin, airways, and some internal organs. This chemical warfare agent has a delayed action and exposure to it may result in blisters on the skin, temporary blindness, and respiratory distress. The casualty will develop a progressive reddening of the affected area, which will gradually develop into large blisters. These blisters are very similar in shape and appearance to those associated with thermal second-degree burns. The fluid within the blisters does not contain any of the agent; however, the skin covering the area is considered to be contaminated until decontamination has been performed.

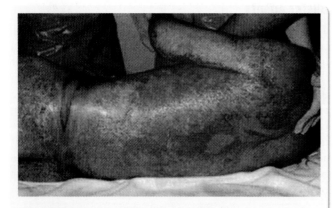

FIGURE 31-4 Skin damage resulting from exposure to sulfur mustard (agent H).

More extensive injury can result in death because of respiratory failure from airway injury or sepsis as a result of bone marrow damage, decrease in white blood cells, and an impaired immune system. As with burns, the primary complication associated with vesicant blisters is secondary infection. If the casualty does survive the initial direct injury from the agent, the depletion of the white blood cells leaves the casualty with a decreased resistance to infections. Although sulfur mustard is regarded as persistent, it does release enough vapors when dispersed to be inhaled. This creates upper and lower airway compromise. The result is damage and swelling of the airways. The airway compromise makes the casualty's condition far more serious.

There is no specific therapy beyond supportive care. Hours later, the casualty may recognize that he or she has been exposed and present to the medical treatment facility (MTF) for evaluation and treatment. The onset time for clinical effects ranges from 2 to 48 hours; most commonly it is between 4 and 8 hours.

Lewisite and Phosgene Oxime

Lewisite (L) and **phosgene oxime (CX)** produce blister wounds very similar to mustard. They are highly volatile and have a rapid onset of symptoms, as opposed to the delayed onset seen with mustard. These agents produce immediate intense pain and discomfort when contact is made. The casualty may have a grayish discoloration at the contaminated site. Although tissue damage also occurs with exposure to these agents, they do not cause the secondary cellular injury that is associated with mustard.

There are no antidotes for mustard or CX exposure. BAL (British anti-Lewisite) is the antidote for agent L. Ensure that the casualty has been decontaminated before ABCs are initiated. The casualty may require prompt airway support if any agent has been inhaled, but this should not occur until after decontamination. Gain IV access and initiate evacuation as soon as possible.

Choking Agents

Choking agents are gases that cause immediate harm to the casualties exposed to them. The primary route of exposure for these agents is through the respiratory tract, which makes them an inhalation or vapor hazard. Once inside the lungs, they damage the lung tissue and fluid leaks into the lungs. Pulmonary edema develops in the casualty, resulting in difficulty breathing due to the inability for air exchange. These agents produce respiratory-related symptoms such as dyspnea, tachypnea, and pulmonary edema. This class of chemical agents consists of chlorine (CL) and phosgene.

Chlorine (CL) was the first chemical used on a large scale in modern warfare; it was used in 1915 in World War I. Most people are familiar with chlorine and its odor because it is used as a disinfectant in swimming pools. It is commonly stored at water treatment plants, and is also widely used in industry; large amounts are shipped by rail and on roadways. During the 1996 Summer Olympics in Atlanta, Georgia, railroad tank cars of it moved past Olympic Village every day.

Chlorine causes irritation to the eyes both as a gas and in solution in swimming pool water. If chlorine gas is inhaled, it causes airway irritation with cough, and a feeling of shortness of breath. Chlorine injures cells by reacting with water to produce hydrochloric acid and oxygen free radicals. It is toxic to any body surface, including the eyes, skin, respiratory tract, and gastrointestinal tract. A high concentration will cause more severe pulmonary damage with both airway and parenchymal damage. Sudden death can result from severe hypoxia and cardiac arrest. After an exposure to a high concentration or a prolonged exposure, chlorine can cause noncardiac pulmonary edema. Intubation should be performed before laryngospasm occurs; oxygen, cool mist, assisted ventilation, the use of positive end expiratory pressure (PEEP), and bronchodilators may be needed. Fluid replacement may be necessary. Toxicity to the eyes and skin should be treated with copious flushing with water.

Phosgene is a common industrial chemical, and was also formerly used as a warfare agent. It has the odor of newly mown hay and becomes a gas at 47°F. It damages primarily the lungs and must be inhaled to cause this damage. At high concentrations, the chlorine part of the molecule irritates the eyes, nose, and upper airways, and may cause fatal laryngospasm. The real damage is done by the carbon double-bond oxygen group (carbonyl group) of the phosgene molecule; this causes severe, though not immediately apparent, lung injury. After phosgene is inhaled, the carbonyl group combines with the components of the membrane dividing the alveoli from the capillaries, and fluid from the blood leaks first into the alveolar septi and then into the alveoli themselves.

Symptoms appear usually from 2 to 12 hours after exposure; the earlier the onset of symptoms, the more severe the effects will be. Dyspnea at exertion worsens to dyspnea at rest after a severe exposure. This is accompanied by a cough productive of frothy, clear sputum. The fluid loss after a severe exposure may be as great as 1 to 2 L per hour. There are two major components to the physical effects of phosgene exposure: hypoxia because of the fluid-filled alveoli, and fluid loss leading to hypovolemia and hypotension. Management of this noncardiac pulmonary edema consists of early intubation if the onset of illness is early; ventilation, oxygen, and positive end expiratory pressure (PEEP); bronchodilators if there is evidence of bronchospasm; and antibiotics after a bacterial pneumonia occurs and an organism can be identified. Steroids may be needed if the usual bronchodilators are not helpful; steroids are not otherwise useful in treating exposures.

TABLE 31-2 ▾ summarizes the chemical agents. The odors of the particular chemicals are provided for informational purposes only. The sense of smell is a poor tool to use to determine whether there is a chemical agent present. Many are unable to smell the agents, and the odor could be derived from another source. This information is useful to you if you receive reports from casualties claiming to smell of bleach or garlic, for example. You should never enter a potentially hazardous area and "smell" to determine whether a chemical agent is present.

TABLE 31-2 Chemical Agents

Class	Military Designations	Odor	Lethality	Onset of Symptoms	Volatility	Primary Route of Exposure
Nerve agents	Tabun (GA) Sarin (GB) Soman (GD) VX	Fruity or none	Most lethal chemical agents can kill within minutes; effects are reversible with antidotes	Immediate	Varies: Moderate (GA, GD) Very high (GB) Low (VX)	Vapor hazard (GB) Both vapor and contact hazard (GA, GD) Contact hazard
Vesicants	Mustard (H) Lewisite (L) Phosgene oxime (CX)	Garlic (H) Geranium (L)	Causes large blisters to form on casualties; may severely damage upper airway if vapors are inhaled; severe intense pain and grayish skin discoloration (L, CX)	Delayed (H) Immediate (L, CX)	Very low (H, L) Moderate (CX)	Primarily contact, with some vapor hazard
Pulmonary agents	Chlorine (CL) Phosgene (CG)	Bleach (CL) Cut grass (CG)	Causes irritation; choking (CL); severe pulmonary edema (CG)	Immediate (CL) Delayed (CG)	Very high	Vapor hazard
Cyanide agents	Hydrogen cyanide (AC) Cyanogen chloride (CK)	Almonds (AC) Irritating (CK)	Highly lethal chemical gases; can kill within minutes; effects are reversible with antidotes	Immediate	Very high	Vapor hazard

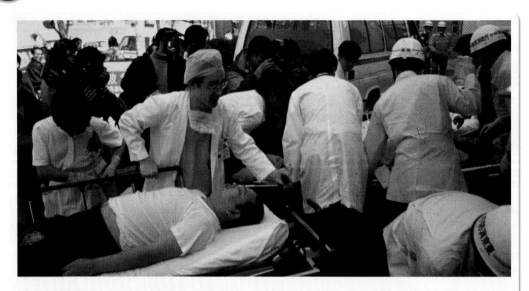

FIGURE 31-5 On March 20, 1995, members of a Japanese cult released sarin (GB) in the Tokyo subway. Ten people died and 5,000 were injured.

The Centers for Disease Control (CDC) categorizes biologic agents into three groups based on the lethality, ease of dissemination, and response required. Category A agents include anthrax, smallpox, botulism, plaque tularemia, and the viral hemorrhagic fevers. Category B agents include ricin, Q-fever, glanders, brucellosis, and food safety threats. Category C agents are emerging infectious diseases.

Biologic agents pose many difficult issues. For one thing, they can be almost completely undetectable. Also, most of the diseases caused by these agents will be similar to other minor illnesses.

Terrorist Use of Chemical Weapons

On March 20, 1995, members of a Japanese cult released sarin (GB) in the Tokyo subway. The affected subway lines intersected at Kasumigaseki station, the office quarters of the Tokyo government. Poisonous gas was found on five trains heading for the station, and the entire city was thrown into confusion for a day. The first arriving medical responders were met with chaos as hundreds and then thousands of people fled the subway system **FIGURE 31-5 ▲**. Many were contaminated and showing signs and symptoms of nerve agent exposure. In the end more than 5,000 people sought medical care for exposure to sarin, and 10 people died. None of the EMS personnel wore protective clothing and most became cross-contaminated. Remember, you can avoid becoming exposed. Don't become a victim.

■ Biologic Agents

Biologic agents are the oldest of the nuclear, biologic, and chemical triad of weapons of mass destruction. References to the use of decaying animal carcasses to contaminate wells go back over 2,000 years. In the Middle Ages, bodies of plague victims were catapulted into cities under siege to cause sickness and death. In North America, during the French and Indian War, blankets contaminated with smallpox were given to Native American tribes to decimate their ranks. During World War I, German agents in Baltimore attempted to infect allied horses with anthrax and glanders as they were being shipped to the front in Europe, because horses were important strategic assets at the time. Prior to the Second World War, Japan was developing a sophisticated biologic warfare research program and reportedly used some of the agents against China.

Dissemination

The most effective delivery method is an aerosol containing biologic agent particles that are in the 1- to 5-micron range. Particles in this size range behave similar to a gas and can be taken into the bronchioles and alveoli during normal respiration. Larger particles either quickly fall out of the biologic aerosol or they become trapped in the upper airway. Smaller particles are breathed into the lungs, but expired out again without retention. The realization of this optimum particle size/infectivity ratio was a major advance in the development of offensive biologic warfare.

The first biologic agents were manufactured as wet slurries of highly concentrated bacterial and viral agents. These slurries were easy and relatively safe to manufacture but were difficult to disseminate in the correct particle size range and had to be refrigerated for storage. After the discovery of the particle size/infectivity relationship, the next significant advance in biologic warfare was the development of biologic agents in freeze-dried powder formulations. Although these were technically difficult and dangerous to manufacture, their low refrigeration requirement, ease of dissemination, and high concentration of infectious agent made them suitable for a variety of covert, tactical, and strategic uses.

Anthrax

<u>Anthrax</u> is the disease caused by *Bacillus anthracis*—a deadly bacteria that lays dormant in a spore-forming stage. When exposed to the optimal temperature and moisture, the germ will be released from the spore (protective shell) and begin to multiply and produce toxins. The routes of entry for anthrax are inhalation, cutaneous **FIGURE 31-6 ▶**, or gastrointestinal (from consuming food that contains spores). The inhalational

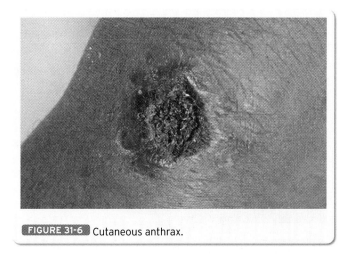

FIGURE 31-6 Cutaneous anthrax.

TABLE 31-3 Characteristics of Anthrax

Dissemination Method	Aerosol
Communicability	Only in the cutaneous form (rare)
Route of entry	Through inhalation of spores, skin contact with spores, or direct contact with skin wound (cutaneous)
Signs and symptoms	Flu-like symptoms, fever, respiratory distress with tachycardia, shock, pulmonary edema, and respiratory failure after 3 to 5 days of flu-like symptoms.
Medical care	Pulmonary/inhalation: BSI precautions, supplemental oxygen, ventilatory support for pulmonary edema or respiratory failure, and transport. Cutaneous: BSI precautions, apply dry sterile dressing to prevent accidental contact with wound and fluids.

form or pulmonary anthrax is the most deadly and often presents as a severe cold. Pulmonary anthrax infections are associated with a 90% death rate if untreated. Antibiotics can be used to treat anthrax successfully. There is also a vaccine to prevent anthrax infections. **TABLE 31-3 ▲** lists the characteristics of anthrax. **TABLE 31-4 ▶** lists the time line of the 2001 Anthrax Attacks.

Smallpox

Smallpox is caused by the *Variola* virus, an orthopox virus, which causes both a major and minor form of the disease. The smallpox virus only causes overt clinical disease in

TABLE 31-4 Anthrax Time Line

Date	Key Event
25 Sep 01	In St. Petersburg, Florida, NBC TV received a letter postmarked September 20, 2001, containing a white powder and notified the FBI.
2 Oct 01	First inhalation anthrax case in 25 years, 63 y/o Robert Stevens.
5 Oct 01	Robert Stevens died of inhalation anthrax. He was the photo editor for American Media.
7 Oct 01	American Media offices were closed after spores are found on Stevens' computer and keyboard. Nasal swipes were obtained from Ernesto Blanco, a 73 y/o mailroom supervisor.
12 Oct 01	An NBC assistant tested positive for cutaneous anthrax. A second letter was sent to NBC in Trenton, New Jersey, postmarked September 18, 2001, which contained a brown granular substance.
13 Oct 01	American Media announced that five people may have been exposed. In New York City (NYC), another NBC employee reported anthrax symptoms.
14 Oct 01	NYC police and two health department technicians tested positive for exposure to anthrax.
15 Oct 01	In NYC, an ABC news worker's son tested positive for cutaneous anthrax.
Oct 01	In Washington, a letter postmarked October 9, 2001, in Trenton, New Jersey sent to Senator Tom Daschle tested positive.
Oct 01	Ernesto Blanco tested positive for inhalation anthrax and spores were found in a Boca Raton, Florida, post office.
17 Oct 01	Anthrax spores were found on a computer keyboard in NYC Governor George Pataki's offices. None of the staff tested positive and his staff began taking Cipro.
18 Oct 01	Dan Rather's assistant tested positive for cutaneous anthrax after penicillin failed to reduce the swelling on her face.
20 Oct 01	Thirteen anthrax hot spots were identified in a Trenton, New Jersey, processing center and three workers tested positive for exposure to anthrax.
21 Oct 01	A 94-year-old woman died of inhalation anthrax.
22 Oct 01	Two workers from the New Jersey processing center visited the doctor for respiratory problems and one died.

(continues)

TABLE 31-4 Anthrax Time Line (*continued*)

Date	Key Event
23 Oct 01	Washington authorities confirmed two postal workers died of inhalation anthrax. The CDC announced that a Trenton, New Jersey, postal worker may have inhalation anthrax.
24 Oct 01	In Washington, three new cases of inhalation anthrax were discovered.
25 Oct 01	The Daschle letter consisted of very pure and highly concentrated anthrax. A handful of countries were capable of manufacturing the grade.
28 Oct 01	A female worker at the Hamilton Township, New Jersey, post office tested positive for inhalation anthrax.
29 Oct 01	Traces of anthrax were found at the Supreme Court.
31 Oct 01	A NYC woman died of inhalation anthrax.
1 Nov 01	As many as 20 federal buildings may have had traces of anthrax.
3 Nov 01	A mailroom processing facility in Camden County, New Jersey, tested positive for the presence of anthrax.
16 Nov 01	Another anthrax-laden letter, similar to the Daschle letter, was addressed to Senator Patrick Leahy.

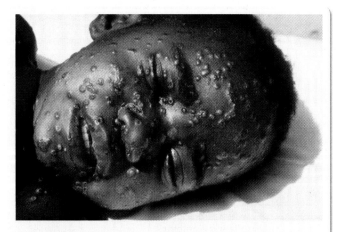

FIGURE 31-7 In smallpox, all the lesions are identical in their development. In other skin disorders, the lesions will be in various stages of healing and development.

TABLE 31-5 Characteristics of Smallpox

Dissemination method	Aerosolized for warfare.
Communicability	High from infected individuals or items (such as blankets used by infected casualties). Person-to-person transmission is possible.
Route of entry	Through inhalation of coughed droplets or direct skin contact with blisters.
Signs and symptoms	Severe fever, malaise, body aches, headaches, small blisters on the skin, and bleeding of the skin and mucous membranes. The incubation period is 10 to 12 days and the duration of the illness is approximately 4 weeks.
Medical care	BSI precautions. There is no specific treatment for smallpox casualties. Casualties should be provided with supportive care (ABCs).

humans, and no animal reservoirs of the virus exist in nature. This was the major reason why the disease was selected for global eradication. The last natural case of smallpox in the world was seen in 1977. Smallpox was declared eradicated in 1980 and it is the only disease to date that has earned this distinction. The United States stopped its civilian vaccination program in 1981. Despite eradication, concerns over clandestine stockpiles of smallpox still remain. The issue for destruction of US laboratory stocks of the virus is under review.

Smallpox is a highly contagious disease. All forms of body substance isolation (BSI) precautions must be used to prevent cross-contamination to health care providers. Simply by wearing examination gloves, a HEPA-filtered respirator, and eye protection, you will greatly reduce your risk of contamination. Before the rash and blisters show, the illness will start with a high fever, body aches, and headaches. The casualty's temperature is usually in the range of 101°F to 104°F.

An easy, quick way to differentiate the smallpox rash from other skin disorders is to observe the size, shape, and location of the lesions. In smallpox, all the lesions are identical in their development. In other skin disorders, the lesions will be in various stages of healing and development. Smallpox blisters also begin on the face and extremities and eventually move toward the chest and abdomen. The disease is in its most con-

tagious phase when the blisters begin to form **FIGURE 31-7 ▲**. Unprotected contact with these blisters will promote transmission of the disease. The characteristics of smallpox are described in **TABLE 31-5 ▲**.

Salmonella

In 1885, pioneering American veterinary scientist, Daniel E. Salmon, discovered the first strain of *Salmonella* in the intestine of a pig. This strain was called *Salmonella choleraesuis*, the designation that is still used to describe the genus and species of this common human pathogen. *Salmonella* is a type of bacteria that causes typhoid fever and many other infections of intestinal origin. Typhoid fever, which is rare in the United States, is caused by a particular strain designated *Salmonella typhi*. However, illness due to other *Salmonella* strains, called salmonellosis, is common in the United States. Today, the number of known strains, technically termed *serotypes* or *serovars*, of these bacteria total over 2,300. Salmonella serotypes *typhimurium* and *enteritidis* are the most common serotypes in the United States. In recent years, concerns have been raised because many strains of *Salmonella* have become resistant to several of the antibiotics traditionally used to treat it, in both animals and humans.

■ Radiologic Devices

Experts say there is enough material and know-how out there for a terrorist to mount a lethal radiologic attack with a dirty bomb, potentially turning a US downtown into a death zone. After the 1993 World Trade Center bombing and the 1995 sarin gas attack of the Tokyo subway, terrorism concerns in general increased, including the possibility that a terrorist would use radiologic weapons. These concerns were realized in 1995 when Chechen rebels buried a container with Cesium-137 in a park in Moscow for purely psychological purposes (ie, to undermine the Russian public's support for the Chechen war). Potential terrorist attack methods could include explosively dispersing a radioactive source, spreading radioactive material on the ground, dispersing the materials in the air, or adding the radioactive material to food or water.

Worldwide Radioactive Sources

In the United States alone, there are about 1.5 million generally licensed sources of radioactive material, and more than 90,000 sources possessed under specific licenses. Other nations make similar uses of radioactive sources. Over 65,000 large gamma sources are in use worldwide, including about 1,600 irradiators, 60,000 gamma processing or radiography sources, and 4,000 radiotherapy or brachytherapy sources. There are at least 638 reactors operating in 68 countries, including 586 research reactors. One hundred and thirty research reactors and 52 multipurpose reactors are actively producing radioisotopes. There are tens of thousands of obsolete radioactive sources worldwide. Obsolete sources have been discovered in schools, old filing cabinets, and office buildings, and purchased at garage sales.

■ Nuclear

Nuclear weapons have only been used on human targets twice: Hiroshima and Nagasaki. These cities had been spared the scourges of the firebomb raids so they could be used as test beds of nuclear weapons' effects. Hiroshima was a bustling city of several hundred thousand people when, on August 6, 1945, a 15-kiloton device was detonated over the city. Destruction was complete. Although the bomb itself did extensive damage, it also initiated a firestorm that essentially destroyed the center of the city and created great numbers of casualties.

For a single bomb, the number of casualties in both cities was large. Over 100,000 people were killed and approximately the same number of people were injured. Survival was hampered by the almost complete destruction of medical assets. Many of those injured had received burns and other injuries; their survival was questionable because there were no medical assets to treat them. That is the real threat of tactical nuclear weapons from a medical perspective—large numbers of casualties with only limited medical assets.

■ High Explosives

High explosives or bomb blasts may be used as the prime mechanism to disseminate nuclear, biologic, and chemical (NBC) materials. When bombs are detonated, the reaction produces an instantaneous chain of events in which the explosive material is rapidly converted into a gas under extremely high pressure and temperature. This gas byproduct is transmitted to the surrounding medium as a blast wave (or shock wave) that travels outward from the explosion.

After the explosion occurs, a mass movement of air (blast and wind) that was originally displaced by the explosive products follows the explosion at speeds that can reach hurricane proportions. This blast wind may be as damaging as the original explosion.

Blast Mechanics

When high-energy explosives are used, such as plastic explosives, TNT, diesel fuel, and fertilizer, they detonate faster than the speed of sound. In low-energy explosives, such as a gunpowder pipe bomb, the pressure within the casing increases so rapidly that it explodes, releasing high-velocity shrapnel as the most deadly byproduct. Low-energy explosives react slower than the speed of sound.

If a solid structure such as a wall or building is present in the path of the explosion, the blast wave will rebound off this structure and generate a reflective force that is magnified almost nine times its original strength. As a result, casualties caught between the blast and the building may suffer injuries two to three times greater than expected for the amount of explosive detonated and the distance from the explosion.

■ National, State, and Local Agencies
Response to a CBRNE Event in the United States

Local response personnel will be the first to respond to a CBRNE incident occurring within the United States. Federal assistance to support crisis and consequence management efforts may not arrive for at least 6 to 10 hours after federal authorities are notified to deploy. The success of the response will be decided by the local emergency responder community training and preparedness program.

Managing a CBRNE Incident Response

In a CBRNE terrorism incident, the federal government will have many responsibilities in an effort to support the state and local community in their response to the incident. Managing CBRNE terrorism incidents requires:

- Planning
- Coordination
- Resources exceeding local assets

The role of each agency is defined in detailed emergency plans, such as the National Response Framework. Medical treatment facilities (MTF) need to have developed plans for responding to CBRNE incidents that occur on and off military reservations.

A CBRNE terrorist incident will involve virtually every type of emergency response and medical asset available in a community, including military MTFs. In addition, it is possible that a CBRNE event could occur on a military installation. Every MTF must be aware of CBRNE agents and the potential threats they pose, and create documented response plans of action involving the entire staff. Every MTF should obtain and maintain equipment and supplies. Conducting periodic CBRNE mass casualty (MASCAL) exercises will maintain readiness. Ideally these plans and exercises will also involve civilian first responder personnel when possible. Awareness, planning, resources (human and equipment), training, and exercise are the keys to CBRNE readiness.

Activating Federal Assistance

Follow established local procedures for notifying local or regional federal agencies, such as your local Federal Bureau of Investigation (FBI) office. Agencies to be notified in the event of a CBRNE terrorism incident include the FBI, Federal Emergency Management Agency (FEMA), and Environmental Protection Agency (EPA), if applicable. A complete list of federal agencies can be found in **TABLE 31-6 ▶**. Make certain to request federal assistance in accordance with your state and local procedures. Normally, the request for federal assistance will be made by the local emergency operations center, through the state emergency operations center, following a disaster declaration by the governor.

Augmentation and Integration Models

Communities may choose from one of two models for their teams: the augmentation model and the integration model. With the augmentation model, personnel are identified as members of the team and are on call. With the integration model, personnel throughout the emergency response community are trained so that there are always enough people on duty to respond. There are MMSTs in the 120 most populated cities in the United States. Funding depends on the size of the city, but averages approximately $350,000 annually.

Focus

Consequence management focuses on measures to protect public health and safety. Efforts such as rescue and medical treatment of casualties, evacuation of people at risk, protection of first responders, and preventing the spread of contamination should be the initial focus. Focus then turns to restoring essential government services and providing emergency relief to government, businesses, and individuals affected by the consequences of terrorism.

TABLE 31-6 Federal Agencies Involved With CBRNE Response	
Agency	**Role**
Federal Emergency Management Agency (FEMA)	The lead federal agency for consequence management response.
Urban search and rescue teams	Have specialized capability for finding and extracting victims from collapsed structures.
Rapid Response Information System (RRIS)	A secure website that can be used as a research vehicle, a training aid, and an overall planning and training resource for preparing to respond to an NBC terrorism incident. The RRIS is accessible at http://rris.fema.gov. Information in the RRIS includes: • Description of federal capabilities • Description of NBC agents and their characteristics • Signs and symptoms • Safety precautions and first aid • Personal protective equipment • Generic munitions information
Metropolitan Medical Strike Team (MMST)	Part of the Metropolitan Medical Response System (MMRS). Although not a federal response agency, it receives its funding for training and equipment from the federal government. Its capabilities include agent detection and identification, patient decontamination, triage and medical treatment, patient transportation to hospitals, and coordination with local law enforcement activities. The personnel on the MMST come from the local emergency response community.
National NBC Medical Response Team (NMRT)	Composed of medical personnel; capable of agent identification, patient decontamination, triage, and medical treatment in support of local health systems. There are four NMRTs that are basically expanded DMATs. They are strategically located in Arlington, Virginia; Los Angeles, California; Denver, Colorado; and Winston-Salem, North Carolina.

(continues)

TABLE 31-6 Federal Agencies Involved With CBRNE Response (continued)

Agency	Role
Environmental Protection Agency (EPA)	Has 275 on-scene coordinators (OSCs) located throughout the United States. It is their decision as to which EPA assets to activate in response to an NBC terrorism incident.
Environmental Response Team (ERT)	Has portable chemical agent instruments capable of detecting and identifying alpha, beta, or gamma radiation in the low and sub parts per million. The teams located in Edison, New Jersey, and Cincinnati, Ohio, have monitoring and entry capability.
Radiological Emergency Response Team (RERT)	Performs radiation monitoring, radionuclide analysis, and radiation health physics and risk assessment. The team has mobile labs.
Environmental Radiation Ambient Monitoring System (ERAMS)	May be able to provide information on the spread of contamination. The EPA has two state-of-the-art radiologic laboratories. By characterizing radiation sources, they can recommend how best to protect public health. There is a lab in Las Vegas, Nevada, and one in Montgomery, Alabama.
Radiological Assistance Program (RAP) within the Department of Energy (DOE)	Provides the initial DOE radiologic emergency response. There are eight program regions under the RAP, each with multiple response RAP teams of approximately 20 people each. These teams have radiation monitoring and detection equipment to assist in identifying the presence of radioactive contamination on personnel, equipment, and property at the accident or incident scene. Some RAP teams have mobile laboratories.

National Guard WMD-CSTs

The National Guard Weapons of Mass Destruction Civil Support Teams' (WMD-CST) mission is to assemble at the designated location within 2 hours, ready to deploy anywhere within a multistate region. The teams are able to be on scene within 24 hours after being alerted. Once the team arrives on scene and has reported to the local incident commander, it will then use its expertise to:

- Detect the unknown CBRNE agent(s)
- Survey and model the hazard
- Advise the incident commander (IC)

The WMD-CST is activated directly by the state's governor. The governor also can delegate activation authority. States can agree to mutually support each other because the National Guard assets can generally be mobilized faster than Department of Defense (DoD) assets. Other DoD units are contacted as needed. The team is made up of Active Guard Reserve (AGR) Army and Air National Guard members who come from various military and civilian backgrounds. The team trains to Army and Emergency First Responder standards and works within the Incident Command System (ICS). Congress has authorized 32 WMD-CSTs. Currently there are 15 teams certified by the Secretary of Defense.

■ Summary

You have learned the meaning of CBRNE, how it relates to homeland security, and the various agencies you may come into contact with during an exercise or an actual event. As a combat medic, you will receive additional training on CBRNE and how to work with and provide medical treatment or casualty decontamination to both military and civilian casualties.

YOU ARE THE
COMBAT MEDIC

Your unit is on patrol in a deserted factory, looking for signs of insurgents. Two soldiers from your unit come across the remains of a campfire and some food debris. It's clear that someone has been in the building recently. Your unit enters further into the building to investigate. Suddenly, you hear the sound of gunfire and yelling. After a few minutes, your commander gives the all clear and then calls, "Medic."

You advance and find three soldiers and one detainee. Two soldiers are securing the detainee while PFC Smith is off to one side, leaning against a wall inside a small room. Before being captured, the detainee threw a glass bottle filled with a clear liquid. When the bottle broke, no one smelled anything. The bottle broke open right in front of PFC Smith.

PFC Smith's eyes are watering and as you approach him, he begins to retch. Immediately, you suspect that PFC Smith has been exposed to a nerve agent. You don the proper personal protective equipment before entering the small room. As you get closer to PFC Smith, you see that his pupils are constricted. This casualty needs to be decontaminated right away. You remove all clothing and equipment from the casualty and wrap him in a clean thermal blanket. You then use the supporting carry to evacuate him from the exposure area. While managing his ABCs, the casualty begins to seize. You administer the two auto-injectors in the Nerve Agent Antidote Kit and call for MEDEVAC.

1. LAST NAME, FIRST NAME Smith, Chris		RANK/GRADE PFC/E3	✓	MALE
				FEMALE
SSN 000-000-0000	SPECIALTY CODE OA			RELIGION Baptist

2. UNIT

FORCE				NATIONALITY		
A/T	AF/A	N/M	MC/M			
	BC/BC	X	NBI/BNC	DISEASE		PSYCH

3. INJURY		X	AIRWAY
FRONT BACK			HEAD
			WOUND
			NECK/BACK INJURY
			BURN
			AMPUTATION
			STRESS
			OTHER (Specify)

Exposure to _____

Nerve Agent _____

4. LEVEL OF CONSCIOUSNESS			
ALERT		PAIN RESPONSE	
VERBAL RESPONSE		X	UNRESPONSIVE

5. PULSE	TIME	6. TOURNIQUET ☐ NO ☐ YES		TIME

7. MORPHINE X NO ☐ YES	DOSE	TIME	8. IV	TIME

9. TREATMENT/OBSERVATIONS/CURRENT MEDICATION/ALLERGIES/NBC (ANTIDOTE)

Watery eyes, vomiting, miosis
No currents meds
No allergies
Exposure to sarin
Admin one NAAK 0425

10. DISPOSITION		RETURNED TO DUTY		TIME
	X	EVACUATED		0435
		DECEASED		

11. PROVIDER/UNIT Lewis, Norm	DATE (YYMMDD)

Aid Kit

Ready for Review

- CBRNE stands for:
  - Chemical agents
  - Biologic agents
  - Radiologic agents
  - Nuclear devices
  - Explosive devices
- CBRNE agents are available and relatively easy to acquire or manufacture.
  - Chemical and biologic agents can be made from readily available components by individuals with the knowledge presented in college-level science courses.
- The most common chemical agents are:
  - Nerve agents: Sarin and VX
  - Blood agents: Cyanide and chloride
  - Blister agents: Mustard and Lewisite
  - Choking agents: Phosgene and chlorine
- Biologic agents are the oldest of the nuclear, biologic, and chemical triad of weapons of mass destruction.
- Experts say there is enough material and know-how out there for a terrorist to mount a lethal radiologic attack with a dirty bomb, potentially turning a US downtown into a death zone.
- High explosives or bomb blasts may be used as the prime mechanism to disseminate NBC materials.

Vital Vocabulary

anthrax A deadly bacteria (*Bacillus anthracis*) that lays dormant in a spore (protective shell); the germ is released from the spore when exposed to the optimal temperature and moisture level. The route of entry can be inhalation, cutaneous, or gastrointestinal (from consuming food that contains spores).

CBRNE Chemical, biologic, radiologic, nuclear, and high yield explosive devices.

chlorine (CL) The first chemical agent ever used in warfare. It has a distinct odor of bleach, and creates a green haze when released as a gas. Initially it produces upper airway irritation and a choking sensation.

cyanide A chemical agent that affects the body's ability to use oxygen. It is a colorless gas that has an odor similar to almonds. The effects begin on the cellular level and are very rapidly seen at the organ system level.

G agents Early nerve agents that were developed by German scientists in the period after WWI and into WWII. There are three such agents: sarin, soman, and tabun.

LD$_{50}$ The amount of an agent or substance that will kill 50% of people who are exposed to it.

Lewisite (L) A blister agent that has a rapid onset of symptoms and produces immediate intense pain and discomfort on contact.

miosis Bilateral pinpoint-constricted pupils.

mutagen A substance that mutates, damages, and changes the structures of DNA in the body's cells.

nerve agent antidote kit (NAAK) Contains two auto-injector medications, atropine and 2-PAM chloride (pralidoxime chloride).

nerve agents A class of chemical called organophosphates; they function by blocking an essential enzyme in the nervous system, which causes the body's organs to become overstimulated and burn out.

off-gassing The emitting of an agent after exposure, for example from a person's clothes that have been exposed to the agent.

phosgene A chemical agent that causes severe pulmonary damage.

phosgene oxime (CX) A chemical blister agent that has a rapid onset of symptoms and produces immediate intense pain and discomfort on contact.

sarin (GB) A nerve agent that is one of the G agents; a highly volatile colorless and odorless liquid that turns from liquid to gas within seconds to minutes at room temperature.

smallpox A highly contagious biologic disease; it is most contagious when blisters begin to form.

soman (GD) A nerve agent that is one of the G agents; twice as persistent as sarin and five times as lethal; it has a fruity odor, as a result of the type of alcohol used in the agent, and is both a contact and inhalation hazard that can enter the body through skin absorption and through the respiratory tract.

sulfur mustard (H) A vesicant chemical agent; it is a brownish-yellowish oily substance that is generally considered very persistent; it has the distinct smell of garlic or mustard and, when released, is quickly absorbed into the skin and/or mucous membranes and begins an irreversible process of damaging the cells.

tabun (GA) A nerve agent that is one of the G agents; it is 36 times more persistent than sarin and approximately half as lethal; it has a fruity smell and is unique because the components used to manufacture the agent are easy to acquire and the agent is easy to manufacture.

V agent (VX) One of the G agents; it is a clear, oily agent that has no odor and looks like baby oil; it is over 100 times more lethal than sarin and is extremely persistent.

vectors Objects used to transfer the agent from the point of release to the target.

vesicants Blister agents; the primary route of entry for vesicants is through the skin.

COMBAT MEDIC *in Action*

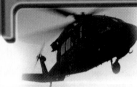

Your unit is on a mission to capture a high-ranking operative. This operative is suspected of being a chemical weapons expert who is only too willing to sell his knowledge to the highest bidder. Your unit receives a tip that he is operating in a water treatment plant on the outskirts of town. Your unit tracks the operative down and captures him in a small office. While the rest of your unit provides cover, two soldiers secure the detainee. A familiar smell lingers in the air, but you cannot immediately place it. While the detainee is being secured, one soldier begins to cough violently. "I can't breathe," he gasps. Now you know what the smell reminds you of—a swimming pool.

1. What could be causing the casualty to cough?
   A. Sarin
   B. Phosgene
   C. Chlorine
   D. VX

2. What is your primary concern for this casualty?
   A. Watery eyes
   B. Seizure
   C. Pulmonary edema
   D. Hypovolemic shock

3. Which mnemonic is used in the diagnosis of a nerve agent?
   A. ABC
   B. NAAK
   C. SLUDGEM
   D. ABCDE

4. Which medication will you administer to this casualty?
   A. NAAK
   B. 2-PAM
   C. Morphine
   D. Bronchodilators

5. True or false? Never intubate a casualty exposed to a choking agent, you could damage the airway.
   A. True
   B. False

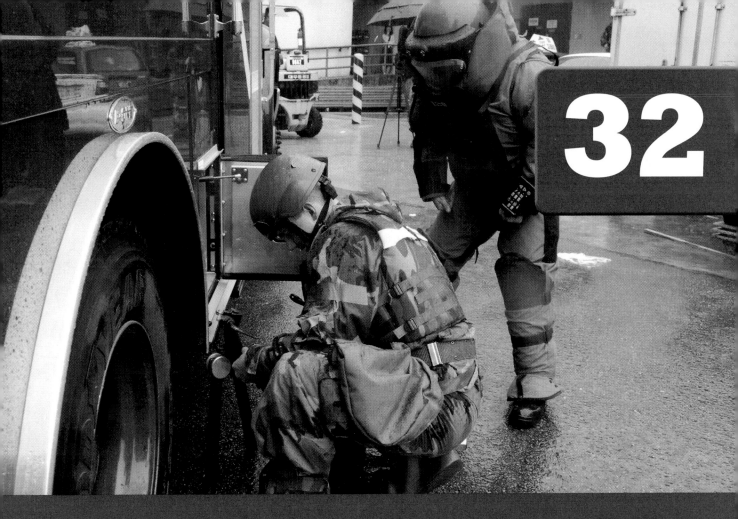

CBRNE Equipment Overview

32

Objectives

Knowledge Objectives
- [ ] Describe the individual protective equipment used in CBRNE incidents.
- [ ] Describe the individual decontamination equipment used in CBRNE incidents.
- [ ] Describe the patient protective equipment used in CBRNE incidents.
- [ ] Describe the detection equipment and alarm systems used in CBRNE incidents.

Introduction

During World Wars I and II, biologic and chemical agents were available and were used. In the decades since, many developed countries and developing countries have achieved the capability to produce both biologic and chemical agents. As a direct result of this, equipment was developed to protect the soldier who may encounter these substances on the battlefield. As a combat medic, it is important for you to know the type of equipment available for chemical protection, detection, and treatment in accordance with FM 3-11.4: *Multiservice TTP for Nuclear, Biological, and Chemical (NBC) Protection* and the *US Army Medical Research Institute of Chemical Defense (USAMRICD) Field Management of Chemical Casualties Handbook*.

Individual Protective Equipment

All soldiers deploying to the battlefield are issued standard A chemical defense equipment to protect them on the integrated battlefield. This equipment includes:

- Chemical protective overgarment
- Chemical protective gloves
- Chemical protective overboots
- Chemical protective mask

The Battle Dress Overgarment

The **battle dress overgarment (BDO)** was issued to all US Army units for chemical protection; however, it is no longer in production and is scheduled for replacement. BDO consists of a pair of trousers and a jacket with a charcoal liner. The outer cloth, made of a 50/50 blend of nylon/cotton, is specially treated with a Scotchgard-type treatment to resist liquid chemical agents **FIGURE 32-1 ▸**. Chemical protective overboots, standard butyl rubber gloves, and glove liners are additional equipment items in the BDO. The BDO adds approximately 11 lb (size medium) to the weight already carried by the soldier.

Once removed from the protective package, which is an uncontaminated environment, the BDO is viable for a maximum of 30 days; however, the unit commander may decide to extend the wear of the BDO past the 30 days. Once exposed to a chemically contaminated environment, the BDO must be replaced within 24 hours.

The Joint Service Lightweight Integrated Suit Technology

The **Joint Service lightweight integrated suit technology (JSLIST)** overgarment **FIGURE 32-2 ▸** is designed to replace the US Army's BDO. As the name suggests, the JSLIST also replaces the US Navy's Chemical Protection Overgarment (CPO) and the US Marine Corps' Saratoga. The JSLIST consists of a pair of trousers and a jacket with an integral hood with a charcoal-impregnated polyurethane foam liner. The outer cloth is made of a 50/50 blend of nylon and cotton with a poplin ripstop. It is also treated with a Scotchgard-type treatment to resist liquid chemical agents. Multipurpose overboots (MULO), standard butyl rubber gloves, and glove liners

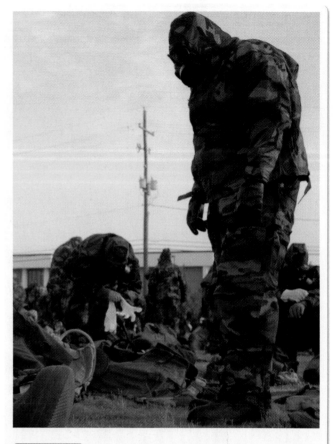

FIGURE 32-1   Battle dress overgarment.

Field Medical Care TIPS

Wearing of the BDO and JSLIST adds 10°F to 15°F to the ambient temperature. Caution must be taken in warmer climates because of the potential for heat-related injuries.

are additional pieces of equipment in the JSLIST. The BDO adds approximately 6 lb (size medium) to the weight already carried by the soldier.

The JSLIST is durable for up to 45 days with up to six launderings and is durable up to 120 days without laundering. Once exposed to a chemical environment, the JSLIST must be replaced within 24 hours.

Chemical Boots

The green vinyl overboot (GVO) or the black vinyl overboot (BVO) is worn with the BDO, over the combat boots to protect feet from contamination by all known agents, vectors, and radiologic particles **FIGURE 32-3 ▸**. In an uncontaminated environment, the boots are good for 14 days. Once inspected for serviceability, the boots may be worn 14 days more if they are found to be serviceable. The multipurpose overboot (MULO) is good for 60 days in an uncontaminated

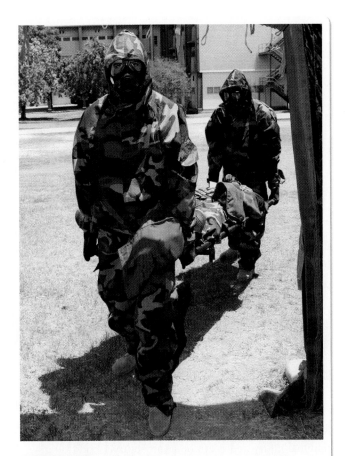

FIGURE 32-2 The Joint Service lightweight integrated suit technology (JSLIST) overgarment.

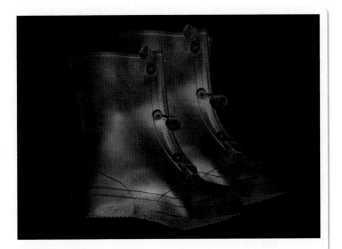

FIGURE 32-3 The green vinyl overboot (GVO) or the black vinyl overboot (BVO) are worn with the BDO.

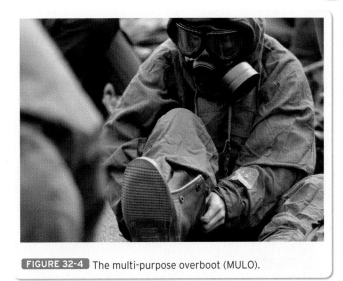

FIGURE 32-4 The multi-purpose overboot (MULO).

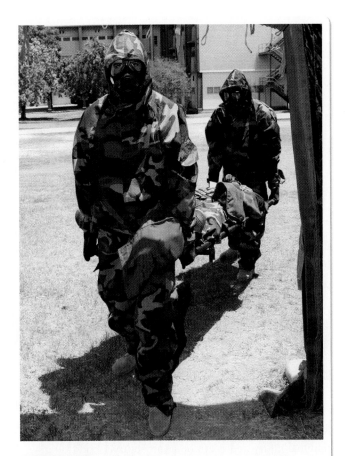

FIGURE 32-5 Chemical protective gloves.

Field Medical Care **TIPS**

The JSLIST Block 1 Glove Upgrade Program is seeking an interim glove to replace the current butyl rubber glove.

Chemical Protective Gloves

Chemical protective gloves are made of butyl rubber with an inner glove made of thin white cotton for use with both the BDO and the JSLIST **FIGURE 32-5 ▲**. These gloves offer no protection against cold weather injuries. In an uncontaminated environment, the gloves can be worn as long as they remain serviceable. In a contaminated environment, the gloves can be worn up to 24 hours. After 24 hours, inspect the gloves, and if they are serviceable, decontaminate the gloves and reuse them. You may repeat this process every 24 hours.

environment **FIGURE 32-4 ▶**. Once inspected for serviceability, the boots may be worn 60 days more if they are found to be serviceable. Both the GVO/BVO and MULO are to be replaced 24 hours after exposure to a contaminated environment. Once inspected and decontaminated, the boots may be worn 24 hours more if they are found to be serviceable.

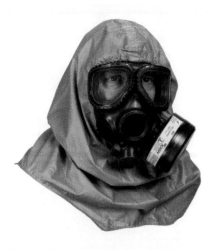

FIGURE 32-6   Chemical protective mask M40A1.

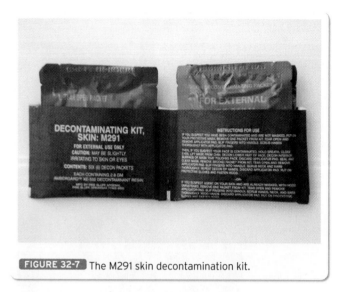

FIGURE 32-7   The M291 skin decontamination kit.

Chemical Protective Mask: M40A1

The M40-series protective masks replaced the M17-series protective mask as the standard Army field mask. The M40A1 is the mask issued to dismounted soldiers and is available in small, medium, and large sizes FIGURE 32-6 ▲. It is designed to protect the wearer from all known chemical, biologic, and riot-control agents (RCA).

The mask consists of a silicone rubber face piece with an in-turned peripheral face seal, a binocular rigid eye lens system, and an elastic head harness. Other features include front and side voicemitters allowing for better communication, particularly when operating FM communications; a drink tube for a drinking capability while being worn; clear and tinted inserts; and a filter canister with NATO-standard threads.

The mask uses a NATO-standard external filter canister with an armor quick disconnect (AQD) for easy change-out. The filter canister may be positioned on the soldier's right or left cheek to allow him or her to fire the M16A2/M4A1 rifles. The filter cannot be exchanged in a contaminated environment. The only optical insert approved for use in the M40A1 mask is a wire-frame type insert.

The M40A1 mask can be worn continuously for 8 to 12 hours and, when worn properly, it will provide protection for the face, eyes, and respiratory tract. While in the theater of operations, filters must be replaced at least every 30 days. The filters must also be replaced whenever any of the following occurs:

- The elements are immersed in water.
- The elements are crushed, cut, or damaged.
- Excessive breathing resistance is encountered.
- After exposure to hydrogen cyanide (blood-type agents).
- When ordered by the unit commander.

■ Individual Decontamination Equipment

The most important and most effective decontamination of any chemical exposure is the self-decontamination done within the first minute or two after exposure. This early action

Field Medical Care TIPS

Protective masks designed for use in tanks and combat vehicles (M40A2) and aircraft (M45) are issued as required.

by the soldier will make the difference between survival or minimal injury and death or severe injury. Good training will always save lives. A soldier operating in a chemically contaminated environment must be able to decontaminate his or her skin and individual equipment.

The M25SA1 personal decontaminating kit, fielded in 1981, provided a skin decontamination capability. With this kit, the soldier's ability to decontaminate his or her individual equipment was still limited. In 1987, the M280 decontamination kit, individual equipment (DKIE) was fielded. The DKIE had various problems, the most significant being that it interfered with the chemical agent monitor (CAM). In November 1989, the US Army adopted the **M291 skin decontamination kit (SDK)**.

The M291 skin decontamination kit consists of a wallet-like carrying pouch containing six individual decontamination packets FIGURE 32-7 ▲, enough to perform three complete skin decontaminations. Each packet contains an applicator pad filled with decontamination powder containing activated resins to absorb and neutralize liquid chemicals on the skin. The operating temperatures are –50°F to 120°F and the storage temperatures are –60°F to 160°F. The M291 allows you to completely decontaminate your skin through physical removal, absorption, and neutralization of toxic agents with no long-term harmful effects. This item is for external use only; it may be slightly irritating to eyes or skin. Be sure to keep the decontamination powder out of eyes, cuts, or wounds, and avoid inhalation of the powder. One applicator pad will decontaminate both hands and face, if necessary.

The purpose of the **M295 decontamination kit, individual equipment (DKIE)** is to decontaminate personal protec-

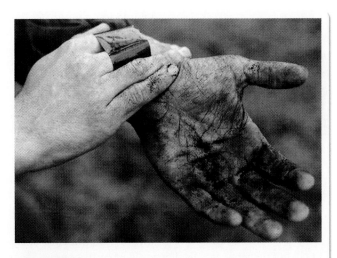

FIGURE 32-8 The M295 decontamination kit, individual equipment (DKIE).

tive equipment such as the M16A2/M4A1, Kevlar helmet, load-bearing equipment (LBE), and M40-series protective mask **FIGURE 32-8▲**. The M295 was developed to replace the M258A1 and M280 decontamination kits. The M295 consists of a kit containing four sealed pouches, each containing an individual wipe-down mitt. Each wipe-down mitt is composed of a decontamination powder contained within a pad material and a polyethylene film backing. The substance found in the mitt is the same substance found in the M291. Two packets are normally required to completely decontaminate all of a soldier's personal equipment, including his or her weapon.

■ Patient Protective Equipment

The purpose of the **patient protective wrap (PPW)** is to protect the patient during evacuation after the BDO or JSLIST has been removed and the casualty has received medical treatment. Medical doctrine calls for the treatment as far forward as possible of casualties from the integrated battlefield. Because treatment will often mandate removal of the BDO or JSLIST and precludes donning replacement chemical protec-

tive gear, the PPW was developed. This wrap protects the casualty from all known chemical agents for up to 6 continuous hours. It is not designed for use by more than one casualty and must be discarded after use.

The protective mask is not needed while the casualty is in the PPW, but should be evacuated with the casualty. Easy casualty insertion into the wrap is provided by one continuous zipper around the outer edge of the top sheet, and observation of the casualty is possible through an impermeable transparent window at the head of the wrap. Below the window, a small transparent pocket is large enough to hold a field medical card or other medical record, and two protected sleeves next to the window permit the passage of IV tubing. The wrap is designed to be used on a litter but can itself become a field-expedient litter if necessary. Along the sides of the wrap are sleeves through which poles can be inserted; these sleeves have handholds for manual carries when poles are not available.

Decontaminable Litter

Contaminated casualties arriving at a medical treatment location will in most cases require decontamination prior to definitive treatment. The **decontaminable litter** was developed to replace the canvas litters **FIGURE 32-9▶**. This litter is made from a monofilament polypropylene honeycomb fabric that does not absorb liquid chemical agents and is not degraded by decontaminating solutions.

The decontaminable litter's carrying handles retract into the metal pole frame, to allow for loading the litter onto the UH-60 helicopter. The handles have two open positions: the first position is a NATO standard and the second position was provided to allow increased gripping comfort by litter bearers.

The purpose of the **resuscitation device, individual chemical (RDIC)** is to ventilate an apneic patient while they are in Mission Oriented Protective Posture (MOPP-4). The RDIC is a ventilatory system comprised of:

- A compressible butyl rubber bag
- A NATO-standard C2 canister filter
- A nonrebreathing valve
- A cricothyroid cannula adapter
- A flexible hose connected to an oropharyngeal mask

The mask is removable from the distal end of the flexible hose for connection of the hose to the cannula adapter. The

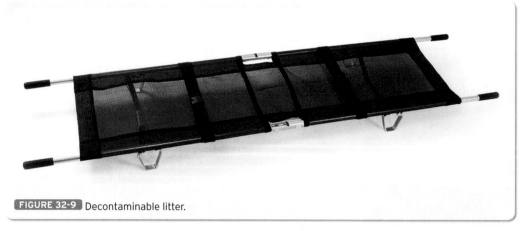

FIGURE 32-9 Decontaminable litter.

Garrison Care TIPS

Resuscitation device, individual chemical (RDIC); NSN: 6665-01-338-6602.

butyl rubber bag resists the penetration of liquid chemical agents that may be on the chemical protective gloves of the combat medic, and is easily decontaminated. The device will deliver up to 600 mL of filtered air per cycle at a rate of 30 cycles per minute.

■ Detection Equipment and Alarm Systems

The purpose of **M8 chemical agent detector paper** is to detect both the presence and specific type of liquid chemical agents. M8 paper is used to test liquid substances for the presence of nerve agents and blister agents. It is similar to the litmus (pH) paper that is found in almost any laboratory in that a test result is indicated in both types of paper by a change in color. The difference is that M8 paper is specifically designed to react to nerve agents and blister agents in liquid form.

Every soldier carries one booklet of M8 paper in the interior pocket of the M40-series protective mask carrier. To use the M8 paper, half of a sheet is blotted onto an unknown liquid. After waiting for 30 seconds, the color change is compared to the colors inside the front cover of the booklet:

- **Yellow:** G (nerve agent)
- **Red:** H (blister agent)
- **Olive green or black:** V (nerve agent)

A false positive may be seen if the M8 paper is exposed to liquid insecticide, antifreeze, or petroleum products, and con-

Garrison Care TIPS

M8 chemical agent detector paper; NSN: 6665-00-050-8529.

tamination should be confirmed with other detection equipment.

The purpose of **M9 chemical agent detector paper** is to detect the presence of liquid chemical agents; however, it will not identify the specific type of agent. M9 paper was developed to enable soldiers to detect nerve and blister agents. It is placed on personnel and equipment to identify the presence of liquid chemical agent aerosols. Each soldier carries one 30′-long by 2″-wide roll of M9 paper. It contains a suspension of an agent-sensitive red indicator dye that will turn a pink, red, reddish brown, or red-purple when exposed to liquid nerve agents and blister agents.

While wearing gloves, one strip is wrapped around the upper arm, the opposite wrist, and then the ankle of the same side as the upper arm, creating a V-shape. After seeing the color change, the soldier must immediately mask, alert others, and, if warranted, proceed with skin decontamination.

Field Medical Care TIPS

False positives may be seen if the M9 paper is exposed to liquid insecticides, antifreeze, or petroleum products. Confirm contamination with other chemical detection equipment.

Field Medical Care TIPS

M9 paper is potentially carcinogenic; therefore, it should not be allowed to come into direct contact with the skin.

Garrison Care TIPS

M9 chemical agent detector paper; NSN: 6665-01-226-5589.

The purpose of the **M256A1 chemical agent detector kit** is to detect and identify chemical agents. The M256A1 chemical agent detector kit entered into military service in 1978. It is used to detect and identify blood, blister, and nerve agents present either as liquid or as vapor. It may also be used for the following:

- To determine when it is safe to unmask
- To locate and identify chemical hazards (reconnaissance)

- To monitor decontamination effectiveness

The M256A1 chemical agent detector kit consists of:

- A plastic carrying case (with nylon strap/belt attachment).
- One booklet of M8 paper (to detect chemical agents in liquid form).
- Twelve disposable sampler-detectors, individually sealed (which detect chemical agents in vapor form). Each sampler-detector contains six crushable ampoules, two crushable heater ampoules, one Lewisite test tablet, a protective strip, and heater pads.
- One set of instruction cards, attached by a lanyard to the carrying case.

A complete test using both the M8 paper and the detector ticket takes approximately 20 minutes to perform. The test kit should not be performed in direct sunlight, because this speeds the evaporation of the reagents. The actual sampler-detectors for the M256A1 are possibly carcinogenic; therefore, trainer sampler-detectors are provided for practical exercises. The vapors from the actual kit are also toxic; a mask and gloves should be worn when using this kit. The M256A1 training devices contain pre-engineered sampler-detectors that show color changes comparable to those seen when the M256A1 detector kit is used in clean or contaminated environments.

> **Garrison Care TIPS**
>
> M256A1 chemical agent detector kit; NSN: 6665-01-133-4964 and M256A1 SIM chemical agent detector kit (tickets) NSN: 6665-01-112-1644.

The purpose of the **chemical agent monitor (CAM)** is to detect nerve and blister agents in vapor form only. It takes in vapors and analyzes the airborne molecules. The CAM is a hand-held device that detects agent vapors drawn by the pump into the sampling chamber of the instrument. The inlet port must not come into contact with a suspected area of evaporating agent on a surface but must nevertheless approach within a few inches of the site of suspected contamination. The CAM displays the intensity of the vapor as a bar code on the front of the CAM, from 1 (low concentration) to 8 (very high concentration).

The purpose of the **improved chemical agent monitor (ICAM)** is to detect chemical agents on personnel and equipment. The ICAM starts up more rapidly and is considered 300% more reliable than the CAM with a 10 times faster start-up time. Its characteristics include:

- Detects G and H agents
- Instantaneous feedback of chemical hazard level

> **Garrison Care TIPS**
>
> Chemical agent monitor: NSN: 6665-01-199-4153.

- Reduces the need for decontamination operations
- Real-time detection of nerve and blister agents.

Operators of these devices should be in MOPP-4.

The purpose of the **M8A1 automatic chemical agent alarm (ACAA)** is to sample the air for the presence of nerve agent vapors only. The M8A1 is the only remote continuous air sampling alarm that the US Army currently possesses. This alarm will sample the air for the presence of the following nerve agent vapors only: GA, GB, GD, and VX. The ACAA detects airborne agent molecules drawn into the sampling chamber by a pump. The operator may specify whether the alarm itself is audible, visual, or both. The system consists of an M43A1 detector and an M42 alarm. The M43A1 is the portion that actually detects the vapor agent. The M42 alarm is connected by WD-1 telephone wire to the M43A1 detector unit. One M43A1 can have as many as five M42 alarms attached.

The M8A1 can be located within a fixed facility. The M43A1 detectors are placed facing into the wind no more than 150 meters outside the unit perimeter, with no more than 300 meters between detectors and, when possible, no more than 400 meters between the detector cells and the alarm units.

> **Garrison Care TIPS**
>
> M8A1 automatic chemical agent alarm; NSN: 6665-01-105-5623.

The purpose of the **M22 automatic chemical agent detection alarm (ACADA)** is to provide detection and warning for nerve and blister agents. The M22 ACADA system is capable of detecting and identifying standard blister and nerve agent vapors simultaneously. The system is soldier-portable, operates with no human interface after system start-up, and provides an audio and visual alarm. It can operate in both hot and cold climates: −30°F to 125°F. The M22 ACADA consists of:

- An M88 detector
- A self-contained alarm and/or remote alarm
- Up to five M42 alarm units

The M22 ACADA is designed to complement the currently fielded M8A1 detector and is deployed in the same manner.

■ Summary

You will either come in contact with or utilize CBRNE equipment while caring for casualties in a contaminated environment, on the integrated battlefield. It is imperative that, for the protection of both you and the casualty, proper methods for wearing and/or operating CBRNE equipment are clearly understood and trained with routinely.

YOU ARE THE
COMBAT MEDIC

It is 0900 hours on a warm and windy morning. You are on sick call in the Battalion Aid Station when a report changes your mission. An unidentified liquid spill has been found in one of the showers. A soldier performing routine maintenance has been exposed. You don your full protective gear and report to the scene. While other combat medics ensure that no one enters the potential hot zone without wearing the proper equipment, you enter the scene.

Assessment

One casualty is sitting on the floor, coughing. "Are you all right?" you ask. You notice that the skin on his hands and forearms is gray.

The casualty coughs, but manages to say, "I'm all right, ma'am." Since the casualty can speak, you know that his airway is patent, for now.

In order to properly decontaminate and treat the casualty, you need to know what you are dealing with. You notice that there is a trail of liquid on the casualty's shirt. Using M8 paper, you test the liquid. After 30 seconds, the paper turns red. Now you know that the casualty has been exposed to a blister agent. You need to get him decontaminated and treated.

"Can you walk?" you ask the casualty. He nods and puts his arm around your shoulder. Using the supporting carry, you evacuate him to the decontamination station where he is thoroughly decontaminated before intubation and IV access are initiated.

1. LAST NAME, FIRST NAME O'Brian, Rory		RANK/GRADE Private E-2	X	MALE	
SSN 000-111-0000	SPECIALTY CODE OA			FEMALE	
				RELIGION Catholic	

2. UNIT

FORCE				NATIONALITY	
A/T	AF/A	N/M	MC/M		
	BC/BC		NBI/BNC	DISEASE	PSYCH

3. INJURY

X	AIRWAY	
	HEAD	
	WOUND	
	NECK/BACK INJURY	
X	BURN	
	AMPUTATION	
	STRESS	
X	OTHER (Specify)	

FRONT   BACK

Exposure to _____

blister agent _____

4. LEVEL OF CONSCIOUSNESS

X	ALERT		PAIN RESPONSE	
	VERBAL RESPONSE		UNRESPONSIVE	

5. PULSE 70 bpm	TIME 0930	6. TOURNIQUET [X] NO [ ] YES		TIME	

7. MORPHINE [X] NO [ ] YES	DOSE	TIME	8. IV ✓	TIME 0935

9. TREATMENT/OBSERVATIONS/CURRENT MEDICATION/ALLERGIES/NBC (ANTIDOTE)

Found coughing with gray skin on hands and forearms.
No current medications, sulfa allergies.

10. DISPOSITION	RETURNED TO DUTY		TIME	
	X	EVACUATED	0945	
		DECEASED		

11. PROVIDER/UNIT Rhodri, Morgan	DATE (YYMMDD)

Aid Kit

Ready for Review

- All soldiers deploying to the battlefield are issued standard A chemical defense equipment to protect the soldier on the integrated battlefield. This equipment includes:
  - Chemical protective overgarment
  - Chemical protective gloves
  - Chemical protective overboots
  - Chemical protective mask
- The most important and most effective decontamination of any chemical exposure is the self-decontamination done within the first minute or two after exposure.
  - This early action by the soldier will make the difference between survival or minimal injury and death or severe injury.
- The purpose of the patient protective wrap (PPW) is to protect the patient during evacuation after the BDO or JSLIST has been removed and the casualty has received medical treatment.
- The detection agents carried by soldiers include:
  - M8 chemical agent detector paper
  - M9 chemical agent detector paper
  - M256A1 chemical agent detector kit
  - Chemical agent monitor (CAM)
  - Improved chemical agent monitor (ICAM)
  - M8A1 automatic chemical agent alarm (ACAA)
  - M22 automatic chemical agent detection alarm (ACADA)

Vital Vocabulary

battle dress overgarment (BDO) Former chemical protection equipment for the US Army.

chemical agent monitor (CAM) Used to detect nerve and blister agents in vapor form only.

decontaminable litter Developed to replace canvas litters; designed not to absorb liquid chemical agents and is not degraded by decontaminating solutions.

improved chemical agent monitor (ICAM) Detects chemical agents on personnel and equipment.

Joint Service lightweight integrated suit technology (JSLIST) Chemical protection equipment designed to replace the US Army's BDO, the US Navy's chemical protection overgarment (CPO), and US Marine Corp's Saratoga.

M22 automatic chemical agent detection alarm (ACADA) Provides detection and warning for nerve and blister agents.

M256A1 chemical agent detector kit Used to detect and identify blood, blister, and nerve agents present either as a liquid or as a vapor.

M291 skin decontamination kit (SDK) Used to decontaminate the skin; a wallet-like carrying pouch containing six individual decontamination packets.

M295 decontamination kit, individual equipment (DKIE) Used to decontaminate personal protective equipment.

M8 chemical agent detector paper Used to detect both the presence and the specific type of liquid chemical agents.

M8A1 automatic chemical agent alarm (ACAA) Samples the air for the presence of nerve agent vapors only.

M9 chemical agent detector paper Used to detect the presence of liquid chemical agents, but does not identify the specific type of agent.

patient protective wrap (PPW) Used to protect the patient during evacuation after the BDO or JSLIST has been removed and the casualty has received medical treatment.

Resuscitation device, individual chemical (RDIC) Used to ventilate an apneic patient while the patient is in MOPP-4.

COMBAT MEDIC *in Action*

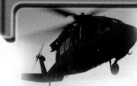

It is a very hot afternoon. You haven't experienced this kind of intense heat since your 68W training. It feels like you are in the middle of a brick oven. The sound of a siren interrupts your thoughts of a nice, cold lemonade. There has been a suspected chemical attack on one of the barracks. You immediately don JSLIST, chemical protective gloves, and the M40A1. Now you are ready to respond to the scene. If you were not hot before, you will be now in all of this protective gear.

1. Wearing of JSLIST adds about _____ °F to _____ °F to the ambient temperature.
   A. 5 to 10
   B. 25 to 30
   C. 15 to 20
   D. 10 to 15

2. The M40A1 is designed to protect against:
   A. all known chemical, biologic, and riot control agents.
   B. all known nerve agents.
   C. all known chemical and nerve agents.
   D. all known biologic agents.

3. The M40AI can be worn continuously for:
   A. 4 to 8 hours.
   B. 24 to 48 hours.
   C. 8 to 12 hours.
   D. 12 to 24 hours.

4. The M256A1 chemical agent detector kit can detect and identify chemical agents and may also be used to:
   A. determine if it is safe to unmask.
   B. locate and identify chemical hazards.
   C. monitor decontamination.
   D. all of the above.

5. The M8A1 automatic chemical agent alarm can detect and identify:
   A. sarin only.
   B. all nerve agents.
   C. GA, GB, GD, and VX only.
   D. chlorine and phosgene only.

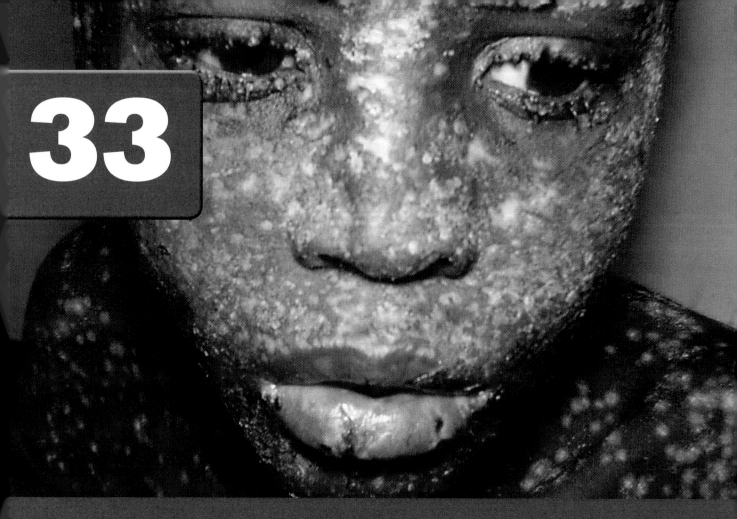

33

Nerve Agents

Objectives

Knowledge Objectives
- [ ] Describe nerve agents.
- [ ] Describe the characteristics of nerve agents.
- [ ] Describe the effects of nerve agents.
- [ ] Describe the treatment steps for nerve agents.
- [ ] Describe the pretreatment for a nerve agent incident.

Introduction

Human beings have always searched for more powerful weapons, whether it is a bigger rock to throw, a better quality bow, or a more powerful bomb. Chemical weapons have been around in less sophisticated forms for decades. They were used extensively in World War I in the form of simple gases such as chlorine and mustard. Today's current crop of chemical weapons are far more dangerous. Among the most dangerous chemical weapons are nerve agents. Nerve agents acquired their name because they affect the transmission of nerve impulses in the nervous system. Nerve agents can be manufactured by fairly simple chemical techniques. The raw materials are inexpensive and readily available. This makes them even more dangerous because they can be made by any irresponsible mind with a laboratory.

Overview of Nerve Agents

Modern **nerve agents** were first developed before World War II in Germany. Germany had stockpiles of nerve agent munitions during World War II, but did not use them for reasons that remain unclear. In the closing days of the war, the United States and its allies discovered these stockpiles, developed these nerve agents, and manufactured their own stockpiles. The United States' nerve agent stockpile contains the agents **sarin (GB)** and the **V agent (VX)** **FIGURE 33-1 ◀**.

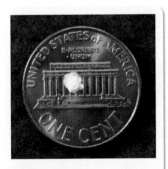

FIGURE 33-1 VX is the most toxic chemical ever produced. The dot on the penny demonstrates the amount needed to achieve a lethal dose.

Nerve agents are considered to be military threat agents. The only known battlefield use of nerve agents was during the Iran-Iraq conflict of 1980 to 1988. Intelligence analysts indicate, however, that many countries have the technology to manufacture nerve agent munitions. In addition, terrorist groups have manufactured and used nerve agents against the public. On March 20, 1995, a Japanese terrorist cult dispersed the sarin nerve agent in a Tokyo subway, which killed 10 people and injured 5,000.

Nerve agents are the most toxic of the currently known chemical agents. They are hazardous in their liquid and vapor states and can cause death within minutes after exposure. Nerve agents can be dispersed from missiles, rockets, bombs, howitzer shells, spray tanks, land mines, and other large munitions.

Actions

Nerve agents inhibit the enzyme **acetylcholinesterase (AChE)**, which is an enzyme present in various body tissues such as muscles, nerve cells, and red blood cells. Inhibition of AChE results in excess acetylcholine in the body at neuromuscular junctions. Nerve impulses originate from the brain and travel as an electrical signal to a target organ to result in a specific action. For example, a motor nerve that innervates skeletal muscle, such as the biceps muscle will cause it to contract. The nerve that stimulates the biceps muscle ends just before reaching the muscle. This electrical signal from the brain stimulates the release of acetylcholine at the end of the nerve. Acetylcholine travels across the synapse or gap between the nerve and the targeted muscle (the biceps) and binds to receptor sites on the muscle. This chemical bond results in the continuation of an electrical impulse across the nerve of the bicep muscle, causing the muscle to contract. For the muscle to stop contracting, acetylcholine must be removed from the receptor sites. This is the job of the enzyme AChE, which removes the acetylcholine from the receptor site and, as a result, prevents further stimulation of the biceps muscle.

Nerve agents bind to part of the AChE molecule. This makes AChE inactive and blocks the action of AChE; therefore, there is no way to stop the action of acetylcholine. Acetylcholine then builds up in the nerve endings and continues to act. In the case of skeletal muscle, the muscles continue to contract because of continued stimulation, causing convulsions. In the case of smooth muscle, the targeted organs continue to contract; for example, sweat glands and salivary glands continue to secrete fluids. Also the smooth muscle of the bowels and urinary tract are continually stimulated, causing them to overact. Glands, such as sweat glands and salivary glands, remain stimulated and continue to secrete fluids. This is why casualties from severe nerve agent exposure have convulsions and fluids are released from every possible location of their bodies (urine, feces, sweat, and saliva). The heart rate in these casualties will also decrease due to overstimulation of the vagus nerve.

Nerve Agent Characteristics

Nerve agents remain in a liquid state unless exposed to extreme cold or heat. Extreme heat will cause the liquid to become a vapor. The volatility of a nerve agent ranges from highly volatile (vapor) to little volatility (liquid or oily state). Nerve agents range in color from clear to light brown and are odorless.

Following release of nerve agents into the air, people may be exposed through skin contact or eye contact, or by breathing air that contains the nerve agent. Some nerve agents can mix with water or foods. Clothing can spread a nerve agent for about 30 minutes after contact, so this could easily lead to the exposure of the nerve agent to masses of people.

Field Medical Care **TIPS**

Sarin is heavier than air, so it sinks to lower lying areas and creates a greater vapor exposure there. Beware of valleys, basements, and subway systems.

◼ Effects of Nerve Agents

The initial effect of exposure to a nerve agent depends on the dosage and the route of exposure. The initial effects from a sublethal amount of nerve agent by vapor exposure are different than the initial effects from a similar amount of liquid nerve agent on the skin.

The levels of exposure range from mild to severe. Mild exposure to small amounts of nerve agent vapor usually cause effects in the eyes, nose, and airway. These effects are from local contact with the vapor, and there may not be a systemic absorption of the nerve agent. A small amount of liquid agent on the skin will cause a systemic effect in the gastrointestinal system. Mild exposure effects include:

- A runny nose worse than a cold or hay fever may be the first indication of nerve agent vapor exposure.
- Frontal headache and eye pain.
- Difficulty in seeing and dimness of vision due to miosis/pupillary constriction. Miosis is usually bilateral in an unprotected individual, but may be unilateral in a masked person with a leak in his or her mask eyepiece.
- Tightness in the chest or difficulty breathing.
- Excessive flow of saliva (drooling).
- Localized sweating at the exposure site.
- Muscular twitching at the exposure site.

With a severe exposure, the signs and symptoms of mild nerve agent exposure may occur. Nausea and vomiting are early signs of liquid exposure on the skin. Diarrhea occurs with exposure to larger amounts of the nerve agent. Severe muscular twitching occurs due to stimulation of the skeletal muscle. After an exposure to a large amount of the nerve agent, fatigue and weakness of the muscles occurs followed by muscle flaccidity. Seizures also can occur. There may be a loss of bowel and bladder control. The casualty may display confused behavior, which may be followed by loss of consciousness. Cessation of respiration occurs within minutes after the exposure to a large amount of nerve agent. Death is usually the result of complete respiratory system failure.

The effects from nerve agent vapor exposure begin within seconds to several minutes after exposure. Loss of consciousness and seizures occur within a minute of exposure. There is no delay period in onset from vapor exposure. Effects from a nerve agent liquid exposure may have a delay in symptoms from 1 to 30 minutes in a large exposure. In a small exposure, the onset of effects may be delayed as long as 18 hours after contact. Generally, the longer the interval, the less severe are the effects to the casualty.

◼ Nerve Agent Treatment

Self-Aid

To perform self-aid, first put on your protective mask and hood. The protective mask and hood protect the face and neck, eyes, mouth, and respiratory tract against nerve agent spray, vapor, and aerosol. Give the alarm for a chemical agent exposure. Perform a hasty self-evaluation for signs and symptoms of nerve agent poisoning and administer an antidote to yourself if signs and/or symptoms are present.

Use one **nerve agent antidote kit (NAAK)** auto-injector set **FIGURE 33-2 ▶**. You should never administer more than one NAAK to yourself. If you have the mental capacity to consider whether you may need more than one NAAK, then you are not experiencing anything more than symptoms of mild exposure.

Alternately, one antidote treatment, nerve agent auto-injector (ATNAA) may be administered **FIGURE 33-3 ▶**. As with the NAAK, you should never administer more than one ATNAA to yourself. Decontaminate your skin if necessary by using the M291 skin decontamination kit. Put on your remaining protective clothing (MOPP level 4) because liquid nerve agents penetrate ordinary clothing rapidly. Seek buddy-aid or medical care.

Each NAAK auto-injector set contains 2.1 mg of atropine, which blocks the effects of acetylcholine and produces relief from most symptoms. A 2-mg IM injection of atropine will be effective in 3 to 10 minutes. NAAK also contains 600 mg (2 mL) of pralidoxime chloride (2-PAM-Cl). 2-PAM-Cl increases the effectiveness of the atropine drug therapy. The role of 2-PAM-Cl is to block and reverse the bonding of the nerve agent to the nerve agent receptor. Think of 2-PAM-Cl as a crowbar that pries nerve agent from AChE. 2-PAM-Cl must be given early in the poisoning, because after a short period of time it may not be effective. Also, 2-PAM-Cl varies in its effectiveness against nerve agents.

Buddy-Aid

If a casualty is unable to care for himself or herself, take immediate steps to protect yourself first, then help the casualty. You cannot help anyone if you are struck down by a nerve agent. Mask the casualty, and if possible have the casualty clear his or her own mask. Check the casualty's pocket flaps and the area around the casualty for expended auto-injectors. This will guide you regarding how much additional treatment may be necessary. Casualties with symptoms of mild nerve agent exposure may self-administer one NAAK/ATNAA, and you may assist as necessary. In casualties exhibiting symptoms of severe nerve agent exposure, administer three NAAK/ATNAA.

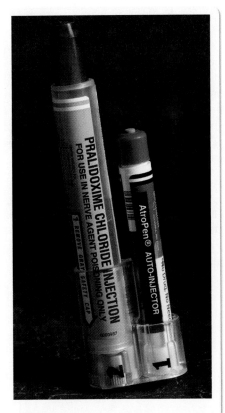

FIGURE 33-2 A nerve agent antidote kit (NAAK) auto-injector set.

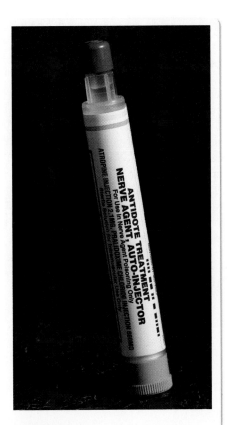

FIGURE 33-3 An antidote treatment, nerve agent auto-injector (ATNAA).

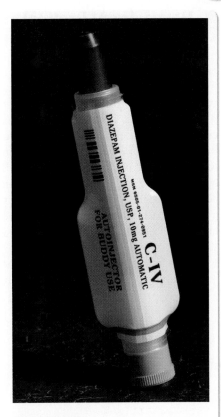

FIGURE 33-4 Convulsant antidote for nerve agent (CANA) injector.

Use your casualty's sets. Remember, each contains two auto-injectors (one atropine and one 2-PAM-Cl).

Administer one convulsant antidote for nerve agent (CANA) injector immediately after the third NAAK/ATNAA FIGURE 33-4 ▲. The CANA injection contains diazepam, which is an antiseizure medication. The CANA should be given to all casualties that require the use of three NAAK/ATNAA kits, regardless of whether the casualty is having detectable seizures. Decontaminate the casualty's exposed skin. Assess the casualty for signs of effectiveness of treatment as evidenced by a heart rate above 90 beats/min, reduced bronchial secretions, reduced salivation, and cessation of convulsions. Administer additional atropine and/or CANA if needed.

Additional atropine may be administered at 15-minute intervals until the casualty's heart rate is above 90 beats/min, bronchial secretions are reduced, and salivation is reduced (atropinization). It may be necessary to administer atropine at intervals of 30 minutes to 4 hours to maintain atropinization

or until the casualty is evacuated to a treatment facility. A second and third CANA may be administered at 5- to 10-minute intervals if convulsions persist.

Secure all used injectors to the casualty's upper left pocket flap of the battle dress overgarment (BDO) or the left pocket on the sleeve of the Joint Service lightweight integrated suit technology (JSLIST) overgarment. Record the number of injections given and all other treatment provided on the casualty's field medical card (FMC). Evacuate and provide assisted ventilations to the casualty if necessary.

Atropine usage will give normal, expected symptoms not related to the nerve agent exposure. The mild side effects include dry mouth, warmth, flushing of skin, minimal drowsiness, and decreased combat performance. The moderate to severe effects include drowsiness, fatigue, blurring of vision, increased heat injury risk, and incapacity of effective combat performance. The side effects of the antidote 2-PAM-Cl include mild visual changes. The side effects of the antidote diazepam (CANA) include decreased combat performance.

■ Nerve Agent Pretreatment

In the late 1990s the US military fielded pyridostigmine bromide as a pretreatment for nerve agent exposure. It is only effective against **soman (GD)**. Surprisingly, it works by acting similarly to a nerve agent. Unlike nerve agents, though, pyridostigmine forms a temporary and reversible bond with AChE. In essence, this pretreatment creates a reserve of this enzyme to combat the effects of nerve agent exposure by binding to about 20% of this enzyme in the body. The pretreatment is discontinued if the soldier is exposed to a nerve agent, thus freeing the AChE to counteract the build-up of acetylcholine that results from nerve agent exposure.

Pyridostigmine is not an antidote, but an antidote enhancer. It should not be taken after nerve agent exposure. It is ineffective unless standard MARK 1 therapy is also used in the appropriate manner. Tens of thousands of US troops took pyridostigmine during the 1990 Gulf War (Gulf War I) conflict. The incidences of side effects, primarily gastrointestinal and urinary, were over 50%, but very few soldiers sought medical care for the side effects. The drug was discontinued in less than 1% of cases.

The nerve agent pyridostigmine pretreatment (NAPP) set contains the pretreatment medication to be taken within 8 hours prior to exposure to nerve agents. Service members are initially issued one NAPP in high-risk environments. Orders to start taking the NAPP will be issued by the proper authority within the chain of command.

■ Summary

Nerve agents are the most toxic of the known chemical agents and are considered major military threat agents. Prompt identification of the signs and symptoms of nerve agent poisoning and immediate treatment are critical tasks.

Your team is searching the abandoned headquarters of a local insurgent group. Intelligence reports that this group may have been manufacturing chemical agents. While searching the building, you identify the presence of a nerve agent with the M256AI chemical agent detection kit. You immediately don your protective mask and hood. Then you sound the alarm to warn the rest of your unit of your findings. They perform self-aid as you perform a quick self-evaluation for signs and symptoms of nerve agent poisoning. You are not exhibiting any signs, so you turn your attention to your unit.

Assessment

Only one soldier does not have his gear on. He is holding his mask and staring into the distance. As you approach him, you notice that the muscles in his face seem to be drooping and his nose is running. His knees begin to buckle as you grab hold of him.

Treatment

"We have to get your mask on," you tell him as you take the mask out of his hands. You immediately mask the casualty and then look around for any expended auto-injectors. There are none. You position the casualty on the ground and administer three NAAK/ATNAA sets to stop the nerve agent symptoms from worsening. Immediately after administering the third set, you administer one CANA to prevent the casualty from seizing. After decontaminating the exposed skin, you assess him. His heart rate is 92 beats/min and his nose is no longer running. You secure all of the used injectors to the casualty's upper left pocket and record your treatment on his FMC. MEDEVAC is notified for immediate evacuation.

1. LAST NAME, FIRST NAME **Martin, David**		RANK/GRADE **SGT/E5**	X	MALE
				FEMALE
SSN **000-111-0000**	SPECIALTY CODE **OZ**	———		RELIGION

2. UNIT				

FORCE				NATIONALITY
A/T	AF/A	N/M	MC/M	
	BC/BC		NBI/BNC	DISEASE	PSYCH

3. INJURY		X	AIRWAY
			HEAD
FRONT BACK			WOUND
			NECK/BACK INJURY
			BURN
			AMPUTATION
			STRESS
		X	OTHER (Specify)

Exposure to

nerve agent

4. LEVEL OF CONSCIOUSNESS			
	ALERT		PAIN RESPONSE
X	VERBAL RESPONSE		UNRESPONSIVE

5. PULSE **92 bpm**	TIME **0455**	6. TOURNIQUET X NO	YES	TIME

7. MORPHINE X NO	YES	DOSE	TIME	8. IV	TIME

9. TREATMENT/OBSERVATIONS/CURRENT MEDICATION/ALLERGIES/NBC (ANTIDOTE)

Exposure to nerve agent
Admin 3 NAAK/ATNAA sets
Admin 1 CANA

10. DISPOSITION	RETURNED TO DUTY		TIME **0507**
	X	EVACUATED	
		DECEASED	

11. PROVIDER/UNIT **Hinkler, Joe**	DATE (YYMMDD)

Aid Kit

Ready for Review

- Chemical weapons have been around in less sophisticated forms for decades.
- Nerve agents are considered to be military threat agents.
- Nerve agents remain in a liquid state, unless exposed to extreme cold or heat.
  - Extreme heat will cause the liquid to become a vapor.
  - The volatility of a nerve agent ranges from highly volatile (vapor) to little volatility (liquid or oily state).
  - Nerve agents range in color from clear to light brown.
  - Nerve agents are odorless.
- To perform self-aid, first put on your protective mask and hood.
  - The protective mask and hood protect the face and neck, eyes, mouth, and respiratory tract against nerve agent spray, vapor, and aerosol.
  - Give the alarm.
  - Perform a hasty self-evaluation for signs and symptoms of nerve agent poisoning.
  - Administer an antidote if signs and/or symptoms are present.

Vital Vocabulary

acetylcholinesterase (AChE) An enzyme present in various body tissues such as muscles, nerve cells, and red blood cells, resulting in excess acetylcholine in the body.

nerve agent antidote kit (NAAK) Contains two auto-injector medications, atropine and 2-PAM-Cl (pralidoxime chloride).

nerve agents A class of chemical called organophosphates; they function by blocking an essential enzyme in the nervous system, which causes the body's organs to become overstimulated and burn out.

sarin (GB) A nerve agent that is one of the G agents; a highly volatile colorless and odorless liquid that turns from liquid to gas within seconds to minutes at room temperature.

soman (GD) A nerve agent that is one of the G agents; twice as persistent as sarin and five times as lethal; it has a fruity odor, as a result of the type of alcohol used in the agent, and is both a contact and inhalation hazard that can enter the body through skin absorption and through the respiratory tract.

V agent (VX) A clear, oily agent that has no odor and looks like baby oil; over 100 times more lethal than sarin and extremely persistent.

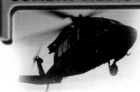

COMBAT MEDIC in Action

Other than military intelligence, there were no signs that warned you about the presence of a chemical agent in the building your unit was searching. Nerve agents are odorless. Thanks to the intelligence you received, you employed your M256AI chemical agent detection kit and quickly donned protection before you were exposed to the nerve agent. By working together as a team, you were able to protect and treat everyone in your unit.

1. Nerve agents inhibit:
   A. ChEa.
   B. AChE.
   C. HcAE.
   D. CEah.

2. When acetylcholine builds up in the nerve endings, the muscles:
   A. contract.
   B. expand.
   C. freeze.
   D. shrink.

3. Nerve agents are in a highly volatile state when they are in this form.
   A. Liquid
   B. Solid
   C. Vapor
   D. Oil

4. Exposed clothing can spread a nerve agent for about _____ after contact.
   A. 2 hours
   B. 10 minutes
   C. 1 hour
   D. 30 minutes

5. Mild exposure to a nerve agent includes the following effects:
   A. Severe muscle twitching
   B. Confused behavior
   C. Rhinorrhea
   D. Vomiting

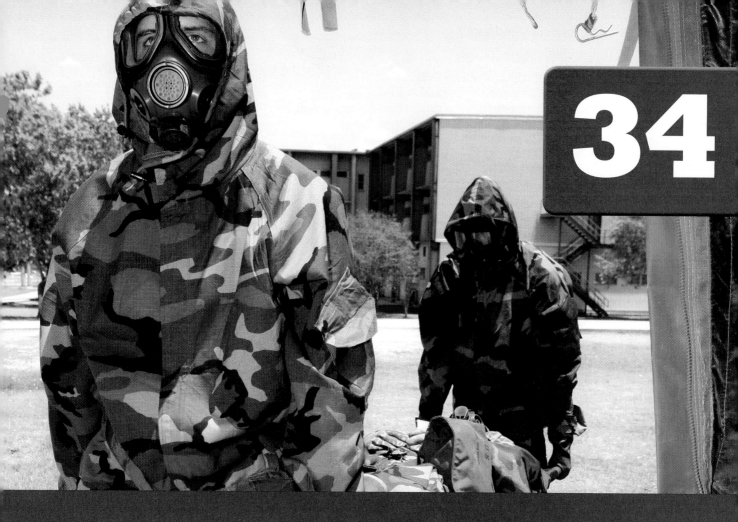

34

Decontamination

Objectives

Knowledge Objectives

- [ ] Describe the medical support objectives in chemical operations.

- [ ] Describe training, equipment, logistics, and evacuation assets.

- [ ] Describe management operations.

- [ ] Describe decontamination station operations.

■ Introduction

Nuclear, biologic, and chemical contamination should not be thought of as an insurmountable problem. On a nonlinear battlefield, soldiers will have to deal with contamination in order to survive, operate, fight, and win. Command will have to modify operations when contamination is present, just as they do for bad weather or a shift in enemy forces. Contamination, like other hazards on a nonlinear battlefield, can kill or injure soldiers and, because of protection measures, degrade the ability of soldiers to fight and operate. Collective protection shelters and individual protective clothing and equipment are only temporary solutions. Decontamination is the only long-term solution.

An important first step in casualty care is decontamination of the casualty; this step needs to occur before treatment in a military treatment facility (MTF). Casualty decontamination includes removal of gross contamination followed by careful removal of all garments. When properly accomplished you will avoid further contamination of the casualty, yourself, or other soldiers.

■ Medical Support Objectives in Chemical Operations

As a combat medic, your goal is to return to duty the maximum number of personnel as soon as possible. You need to manage casualties so that chemical agent injuries are minimized and any other injuries or illnesses are not aggravated. You also need to protect soldiers handling contaminated casualties or working in contaminated areas by ensuring that they are wearing the proper protective equipment. Avoid spreading contamination in ambulances, other evacuation vehicles, MTFs, and adjoining areas. Continue the MTF operations so that normal services unrelated to the medical treatment of chemical agent injuries are maintained at all times. Your job is to treat all casualties at all times.

■ Planning Factors

The initial management and treatment of casualties contaminated with a chemical agent will vary based on the tactical situation and the nature of the contaminant. Therefore, each MTF must have a plan and put it into effect immediately, and then modify it to meet each specific situation. Casualty decontamination sites are co-located with an MTF. This ensures that medical supervision of casualty decontamination is available. Specifics on the management of chemically contaminated casualties at the MTF are found in FM 8-10-7.

Each MTF has identical medical equipment sets (MES) for chemical agent patient decontamination and treatment. The numbers of each type of MES vary, depending on the echelon of care. For example, the Battalion Aid Station (BAS) has one chemical agent casualty decontamination MES and two chemical agent casualty treatment MES. Each MTF must be prepared to treat chemical agent casualties generated in the geographic area of the MTF. Casualties are received from a forward and, in some cases, a lateral MTF. The accomplishment of the medical objectives plus casualty decontamination will require augmentation of the BAS and Forward Support Medical Company (FSMC) by 8 to 20 personnel from the supported unit.

Heat Index

The garments designed to protect you from contamination also raise your body temperature very quickly. The wet bulb globe thermometer (WBGT) index determines the heat condition, which is assigned a number (1–5) or a corresponding color code (white, green, yellow, red, black) that can be displayed with flags or other devices. Mission-oriented protective posture (MOPP) gear increases the ambient WBGT index by 10°F; that is, 10°F is added to WBGT reading before the heat condition is designated. Soldiers wearing butyl rubber aprons on the decontamination line while at MOPP-4 may experience an even greater heat load. For someone at MOPP-4, a relatively comfortable WBGT of 82°F (heat category 2, green) would increase to a level of over 92°F (heat category 5, black), the most severe and debilitating level of heat stress. Therefore, frequent rotation of personnel to reduce the occurrence of heat injuries is another factor to consider when determining total personnel requirements.

■ Training, Equipment, Logistics, and Evacuation Assets

Training

Commanders must ensure that medical personnel and the decontamination team members provided by the supported unit are trained to manage, decontaminate, and treat chemical agent–contaminated casualties. Soldiers must be trained to protect themselves from chemical agent injuries. In addition, provisions must be made for practice exercises that will enable them to accomplish their responsibilities with speed and accuracy during an incident.

Decontaminating a casualty with speed is achieved through practice. Training emphasis should be placed on the following subjects:

- Employing individual protection
- Practicing personal decontamination
- Using chemical agent detection paper and the chemical agent monitor (CAM) to monitor for and detect chemical agents
- Providing emergency medical treatment (EMT)
- Performing casualty decontamination
- Evacuating decontaminated casualties
- Evacuating contaminated casualties
- Sorting and receiving contaminated casualties into a system designed for the treatment of both contaminated and noncontaminated casualties
- Casualty lifting and transfer techniques

CBPS

The **chemical and biologic protective shelter (CBPS)** is a direct replacement for the M51 chemical agent/biologic agent shelter, which eliminates the excessive erection and striking time, insufficient floor space, lack of natural ventilation, and unavailability of prime movers, which were the problems with the M51. The CBPS can be set up or struck three times daily when operating as a Battalion Aid Station. Setup times of the inflatable rib tent have been established at 15 to 20 minutes, and tear-down times at approximately 30 minutes.

The CBPS consists of a power support system and inflatable tent. The primary power source is the engine of a high-mobility multipurpose wheeled vehicle (HMMWV) variant and a backup generator mounted in a high-mobility multipurpose trailer. This system provides air conditioning or heating and electricity for lighting, equipment, and filtered air.

A crew of four, who are carried in the HMMWV, staff the CBPS. The inflatable rib tent provides 300 square feet of usable floor space, with a litter casualty airlock and optional ambulatory casualty airlock. The CBPS has removable side entrances to allow side-to-side setup of additional CBPS.

Detection Equipment

Before you can decontaminate, you need to know which chemical agent has been released. Point detectors sample the immediate area to determine the presence of any chemical agents. The sample is most often taken from the atmosphere; however, specialized detection kits can be used to sample the soil or water. In addition to monitoring the atmosphere, the point detectors provide monitoring after an attack, identify the contaminated area, monitor collective protection areas, monitor the effectiveness of decontamination, and monitor chemical contamination during reconnaissance efforts.

M8 chemical agent detection paper detects and identifies liquid chemical agents. It is tan in color and comes in a booklet containing 25 perforated sheets, which are heat sealed in a polyethylene envelope. M9 chemical agent detection paper is a portable single roll of paper that comes with a Mylar adhesive back and coated tape. The agent-sensitive dyes will turn pink, reddish brown, or red-purple when exposed to an agent, but the paper does not identify the specific agent. The M256A1 chemical agent detector kit is a portable expendable item capable of detecting and identifying hazardous concentrations of nerve and blister agents and cyanide.

Chemical Agent Alarms

The **M8A1 automatic chemical agent alarm** is an automatic chemical agent detection and warning system designed to provide real-time detection of the presence of nerve agent vapors or inhalable aerosols.

The **M22** is an "off-the-shelf" automatic chemical agent alarm system capable of detecting and identifying standard blister and nerve agents. The M22 system is portable, operates independently after system start-up, and provides an audible and visual alarm. The M22 system also provides a communications interface for automatic battlefield warning and reporting.

The **chemical agent monitor (CAM)** and **improved chemical agent monitor (ICAM)** are hand-held, soldier-operated devices designed for monitoring chemical agent contamination on personnel, equipment, and surfaces.

Logistics

Provisions must be made to ensure that medical personnel are supplied and equipped to manage and treat contaminated casualties. Also, supplies and equipment must be provided for protection of personnel manning the contaminated areas. Medical supplies are stored or stocked in a manner that reduces potential loss from chemical contamination.

Patient protective wraps (PPWs) must be available for casualties whose injuries require decontamination (clothing removal) for treatment in the clean treatment area. After treatment, decontaminated casualties must be placed in PPWs before they are moved to the evacuation point.

Site Location

A decontamination area is established on the downwind side of the MTF. It is provided with overhead protection such as plastic sheeting, trailer covers, ponchos, or tarpaulins. The site may have been designated in the operation order or selected based on the current Mission, Enemy, Terrain and weather, Troops and support available, Time available, Civil considerations (METT-TC). If at all possible, the site is off the main route but is easy to access. It needs to be a large enough area to support the operation and must have good overhead concealment and a good water source. Finally, it needs to have good drainage. A personnel decontamination station may be used by decontamination teams to reduce their MOPP levels for resting as well as for the ambulatory casualty.

Evacuation Assets

On the modern battle space, there are three basic modes of evacuating casualties: personnel, ground vehicles, and aircraft. Personnel who physically carry casualties incur a great deal of inherent stress. Cumbersome MOPP gear, climate, increased workloads, and fatigue will greatly reduce the effectiveness of unit personnel. Once a vehicle has entered a contaminated area, it is highly unlikely that it can be spared long enough to undergo a complete decontamination. This will depend on the contaminant, the tempo of the battle, and the resources available for casualty evacuation. Ground ambulances should be used instead of air ambulances in the contaminated area because they are more plentiful and easier to decontaminate, and can be replaced more easily. However, this does not preclude use of aircraft if required.

■ Management Operations

Medical facilities treating chemical casualties must divide their operations into two categories—contaminated and uncontaminated. Contaminated operations include triage, emergency treatment, and patient decontamination. Uncontaminated operations include treatment and final disposition. Any MTF that receives contaminated casualties will have a casualty receiving area that consists of a dirty side and a clean side separated by a hot line that must not be crossed by contaminated casualties, garments, or equipment. The area where casualties are received, on the dirty side of the hot line,

---

Field Medical Care TIPS

Every soldier entering the decontamination area, including casualties, must be masked or have other respiratory tract protection in place.

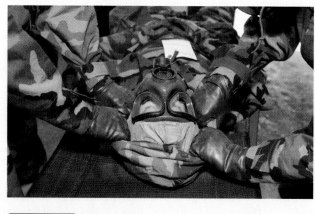

FIGURE 34-1 Hood removal.

is where initial triage is done, emergency medical care is provided, and the casualty is decontaminated.

■ Decontamination Station Operations

The dirty dump should be established at a minimum of 100 meters or 75 yards from the processing station. The dirty dump is marked with the standard NATO nuclear, biologic, chemical (NBC) marker. Once the site is closed, higher headquarters (HQ) is notified by sending an NBC 5 Report.

Arrival Point

The entry point is a clearly delineated area into which all casualties arrive. Ambulances unload casualties at this point and ambulatory casualties report to this point. The entry and exit roads must be clearly marked. Organic staffing in this area may be minimal and all casualties arriving in this area will be sent to the triage station. All personnel should be in MOPP-4.

Most contaminants are removed by carefully removing all of the casualty's clothing. The casualty's protective mask is not removed during the decontamination process. Remove the casualty's mask hood, overgarments, booties and boots, the Army Combat Uniform (ACU), and undergarments.

Triage

The triage officer sorts each casualty into one of four categories: immediate, minimal, delayed, or expectant. At lower echelons of care, the triage officer may be a senior medic; at higher echelons, he or she may be a physician's assistant, dentist, or physician. Triage categories for casualties of chemical warfare agents are:

- **Immediate:** A casualty in the immediate category needs to have a medical procedure performed within an hour or so to save his or her life.
- **Minimal:** A casualty in the minimal category needs minor care and is expected to return to duty within hours after that care is provided.
- **Delayed:** A casualty in the delayed category has a serious injury, but can wait for care. The delay will not change the ultimate outcome.
- **Expectant:** A casualty in the expectant category needs care that is beyond the capability of that MTF to provide. In addition, the needed care is required before the casualty can be evacuated to the MTF that can provide such care.

The triage officer will send casualties to one of the following:

- Back to duty
- The emergency treatment station
- The decontamination area
- The dirty evacuation area

Emergency Treatment Station

In the emergency treatment station, the casualty is provided emergency lifesaving medical care and is stabilized for the 10- to 20-minute decontamination procedure that is necessary before he or she can enter the clean area of the MTF for more elaborate treatment. Casualties with minor injuries might be treated here if they can be returned to duty.

Clothing Removal

Move the casualty to the clothing removal station. After the casualty has been triaged and stabilized (if necessary) by the senior medic in the decontaminated area, move the casualty to the litter stands at the clothing removal station.

Hood Removal

Decontaminate the hood using an individual equipment decontamination kit (IEDK) or 5% chlorine solution to wipe down the front, sides, and top of the hood. Remove the hood by cutting it with scissors or by loosening it from the mask attachment points for the quick-doff hood or other similar hoods FIGURE 34-1 ▲. Before cutting the hood, dip the scissors in a 5% chlorine solution. Decontaminate the protective mask and exposed skin by using the M291 skin decontamination kit (SDK) or a 0.5% chlorine solution to wipe the external parts of the mask. Continue by wiping the exposed areas of the casualty's face, including the neck and behind the ears. Do not remove the face mask. Remove gross contaminations from the casualty's overgarment with an M291 SDK or a 5% chlorine solution.

Field Medical Card

Remove the field medical card by cutting the tie wire, allowing the FMC to fall into a plastic bag FIGURE 34-2 ▶. Seal the plastic bag and rinse the outside of the bag with a 5% chlo-

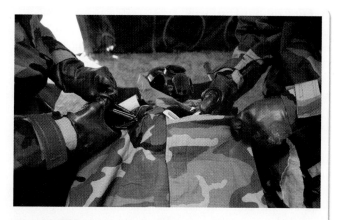

FIGURE 34-2 Remove the field medical card by cutting the tie wire, allowing the FMC to fall into a plastic bag.

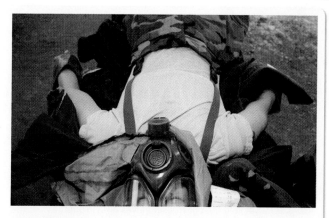

FIGURE 34-4 Continue tucking the clothing between the arm and chest. Roll the cut sleeves away from the arms, exposing the black liner.

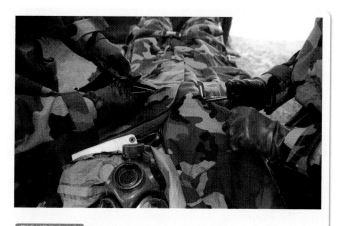

FIGURE 34-3 Cutting the overgarment jacket.

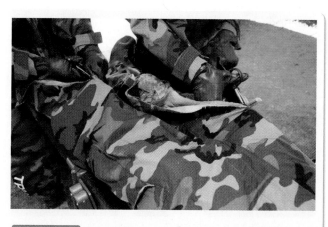

FIGURE 34-5 Cut and remove the overgarment trousers.

rine solution. Place the plastic bag under the back of the protective mask's head straps. The FMC will remain with the casualty in the contaminated area and a clean copy will be made before the casualty is moved into the clean area. Remove the casualty's personal effects and place in a plastic bag labeled with the casualty's identification and seal the bag.

Overgarment Jacket

Cut and remove the overgarment jacket FIGURE 34-3 ▲. Before cutting the overgarment jacket and trousers, dip the scissors in 5% chlorine solution to prevent contamination of the casualty's ACU or undergarments. Make two cuts, one up each sleeve from the wrist up to the shoulder and then across the shoulder through the collar. Cut around bandages, tourniquets, and splints leaving them in place. Do not allow your gloves to touch the casualty along the cut line. Keep the cuts close to the inside of the arm so that most of the sleeve material can be folded outward. Unzip the jacket and roll the chest sections to the respective sides, with the inner surface outward. Continue tucking the clothing between the arm and chest. Roll the cut sleeves away from the arms, exposing the black liner FIGURE 34-4 ▶.

Overgarment Trousers

Cut and remove the overgarment trousers FIGURE 34-5 ▲. Cut both trouser legs starting at the ankle. Keep the cuts near the inside of the legs, along the inseam, to the crotch. With the left leg, cut all the way to the waist, avoiding the pockets. With the right leg, cut across at the crotch to the left leg cut. Cut around bandages, tourniquets, and splints leaving them in place. Place the scissors in a 5% chlorine solution. Fold the cut trouser halves away from the casualty and allow the halves to drop to the litter with the contaminated (green) side down. Roll the inner leg portion under and between the legs FIGURE 34-6 ▶.

Gloves

Remove the casualty's gloves. Before touching the casualty, the decontamination team decontaminates its gloves with a 5% chlorine solution. Lift the casualty's arms up and out of the cutaway sleeves unless this is detrimental to his or her condition. Grasp the fingers of the gloves, roll the cuffs over the fingers, and turn the gloves inside out FIGURE 34-7 ▶. Do not remove the inner cotton gloves at this time. Carefully lower the casualty's arms across his or her chest after the outer

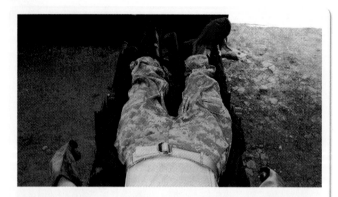

FIGURE 34-6 Fold the cut trouser halves away from the casualty and allow the halves to drop to the litter with the contaminated (green) side down. Roll the inner leg portion under and between the legs.

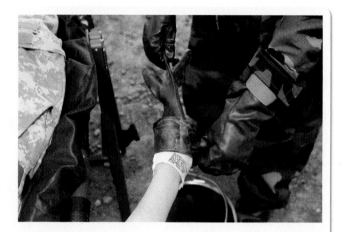

FIGURE 34-7 Grasp the fingers of the gloves, roll the cuffs over the fingers, and turn the gloves inside out.

gloves have been removed. Do not allow the casualty's arms to come into contact with the exterior of his or her overgarment. Drop the gloves into the contaminated waste bag. The team members then must decontaminate their gloves with the 5% chlorine solution.

Overboots

Remove the overboots. Cut the overboot laces and fold the lacing eyelets flat outward. While standing at the foot of the litter, hold the casualty's heel with one hand. Pull the overboot downward, then toward you to remove it. Remove the two overboots simultaneously. This reduces the likelihood of contaminating one of the combat boots.

While holding the casualty's heels off the litter, have a team member wipe the end of the litter with a 5% chlorine solution to neutralize any contamination that was transferred to the litter from the overboots. Lower the casualty's heels onto the decontaminated litter. Place the overboots in the contaminated waste bag. The team members then must decontaminate their gloves with the 5% chlorine solution.

Army Combat Uniform

Cut and remove the ACU. To cut and remove the ACU jacket and trousers, follow the procedures for removing the protective overgarment. Cut and remove the combat boots by cutting the bootlaces along the tongue. Remove the boots by pulling them toward you and place the boots in the contaminated waste bag. Do not touch the casualty's skin with your contaminated gloves when removing his or her boots.

Cut and remove the undergarments. Follow the procedures for cutting away the protective overgarment and rolling it away from the casualty. If the casualty is wearing a brassiere, cut it between the cups. Cut both shoulder straps where they attach to the cups and lay them back off of the shoulders. Remove the socks and cotton gloves. Do not remove the identification tags.

Casualty Transfer

After the casualty's clothing has been cut away, transfer the casualty to a decontaminated litter or a canvas litter with a plastic sheeting cover. Three decontamination team members then decontaminate their gloves and aprons with a 5% chlorine solution. One team member places his or her hands under the casualty's legs at the thighs and Achilles tendons, a second member places his or her arms under the casualty's back and buttocks, and a third member places his or her arms under the casualty's shoulders and supports the head and neck. They carefully lift the casualty using their knees and not their backs to minimize back strain. While the casualty is elevated, another team member removes the litter from the litter stands and replaces it with a decontaminated (clean) litter. The team members carefully lower the casualty onto the clean litter. The clothing and overgarments are placed in a contaminated waste bag and moved to the contaminated waste dump. The dirty litter is rinsed with the 5% chlorine solution and placed in the litter storage area.

Spot Decontamination

With the casualty in a supine position, spot decontaminate the skin by using an SDK or a 0.5% chlorine solution. Decontaminate areas of potential contamination, including areas around the neck, wrists, and lower parts of the face. Decontaminate the casualty's identification tags and chain, if necessary. A complete body wash is not appropriate and may be harmful to the casualty. During a complete body wash, the casualty would have to be rolled over to reach all areas of the skin. This is not necessary for an adequate decontamination.

To perform a spot decontamination, first gently cut away any bandages. Then decontaminate the area around the wound and irrigate it with a 0.5% chlorine solution. If bleeding begins, replace the bandage with a clean one. Replace any old tourniquet by placing a new one ½″ to 1″ above the old one. Then remove the old tourniquet and decontaminate the casualty's skin with an SDK or a 0.5% chlorine solution. Do not remove any splint. Decontaminate the splint by thoroughly rinsing it, including the padding and cravats, with a 0.5% chlorine solution.

Finally, ensure the completeness of decontamination. Check the casualty with M8 detector paper or the CAM for completeness of decontamination. Dispose of contaminated bandages and coverings by placing them in a contaminated waste bag. Seal the bag and place it in the contaminated waste dump.

Moving Over the Hot Line

Once the casualty's clothing has been cut away and his or her skin, bandages, and splints have been decontaminated, transfer the casualty to the shuffle pit and place the litter on the litter stands. The shuffle pit is wide enough to prevent the decontamination team members from straddling it while carrying the litter. A third team member will assist with transferring the casualty to a clean treatment litter in the shuffle pit. Then the decontamination personnel rinse or wipe down their aprons and gloves with a 5% chlorine solution. The three team members lift the casualty off the decontaminated litter. While the casualty is elevated, another team member removes the litter from the stands and returns it to the decontamination area. A medic from the clean side of the shuffle pit replaces the litter with a clean one. The casualty is lowered onto the clean litter. Two medics from the clean side of the shuffle pit move the casualty to the clean treatment area. The casualty is treated in this area or awaits processing. The litter is wiped down with a 5% chlorine solution in preparation for reuse. Once the casualty is in the air lock of the CPS and the air lock has been purged, his or her protective mask is removed. Place the mask in a plastic bag and seal it.

Treatment Area

The capability to care for casualties increases greatly from the lower echelon of care to the highest. The BAS will have a physician's assistant, a physician, or both and several medics. The higher echelons, the hospitals, will have a full surgical staff including subspecialists, surgical facilities, and full support capabilities to provide all needed immediate care.

With limited resources available, the major tasks for a BAS are to provide lifesaving care and to prepare the casualty for evacuation. By necessity these must be short, simple procedures. At higher echelons, the treatment area will be located in a collective protection shelter; otherwise, it should be at least 100 meters upwind from the receiving area.

Evacuation

After receiving care in a low echelon MTF, the casualty is evacuated in a clean vehicle to a higher echelon for further care. If a clean vehicle is not available, the casualty may be placed in a patient protective wrap (PPW) and evacuated in a dirty vehicle.

Decontaminating Ambulatory Casualties

All ambulatory casualties requiring medical care in the clean treatment area of the BAS will be decontaminated. Stable casualties not requiring treatment at the BAS, but requiring evacuation to the medical company's clearing station or a corps hospital for treatment (eg, a casualty with a broken arm) should be evacuated in their protective overgarments

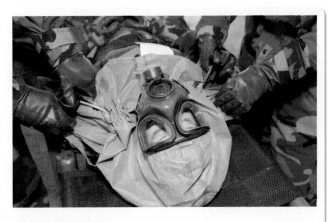

FIGURE 34-8 Removing the hood.

and masks by any available transportation. However, before evacuation, spot remove all thickened agents from their protective clothing. The ambulatory casualty is decontaminated and undressed. Some procedures in the following steps can be done by one soldier, whereas others require more than one.

Remove the Load Carrying Equipment (LCE)

Remove the load carrying equipment (LCE) by unfastening/ unbuttoning all connectors or tie straps, and then place the equipment in a plastic bag. Place the plastic bag in the designated storage area for later decontamination.

Decontaminate the Mask and Hood

Begin the clothing removal process. After the casualty has been triaged and treated, if necessary, by the senior medic in the casualty decontamination station, the clothing removal process begins. Use either an IEDK or a 5% chlorine solution or household bleach to wipe down the front, sides, and top of the hood. Remove the hood by cutting it with scissors or by loosening it from the mask attachment points for the quick-doff hood or other similar hoods. Before cutting the hood, dip the scissors in a 5% chlorine solution. Cut the neck cord and the small string under the voicemitter. Release or cut the hood shoulder straps and unzip the hood zipper. Cut the hood upward to the top of the eye lens outsert, staying close to the filter inlet cover and eye lens outsert, then across the forehead to the outer edge of the other eye lens outsert. Proceed downward toward the casualty's shoulder, staying close to the eye lens outsert and filter inlet cover, then across the lower part of the voice mitter to the zipper. After dipping the scissors in the 5% chlorine solution, cut the hood from the center of the forehead over the top of the head. Fold the left and right sides of the hood away from the casualty's head and remove the hood FIGURE 34-8 ▲.

Decontaminate the mask and the casualty's face by using an SDK or a 0.5% chlorine solution. Cover the mask's air inlets with gauze or your hands to keep the mask filters dry. Continue by wiping the exposed areas of the casualty's face, including the neck and behind the ears. Do not remove the protective mask.

Cut the casualty's FMC tie wire, allowing the FMC to fall into a plastic bag. Seal the plastic bag and rinse the outside of the bag with a 5% chlorine solution. Place the plastic bag under the back of the protective mask's head straps. The FMC will remain with the casualty in the contaminated area and a clean copy will be made before the casualty is moved to the clean area.

Gross Contamination

Remove gross contamination from the casualty's protective overgarment FIGURE 34-9 ▼ . Remove all visible contamination spots from the overgarment by using an SDK (preferred method) or a 0.5% chlorine solution.

Overgarment Removal

Remove the casualty's personal effects from his or her protective overgarment and ACU pockets. Place the articles in a plastic bag, label the bag with the casualty's identification, and seal the bag. If the articles are not contaminated, they are returned to the casualty. If the articles are contaminated, place them in the contaminated holding area until they can be decontaminated, and then return them to the casualty.

Remove the overgarment jacket. Have the casualty stand with his or her feet spread apart at shoulder width. Unsnap the front flap of the jacket and unzip the jacket. If the casualty can extend his or her arms, have him or her clench both fists and extend his or her arms backward at about a 30° angle. Move behind the casualty, grasp his or her jacket collar at the sides of the neck, and peel the jacket off the shoulders at a 30° angle down and away from the casualty FIGURE 34-10 ▶ . Avoid any rapid or sharp jerks, which spread contamination. Gently pull the inside sleeves over the casualty's wrists and hands.

If the casualty cannot extend his or her arms, you must cut the jacket to aid in its removal. Before cutting the overgarment jacket, dip the scissors in a 5% chlorine solution to prevent contamination of the casualty's ACU or underclothing. As with the litter casualty, make two cuts, one up each sleeve from the wrist up to the shoulder and then across the shoulder through the collar. Cut around bandages, tourniquets,

and splints, leaving them in place. Do not allow your gloves to touch the casualty along the cut line. Peel the jacket back and downward to avoid spreading contamination. Ensure that the outside of the jacket does not touch the casualty or his or her inner clothing.

Cut and remove the overgarment trousers. Unfasten or cut all ties, buttons, or zippers before grasping the trousers at the waist and peeling them down over the casualty's combat boots FIGURE 34-11 ▼ . Again, the trousers are cut to aid in removal. If necessary, cut both trouser legs starting at the ankle. Keep the cuts near the inside of the legs, along the inseam, to the crotch. Cut around all bandages, tourniquets, and splints. Continue to cut up both sides of the zipper to the waist and allow the narrow strip with the zipper to drop between the legs. Peel or allow the trouser halves to drop to the ground. Have the casualty step out of the trouser legs one at a time. Place the trousers in the contaminated waste bag. Place the scissors in a 5% chlorine solution.

Remove the outer gloves. Grasp the fingers of the gloves, roll the cuffs over the fingers, and turn the gloves inside out. Do not remove the inner cotton gloves at this time. Drop the gloves into the contaminated waste bag. Do not allow the

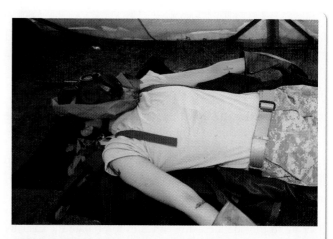

FIGURE 34-10 Remove the overgarment jacket.

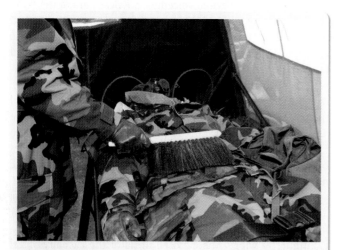

FIGURE 34-9 Remove gross contamination from the casualty's protective overgarment.

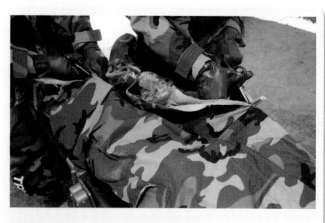

FIGURE 34-11 Remove the overgarment trousers.

casualty to touch his or her clothing or other contaminated objects with his or her hands.

Remove the overboots. Cut the overboot laces and fold the lacing eyelets flat on the ground. Step on the toe and heel eyelets to hold the overboot on the ground and have the patient step out of it. Repeat this procedure for the other overboot. If the overboots are in good condition, they can be decontaminated and reissued.

Remove the casualty's cotton glove liners. Instruct the casualty to remove his or her own cotton glove liners to reduce the possibility of spreading contamination. Have the casualty grasp the heel of one glove liner with the other gloved hand, peeling it off of the hand. Hold the removed glove by the inside and grasp the heel of the other glove, peeling it off of his or her hand **FIGURE 34-12 ▾**. Place both gloves in the contaminated waste bag.

Check for Contamination

After the casualty's overgarment has been removed, check his or her ACU by using M8 detector paper or the CAM. Carefully survey the casualty, paying particular attention to discolored areas, damp spots, and tears on the uniform; areas around the neck, wrists, and ears; and bandages, tourniquets, and splints **FIGURE 34-13 ▸**. Remove any contaminated spots by using an SDK or a 0.5% chlorine solution or, if possible, by cutting away the contaminated area. Always dip the scissors in a 5% chlorine solution after each cut. Recheck the area with the detection equipment. If significant contamination is found on the ACU, then remove it and spot decontaminate the skin. Do not remove the casualty's identification tags.

Spot Decontamination

Use an SDK or a 0.5% chlorine solution to spot decontaminate the skin and areas of potential contamination, including areas around the neck, wrists, and lower parts of the face. Decontaminate the casualty's identification tags and chain, if necessary. Have the casualty hold his or her breath, close his or her eyes, and lift, or assist him or her with lifting, the mask at the chin. Wipe his or her face and exposed areas of the skin with an SDK or a 0.5% chlorine solution. Starting at the top of the ear and quickly wiping downward, wipe all folds in the skin, ear lobes, upper lip, chin, dimples, and nose. Continue up the other side of the face to the top of the other ear. Wipe the inside of the mask where it touches the face. Have the casualty reseal and check his or her mask.

Gently cut away any bandage. Decontaminate the area around the wound and irrigate it with a 0.5% chlorine solution. If bleeding begins, replace the bandage with a clean one. Replace any old tourniquet by placing a new one ½″ to 1″ above the old one. Remove the old tourniquet and decontaminate the casualty's skin with an SDK or a 0.5% chlorine solution. Do not remove any splint. Decontaminate the splint by thoroughly rinsing it, including the padding and cravats, with a 0.5% chlorine solution. Dispose of contaminated bandages and coverings by placing them in a contaminated waste bag. Seal the bag and place it in the contaminated waste dump.

Clean Treatment Area

Have the decontaminated casualty proceed through the shuffle pit to the clean treatment area. To ensure that the casualty's boots are well decontaminated, have him or her stir the contents of the shuffle pit with his or her boots as he or she crosses it. The casualty's combat boots and protective mask will be removed at the entrance of the CPS or clean treatment area.

■ Summary

We have come a long way since 1984. The emphasis today is on the concept of partial decontamination (that which is essential to sustain the fight). This means that most decontamination will be at or near the areas of operations with internal resources and with only minimal support by external resources, such as the Chemical Corps' decontamination resources. It will not be until a unit's combat potential must be restored that complete decontamination will be done. Under this doctrine, it is apparent that commanders will have to plan for decontamination operations and concentrate their resources where their priorities dictate in order to operate on the air/land battlefield.

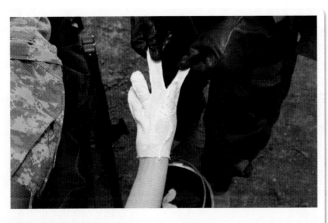
FIGURE 34-12 Remove the casualty's cotton glove liners.

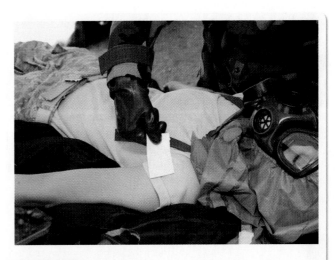
FIGURE 34-13 Check the casualty for contamination.

YOU ARE THE
COMBAT MEDIC

It is a hot and dry morning when you get word that a unit has been exposed to a chemical agent in the field. When the alarm sounded that there was a chemical agent exposure, the unit all donned their personal protective equipment. As a combat medic, you are assigned to a decontamination team to decontaminate the exposed casualties in the field. After donning the proper personal protective equipment, you report to the decontamination station to assist.

The first casualty is having difficulty breathing and there is concern over the patency of his airway. This casualty needs to be decontaminated and evacuated to the MTF. He has been through the emergency treatment station, where he was stabilized in preparation for the decontamination procedure. The decontamination procedure will take about 10 to 20 minutes; then the casualty will be ready to enter the clean area of the MTF for advanced medical care.

The casualty is lying on a decontamination litter propped up on litter stands. First, you decontaminate the hood with a solution and then cut the hood off of the casualty, keeping the face mask in place. Then you remove what appears to be dust from his overgarment with an M291 SDK. The FMC is cut off and placed into a sealed plastic bag that is rinsed with a 5% chlorine solution. A clean copy of the FMC will be made before the casualty enters the clean area.

Now that the gross contamination has been removed, you can now cut and remove the overgarment jacket and trousers. After you have cut and rolled away the overgarments, you roll and remove the casualty's outer gloves only, making certain that the casualty's arms do not touch the overgarment. The goal is to prevent secondary contamination. The overboots are then removed and the end of the litter is wiped down with a 5% chlorine solution.

You remove the casualty's BDU in the same manner as the overgarments. Then the casualty is transferred to a decontaminated litter and a spot decontamination is performed. Finally, you check the casualty with M8 detector paper and ensure that the casualty is clean. The casualty is ready to be transferred across the shuffle pit and be treated in the clean treatment area.

1. LAST NAME, FIRST NAME		RANK/GRADE	X	MALE
Callas, Mario		CPL		FEMALE

SSN	SPECIALTY CODE	RELIGION
000-111-0000	OA	Catholic

2. UNIT

FORCE				NATIONALITY	
A/T	AF/A	N/M	MC/M		
	BC/BC		NBI/BNC	DISEASE	PSYCH

3. INJURY		AIRWAY
		HEAD
FRONT	BACK	WOUND
		NECK/BACK INJURY
		BURN
		AMPUTATION
		STRESS
		X OTHER (Specify)

Exposed to

chemical agent

4. LEVEL OF CONSCIOUSNESS			
ALERT		X	PAIN RESPONSE
VERBAL RESPONSE			UNRESPONSIVE

5. PULSE	TIME	6. TOURNIQUET			TIME
60 bpm	0515	[X] NO	☐ YES		

7. MORPHINE		DOSE	TIME	8. IV	TIME
[X] NO ☐ YES				—	

9. TREATMENT/OBSERVATIONS/CURRENT MEDICATION/ALLERGIES/NBC (ANTIDOTE)

Exposed to a chemical agent
28 breaths/min, labored

10. DISPOSITION		RETURNED TO DUTY	TIME
	X	EVACUATED	0535
		DECEASED	

11. PROVIDER/UNIT	DATE (YYMMDD)
Verdi, Richard	

Ready for Review

- Nuclear, biologic, and chemical contamination should not be thought of as an insurmountable problem.
  - On a nonlinear battlefield, soldiers will have to deal with contamination in order to survive, operate, fight, and win.
- As a combat medic, your goal is to return to duty the maximum number of personnel as soon as possible.
- You need to manage casualties so that chemical agent injuries are minimized and any other injuries or illnesses are not aggravated.
- You also need to protect soldiers handling contaminated casualties or working in contaminated areas by ensuring that they are wearing the proper protective equipment.
- Commanders must ensure that medical personnel and the decontamination team members provided by the supported unit are trained to manage, decontaminate, and treat chemical agent-contaminated casualties.
- Soldiers must be trained to protect themselves from chemical agent injuries.
- Medical facilities treating chemical casualties must divide their operations into two categories—contaminated and uncontaminated.
  - Contaminated operations include triage, emergency treatment, and patient decontamination.
  - Uncontaminated operations include treatment and final disposition.

Vital Vocabulary

chemical agent monitor (CAM) A hand-held, soldier-operated device designed for monitoring chemical agent contamination on personnel, equipment, and surfaces.

chemical and biologic protective shelter (CBPS) A direct replacement for the M51 chemical agent/biologic agent shelter.

delayed A casualty who has a serious injury, but who can wait for care; the delay will not change the ultimate outcome.

expectant A casualty who needs care that is beyond the capability of an MTF to provide; the needed care is required before the casualty can be evacuated to an MTF that can provide such care.

immediate A casualty who needs to have a medical procedure performed within an hour or so to save his or her life.

improved chemical agent monitor (ICAM) A hand-held, soldier-operated device designed for monitoring chemical agent contamination on personnel, equipment, and surfaces.

M8A1 automatic chemical agent alarm An automatic chemical agent detection and warning system designed to provide real-time detection of the presence of nerve agent vapors or inhalable aerosols.

M22 An off-the-shelf automatic chemical agent alarm system capable of detecting and identifying standard blister and nerve agents.

minimal A casualty who needs minor care and who is expected to return to duty within hours after that care is provided.

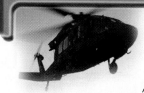

COMBAT MEDIC *in Action*

It is a very hot day with the midday sun burning up the sky and heating up every square inch of earth. After removing a group of insurgents from the area last week, a unit is patrolling a rural village to ensure that the civilians are safe. During the patrol, the unit is exposed to a chemical agent. As the combat medic, you are assigned to assist in decontaminating and treating this unit. Before you can decontaminate any casualties, you have to properly set up a decontamination station. The exposure took place near a well and three houses. What equipment will you need? How will you keep the civilians and the environment safe?

1. The triage officer sorts each casualty into one of which four categories?
   A. Hot, warm, cold, clean
   B. Nerve, biologic, chemical, radiation
   C. Immediate, minimal, delayed, expectant
   D. Red, orange, yellow, green

2. Which piece of equipment is NOT used to detect a chemical agent?
   A. Point detectors
   B. CBPS
   C. CAM
   D. ICAM

3. After decontamination, what does the casualty don?
   A. BDU
   B. Overgarments
   C. PPW
   D. Scrubs

4. Medical facilities treating chemical casualties are divided into what two categories?
   A. Untreated and treated
   B. Serious and ambulatory
   C. Evacuated and return to duty
   D. Contaminated and uncontaminated

5. Why is frequent rotation of personnel necessary in a decontamination station?
   A. Equipment is heavy
   B. Danger of heat stress
   C. Danger of hypothermia
   D. Tradition

Convention

pour l'amélioration du sort des Militaires blessés dans les armées en campagne.

La Confédération Suisse, Son Altesse Royale le Grand-Duc de Bade; Sa Majesté le Roi des Belges, Sa Majesté le Roi de Danemark; Sa Majesté la Reine d'Espagne, Sa Majesté l'Empereur des Français; Son Altesse Royale le Grand-Duc de Hesse; Sa Majesté le Roi d'Italie, Sa Majesté le Roi des Pays-Bas; Sa Majesté le Roi de Portugal et des Algarves; Sa Majesté le Roi de Prusse, Sa Majesté le Roi de Wurtemberg, également, animés du désir d'adoucir, autant qu'il dépend d'eux, les maux inséparables de la guerre, de supprimer les rigueurs inutiles et d'améliorer le sort des militaires blessés sur les champs de bataille, ont résolu de conclure une Convention à cet effet et ont nommé pour leurs Plénipotentiaires, savoir:

La Confédération Suisse:

le Sieur Guillaume-Henri Dufour, Grand-Officier de l'Ordre Impérial de la Légion

© IC

International Humanitarian Law

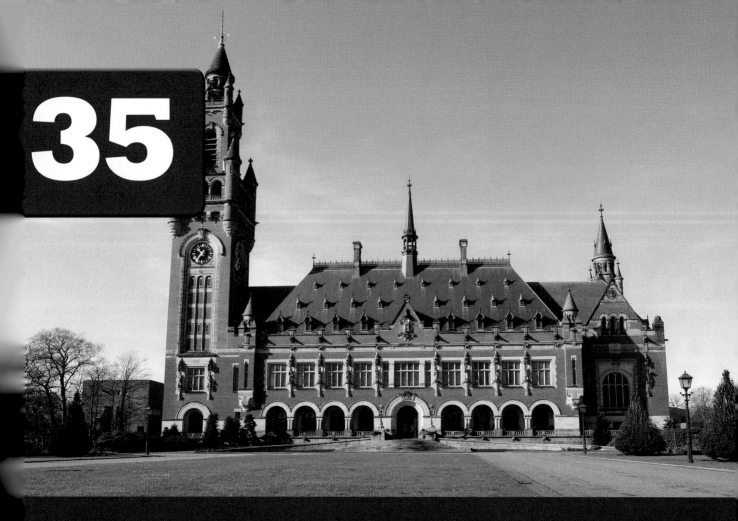

35

International Humanitarian Law for Combat Medics

Thomas F. Ditzler, MA, PhD, FRSPH, FRAI
Director of Research, Department of Psychiatry
Tripler Army Medical Center, Honolulu

Patricia R. Hastings, DO, RN, MPH, NREMT, FACEP
Colonel, Medical Corps
Director, US Army EMS

Objectives

Knowledge Objectives

- [ ] Define international humanitarian law.
- [ ] Describe how international humanitarian law was formed.
- [ ] List the general principles of the Geneva Conventions.
- [ ] Define the term *noncombatants* under the Geneva Conventions.
- [ ] List the two types of protection that medics have under the Geneva Conventions.
- [ ] List the protective signs and symbols of international humanitarian law.

Knowledge Objectives
(continued)

- ☐ Define *medical personnel*.
- ☐ Identify the types of protected medical facilities and transports.
- ☐ Describe self-defense and the defense of patients.
- ☐ Describe the duties and rights of medics.
- ☐ Describe how to treat detainees.
- ☐ Discuss the medic's role in compliance with the Geneva Conventions.

■ Introduction

Customary international law and lawmaking treaties such as the Geneva and Hague **Conventions** regulate the conduct of hostilities on land. The rights and duties set forth in the conventions are part of the supreme law of the land. The United States is obligated to adhere to these conventions even when an opponent does not.

Department of Defense (DoD) and US Army policies require that we conduct operations in a manner consistent with the obligations set forth by these conventions. During all military operations, members of the US armed forces must be prepared to detain personnel who are no longer willing or able to continue fighting, and other personnel based on detention criteria such as being a threat to US forces or to members of the local population, and other security interests. For the medical community, this also means being prepared to take into custody, protect, and medically care for all categories of potential detainees. It is imperative that all individuals detained by US forces are treated in accordance with DoD policies and domestic and international law. Be aware of your responsibility to adhere to and maintain the DoD and Army policies in a manner consistent with these obligations.

Please note, for the purposes of this chapter, we will use the term *medic* to represent medical personnel in general.

■ What Is International Humanitarian Law and What Is Its History?

Today, medics and the US military work under the protections of **international humanitarian law (IHL)**, sometimes referred to as the law of armed conflict (LOAC) or law of war. The Geneva Conventions are central to these laws. The Geneva Conventions (sometimes called humanitarian law proper) consist of four conventions (treaties) and two protocols (additional agreements). They are specifically designed to protect persons who are noncombatants, including military personnel who are wounded, captured, or otherwise out of combat.

Garrison Care **TIPS**

The rule of law is better than the rule of any individual.

–Aristotle of Stragira, Greek philosopher (384-322 BCE)

Garrison Care **TIPS**

In ancient China, it was forbidden to wage war during the planting or harvesting seasons. This prevented famine.

Garrison Care **TIPS**

The Greeks and Romans considered women and children to be noncombatants.

A closely related body of laws, called Hague Law (or the law of war), establishes methods of warfare. It consists of treaties that state what is and is not allowed in armed conflict or war.

■ What Are the Geneva Conventions About?

International law and treaties such as the Geneva and Hague Conventions regulate the conduct of hostilities. The Geneva Conventions specifically assert the protections accorded to noncombatants during periods of armed conflict. The rights and duties set forth in these conventions are incorporated into DoD and Army policies. The United States is obligated to adhere to these standards even when an opponent does not.

The Origins of International Humanitarian Law

Humans have tried to bring order to conflict for thousands of years. Some of the first written laws were from Hammurabi, the sixth king of ancient Babylon (1792-1750 BCE). Some of his laws covered the issues of conflict and war **FIGURE 35-1 ▶**. The 284 laws called the Code of Hammurabi were chiseled into a stele (stone monument) and placed in public so that all could see the laws. The stele was rediscovered in 1901 and now resides in the Louvre Museum in Paris, France.

The laws were very specific, and each offense was assigned a particular punishment. Punishments were harsh by modern standards, with many offenses resulting in death or maiming. Punishments were based upon the "an eye for an eye and a tooth for a tooth" philosophy. Although the penalties of Hammurabi's laws may seem cruel today, the fact that this ancient king put into writing the laws of his kingdom and attempted to make them a system was significant.

The Code of Hammurabi contained the concept of presumption of innocence and it also suggested that the accused and accuser have the opportunity to provide evidence. However, there is no provision for extenuating circumstances to mitigate or change the punishment of the offender.

One law in the Code of Hammurabi covered the subject of prisoners of war (POWs):

> If a chieftain or a man is captured on the "Way of the King" [in war], and a merchant buy him free, and bring him back to his place; if he have the means in his house to buy his freedom, he shall buy himself free; if he have nothing in his house with which to buy himself free, he shall be bought free by the temple of his community; if there be nothing in the temple with which to buy him free, the court shall buy his freedom. His field, garden, and house shall not be given for the purchase of his freedom.

Hammurabi's reputation as a lawgiver has caused his depiction to be placed on several US government buildings. Hammurabi is seen in the US House of Representatives and an image of Hammurabi receiving the laws from the Babylonian sun god is on the south wall of the US Supreme Court building.

The Code of Hammurabi is often cited as the first example of the concept that some laws are basic and are part of our basic human rights and duties. These basic human rights are beyond the capacity of even a king to change. By having the laws inscribed in stone, Hammurabi Code's was immutable and absolute.

Other cultures also established rules of war. The Chinese warrior, General Sun Tzu (544-496 BCE), wrote *The Art of War*, which suggested putting limits on the way in which wars were conducted. Around 200 BCE, the concept of war crimes emerged in the Hindu *Code of Manu*. In 1305, the Scottish hero Sir William Wallace, made famous in the film *Braveheart* (1995), was tried by the English for the wartime murder of civilians. And in 1625, the Dutch jurist Hugo Grotius laid some of the early foundations for international law in *On the Law of War and Peace*, which discussed the humanitarian treatment of civilians in war.

During the time of President George Washington, King Kamehameha I (c. 1758-1819) conquered the Hawaiian Islands and formally established the Kingdom of Hawaii in 1810. King Kamehameha is remembered for the Law of the Splintered Paddle (Mamalahoe Kanawai), which protected the rights of noncombatants in times of battle **FIGURE 35-2 ▶**. The law, "Let every elderly person, woman, and child lie by the roadside in safety," is enshrined in the state constitution, and is a model for modern humanitarian law regarding the treatment of civilians and other noncombatants during battle. It was created when King Kamehameha was fighting on Oahu. His leg became caught in a reef. A terrified fisherman came upon him and hit King Kamehameha on the head with a paddle in order to protect his family. Despite the violent blow, King Kamehameha escaped from the reef with his injury. The fisherman was found and brought before King Kamehameha. Instead of ordering for him to be killed, King Kamehameha ruled that the fisherman was a noncombatant. This became known as the Law of the Splintered Paddle. It stated that noncombatants should not be attacked.

The complete original 1797 law in Hawaiian and translated to English is:

Māmalahoe Kānāwai:
E nā kānaka, E mālama 'oukou i ke akua
A e mālama ho'i ke kanaka nui a me kanaka iki;
E hele ka 'elemakule, ka luahine, a me ke kama
A moe i ke ala
'A'ohe mea nāna e ho'opilikia.
Hewa nā - Make.

Law of the Splintered Paddle:
O my people, Honor thy god;
Respect alike [the rights of] men great and humble;
See to it that our aged, our women, and our children
Lie down to sleep by the roadside
Without fear of harm.
Disobey, and die.

King Kamehameha's final words were "E na'i wale no 'oukou, i ke kupono a'ole au," roughly translated as, "Continue my just deeds, they are not yet finished."

On April 4, 1863, President Lincoln signed General Order Number 100, Instructions for the Government of the Armies of the United States in the Field. It was also called the Leiber Code and was his instruction to the Union Army as to how soldiers should conduct themselves in wartime. This code, named after Francis Leiber, a lawyer and early political scientist, specified humane treatment for civilians and additionally was the first US law that prohibited killing prisoners of war.

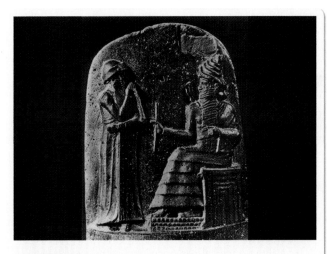

FIGURE 35-1 The upper part of the stele of Hammurabi's code of laws.

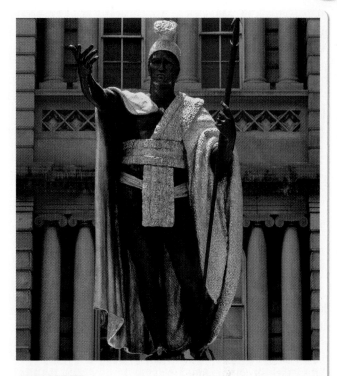

FIGURE 35-2 King Kamehameha I established the Law of the Splintered Paddle, which protected noncombatants from the dangers of battle.

Following are a number of principles that provide the superstructure or guide for the specific articles of the Geneva Conventions. These may be viewed as recurrent themes in each of the conventions and provide an executive summary of the overall intent of the conventions:

- The wounded and sick must be collected and cared for by the group involved in the conflict that has them in its power.
- Conduct toward persons who do not or can no longer fight is dictated by the following essential protections:
  - Respect for their life, both physically and mentally.
  - Provision of humane treatment, without discrimination.
  - Protection from acts of violence or reprisal.
  - The right to exchange news with their families and receive aid.
  - It is forbidden to kill or wound an adversary who surrenders or is unable to resist.
  - No one may be held responsible for an act he or she did not commit.
  - No one may be subjected to cruel or degrading punishment or other treatment including rape or enforced prostitution.
  - Collective punishment is prohibited.
  - Taking of hostages is prohibited.
  - Pillage (theft of property or goods) is prohibited.
  - Enslavement is prohibited.

■ History of the Geneva Conventions

The evolution of the Geneva Conventions began in Europe in the same time frame as the US Civil War. In 1859, Henry Dunant, a Swiss businessman, witnessed the French and Austrians fighting at the Battle of Solferino in Italy

FIGURE 35-3 ▼. The battle was horrific; it involved 200,000 troops, lasted 9 hours, and produced 40,000 casualties. Many of the wounded were either shot or bayoneted. In response to the carnage, Dunant quickly mobilized inhabitants of the local area to assist in attending to the remaining survivors. He later wrote a book about his experiences in Solferino and embarked on an initiative to establish limitations on the conduct of armed conflict. Dunant then formed a working group in Geneva, Switzerland to assist him in his efforts. This was the beginning of the International Committee of the Red Cross.

In 1864 the Swiss government convened an international conference attended by 16 nations who adopted the first "Geneva Convention for the Amelioration of

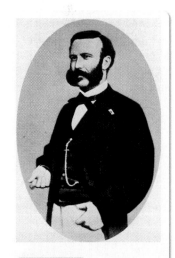

FIGURE 35-3 The horrors of the Battle of Solferino caused Henry Dunant to write *A Memory of Solferino*, which provided the motivation to create the International Committee of the Red Cross.

the Condition of Wounded in Armies in the Field." Over the next 8 decades, changes in the methods of warfare necessitated additions and refinements to the Geneva Conventions. By 1949 protections were extended to include:

- Wounded and sick members of the armed forces on land and sea
- Shipwrecked members of armed forces
- Medical personnel
- Medical facilities and equipment
- Support personnel accompanying the armed forces
- Military chaplains
- Civilians who spontaneously take up arms to repel an invasion
- Hospital ships
- Prisoners of war (POWs)
- Enemy prisoners of war (EPW)
- Civilians

The International Community of the Red Cross, which has the official role in protecting victims of war, uses **protecting powers** to enforce the Geneva Conventions and to document offenses against the Geneva Conventions. An example of a protecting power is the International Committee of the Red Cross itself or an appointed neutral nation documenting compliance with the Geneva Conventions during a conflict. Additionally, nations that are signatories to the Geneva Conventions are required to enforce the rules of the Geneva Conventions themselves and publicize serious violations, known as **grave breaches** or war crimes. In addition, all signatories are required to educate their respective militaries and their citizens about these laws. Today, the Geneva Conventions have been signed by all 194 nations in the United Nations. **FIGURE 35-4 ▾** and **FIGURE 35-5 ▾** show the relationship between the Geneva Conventions and other bodies of international law.

■ Who Are the Noncombatants Entitled to Protected Status?

Under the law of war, certain persons are protected as noncombatants. At a minimum, the groups of noncombatants entitled to protected status include those persons who are:

- Wounded, shipwrecked, or sick military personnel, who are out of combat
- Civilians, including delegates of the International Committee of the Red Cross (ICRC) and humanitarian agencies
- Military medical personnel, including nonclinical personnel assigned to medical activities
- Chaplains/clergy
- War correspondents
- Retained persons, including civilians authorized to accompany the military

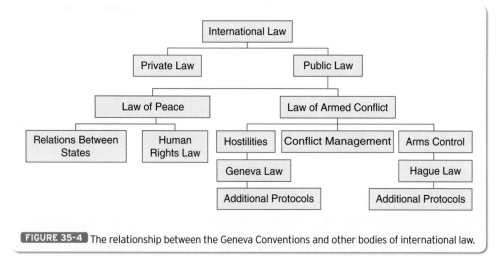

FIGURE 35-4 The relationship between the Geneva Conventions and other bodies of international law.

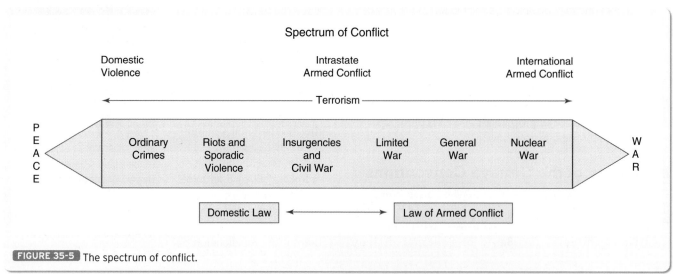

FIGURE 35-5 The spectrum of conflict.

Captors must respect (not attack) and protect (care for) all persons who are noncombatants, specifically including military medical personnel. According to the First Geneva Convention, medical personnel are specifically defined as:

> . . . personnel exclusively engaged in the search for, or the collection, transport, or treatment of the wounded and the sick . . . (they) shall be respected and protected in all circumstances.

This definition includes permanent medical personnel such as physicians, nurses, physician assistants, and medics. It is important to note that personnel who look after the administration and maintenance of medical units and establishments are also protected. This is true because their responsibilities are an integral part of military medical service, which could not function properly without them.

Protection from Attack

The Geneva Conventions protects medical personnel because they are noncombatants. Medical personnel who perform nonmedical duties harmful to the enemy lose their protective status. For example, being assigned to guard a nonmedical facility would jeopardize protective status. Medical personnel should only be assigned to administrative duties that are directly connected with the operation and administration of the medical unit. Does this mean that medical personnel cannot do anything other than treat patients? No. Because the rule is that they may not perform acts that are harmful to the enemy, they can perform various administrative and medical duties that do not harm the enemy, such as accompany a unit on a mission. Medical personnel may respond if hostilities arise; however, medical personnel should not engage the enemy as an aggressor.

Protection for Medical Personnel Upon Capture

If captured, medical personnel are considered to be retained personnel and not POWs. As retained personnel they can only be required to perform medical duties and must receive at least all the benefits conferred on POWs. During their retention, medical personnel must obey all POW camp rules, but may only be retained as long as needed to tend to prisoners of war who are sick and wounded. Retained medical personnel must be returned to their units when their "retention is not indispensable."

■ Protective Signs and Symbols

The Geneva Conventions recognize the red cross, red crescent, or red crystal on a white background as a protective sign; all persons and property and assets bearing one of the symbols must be spared. In addition to these three symbols, the red Star of David is recognized in practice, but the emblem has not been officially authorized by the Geneva Conventions. To ensure compliance, one of these signs must be conspicuously displayed on all medical units, facilities, personnel, equipment, transport, and hospitals, and in other places as necessary to adequately identify them as medical. In December 2005 the International Committee of the Red Cross added the red crys-

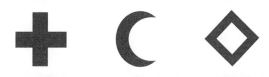

FIGURE 35-6 The red cross, the red crescent, and the red crystal.

tal for those organizations that perceive the red cross or red crescent as having a cultural, religious, or political connotation. The red crystal is free from those issues, and has the same legal status as the red cross and red crescent and may be used in the same way or under the same conditions. Like the red cross and red crescent, it may be used on a temporary basis by medical services attached to armed forces in place of their own emblems when used for identification as a protected entity. The red crystal is not a replacement for the other symbols, but may be seen in areas of conflict or humanitarian work. The red crystal may also be seen with another legitimate symbol inside it; for example, a red cross, red crescent, or red Star of David. Other countries have applied to the International Committee of the Red Cross to use their particular symbol instead of the red cross, crescent, or crystal (for example, a red flame or a red elephant on a white background), but these applications have been declined. The move is toward using a limited number of emblems for the sake of clarity.

The United States uses only the red cross to denote medical assets. It is important to note that the red cross is *not* a religious symbol. The symbol of the red cross on a white background is the reverse of the Swiss national flag in honor of the role of Switzerland in the development of the Geneva Conventions.

The red cross, red crescent, and red crystal emblems are visible symbols of the protections of war victims under the Geneva Conventions **FIGURE 35-6 ▲**. These also represent the neutrality of those who wear or display them. Misuse of these symbols is counter to the rules of international humanitarian law. The unauthorized use of the emblems for commercial enterprises, medical offices, or pharmacies, or for purposes that are inconsistent with IHL is illegal. **Perfidy** is use of the symbols during armed conflict to protect combatants and/or military equipment and with the intent to deceive the enemy. If this perfidious use of the emblem causes death or serious injury, the use of these symbols is considered a war crime.

■ Definition of Medical Personnel

Because of their unique role and responsibilities, it is important for Army medics to be clear about who is considered medical personnel. According to the Geneva (I) Convention for the Amelioration of the Condition of the Wounded and Sick in Armed Forces in the Field, chapter IV, Articles 24 and 25:

> Medical personnel are personnel exclusively engaged in the search for, or the collection, transport or treatment of the wounded or sick, or in the prevention of disease, staff

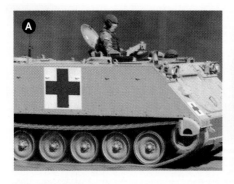 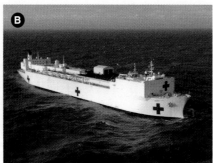 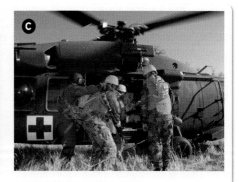

FIGURE 35-7 Transports of the wounded and sick or of medical equipment should not be attacked. Medical transports include: (**A**) ambulances, (**B**) medical ships, and (**C**) medical aircraft.

exclusively engaged in the administration of medical units and establishments, as well as chaplains attached to the armed forces, shall be respected and protected in all circumstances. Members of the armed forces specially trained for employment, should the need arise, as hospital orderlies, nurses or auxiliary stretcher-bearers, in the search for or the collection, transport or treatment of the wounded and sick shall likewise be respected and protected if they are carrying out these duties at the time when they come into contact with the enemy or fall into his hands.

This definition obviously includes the duties of medics.

Prohibition Against Targeting of Medical Facilities

The Geneva Conventions provide that a fixed or mobile medical establishment ". . . shall at all times be respected and protected . . . and that medical supplies may not be intentionally destroyed. The protection will not cease, unless such facilities are used to commit . . . acts harmful to the enemy." If at all possible, do not place medical facilities near military objectives in order to minimize collateral damage to the medical facility in the event the military objective is attacked.

<u>Collateral damage</u> is damage or loss caused incidentally during an attack undertaken despite all necessary precautions designed to prevent or minimize loss of civilian life, injury to civilians, and damage to civilian objects.

Could a commander order the removal of the red cross and still use the facility or a vehicle for a medical purpose? Yes, there is no requirement to affix a red cross. However, this may jeopardize the protection the facility or vehicle would be entitled to, because the enemy may not recognize it as part of a medical unit. Also, to be protected under the Geneva Conventions, the emblem must be red upon a white background.

If a commander wants to use an ambulance for a nonmedical purpose, such as for transporting combat troops, he or she may do so, but first must cover the red cross or other protective emblem. This will result in the ambulance being a legitimate target. A red cross cannot be placed on a combat vehicle so it will not be attacked while it is performing a non-

medical function. As mentioned earlier, misuse of the medical emblem in this manner is a war crime.

Transports of the wounded and sick or of medical equipment should not be attacked. Medical transports include ambulances, medical ships, and medical aircraft **FIGURE 35-7 ▲**. Medical aircraft used exclusively for the removal of the sick and wounded and for the transport of medical personnel and equipment should not be attacked, but should be respected by the enemy while it is marked with a distinctive medical emblem and is flying at heights, times, and on routes specifically agreed upon between the parties concerned.

All means of military medical transport, whether permanent or temporary, must be exclusively assigned to medical purposes in order to be entitled to protection. A convoy carrying both wounded and able-bodied soldiers or arms, for example, would lose this right, to the detriment of the wounded. Medical aircraft must bear, clearly marked, the distinctive red emblem together with their national colors on their lower, upper, and lateral surfaces. Unless agreed to otherwise, flights over enemy or enemy-occupied territory are prohibited. Medical aircraft shall obey every summons to land. In the event that a landing is thus imposed, the aircraft with its occupants may continue its flight after examination, if any. In the event of involuntary landing in enemy or enemy-occupied territory, the wounded and sick as well as the crew of the aircraft may be prisoners of war; medical personnel will be treated as designated in the Geneva Conventions.

Self-Defense and Defense of Patients

In combat operations, medical personnel are entitled to defend themselves and their patients. They are only permitted to use small defensive arms against an enemy who might attack them in violation of the Geneva Conventions. If medical personnel start acting as combatants, the enemy will respond accordingly. So long as the enemy is complying with the law of war, medical personnel may not use weapons in an offensive mode. It is only when the enemy violates the law of war that medical personnel may use these defensive weapons in combat; otherwise, you will lose your protected status.

The use of or mounting of offensive weapons on dedicated medical evacuation vehicles and aircraft jeopardizes the protections afforded by the Geneva Conventions. These offensive weapons can include, but are not limited to:

- Machine guns
- Grenade launchers
- Hand grenades
- Antitank weapons

If medical personnel are carrying grenades and have machine guns it would be hard to argue that these weapons are defensive, and this could jeopardize the protection of the medical establishment.

Duties and Rights of Medics

In *The Manual on the Rights and Duties of Medical Personnel in Armed Conflict*, Dr. Baccino-Astrada points out medical personnel must be fully aware of their duties, as well as the rights to which they are entitled in the performance of their tasks.

Medic Duties

In general, a medic's duties may be thought of as duties of action and duties of abstention. Not surprisingly, duties of action are directly linked to the rights of persons who are entitled to their care; they generally concern medical care that must be performed to meet the needs of persons requiring such services; for example, applying a tourniquet to a severely bleeding patient. Duties of abstention may be thought of as those things that the medic consciously avoids because they are against the patients' best interest, such as avoiding any practices that would be considered unethical; for example, using an ambulance marked with a red cross to transport weapons.

Medic Rights

The rights of medical personnel, including medics, are connected to the obligations incumbent on the states who are parties to the conflict and to the state to which the medical personnel belong (whether that state is a party to the conflict or not). Dr. Baccino-Astrada comments:

> Among the recognized rights of medical personnel, a distinction can likewise be made between those which imply action, by the parties to the conflict, such as providing medical personnel with all the help needed for them to accomplish their . . . mission as well as possible, and those which only imply a duty to abstain from taking action, such as not taking retaliatory measures against medical personnel.

In other words, because the United States is a signatory of the Geneva Conventions, the Geneva Conventions apply to you, the American soldier medic.

Detainee Care

During all military operations, members of the United States armed forces must be prepared to detain personnel who are no longer willing or able to continue fighting, as well as other personnel based on detention criteria: threat to US forces, threat to members of the local population, and other security interests. For the medical community, this also means being prepared to take into custody, protect, and medically care for all categories of potential detainees. It is imperative that all individuals detained by US forces are treated in accordance with DoD policies and domestic and international law. The medic should be aware of his or her responsibility to adhere to and maintain the DoD and Army policies in a manner consistent with these obligations.

Remember, IHL is the body of rules that, in wartime, protects people who are not or are no longer participating in the hostilities. Its central purpose is to limit and prevent human suffering in times of armed conflict. This specifically applies to detainees.

The term **detainee** refers to any person captured or otherwise detained by an armed force. US Army policy dictates that all detainees will be treated humanely in accordance with the applicable principles of the Geneva Conventions. These principles are reinforced with many Department of the Army references. If the number of regulations denotes the importance of a topic, then proper detainee care is critical. Some of these regulations include:

- AR 190-8, Enemy Prisoners of War Retained Personnel, Civilian Internees, and Other Detainees
- DoD Directive 2310.1, DoD Program for Enemy Prisoners of War (EPW) and Other Detainees
- The Declaration of Tokyo (1975)
- DoD Directive 5100.77, DoD Law of War Program
- DoD 6025.18-R, DoD Health Information Privacy Regulation, Jan 03, c7.11.4
- FM 27-10, The Law of Land Warfare
- FM 8-10-5, Brigade and Division Surgeons' Handbook

Military Medical Ethics

The military physician advises the commander on **medical ethics**. Medical ethics are the application of values and judgments as they apply to the care of patients. Important values are:

- **Beneficence:** Acting in the best interest of the patient.
- **Nonmaleficence:** "First, do no harm."
- **Autonomy:** The patient has the right to choose or refuse treatment unless there are compelling issues, such as public health needs.
- **Justice:** Scarce health resources will be triaged fairly and equally for care.
- **Dignity:** The patient has a right to dignity.
- **Truthfulness:** Encompasses the concepts of informed consent and disclosure of information.

Similar to our noncombat roles, all military health care providers, including medics, are expected to act as patient advocates for detainees. Medics are often the caretakers for detainees and must refrain from participating in any action adverse to a detainee's health.

There are four categories of detainees listed in the Geneva Conventions. All are entitled to the privileges of the Geneva Conventions and the protections afforded in other Army regulations.

1. **Enemy prisoner of war (EPW):** An EPW is a detained person as described in the Geneva Conventions. In particular, an EPW is someone who, while engaged in combat under orders of his or her government, is captured by the opposing armed forces.

2. **Civilian internee (CI):** A CI is confined to a specific area during armed conflict for reasons of security or protection, or due to commission of an offense (insurgent, rebellious, or criminal) against the detaining power. During World War II, the United States interned Americans of Japanese descent because of unfounded beliefs that these individuals would act as spies or commit sabotage. As we now know, this was untrue. In fact, the 100th Battalion/442nd Regimental Combat Team, which fought in the European theater, was composed of Japanese-Americans and was the most highly decorated unit in the history of the United States. Twenty-one of its members earned the Medal of Honor. Despite their patriotism and sacrifice, the families of many of the 442nd infantry soldiers were interned in the United States. Today, the Geneva Conventions state that civilians should be allowed to live as normally as possible and internment should be for valid security reasons only.

3. **Retained person (RP):** Captured personnel who are medical, chaplains, or in voluntary aid societies (eg, Red Cross) are considered retained personnel. They are to be allowed to work in their capacity as caregivers and be repatriated (returned) as soon as their services are no longer needed.

4. **Other detainees (OD):** This is any person in the custody of US armed forces who has not yet been classified as an EPW, CI, or RP.

As part of the global war on terror, the United States has added an additional classification for detainees who do not specifically fall into one of the above categories: **enemy combatants (EC)**. Persons classified as EC are still entitled to be treated humanely.

Care and Treatment of Detainees

Our nation's laws require that we give certain rights to people captured on the battlefield. These are basic rights, and soldiers are expected to be aware of them. In addition, affording these protections has military value. If the enemy knows we will treat them (and/or their family) with dignity and respect, he or she is more likely to surrender. It is also more likely that

the enemy will reciprocate by extending such rights to our soldiers if they should become prisoners of war. Although some terrorist groups will not adhere to the Geneva Conventions, it is dangerous to think that reprisal will help. As we have seen from past incidents of soldiers' flawed judgment, ignoring the Geneva Conventions only establishes an environment of distrust, encourages escalating reactions, and creates more sympathy for the enemy. We have seen this in the Vietnam War in the My Lai massacre (1968) and in the mistreatment of detainees at Abu Ghraib prison in Iraq (2004).

Why should we care about the welfare of the enemy? After the 1991 Gulf War, many Iraqi prisoners were reluctant to leave, and asked to remain in our POW facilities. Think of all of the lives that were saved when thousands of Iraqi soldiers gave up. Which would you rather have: 10,000 enemy soldiers surrendering or 10,000 enemy soldiers wanting to shoot you? If the enemy thinks we will kill him or her if they surrender, why would they surrender? We want to encourage the enemy to surrender, so we want the enemy to know that we will care for them and their families with dignity and in a humane manner.

Initial actions upon capture of a person considered to be an EPW, even if later they fall into another category, include the five Ss. This is a safety issue for you, your unit, and the individual(s) detained. The five Ss are:

1. *Search* immediately for weapons, ammunition, equipment, and documents with intelligence value. EPW/RP will be allowed to retain personal effects of sentimental or religious value.

2. *Segregate* them into groups of enlisted, noncommissioned officers, officers, civilians, or undetermined status. Individuals presumed to have intelligence value should be separated immediately from other EPWs. Depending on the situation, women and children may be involved. Additionally, warring factions may need to be separated.

3. *Silence* is critical. Communication among the captured personnel is dangerous for all concerned. Segregation prevents prisoners from communicating verbally or with signals.

4. *Safeguard* those captured. While they are your prisoner, you are responsible for them. Do not use those captured as a shield.

5. *Speed* them to the rear. The wounded EPW patient is evacuated to the rear as soon as their medical condition permits. The evacuation is made based on medical need, not the uniform worn or the actions taken. All personnel should be given documentation and/or a triage tag noting any information needed in transport.

Accomplishment of the military mission requires that we treat those who are captured humanely. Many of these people will be victims of war, and some may be enemy soldiers, but once captured, they are entitled to the same humane treatment. Medical standards for detainees are the same as for US

Garrison Care TIPS

There is a comprehensive list of terrorists and terrorist groups identified under Executive Order 13224 located at www.treas.gov/ofac/. Most personnel affiliated with these organizations will be classified as EC.

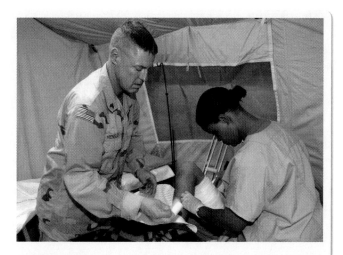
FIGURE 35-8 Medical care for soldiers and for detainees is exactly the same and of the highest quality.

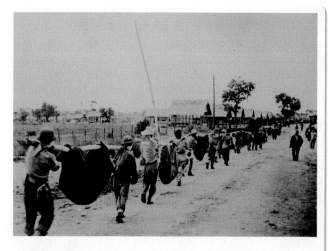
FIGURE 35-9 At least 6,000 to 11,000 Allied soldiers died during the Bataan Death March in 1942.

forces FIGURE 35-8 ▲. As noted in the Geneva Conventions, "Members of the armed forces . . . who are wounded or sick shall be respected and protected in all circumstances."

In addition to being treated humanely, detainees must be cared for without adverse distinction founded on sex, race, nationality, religion, or similar criteria, and attempts on their lives are strictly prohibited. The Geneva Conventions further require that detainees will not be left without medical assistance and care. Priority for medical treatment is based on the severity of the wound or injury. The most urgent wounded or sick soldiers will be treated first, regardless of the uniform they are wearing.

Initial Actions Upon Capture

There are almost 100 articles in the Geneva Conventions that deal with conditions for detainees. These cover the things we often hear in movies, such as "name, rank, serial number, and age" questions. The prohibition on asking for information other than identification was added after World War II to prevent inhumane coercive methods used to extract information. Additionally, these articles cover medical care, hygiene, sanitation, work (and pay), relief parcels, retained medical personnel, living conditions, discipline, and punishment. Anyone who tortures a detainee in any status is committing a war crime.

Detainees without injury are to be evacuated from the combat zone and into appropriate channels as quickly as possible. This must be carried out humanely. Although detainees may travel on foot, they may not be subjected to forced marches. The most glaring example of such an abuse was the Bataan Death March that occurred in the Philippines during World War II FIGURE 35-9 ▶. Such activities are considered war crimes. As noted earlier, ill or injured detainees must be evacuated separate from, but in the same manner as, US and allied forces. For those requiring care, treatment will be given based on need at the appropriate medical facility.

At any time during or after evacuation, physical abuse, including deprivation of sleep, food, or water; stress positions; intentional humiliation; and verbal abuse are prohibited. Detainees must not be completely stripped of clothing at any time. Intelligence value remains secondary to treating all detainees humanely with a view to their ultimate release and reconciliation. To act otherwise creates deep-seated hatreds and prolongs the conflict.

Body cavity exams or searches may be performed for valid medical reasons with the verbal consent of the detainee. However, these exams should not be performed as part of a routine intake physical examination. Body cavity searches without consent are conducted only when there is a reasonable belief or evidence that the detainee is concealing an item that presents a security risk. If possible, a body cavity exam will be conducted by personnel of the same gender.

No medics or other medical personnel involved in the care of detainees will assist with interrogations. Further advice on how to conduct interrogations or interpret medical data for the purposes of interrogations is prohibited. Interrogations are performed only by trained and certified military intelligence personnel. The concept of using medics to "soften up" detainees or inform interrogators of medical issues to assist with interrogations is prohibited.

Living conditions will of necessity limit the mobility of the detainee; however, detainees are not criminals and therefore they must be housed in conditions similar to the soldiers of the detaining authority. Recreational sports, religious services, and food services must be provided and take into account the culture of the detainee. All are important for the detainee's well-being.

Food is an important issue. Withholding of food is never allowed. However, one would think that a diet high enough in calories is all that is required. This is not necessarily true. During World War II, many Allied soldiers in the Pacific theater became malnourished on a diet of rice, because it had too few nutrients. Similarly, Japanese soldiers were unable to tolerate European diets in POW camps. The detaining authority must also consider that exposures to unfamiliar microbes may cause severe problems.

Humiliation or embarrassment of detainees is absolutely prohibited. Taking of photographs for the purpose of humiliating detainees also is prohibited. The need for photographs for documentation of injuries or conditions will be determined by the command or medical authorities.

Evacuation and Care of Detainees

Those units designated to hold and evacuate detainees must categorize sick and wounded detainees in their custody as walking or nonwalking (litter) wounded. Ill or injured detainees are taken to the nearest medical treatment facility (MTF) and evacuated through medical channels. Detainees will be transferred to another MTF only if medically stable, and will never be transferred out of the country without the secretary of defense's (SECDEF) approval. Provision of medical care for detainees is in accordance with the Geneva Conventions and Army regulations. In-processing medical requirements are similar to a soldier readiness program (SRP), which most soldiers have experienced.

After arrival at the detention facility, detainees will in-process and receive a medical examination that will include a height and weight check, dental exam, mental health screening, chest x-ray, and screening for communicable diseases such as tuberculosis or sexually transmitted diseases. The overall health, hygiene, and nutritional status of the detainee will be noted. Detainees will be immunized against diseases as recommended by the theater surgeon. Any immediate medical needs will be addressed and routine care will be noted to be scheduled for medical care later. Sick call will be available each day and each detainee will be reweighed every month. Any detainee unable to be cared for in the detention facility will be moved to an appropriate facility for care. The living conditions must be sanitary and hygiene must be maintained. As previously discussed, the medical in-processing will not include a body cavity search unless medically indicated.

A record for each detainee will be created during in-processing, and all of the screening information will be recorded. Medical records will accompany detainees throughout the medical system. Though not included under the Health Insurance Portability and Accountability Act (HIPAA), detainee health care information is protected by regulation; only those with a need to know are to have access to the information. This will be documented on a DA 4254, and only specific information to satisfy a legitimate request will be released. The medical treatment facility commander determines what information is applicable.

Detainees are entitled to a copy of these records on their release. The health care provider names are stricken from the copied records. The original records are retained by the United States.

Some medical information may be required for safety in the detention facility. For example, those with communicable diseases such as tuberculosis may require separation from

Per DoD policy, as a general rule the ICRC is the only such organization authorized access to detainees.

other detainees. Additionally, guards will need to be informed of how to mitigate the risks of contamination.

Detainees will receive copies of the applicable portions of the Geneva Conventions in their own language. Representatives of the International Committee of the Red Cross (ICRC) may be in attendance to review in-processing procedures. The ICRC receives a list of all detainees in our custody and has access to detainees for interviews.

Outpatient Care

As noted, detainee sick call needs to be held daily for those in need of medical care. Enemy Prisoners of War (EPWs), Retained Persons (RPs), and Civilian Internees (CIs) are not to be denied medical care. When possible, detainees will be cared for separately from others. There also are cultural issues that must be considered. As much as feasible, female health care providers and medics screen and care for female detainees.

It should not have to be stated, but all MTF staff, including security personnel, working with detainees must maintain a professional appearance and military bearing at all times. It is necessary to provide humane treatment, but care must also be given to not identify too closely with the detainees or their situation. In conflict, as in humanitarian, disaster, and refugee situations, one must maintain a professional bearing and not lose objectivity. One of the best ways to guard against dehumanization of the detainees or loss of objectivity about the situation is maintenance of military bearing. It is *never* appropriate to use your position as a soldier for personal gain. Remember the "family rule": how would you hope another soldier would care for your family?

The detaining authority is required to provide any necessary medical support to EPWs, RPs, CIs, and other detainees. This medical support includes first aid, a sanitary food service, preventive medicine, sanitation, medical services, and medical supplies, such as glasses, prosthetics, and medications.

The detaining authority also coordinates the use of medically trained EPW, CI, and RP personnel, and any captured medical materials. Special considerations and precautions must be observed, but consider that, just as you would want to provide care to your colleagues and fellow soldiers if captured, very likely they feel the same.

Detainees will not be handcuffed or tied, except to ensure safe custody or when prescribed by a responsible medical officer as needed to control a medical case requiring restraint.

The detaining authority (in our case the United States) is bound to take all sanitary measures necessary to ensure clean camps to prevent epidemics. Every camp must have an infirmary. Any detainee with a contagious disease, mental condi-

Garrison Care **TIPS**

Detainees have the right and must receive the basic necessities to stay in good health. Additionally, the cultural and social norms and situation must be considered. The detaining authority has an obligation to reasonably accommodate the food habits of detainees; for example, one should not provide a person of the Muslim faith with pork. There may be gender, religious, or other beliefs that need to be taken into account.

Shelter and clothing should be consistent with the climate of the region. For example, if you capture a detainee in a cold region during the winter, the US has an obligation to ensure that the detainee is properly clothed. This does not mean that you must give up equipment to comfort the detainee, but you must find adequate clothing or tell your chain of command of this need.

tion, or other illness as determined by the medical officer will be isolated from the other patients.

Detainees suffering from serious diseases or whose condition necessitates special treatment, surgery, or hospital care must be admitted to any military or civilian medical unit where treatment can be given. Special facilities need to be available for the care and rehabilitation of the disabled. As mentioned before, detainee evacuation outside the theater of operations requires SECDEF approval.

The detaining authorities shall, upon request, issue to every detainee who has undergone treatment an official certificate indicating the nature of the injury or illness and the duration and type of treatment received. Duplicate certificates are sent to the International Committee of the Red Cross. At the same time, medics and other medical personnel must complete the appropriate medical records: SF 88 (Report of Medical Examination), SF 600 (Chronological Record of Medical Care), and DA Form 3444 (Treatment Record). Medical care documentation occurs at every level of medical care and is transferred with the detainee.

Medical inspections are held once a month; the height and weight of each detainee is recorded. These inspections monitor the general state of health, nutrition, and cleanliness of detainees and are intended to detect communicable diseases (eg, TB, STDs, HIV, lice).

Commanders are responsible for the sanitary conditions of the camp and inspections of the camp. Detainees are to be provided with sanitary supplies, service, and facilities necessary for their personal cleanliness and sanitation. Separate latrine facilities need to be provided for each gender.

The inhumane treatment of detainees is prohibited and not justified by the stress of combat or deep provocation. At no time will detainee medical information be available for interrogation purposes. Medical personnel are obliged, however, to report any information obtained during the course of

medical care that could affect the safety and security of other detainees or of Allied Forces. Detainees are to be protected against all acts of violence including rape, forced prostitution, assault, theft, and bodily injury. Research, medical, or scientific experiments are prohibited.

During transport, detainees need to have sufficient food and drinking water to keep them in good health, and should be provided adequate clothing, shelter, and medical attention.

Personnel resources to guard detainee medical patients are provided by the echelon commander; medical personnel do not guard detainee patients.

■ Army Values and Compliance With the Geneva Conventions

As mentioned earlier, the United States is a party to and signatory of the Geneva Conventions, which afford protection for medical personnel, facilities, and evacuation platforms (including aircraft on the ground). Violation of the Geneva Conventions can result in the loss of protection afforded by them.

Obligation to Report Violations

Suppose you are given an order such as, "Shoot every man, woman, and child in sight." Although every soldier is taught to obey the commands of a military superior under threat of military legal action, obviously this is an unlawful order. What should you do? If the soldier obeys the order to commit an illegal act, he or she may be charged with a war crime; however, if he or she disobeys the order, the soldier may face the Uniform Code of Military Justice (UCMJ). There may even be a risk of violence against you for the refusal. First, try to get the order rescinded. Remind the person who gave the order that it violates the law of war. If the person persists, you must disregard that order. This takes courage, but if you follow a criminal order, you are responsible for, and can be tried and punished for, committing the crime under the law of war. Remember, no one can force you to commit a crime, and you cannot be court-martialed or punished for refusing to obey an unlawful order.

The lack of courage to disregard a criminal order, or a mistaken fear that you could be court-martialed for disobedience of an order, is no excuse. The Code of Conduct says, "I am an American fighting [soldier], responsible for my actions and dedicated to the principles [that] make my country free." The soldier who follows the Code of Conduct should have no problem identifying and disobeying criminal orders. If a criminal order results in a violation of the law of war, then you must report the violation to the appropriate authorities. Your first and best option is to report through your chain of command.

You must report any known or suspected violation of the laws of war. Your first and best option is to report through your chain of command. Your commander has established regulations governing reporting procedures. If you fail to follow these procedures, you could be prosecuted under the UCMJ.

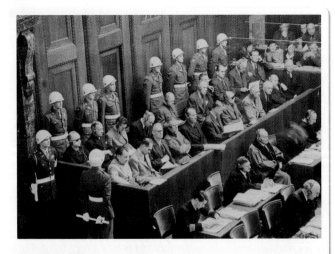

FIGURE 35-10 The concept "plea of superior orders" was used by Nazis accused of war crimes in World War II, but was rejected by the Nürnberg Tribunal.

But what do you do if you must report a known or suspected violation by someone in your chain of command? Other reporting options include:

- Local office of the Inspector General
- Office of the Provost Marshal (military police)
- Judge Advocate (military lawyer)
- A chaplain, who can help you report through official channels

Regardless of how you decide to report a violation of the law of war, you should do it immediately. Evidence and witnesses disappear quickly. Also, a prompt investigation is more likely to dispel any mistaken charges. Even the perception of impropriety can be detrimental to the mission and US interests. In the past, people have violated these rules and have been tried and sentenced for such violations.

Each soldier is held accountable for the atrocities and crimes they commit **FIGURE 35-10 ▲**. The concept "plea of superior orders" was used by Nazis accused of war crimes in World War II, but was rejected by the Nürnberg Tribunal, which stated, "The fact that the defendant acted pursuant to the orders of the government or of a superior shall not free him from responsibility, but may be considered in mitigation of punishment if the Tribunal determines that justice so requires."

Superiors must be cognizant at all times that they may be held responsible for the actions of their subordinate soldiers. Similarly, they must use care not to utter words that could be perceived as, or in fact be, unlawful orders. Additionally, superiors cannot stand by or condone war crimes. The case of General Yamashida of Japan demonstrates this concept. In 1944, the general was in control of the Philippines. Although General Yamashida never gave any unlawful orders, he was held accountable for the atrocities and brutalities committed by his forces. The Manila Massacre of February 1945 was responsible for the deaths of at least 100,000 Philippine citizens. The military commission found:

> . . . where murder and rape and vicious, vengeful actions are widespread offences, and there is no effective attempt by a commander to discover and control the criminal acts, such a commander may be held responsible, even criminally liable, for the lawless acts of his troops, depending upon their nature and the circumstances surrounding them.

Protecting Civilians in Wartime

Protection for civilians is a basic principle of humanitarian law: civilians not taking part in the fighting must on no account be attacked and must be spared and protected. The Geneva Conventions contain specific rules to protect civilians, including the following:

- Pillage, reprisals, indiscriminate destruction of property, and the taking of hostages is prohibited. Civilians are not to be subject to collective punishment or deportation.
- The safety, honor, family rights, religious practices, manners, and customs of civilians are to be respected.
- Civilians are to be protected from murder, torture or brutality, and discrimination on the basis of race, nationality, religion, or political opinions.
- Children who are orphaned or separated from their families must be cared for.
- If security allows, civilians must be permitted to lead normal lives.

Accountability

The law is a system of rules enforced through institutions. It is generally understood to be the collection of written or understood rules and codes designed to govern behaviors or actions of a defined group of people. The law also concerns appropriate consequences for deviations from acceptable behavior. War crimes (violations of laws governing armed conflict) and crimes against humanity constitute a special area of the law. These crimes are considered international; however, they may be prosecuted by the country that has suffered from the crime, the victor in the conflict, or the nation that had control of the soldier. Many World War II war crimes trials were conducted by military tribunals or national courts.

Laws, and the larger legal systems of which they are a part, attempt to codify important values about equity, fairness, and justice, and generally reflect the cultural themes and beliefs of the society they represent. Most legal systems are divided into areas that address specific concerns. In the United States, for example, our legal system is divided into groups of laws that address property, contracts, trust, tort, criminal, constitutional, maritime, administrative, and international issues. In time of peace in the United States, medical personnel function under civilian tort law, which allows claims for compensation when someone or their property is harmed. If the harm involves criminality, the state prosecutes and, in the event of conviction, the court may punish the offender. In times of war or armed conflict, military medical personnel and civilians working with them function under the umbrella of international humanitarian law. Violations may be prosecuted as war crimes. For the most part, the United States government has retained the right to prosecute crimes committed by its military members under the Uniform Code of Military Justice.

What Are the Benefits of International Humanitarian Law?

Armed conflicts of the 20th and early 21st centuries have made it clear that parties to a conflict do not necessarily abide by the standards set forth in international humanitarian law. Understandably, people may ask why the United States perseveres in its adherence to IHL when other parties do not. The following are a few reasons that are commonly cited to justify our investment in limiting the methods of war:

- Prevents unnecessary suffering and destruction
- Does not impede legitimate warfare
- Speeds war termination and simplifies posthostilities reconciliation
- Enhances reciprocity for our forces
- Supports international values
- Decreases the likelihood of injury and the destruction of noncombatants through proportionality of response
- With necessity, targeting must offer a military advantage
- Collateral damage is decreased, and commanders are obliged to minimize damage

Summary

We have discussed the evolution and general principles of the Geneva Conventions, international humanitarian law, and the specific applications of the law to combat medics. The guiding principle is humanity; although nations still engage in war, many nations have set rules to make warfare more humane and to decrease the terrible sufferings caused by war. The rules recognize that everyone involved in war is a human being, with rights and dignity. This includes enemy prisoners of war, American prisoners of war, detained civilians, or captured persons; all are human beings and all deserve to be treated humanely. The humanitarian provisions of the law of war protect everyone caught up in the conflict, whether friend, foe, or bystander.

As American soldiers, it is our duty to avoid inflicting any unnecessary suffering or destruction. We must treat all prisoners of war, other captured or detained persons, and civilians humanely. We will refuse to obey any order that requires us to commit an act that violates the law of war. We will report any violation of the law of war to appropriate authorities. Above all, we must remember that each of us is personally responsible for any unlawful act we commit.

By knowing our rights and responsibilities as human beings and as US soldiers, by reporting all suspected war crimes to the proper authorities, and by knowing the rights of our enemy and of the civilian population, we play an important part in mission success and a return to peace.

Aid Kit

Ready for Review

- Medics and the United States military work under the protections of international humanitarian law (IHL), sometimes referred to as the law of armed conflict (LOAC) or law of war.
  - The Geneva Conventions are central to these laws.
- International law and treaties such as the Geneva and Hague Conventions regulate the conduct of hostilities.
  - The Geneva Conventions specifically assert the protections accorded to noncombatants during periods of armed conflict.
  - The rights and duties set forth in these conventions are incorporated into DoD and Army policies.
  - The United States is obligated to adhere to these standards even when an opponent does not.
- At a minimum, the groups of noncombatants entitled to protected status include those persons who are:
  - Wounded, shipwrecked, or sick military personnel, who are out of combat
  - Civilians, including delegates of the International Committee of the Red Cross (ICRC) and humanitarian agencies
  - Military medical personnel, including nonclinical personnel assigned to medical activities
  - Chaplains/clergy
  - War correspondents
  - Retained persons, including civilians authorized to accompany the military
- The Geneva Conventions recognize the red cross, red crescent, or red crystal on a white background as a protective sign; all persons, property, and assets bearing one of the symbols must be spared.
  - To ensure compliance, one of these signs must be conspicuously displayed on all medical units, facilities, personnel, equipment, transport, and hospitals, and in other places as necessary to adequately identify them as medical.
- If at all possible, do not place medical facilities near military objectives in order to minimize collateral damage to the medical facility in the event the military objective is attacked.
- During all military operations, members of the US armed forces must be prepared to detain personnel who are no longer willing or able to continue fighting, and other personnel based on detention criteria: threat to US forces, threat to members of the local population, and other security interests.
  - For the medical community, this also means being prepared to take into custody, protect, and medically care for all categories of potential detainees.
- The United States is a party to and signatory of the Geneva Conventions.
  - The Geneva Conventions afford protection for medical personnel, facilities, and evacuation platforms (including aircraft on the ground).
  - Violation of the Geneva Conventions can result in the loss of protection afforded by them.

Key Terms

civilian Person who is not a member of the enemy's armed forces and does not take part in the hostilities.

civilian internee (CI) A person interned during an international armed conflict for security reasons, for protection, or because they have committed an offense (insurgent or criminal) against the detaining power.

collateral damage Unintentional or incidental injury or damage to persons or objects that would not be lawful military targets in the circumstances ruling at the time. Such damage is not unlawful so long as it is not excessive in light of the overall military advantage anticipated from the attack (from Joint Publication 3-60).

convention A binding agreement between states. Generally used for formal multilateral instruments with a broad number of parties.

detainee Any person captured or otherwise detained by an armed force.

enemy prisoner of war (EPW) detained person as described in the Geneva Conventions who, while engaged in combat under orders of his or her government, is captured by the armed forces of the enemy.

grave breach A gross violation of the basic principles of the Geneva Conventions; also known as a war crime.

international humanitarian law (IHL) The body of rules that protects people who are not or who are no longer participating in hostilities in wartime.

medical ethics The application of values and judgments as they apply to the care of patients.

other detainee (OD) A person in the custody of US armed forces that has not yet been classified.

perfidy A calculated violation of trust; treachery. As applied to the Geneva Conventions, it usually means the deliberate use of the protective emblem of the Red Cross under false pretenses. Referred to as "perfidious use," this act is a war crime.

protecting power An entity such as the International Committee of the Red Cross or a nation appointed to document compliance with the Geneva Conventions during conflict. The protecting power is recognized as empowered to represent the other country and protect its interests. Poland was the protecting power for the United States in Iraq after the first Gulf War.

retained person (RP) Enemy who is medical personnel, a chaplain, or is in a voluntary aid society.

Review Questions

1. **What kind of human rights are commonly violated in an armed conflict?**

   Answer: Armed conflict can result in a violation of a wide range of laws. In modern armed combat, there are restrictions on who can be targeted: only combatants in opposing forces and military objects. Unfortunately, very often woman and children suffer disproportionately, and are specifically targeted for abuse and attack. Sometimes, members of groups are targeted on racial, religious, or ethnic grounds–this is also prohibited. The rules are to be observed by governments, their armed forces, armed opposition groups, and any other parties to a conflict. The four Geneva Conventions of 1949 establish the humanitarian protections that we apply during armed conflict.

2. **Under the laws of war, noncombatants are afforded protected status under the Geneva Conventions. Can you name these protections?**

   Answer:

   A. Civilians and civilian property may not be the subject of a military attack. Civilians are people who are not members of the enemy's armed forces and do not take part in the hostilities. Journalists and members of the International Committee of the Red Cross (ICRC) are also given protection as civilians.

   B. Wounded and sick in the field and at sea. Soldiers who have fallen by reason of sickness or wounds and who cease to fight are to be respected and protected.

   C. Prisoners of war. Surrender may be made by any means that communicates the intent to give up. There is no clear-cut rule as to what constitutes surrender. However, most agree that surrender constitutes a cessation of resistance and placement of one's self at the direction of the captor. Captors must respect (not attack) and protect (care for) those who surrender.

   D. Chaplains are considered protected persons.

   E. Medical personnel are specifically identified in the First Geneva Convention to include permanent medical personnel (doctors, nurses, physician's assistants, and combat medics) and support personnel.

   F. Protection for civilians is a basic principle of humanitarian law: Civilians not taking part in the fighting must on no account be attacked and must be spared and protected. The Geneva Conventions contain specific rules to protect civilians, including the following:

      • Pillage, reprisals, indiscriminate destruction of property, and the taking of hostages is prohibited. Civilians are not to be subject to collective punishment or deportation.

      • The safety, honor, family rights, religious practices, manners, and customs of civilians are to be respected.

      • Civilians are to be protected from murder, torture or brutality, and discrimination on the basis of race, nationality, religion, or political opinions.

      • Children who are orphaned or separated from their families must be cared for.

      • If security allows, civilians must be permitted to lead normal lives.

3. **Under the Geneva Conventions, medical personnel receive two forms of protection: protection from attack and protection upon capture. Are medical support personnel who do not directly treat patients in this protected status?**

   Answer: Yes. Those who look after the administration of medical units and establishments are similarly protected, because they are an integral part of the medical service of the military, which could not function without them. However, medical personnel who perform nonmedical duties harmful to the enemy lose their protective status.

4. **In addition to medical care, what types of duties may a medic perform and remain in protected status under the Geneva Conventions?**

   Answer: The rule is that medical personnel may not perform acts that are harmful to the enemy, because this will jeopardize their protected status. They can do various administrative or other duties that do not harm the enemy.

5. **What if medical personnel are assigned to guard a nonmedical facility?**

   Answer: This will jeopardize their protective status. Medical personnel should not be assigned to administrative duties not directly connected with the operation or administration of the medical unit.

6. **If captured, medical personnel are considered to be Retained Personnel and not POWs. What are the basic protections of Retained Personnel?**

    Answer: Retained Personnel can be required to perform only medical duties; they must receive at least all the benefits conferred on POWs and may be retained only as long as needed to tend to POWs who are sick and wounded. During the period of retention, however, they must obey POW camp rules.

7. **In combat operations, medical personnel are entitled to defend themselves and their patients. What types of weapons may a medic carry and still be considered protected under the Geneva Conventions?**

    Answer: Medics are permitted to use only small defensive arms to protect themselves and/or their patients against an enemy who might attack them in violation of the Geneva Conventions.

8. **What happens if medical personnel use these defensive weapons to fire at enemy soldiers?**

    Answer: If you start acting as combatants, the enemy will respond accordingly. So long as the enemy is complying with the law of war, medical personnel may not use weapons in an offensive mode. It is only when the enemy violates the law of war that medical personnel may use these defensive weapons in combat; otherwise, you will lose your protected status. The use of or mounting of offensive weapons on dedicated medical evacuation vehicles and aircraft jeopardizes the protections afforded by the Geneva Conventions. These offensive weapons can include, but are not limited to, machine guns, grenade launchers, hand grenades, or antitank weapons.

9. **What if medical personnel are carrying grenades and have machine guns?**

    Answer: It would be hard to argue that these weapons are defensive, and this could jeopardize the protection of the medical establishment.

10. **Could a commander order the removal of the red cross and still use a vehicle for a medical purpose?**

    Answer: Yes, there is no requirement to affix a red cross to anything. However, this may jeopardize the protection the vehicle would be entitled to because the enemy may not recognize it as a medical asset.

11. **In order to enhance OPSEC, can the emblem be camouflaged (eg, use a dark brown cross with a light sand-colored background)?**

    Answer: To be protected under the Geneva Conventions, the emblem must be red upon a white background.

12. **Suppose a commander wants to use an ambulance for a nonmedical purpose (eg, transport combat troops). Can he or she do so?**

    Answer: Yes, but he or she must cover up the red cross or other protective emblem. This will result in the ambulance being a legitimate target.

13. **How about the opposite situation: Can a commander take a combat vehicle and put a red cross on it so it won't be attacked while it is performing a nonmedical function?**

    Answer: No. Misuse of the medical emblem in this manner is a war crime. All means of military medical transport, whether permanent or temporary, must be exclusively assigned to medical purposes in order to be entitled to protection. Medical aircraft shall bear, clearly marked, the distinctive emblem together with their national colors on their lower, upper, and lateral surfaces. A convoy carrying both wounded and able-bodied soldiers or arms, for example, would lose any protection, to the detriment of the wounded.

14. **Why should we care about the welfare of the enemy?**

    Answer: After the 1991 Gulf War, many Iraqi prisoners were reluctant to leave and asked to remain in our POW facilities. Think of all of the lives that were saved when thousands of Iraqi soldiers gave up. Which would you rather have: 10,000 enemy soldiers surrendering or 10,000 enemy soldiers wanting to shoot you? If the enemy thinks we will kill them if they surrender, then why would they surrender? We want to encourage the enemy to surrender, so we do not want enemy prisoners dying in our custody.

15. **Suppose wounded and hungry enemy soldiers are under your medical care. You think that they know the locations of enemy units in the area. Can you deny them medical treatment or food until they tell interrogators what the interrogators want to know?**

    Answer: No. The Geneva Conventions that protect EPWs prohibit forcing a prisoner into giving information of any kind, whatsoever.

16. **Your unit is conducting a search in a built-up area. As they go from building to building, a few weapons are discovered. But in one home, they find some interesting art objects and decide to take them. Would this be a crime?**

    Answer: Yes, by taking the objects, you are violating the law of war. They have no right to the property. If, during the same search, they deliberately smash dishes, burn books, and destroy clothing, they would also be violating the law of war by destroying property when it is militarily unnecessary.

17. **Describe the ways a soldier may report a suspected war crime. To whom could you report a suspected war crime?**

    Answer: Reporting should occur as soon as possible and use the chain of command if possible. Other reporting options include:
    - Local office of the Inspector General
    - Office of the Provost Marshal (military police)
    - Judge Advocate (military lawyer)
    - A chaplain, who can help you report through official channels

18. **Describe the medical standard of care utilized with EPWs.**

    Answer: The detaining authority is required to provide any necessary medical support to enemy prisoners of war (EPW), retained personnel (RP), civilian internees (CI), and other detainees. This medical support includes first aid, a sanitary food service, preventive medicine, sanitation, medical services, and medical supplies, such as glasses, prosthetics, and medications.

19. **When do we conduct body cavity searches on EPWs?**

    Answer: Body cavity exams or searches may be performed for valid medical reasons with the verbal consent of the patient. However, these exams should not be performed as part of a routine intake physical examination. Body cavity searches without consent are conducted only when there is a reasonable belief or evidence that the detainee is concealing an item that presents a security risk. If possible, a body cavity exam will be conducted by personnel of the same gender.

20. **Under what medical conditions do we isolate detainees?**

    Answer: The detaining authority (in our case the United States) is bound to take all sanitary measures necessary to ensure clean camps to prevent epidemics. Every camp must have an infirmary. Any detainee with a contagious disease, mental condition, or other illness as determined by the medical officer needs to be isolated from the other patients.

Glossary

abduction Movement away from the midline of the body.

abrasion An injury in which a portion of the body is denuded of epidermis by scraping or rubbing.

access port A sealed hub on an administration set designed for sterile access to the IV fluid.

acetabulum The cup-shaped cavity in which the rounded head of the femur rotates.

acetylcholinesterase (AChE) An enzyme present in various body tissues such as muscles, nerve cells, and red blood cells, resulting in excess acetylcholine in the body.

acidosis A pathologic condition resulting from the accumulation of acids in the body.

acromion Lateral extension of the scapula that forms the highest point of the shoulder.

action The expected therapeutic effect of a medication on the body.

active immunity Protection produced by the person's own immune system that is usually permanent.

active transmission A disease-causing agent undergoes some change in the body of an arthropod before being transmitted.

acute mountain sickness (AMS) An altitude illness characterized by headache plus at least one of the following: fatigue or weakness, gastrointestinal symptoms (nausea, vomiting, or anorexia), dizziness or lightheadedness, or difficulty sleeping.

adduction Movement toward the midline of the body.

adenoids Lymphatic tissues located on the posterior nasopharyngeal wall that filter bacteria.

adhesion A band of scar tissue that binds together two anatomical surfaces normally separated.

adipose Referring to fat tissue.

adipose tissue Fat tissue.

alkalosis A pathologic condition resulting from the accumulation of bases in the body.

allergic reaction An unpredictable response to a medication.

altered mental status A change in the way a casualty thinks and behaves that may signal damage in the central nervous system.

altitude illnesses Conditions caused by the effects from hypobaric (low atmospheric pressure) hypoxia on the CNS and pulmonary systems as a result of unacclimatized people ascending to altitude; they range from acute mountain sickness (AMS) to high-altitude cerebral edema (HACE) and high-altitude pulmonary edema (HAPE).

alveolar air The amount of air that reaches the alveoli and participates in gas exchange with capillary blood, about 350 cc.

alveoli Balloon-like clusters of single-layer air sacs that are the functional site for the exchange of oxygen and carbon dioxide in the lungs.

ampules Small glass containers that are sealed and the contents sterilized.

amputation An injury in which part of the body is completely severed.

anaerobic metabolism The metabolism that takes place in the absence of oxygen; the principal product is lactic acid.

anaphylactic A severe hypersensitivity reaction that involves bronchoconstriction and cardiovascular collapse.

anaphylactic shock An unusual or exaggerated allergic reaction to foreign protein or other substances.

anaphylaxis An extreme, life-threatening systemic allergic reaction that may include shock and respiratory failure.

angioedema Diffuse swelling following the administration of a medication; may start with the lips, hands, feet, or mucous membranes and may progress to the airway.

angle of Louis Prominence on the sternum that lies opposite the second intercostal space.

anion An ion that contains an overall negative charge.

anterior tibial artery The artery that travels through the anterior muscles of the leg and continues to the foot as the dorsalis pedis.

anthrax A deadly bacteria (*Bacillus anthracis*) that lays dormant in a spore (protective shell); the germ is released from the spore when exposed to the optimal temperature and moisture level. The route of entry can be inhalation, cutaneous, or gastrointestinal (from consuming food that contains spores).

antibody Protein molecules (immunoglobulin) produced to help eliminate an antigen.

antidiuretic hormone (ADH) A hormone produced by the pituitary gland that signals the kidneys to prevent excretion of water.

antigen A live or inactivated substance (eg, protein, polysaccharide) capable of producing an immune response.

anuria Absence of urine production.

aorta The principal artery leaving the left side of the heart and carrying freshly oxygenated blood to the body.

aortic pulsations Pulsations of the aorta.

aphonia Inability to speak.

appendicular skeleton The part of the skeleton comprising the upper and lower extremities.

arachnoid The middle membrane of the three meninges that enclose the brain and spinal cord.

arterial air embolism Air bubbles in the arterial blood vessels.

arteries The blood vessels that carry blood away from the heart.

arteriole The smallest branch of an artery leading to the vast network of capillaries.

articulations The locations where two or more bones meet; joints.

arytenoid cartilages Pyramid-like cartilaginous structures that form the posterior attachment of the vocal cords.

asepsis Practices that minimize or eliminate microorganisms that can cause infection and disease.

aseptic technique A method of cleansing used to prevent contamination of a site when performing an invasive procedure, such as inserting an IV line.

Asherman Chest Seal A commercial occlusive bandage used to close open chest wounds.

aspiration Entry of fluids or solids into the trachea, bronchi, and lungs.

ataxia A staggered walk or gait caused by injury to the brain or spinal cord.

atelectasis Alveolar collapse that prevents use of that portion of the lung for ventilation and oxygenation.

atrophy Wasting away of a tissue.

auricle Part of the external ear that is shaped to collect sound waves and direct them toward the external auditory meatus.

autoclave A pressure steam sterilizer.

autonomic nervous system Consists of nerves, ganglia, and plexus that carry impulses to all smooth (involuntary) muscles, secretory glands, and the heart.

AVPU scale A method of assessing a casualty's level of consciousness by determining whether a casualty is Awake and alert, responsive to Verbal stimuli or Pain, or Unresponsive; used principally in the initial assessment.

avulsion An injury that leaves a piece of skin or other tissue partially or completely torn away from the body.

axial skeleton The part of the skeleton comprising the skull, spinal column, and rib cage.

axillary artery The artery that runs through the axilla, connecting the subclavian artery to the brachial artery.

bacteremia Blood infection.

bacteria Single-celled organisms without a nucleus.

bacterial infection When bacterial pathogens invade the body.

bag-valve-mask (BVM) device Manual ventilation device that consists of a bag, mask, reservoir, and oxygen inlet; capable of delivering up to 100% oxygen.

ballistics The study of the dynamic properties and characteristics of bullets or projectiles.

Battalion Aid Station (BAS) Provides combat health support for the maneuver battalions of the brigade as a medical platoon and utilizes combat medics in direct support of the maneuver companies of the battalion.

battalion surgeon Physician who is a special staff officer and advisor to the Battalion Commander regarding the employment of the medical platoon and the health of the battalion.

battle buddy A soldier's fighting buddy.

battle dress overgarment (BDO) Former chemical protection equipment for the US Army.

battle fatigue A broad group of physical, mental, and emotional signs that naturally result from the heavy mental and emotional work of facing danger under difficult conditions.

Battle's sign Bruising over the mastoid bone behind the ear commonly seen following a basilar skull fracture; also called retroauricular ecchymosis.

bed rest The patient is restricted to bed, with allowances for necessary travel to the dining facility and latrine.

blast front The leading edge of the shock wave.

blood The fluid tissue that is pumped by the heart through the arteries, veins, and capillaries; consists of plasma and formed elements or cells, such as red blood cells, white blood cells, and platelets.

blunt trauma Injury resulting from compression or deceleration forces, potentially crushing an organ or causing it to rupture.

body substance isolation (BSI) An infection control concept and practice that assumes that all body fluids are potentially infectious.

bolus A term used to describe "in one mass"; in medication administration, a single dose given by the IV route; may be a small or large quantity of the medication.

brachial artery The artery that runs through the arm and branches into the radial and ulnar arteries.

bradycardia A slow heart rate, less than 60 beats/min.

brain Part of the central nervous system located within the cranium; contains billions of neurons that serve a variety of vital functions.

brain stem The portion of the brain that connects the spinal cord to the rest of the brain, and contains the medulla, pons, and midbrain.

brisance The shattering effect of a shock wave and its ability to cause disruption of tissues and structures.

bronchioles Subdivision of the smaller bronchi in the lungs; made of smooth muscle; dilate or constrict in response to various stimuli.

buffer A substance or group of substances that controls the hydrogen levels in a solution.

bulla An elevated lesion (> 1 cm) containing serous fluid.

burn An injury to the body that occurs when the body or a body part receives more energy than it can absorb without injury.

bursa A fluid-filled sac located adjacent to joints that reduces the amount of friction between moving structures.

bursitis Inflammation of a bursa.

butterfly catheter A rigid, hollow, venous cannulation device identified by its plastic "wings" that act as anchoring points for securing the catheter.

calcaneus The heel bone; the largest of the tarsal bones.

cannulation The insertion of a hollow tube into a vein to allow for fluid flow.

canthus The corner of the eye.

capillary The fine end-divisions of the arterial system that allow contact between cells of the body tissues and the plasma and red blood cells.

capillary beds The terminal ends of the vascular system where fluids, food, and wastes are exchanged between the vascular system and the cells of the body.

capnographer Device that attaches in between the endotracheal tube and bag-valve-mask device; contains colorimetric paper, which should turn yellow during exhalation, indicating proper tube placement.

cardiac output The volume of blood delivered to the body in 1 minute.

cardiac tamponade A life-threatening accumulation of excess fluid or blood in the pericardial sac to the extent that it interferes with cardiac function.

cardiogenic shock Shock caused by inadequate function of the heart, or pump failure.

Care Under Fire Phase of care when the medic and casualty are under enemy fire.

carina Point at which the trachea bifurcates (divides) into the left and right mainstem bronchi.

carpals The eight small bones of the wrist.

cartilage Tough, elastic substance that covers opposable surfaces of moveable joints and forms part of the skeleton.

cartilaginous joints Joints that are spanned completely by cartilage and allow for minimal motion.

casualty collection point (CCP) Term used to refer to the area where a casualty is collected by a medical evacuation team.

casualty evacuation (CASEVAC) Term used by nonmedical units to refer to the movement of casualties aboard nonmedical vehicles or aircraft.

cathecholamines Epinephrine and norepinephrine.

catheter A flexible, hollow structure that delivers fluid.

cation An ion that contains an overall positive charge.

cauda equina The location where the spinal cord separates; composed of nerve roots.

cavitation A temporary cavity that forms from the pressure wake from a bullet that stretches the skin outward.

CBRNE Chemical, biologic, radiologic, nuclear, and high yield explosive devices.

cellular perfusion The ability of a cell to take in oxygen and remove carbon dioxide.

cellulitis Infection of the skin characterized by heat, pain, redness, and edema.

central nervous system (CNS) The system containing the brain and spinal cord.

cerebrospinal fluid (CSF) Fluid produced in the ventricles of the brain that flows in the subarachnoid space and bathes the meninges.

chemical agent monitor (CAM) A hand-held, soldier-operated device designed for monitoring chemical agent contamination on personnel, equipment, and surfaces.

chemical and biologic protective shelter (CBPS) A direct replacement for the M51 chemical agent/biologic agent shelter.

chemoprophylaxis The use of a drug or a chemical to prevent a disease.

chief complaint Reason for the patient's visit; typically one sentence in length.

chlorine (CL) The first chemical agent ever used in warfare. It has a distinct odor of bleach, and creates a green haze when released as a gas. Initially it produces upper airway irritation and a choking sensation.

civilian Person who is not a member of the enemy's armed forces and does not take part in the hostilities.

civilian internee (CI) A person interned during an international armed conflict for security reasons, for protection, or because they have committed an offense (insurgent or criminal) against the detaining power.

clavicle An S-shaped bone, also called the collarbone, that articulates medially with the sternum and laterally with the shoulder.

closed abdominal injury An injury in which there is soft tissue damage inside the body, but the skin remains intact.

closed (suction) drains Self-contained suction units that connect to drainage tubes within the wound.

closed fracture A fracture in which the skin is not broken.

closed wound An injury in which damage occurs beneath the skin or mucous membrane but the surface remains intact.

collateral damage Unintentional or incidental injury or damage to persons or objects that would not be lawful military targets in the circumstances ruling at the time. Such damage is not unlawful so long as it is not excessive in light of the overall military advantage anticipated from the attack (from Joint Publication 3-60).

colloids Solutions that contain proteins that are too large to pass out of the capillary membranes and therefore remain in the vascular compartment.

combat arms earplug (CAEP) Double-ended earplug designed for two different types of hearing protection; for use in military environments.

combat lifesavers (CLS) Nonmedical personnel in the unit who have been trained in bandaging, splinting, and IV initiation.

Combat/Operational Stress Control (COSC) Encompasses programs developed and actions taken by military leadership to prevent, identify, and manage adverse combat stress reactions in units to optimize mission performance, conserve fighting strength, prevent or minimize adverse affects of combat stress on soldiers' physical, psychological, intellectual, and social health, and return the unit or service member to duty expeditiously.

Combat Pill Pack Small pack of pain control medications and an antibiotic tablet that can be self-administered by the injured soldier.

combat stress The individual soldier's internal psychological and physiological processes of reacting to and dealing with combat stressors.

combat stress casualty A soldier who is rendered combat ineffective due to battle fatigue.

combat stressors Any stressors that occur in the context of performing one's combat mission.

Combitube Multilumen airway device that consists of a single tube with two lumens, two balloons, and two ventilation ports; an alternative device if endotracheal intubation is not possible or has failed.

compartment syndrome An increase in tissue pressure in a closed fascial space or compartment that compromises the circulation to the nerves and muscles within the involved compartment.

compensated shock The early stage of shock, in which the body can still compensate for blood loss.

compliance The ability of the lungs and chest wall to expand and contract in response to the application of force.

concentration The total weight of a medication contained in a specific volume of liquid.

concentration gradient The natural tendency for substances to flow from an area of higher concentration to an area of lower concentration, either within the cell or outside the cell.

conduction Transfer of heat to a solid object or a liquid by direct contact.

conjunctiva A thin, transparent membrane that covers the sclera and internal surfaces of the eyelids.

conjunctivitis Inflammation of the conjunctiva.

constipation Inability to have a bowel movement, or a painful straining bowel movement with firm, hard stools.

contact dermatitis Skin inflammation caused by exposure to irritants or allergens.

contaminated Containing microorganisms.

contraindications Situations in which a medication should not be given because it would not help or may actually harm.

contusion A bruise; an injury that causes bleeding beneath the skin but does not break the skin.

convection Mechanism by which body heat is picked up and carried away by moving air currents.

convention A binding agreement between states. Generally used for formal multilateral instruments with a broad number of parties.

cornea The transparent anterior portion of the eye that overlies the iris and pupil.

coronary sinus Veins that collect blood that is returning from the walls of the heart.

cranial nerves Carry impulses to and from specialized organs and the brain.

crepitus A grating or grinding sensation caused by fractured bone ends or joints rubbing together; also air bubbles under the skin that produce a crackling sound or crinkly feeling.

cricoid cartilage Forms the lowest portion of the larynx; also referred to as the cricoid ring; it is the first ring of the trachea and the only upper airway structure that forms a complete ring.

cricothyroid membrane A thin, superficial membrane located between the thyroid and cricoid cartilages that is relatively avascular and contains few nerves; the site for emergency surgical access to the airway.

cricothyrotomy Surgical procedure to provide an emergency airway by opening the cricothyroid membrane.

crushing the vector When the vector is smashed into the skin of the host and the host wipes off the dead bug, the pathogen is rubbed into the skin.

crusting Also called scabs; skin lesions that consist of dried serum, blood, or pus.

crystalloids Solutions of dissolved crystals (salt or sugar) in water.

crystalloid solution A type of intravenous solution that contains compounds that quickly disassociate in solution and can cross membranes; considered the best choice for prehospital care of injured casualties who need fluids to replace lost body fluid.

cutaneous Pertaining to the skin.

cutaneous abscess A deep, tender, red papule that becomes pus-filled.

cyanide A chemical agent that affects the body's ability to use oxygen. It is a colorless gas that has an odor similar to almonds. The effects begin on the cellular level and are very rapidly seen at the organ system level.

cystitis Also known as urinary tract infection (UTI); an infection of the urinary bladder.

D_5W An intravenous solution made up of 5% dextrose in water.

DCAP-BTLS Mnemonic standing for Deformities, Contusions, Abrasions, Penetrations, Burns, Tenderness, Lacerations, and Swelling.

dead air space Any portion of the airway that does not contain air and cannot participate in gas exchange.

decerebrate (extensor) posturing Abnormal posture characterized by extension of the arms and legs; indicates pressure on the brain stem.

decompensated shock The late stage of shock, when blood pressure is falling.

decontaminable litter Developed to replace canvas litters; designed not to absorb liquid chemical agents and is not degraded by decontaminating solutions.

decorticate (flexor) posturing Abnormal posture characterized by flexion of the arms and extension of the legs; indicates pressure on the brain stem.

deep fascia A dense layer of fibrous tissue below the subcutaneous tissue; composed of tough bands of tissue that ensheath muscles and other internal structures.

deep frostbite A type of frostbite in which the affected part looks white, yellow-white, or mottled blue-white and is hard, cold, and without sensation.

dehiscence Separation of a surgical incision or rupture of a wound closure.

dehydration Condition where the body loses too much fluid, salt, and minerals.

delayed Triage category for casualties who have less risk of losing life or limb due to delayed treatment.

delayed primary closure (tertiary intention) A combination of the primary and secondary intentions. The wound is initially cleaned, debrided, and irrigated, and then is observed for a period of time before closure.

depolarization The rapid movement of electrolytes across a cell membrane that changes the cell's overall charge. This rapid shifting of electrolytes and cellular charges is the main catalyst for muscle contractions and neural transmissions.

depression A sad or unhappy mood that you cannot control.

dermis The inner layer of skin containing hair follicle roots, glands, blood vessels, and nerves.

desquamation The continuous shedding of the dead cells on the surface of the skin.

detainee Any person captured or otherwise detained by an armed force.

diabetes insipidus A form of diabetes characterized by polyuria and polydipsia (excessive thirst) that often results from decreased or absent ADH production.

diaphoresis Excessive secretion of sweat.

diaphragm The major muscle of breathing. It is the anatomic point of separation between the thoracic cavity and the abdominal cavity.

diarrhea Liquid stool.

diffusion A process in which molecules move from an area of higher concentration to an area of lower concentration.

digital arteries The arteries that supply blood to the fingers and toes.

direct exposure The effect of being exposed to situations or circumstances that directly cause a stressful or emotional reaction.

disinfectants Destroy most pathogens but not necessarily their spores.

dislocation The displacement of a bone from its normal position within a joint.

dorsal Referring to the back or posterior side of the body or an organ.

dose The amount of medication given on the basis of the casualty's size and age.

drain A device that is used to remove excess fluid from a wound or body part.

drip chamber The area of the IV administration set where fluid accumulates so that the tubing remains filled with fluid.

drip rate Number of drops per minute.

drip set Another name for an administration set.

drug interaction When one medication modifies the action of another medication.

drug reconstitution Injecting sterile water (or saline) from one vial into another vial containing a powdered form of the drug.

drug tolerance A progressive decrease in the effectiveness of a medication.

drugs Chemical agents used in the diagnosis, treatment, and prevention of disease.

dura mater The outermost of the three meninges that enclose the brain and spinal cord; it is the toughest membrane.

duty Patient is returned to his or her unit for full duty without any restrictions.

dysphagia Difficulty swallowing.

dysphasia Impairment of speech.

dysphonia Difficulty speaking.

dyspnea Any difficulty in respiratory rate, regularity, or effort.

ecchymosis Bruising or discoloration associated with bleeding within or under the skin.

Echelon I Medical treatment is provided by designated combat medics or by treatment squads in Battalion Aid Stations.

Echelon II Medical treatment is provided at the clearing stations operated by treatment platoons of the medical company.

Echelon III Medical treatment is provided in a medical treatment facility.

Echelon IV Medical treatment is provided in a hospital.

Echelon V Medical treatment is provided by support base hospitals.

electrolyte A charged atom or compound that results from the loss or gain of an electron. These are ions the body uses to perform certain critical metabolic processes.

emergency bandage Commercial bandage used as a pressure bandage to control hemorrhage.

emergency medical technician (EMT) An EMS professional who is trained and licensed by the state to provide emergency medical care in the field.

emergent Alternative triage category that denotes a casualty who requires attention within minutes to several hours to avoid death or major disability.

empiric antibiotics The usage of an antibiotic prior to the establishment of the type of bacteria causing the illness.

endemic When a disease exists at low levels among the local population who have a degree of immunity.

endosteum The inner lining of a hollow bone.

endotracheal tube (ET) A tube designed to be placed into the trachea for the purpose of airway management.

enemy prisoner of war (EPW) A detained person as described in the Geneva Conventions who, while engaged in combat under orders of his or her government, is captured by the armed forces of the enemy.

envenomation The poisonous effects of the bites or stings of arthropods or snakes.

environmental emergencies Medical conditions caused or exacerbated by the weather, terrain, or unique atmospheric conditions such as high altitude or underwater.

epidermis The outermost layer of the skin.

epiglottis Leaf-shaped cartilaginous structure that closes over the trachea during swallowing.

epinephrine A hormone (adrenaline) produced by the body and a drug produced by pharmaceutical companies to increase pulse and blood pressure; the drug of choice for an anaphylactic reaction.

epistaxis Nosebleed.

escharotomy A surgical cut through the eschar or leathery covering of a burn injury to allow for swelling and minimize the potential for development of compartment syndrome in a circumferentially burned limb or the thorax.

eustress The degree of stress necessary to sustain and improve tolerance to stress without overstraining and disrupting the human system.

evacuation asset Usually either an air or a ground ambulance, but it may be a vehicle of opportunity to evacuate casualties to a medical treatment facility.

evaporation The conversion of a liquid to a gas.

evisceration Protrusion of an internal organ through a wound or surgical incision.

exhalation Passive movement of air out of the lungs.

expectant Triage category for casualties so critically injured that only complicated and prolonged treatment would offer any hope of improving life expectancy.

expiration Passive movement of air out of the lungs; also called exhalation.

exsanguination Total blood loss leading to death.

external ballistics The study of projectiles in the phase between the weapon and the intended target. This includes velocity, trajectory, and many other factors.

extravasation Passage or escape into the tissues, usually of blood, serum, or lymph.

extubation The process of removing the tube from an intubated patient.

exudate Fluid that has penetrated from blood vessels into the surrounding tissues resulting from inflammation; pus.

eyelash reflex Contraction of the patient's lower eyelid when upper eyelashes are stroked; fairly reliable indicator of the presence or absence of an intact gag reflex.

facet joint The joint on which each vertebra articulates with adjacent vertebrae.

fascia The fiber-like connective tissue that covers arteries, veins, tendons, and ligaments.

FAST1 device A sternal IO device used in adults; stands for First Access for Shock and Trauma.

fatigue The distress and impaired performance that come from doing something too hard or for too long.

fecal contamination When the vector defecates into a wound on the host.

fecalith Hardened feces.

femoral artery The main artery supplying the thigh and leg.

femur The proximal bone of the leg that extends from the pelvis to the knee.

fibrous joints Joints that contain dense fibrous tissue and allow for no motion.

fibula The smaller of the two bones of the lower leg.

field medical assistant Medical service corps officer who is the operations/readiness officer of the platoon; the principle assistant to the battalion surgeon for operations, administration, and logistics.

Field Medical Card (DD Form 1380) Designed to provide medical information about the casualty's injury or illness and the medical treatment provided; records the casualty's entire disposition.

first-degree burn A burn involving only the epidermis, producing very red, painful skin.

flail chest An injury that involves two or more adjacent ribs fractured in two or more places, allowing the segment between the fractures to move independently of the rest of the thoracic cage.

flash chamber The area of a catheter that fills with blood to help indicate when a vein is cannulated.

flat bones Bones that are thin and broad, such as the scapula.

flexion injury A type of injury that results from forward movement of the head, typically as the result of rapid deceleration, such as in a car crash, or with a direct blow to the occiput.

folliculitis Inflammation of a hair follicle caused by infection, chemical irritation, or minor physical injury.

foramen magnum A large opening at the base of the skull through which the spinal cord exits the brain.

Forward Aid Station (FAS) At this location, patients are evaluated, treated for immediate life-threatening injuries, and stabilized for transport to a higher level treatment facility. The primary care provider is the battalion physician assistant.

frostbite Localized damage to tissues resulting from prolonged exposure to extreme cold.

G agents Early nerve agents that were developed by German scientists in the period after WWI and into WWII. There are three such agents: sarin, soman, and tabun.

gag reflex Automatic reaction when something touches an area deep in the oral cavity; helps protect the lower airway from aspiration.

gallbladder A sac on the undersurface of the liver that collects bile from the liver and discharges it into the duodenum through the common bile duct.

gastritis Inflammation of the stomach.

gastroenteritis Stomach and intestinal inflammation.

generic name The original chemical name of a medication (in contrast with one of its trade names); not capitalized.

Glasgow Coma Scale (GCS) A widely accepted method of assessing level of consciousness that is based on three independent measurements: eye opening, verbal response, and motor response.

glottis The space between the vocal cords that is the narrowest portion of the adult's airway; also called the glottic opening.

grave breach A gross violation of the basic principles of the Geneva Conventions; also known as a war crime.

gtt A measurement that indicates drops.

head tilt–chin lift maneuver Manual airway maneuver that involves tilting the head back while lifting up on the chin; used to open the airway of a semiconscious or unconscious nontrauma patient.

heart A hollow muscular organ that receives blood from the veins and propels it into the arteries.

heat cramps Acute and involuntary muscle pains, usually in the lower extremities, the abdomen, or both, that occur because of profuse sweating and subsequent sodium losses in sweat.

heat exhaustion A clinical syndrome characterized by volume depletion and heat stress that is thought to be a milder form of heat illness and on a continuum leading to heat stroke.

heat illness The increase in core body temperature due to inadequate thermolysis.

heat stroke The least common and most deadly heat illness, caused by a severe disturbance in thermoregulation, usually characterized by a core temperature of more than 104°F (40°C) and altered mental status.

Heimlich maneuver Abdominal thrusts performed to relieve a foreign body airway obstruction.

hematemesis Vomiting up blood.

hematoma A localized collection of blood in the soft tissues as a result of injury or a broken blood vessel.

hemoglobin An iron-containing pigment found in red blood cells; carries 97% of oxygen.

hemopneumothorax An injury to the chest cavity causing blood and air to collect in the chest cavity.

hemoptysis Coughing up blood.

hemorrhage The escape of blood and plasma from capillaries, veins, and arteries; bleeding.

hemorrhoids Varicose veins in the lower rectum or anus.

hemostasis Control of bleeding by formation of a blood clot.

Hemovac A drainage system used for larger amounts, up to 500 mL, of drainage.

hepatitis Inflammation of the liver.

herpes simplex An infection from the herpes simplex virus (HSV).

herpes zoster Also called shingles; an infection caused by the chicken-pox virus.

herpetic whitlow An HSV infection of the fingers, resulting from the inoculation of HSV through a skin break.

high-altitude cerebral edema (HACE) An altitude illness in which there is a change in mental status and/or ataxia in a person with AMS or the presence of mental status changes and ataxia in a person without AMS.

high-altitude pulmonary edema (HAPE) An altitude illness characterized by dyspnea at rest, cough, severe weakness, and drowsiness that may eventually lead to central cyanosis, audible rales or wheezing, tachypnea, and tachycardia.

hilum Point of entry of all of the blood vessels and the bronchi into each lung.

homeostasis The balance of all systems of the body; also known as homeostatic balance.

host resistance Some naturally occurring body flora have an antibiotic relationship with pathogens and contribute to a person's health.

humerus The bone of the upper arm.

hydrophilic Water-loving.

hydrophobic Water-fearing.

hyoid bone A small, horseshoe-shaped bone to which the jaw, tongue, epiglottis, and thyroid cartilage attach.

hypercalcemia High serum calcium levels.

hyperextension Extension of a limb or other body part beyond its usual range of motion.

hyperkalemia High serum potassium levels.

hyperresonance A high-pitched sound heard when percussing the chest of a casualty with a tension pneumothorax.

hypertonic solution A solution that has a greater concentration of sodium than does the cell; the increased extracellular osmotic pressure can draw water out of the cell and cause it to collapse.

hypertrophy An increase in size.

hyperventilation Occurs when CO_2 elimination exceeds CO_2 production; also the increase in the number of respirations per minute above the normal range.

hypocalcemia Low serum calcium levels.

hypokalemia Low serum potassium levels.

hypothermia A condition in which the internal body temperature falls below 95°F (35°C), usually as a result of prolonged exposure to cool or freezing temperatures.

hypotonic solution A solution that has a lower concentration of sodium than does the cell; the increased intracellular osmotic pressure lets water flow into the cell, causing it to swell and possibly burst.

hypoventilation Occurs when CO_2 production exceeds the body's ability to eliminate it by ventilation; also the decrease in the number of respirations per minute that falls below the normal range.

hypovolemia A large drop in body fluids.

hypovolemic shock A condition in which low blood volume, due to massive internal or external bleeding or extensive loss of body fluids, results in inadequate perfusion.

hypoxia A lack of oxygen to the body's cells and tissues.

ilium The broad, uppermost bone of the pelvis.

immediate Triage category for casualties whose condition demands immediate resuscitative treatment.

immersion syndrome A process similar to frostbite but caused by prolonged exposure to cool, wet conditions.

immunization Taking substances related to a biologic agent to develop resistance or antibodies in the body.

impetigo A superficial bacterial skin infection.

improved chemical agent monitor (ICAM) A hand-held, soldier-operated device designed for monitoring chemical agent contamination on personnel, equipment, and surfaces.

improved first aid kit (IFAK) New first aid kit carried by every soldier in the Army.

inactivated vaccines Produced from a form of the virus or bacteria that cannot replicate, they are generally not as effective as live vaccines and often require three to five doses and/or require booster shot(s).

incision A wound usually made deliberately, as in surgery; a clean cut, as opposed to a laceration.

indications Therapeutic uses for a specific medication.

indirect exposure The effect of being exposed to situations or circumstances that others may experience that indirectly cause a stressful or emotional reaction.

inferior vena cava One of the two largest veins in the body; carries blood from the lower extremities and the pelvic and abdominal organs into the heart.

infiltration The escape of fluid into the surrounding tissue.

inhalation The active process of moving air into the lungs.

inoculation When a vector injects the pathogen into the host with its saliva while it feeds on the host.

inspiration The active process of moving air into the lungs; also called inhalation.

insufflation Inhaling oxygen into the body cavity.

integument The skin.

intercostal space The space between two ribs, named according to the number of the rib above it, that contains the intercostal muscles and neurovascular bundle.

internal ballistics The study of projectiles and their effect on human tissue.

international humanitarian law (IHL) The body of rules that protects people who are not or who are no longer participating in hostilities in wartime.

interstitia Water between the vascular system and the surrounding cells (for example, between the membranes of two cells located outside the vascular compartment in the body).

intradermal (ID) injection A method of delivering a medication into the skin.

intramuscular (IM) injection A method of delivering a medication into the muscle of the body by placing a needle into a muscle space and injecting the medication into the tissue.

intramuscular (IM) route Injection into a muscle; a medication delivery route.

intraosseous (IO) infusion A technique of administering fluids, blood and blood products, and medications into the intraosseous space of a long bone.

intraosseous (IO) route Injection into the bone; a medication delivery route.

intravascular The water portion of the circulatory system surrounding the blood cells (for example, in the heart, arteries, or veins).

intravenous (IV) route Injection directly into a vein; a medication delivery route.

ion A charged atom or compound that results from the loss or gain of an electron.

ionic concentration The amount of charged particles found in a particular area.

iris The colored portion of the eye.

irregular bones Bones with unique shapes that allow them to perform a specific function and that do not fit into the other categories based on shape.

irreversible shock The final stage of shock, resulting in death.

ischium The lowermost dorsal bone of the pelvis.

isotonic solution A solution that has the same concentration of sodium as does the cell. In this case, water does not shift, and no change in cell shape occurs.

Jackson-Pratt A drainage device that is used when small amounts (100 to 200 mL) of drainage is anticipated.

jaw-thrust maneuver Manual airway maneuver that involves stabilizing the patient's head and thrusting the jaw forward; the preferred method of opening the airway of a semiconscious or unconscious trauma patient.

joint The point at which two or more bones articulate, or come together.

joint capsule A saclike envelope that encloses the cavity of a synovial joint.

Joint Service lightweight integrated suit technology (JSLIST) Chemical protection equipment designed to replace the US Army's BDO, the US Navy's chemical protection overgarment (CPO), and US Marine Corp's Saratoga.

kidneys Two retroperitoneal organs that excrete the end products of metabolism as urine and regulate the body's salt and water content.

kinetic energy The energy of motion; this energy is transferred to anything that the projectile comes in contact with.

KING LT-D A disposable supraglottic airway used as an alternative to tracheal intubation or mask ventilation.

laceration A wound made by tearing or cutting tissues.

lacrimal glands The structures in which tears are secreted and drained from the eye.

lactated Ringer's (LR) solution A sterile crystalloid isotonic intravenous solution of specified amounts of calcium chloride, potassium chloride, sodium chloride, and sodium lactate in water.

lactic acid A metabolic end product of the breakdown of glucose that accumulates when metabolism proceeds in the absence of oxygen.

lamina Components of the spine that rise from the posterior pedicles and fuse to form the posterior spinous processes.

laryngospasm Spasmodic closure of the vocal cords.

larynx A complex structure formed by many independent cartilaginous structures that all work together; where the upper airway ends and the lower airway begins.

LD$_{50}$ The amount of an agent or substance that will kill 50% of people who are exposed to it.

lens A transparent body within the globe of the eye that focuses light rays.

Lewisite (L) A blister agent that has a rapid onset of symptoms and produces immediate intense pain and discomfort on contact.

ligaments Tough bands of tissue that connect bone to bone around a joint or support internal organs within the body.

liver A large solid organ that lies in the right upper quadrant immediately below the diaphragm; it produces bile, stores sugar for immediate use by the body, and produces many substances that help regulate immune responses.

live (attenuated) vaccines Produced from a weakened form of the virus or bacteria that must replicate to be effective, they have an immune response similar to natural infection, are usually effective with one dose, can produce severe reactions, and are unstable.

local reaction Mild to moderate allergic reaction occurring in a localized area.

long bones Bones that are longer than they are wide.

lung compliance The ability of the alveoli to expand when air is drawn into the lungs during either negative-pressure ventilation or positive-pressure ventilation.

lysis The rupturing of a cell caused by either the presence of certain enzymes or the uncontrolled influx of material into the cell.

M22 automatic chemical agent detection alarm (ACADA) Provides detection and warning for nerve and blister agents.

M256A1 chemical agent detector kit Used to detect and identify blood, blister, and nerve agents present either as a liquid or as a vapor.

M291 skin decontamination kit (SDK) Used to decontaminate the skin; a wallet-like carrying pouch containing six individual decontamination packets.

M295 decontamination kit, individual equipment (DKIE) Used to decontaminate personal protective equipment.

M8 chemical agent detector paper Used to detect both the presence and the specific type of liquid chemical agents.

M8A1 automatic chemical agent alarm (ACAA) An automatic chemical agent detection and warning system designed to provide real-time detection of the presence of nerve agent vapors or inhalable aerosols.

M9 chemical agent detector paper Used to detect the presence of liquid chemical agents, but does not identify the specific type of agent.

macrodrip set An administration set named for the large orifice between the piercing spike and the drip chamber; allows for rapid fluid flow into the vascular system.

macule A flat, small (< 1 cm) skin lesion colored white to brown to red to purple.

Main Aid Station (MAS) Consists of the battalion surgeon, combat medics, and ambulances. At this location, patients are evaluated, treated for immediate life-threatening injuries, and stabilized for transport to a higher level treatment facility.

malleolus The large, rounded bony protuberance on either side of the ankle joint.

manubrium The superior segment of the sternum; its lower border defines the angle of Louis.

mass casualty (MASCAL) situation When the number of casualties exceeds the available medical capability to rapidly treat and evacuate.

mechanism of action A predictable chemical reaction or how the medication works.

mechanism of injury (MOI) The way in which traumatic injuries occur; the forces that act on the body to cause damage.

mediastinum Space within the chest that contains the heart, major blood vessels, vagus nerve, trachea, and esophagus; located between the two lungs.

medical asepsis Practices that minimize the number of microorganisms or prevent the transmission of microorganisms from one person to another.

medical ethics The application of values and judgments as they apply to the care of patients.

medical evacuation (MEDEVAC) The transportation of casualties to medical facilities, performed by dedicated medical vehicles and aircraft staffed with medical personnel who provide care en route.

medical intelligence The process of gathering essential medical information before an operation begins, allowing unit leaders and combat medics to tailor their operational plans.

medical regulating Tool used to identify the casualties awaiting evacuation to the next echelon of medical care.

medical treatment facility (MTF) A medical facility used for treatment of casualties; varies in size from a battalion aid station to a combat support hospital.

medullary canal The hollow center portion of a long bone.

melena Passing of feces with a black, tarry appearance.

metabolic The breakdown of ingested foodstuffs into smaller and smaller molecules and atoms that are used as energy sources for cellular function.

metacarpals The five bones that form the palm and back of the hand.

metatarsals The five long bones extending from the tarsus to the phalanges of the foot.

metric system A decimal system based on tens for the measurement of length, weight, and volume.

METT-T Mnemonic standing for Mission, Enemy, Terrain, Troops and equipment, and Time available.

microdrip set An administration set named for the small orifice between the piercing spike and the drip chamber; allows for carefully controlled fluid flow and is ideally suited for medication administration.

microorganisms Microscopic living cells found almost everywhere in the environment.

minimal Triage category for casualties with superficial wounds who can utilize self-aid or buddy-aid.

miosis Bilateral pinpoint-constricted pupils.

muscle fatigue The condition that arises when a muscle depletes its supply of energy.

mutagen A substance that mutates, damages, and changes the structures of DNA in the body's cells.

myocardial contusion Blunt force injury to the heart that results in capillary damage, interstitial bleeding, and cellular damage in the area.

myoglobin A protein found in muscle that is released into the circulation after crush injury or other muscle damage and whose presence in the circulation may produce kidney damage.

nasal septum A rigid partition composed of bone and cartilage; divides the nasopharynx into two passages.

nasopharyngeal airway (NPA) An airway adjunct inserted into the nostril of a casualty who is not able to maintain a viable airway.

nasopharynx The nasal cavity; formed by the union of the facial bones.

needle decompression Also referred to as a needle thoracostomy or needle thoracentesis, this procedure introduces a needle or angiocath into the pleural space in an attempt to relieve a tension pneumothorax.

needle thoracostomy The introduction of a needle catheter unit into the chest cavity to remove air under pressure.

negative-pressure ventilation Drawing of air into the lungs; airflow from a region of higher pressure (outside the body) to a region of lower pressure (the lungs); occurs during normal (unassisted) breathing.

negative wave pulse The phase of an explosion in which pressure from the blast is less than atmospheric pressure.

neoplasm Cancerous process.

nephrolithiasis Kidney stones.

nerve agent antidote kit (NAAK) Contains two auto-injector medications, atropine and 2-PAM-Cl (pralidoxime chloride).

nerve agents A class of chemical called organophosphates; they function by blocking an essential enzyme in the nervous system, which causes the body's organs to become overstimulated and burn out.

neurogenic shock The malfunction of the automatic nervous system in regulating blood vessel tone and cardiac output.

neurovascular bundle A closely placed grouping of an artery, a vein, and a nerve that lies beneath the inferior edge of a rib.

nodule A palpable, solid lesion, 1–2 cm, and elevated.

nonemergent Alternative triage category that denotes a casualty who does not require the attention of the emergent group although they may require surgery; also lack significant potential for loss of life, limb, or eyesight.

nonprogressive shock A synonym for compensated shock.

normal saline (NS) 0.9% sodium chloride; an isotonic crystalloid.

nosocomial infection An infection that patients acquire while in a medical care facility.

occlusion Blockage, usually of a tubular structure such as a blood vessel.

off-gassing The emitting of an agent after exposure, for example from a person's clothes that have been exposed to the agent.

oliguria Decreased urine output.

open abdominal injury An injury in which there is a break in the surface of the skin or mucous membrane, exposing deeper tissue to potential contamination.

open drains Drainage that passes through an open-ended tube into a receptacle or out onto the dressing.

open fracture Any break in a bone in which the overlying skin has been damaged.

open pneumothorax The result of a defect in the chest wall that allows air to enter the thoracic space.

open wound An injury in which there is a break in the surface of the skin or the mucous membrane, exposing deeper tissue to potential contamination.

orientation The mental status of a casualty as measured by memory of casualty: name, place (current location), time (current year, month, and approximate date), and event (what happened).

oropharyngeal airway (OPA) An airway adjunct inserted into the mouth to keep the tongue from blocking the upper airway.

oropharynx Forms the posterior portion of the oral cavity, which is bordered superiorly by the hard and soft palates, laterally by the cheeks, and inferiorly by the tongue.

osmolarity The ability to influence the movement of water across a semipermeable membrane.

osmosis The movement of water across a cell membrane from an area of lower to higher solute molecules.

osmotic pressure Pressure created against the cell wall by the presence of water.

ossicles Three small bones in the middle ear.

other detainee (OD) A person in the custody of US armed forces who has not yet been classified.

otitis externa Swimmer's ear.

otitis media Middle ear infection.

otoscopic examination Medical examination of the inner ears.

ovarian torsion A condition whereby an ovary twists upon itself.

over-the-needle catheter The prehospital standard for IV cannulation. It consists of a hollow tube over a lasersharpened steel needle; also referred to as an angiocath.

palate Forms the roof of the mouth and separates the oropharynx and nasopharynx.

pallor Absence of color.

pancreas A flat, solid organ that lies below the liver and the stomach; it is a major source of digestive enzymes and produces the hormone insulin.

papule A solid, raised lesion (< 1 cm).

paradoxical motion The motion of the chest wall that is detached in a flail chest; the motion is exactly the opposite of normal motion during breathing: in during inhalation, out during exhalation.

paranasal sinuses Air-filled, paired extensions of the nasal cavity within the bones of the skull.

parenteral Drug administration through any route other than the gastrointestinal tract; parenteral routes include intravenous, intramuscular, intraosseous, subcutaneous, transdermal, intrathecal, inhalation, intralingual, intradermal, and umbilical.

paresthesia Sensation of tingling, numbness, or "pins and needles" in a body part.

parietal pleura Thin membrane that lines the chest cavity.

Parkland formula A formula that recommends giving 4 mL of normal saline for each kilogram of body weight, multiplied by the percentage of body surface area burned; sometimes used to calculate fluid needs during lengthy transport times.

passive immunity Protection transferred from another person or animal via an antibody.

passive transmission When an arthropod carries a pathogen from one host to another.

past medical history (PMH) Significant past or ongoing medical conditions.

past surgical history (PSH) Any surgeries the patient has had.

patch A large macule (> 1 cm), such as freckles, flat moles, and tattoos.

patella The kneecap.

patent Open.

patient protective wrap (PPW) Used to protect the patient during evacuation after the BDO or JSLIST has been removed and the casualty has received medical treatment.

pectoral girdle The shoulder girdle.

pedicle A narrow strip of tissue by which an avulsed piece of tissue remains connected to the body.

pedicles Thick lateral bony struts that connect the vertebral body with spinous and transverse processes and make up the lateral and posterior portions of the spinal foramen.

pelvic girdle The large bone that arises in the area of the last nine vertebrae and sweeps around to form a complete ring.

penetrating trauma An injury in which the skin is broken; direct contact results in laceration of the structure.

Penrose drain A soft tube that may be advanced or pulled out in stages as the wound heals from the inside out.

peptic ulcer disease (PUD) Abrasion of the stomach or small intestine.

perfidy A calculated violation of trust; treachery. As applied to the Geneva Conventions, it usually means the deliberate use of the protective emblem of the Red Cross under false pretenses. Referred to as "perfidious use," this act is a war crime.

perfusion The circulation of blood within an organ or tissue in adequate amounts to meet the cells' current needs.

pericardium Double-layered sac containing the heart and the origins of the superior vena cava, inferior vena cava, and pulmonary artery.

periosteum The fibrous tissue that covers bone.

peripheral nervous system All the nerves outside of the central nervous system.

peritonitis Inflammation of the lining around the abdominal cavity (peritoneum) that results from either blood or hollow organ contents spilling into the abdominal cavity.

pH A measure of the acidity of a solution; potential of hydrogen.

phospholipid bilayer The cell membrane's double layer, consisting of a hydrophilic outer layer composed of phosphate groups and a hydrophobic inner layer made up of lipids, or fatty acids. It is this structure and composition that allows the cell membrane to have selective permeability.

phalanges The bones of the fingers or toes.

pharmacology The study of the properties and effects of medications.

pharynx Throat.

phosgene A chemical agent that causes severe pulmonary damage.

phosgene oxime (CX) A chemical blister agent that has a rapid onset of symptoms and produces immediate intense pain and discomfort on contact.

physical stressors Evoke specific stress reflexes such as shivering or sweating.

physician's assistant (PA) Health care professional who performs general technical health care and administrative duties.

physiological dependence When the body has developed a physical need for the medication.

physis The growth plate in long bones.

pia mater The innermost of the three meninges that enclose the brain and spinal cord; it rests directly on the brain and spinal cord.

piggyback administration The addition of a second IV administration set to a primary line via an access port.

plantar Referring to the sole of the foot.

plaque A papule > 1 cm or a group of papules.

plasma A sticky, yellow fluid that carries the blood cells and nutrients and transports cellular waste material to the organs of excretion.

platelets (thrombocytes) Tiny, disk-shaped elements that are much smaller than the cells; they are essential in the initial formation of a blood clot, the mechanism that stops bleeding.

platoon sergeant Assists the platoon leader and supervises the operations of the platoon.

pleura Membrane lining the outer surface of the lungs (visceral pleura), the inner surface of the chest wall, and the thoracic surface of the diaphragm (parietal pleura).

PMS Mnemonic standing for pulse, motor function, sensory function.

point tenderness Tenderness that is sharply localized at the site of an injury; found by gently palpating along the bone with the tip of one finger.

polydipsia Excessive thirst.

polyuria The passage of an unusually large volume of urine in a given period. In diabetes, polyuria can result from excreting excess glucose in the urine.

popliteal artery The artery in the area or space behind the knee joint.

portal of exit Where the microorganism leaves the reservoir.

portals of entry Where the microorganism can enter the host.

positive-pressure ventilation Forcing of air into the lungs.

positive wave pulse The phase of an explosion in which there is a pressure front with a pressure higher than atmospheric pressure.

posterior tibial artery The artery that travels through the calf muscles to the plantar aspect of the foot.

posttraumatic stress disorder (PTSD) Symptoms such as painful memories, anxiety, guilt, and unpleasant dreams that are normal responses after extremely abnormal and distressing events.

postural hypotension Symptomatic drop in blood pressure related to the casualty's body position, detected by measuring pulse and blood pressure while the casualty is lying supine, sitting up, and standing. An increase in pulse rate and a decrease in blood pressure in any one of these positions is considered a positive sign for this condition.

priapism An abnormal, continuing erection of the penis caused by spinal trauma.

primary blast injury Injuries caused by an explosive pressure wave on the gas-containing organs of the body.

primary healing Wound closure immediately following the injury and prior to the formation of granulation tissue.

Priority I–Urgent MEDEVAC category assigned to casualties who should be evacuated as soon as possible and within a maximum of 2 hours.

Priority IA–Urgent Surgical MEDEVAC category assigned to casualties who must receive far forward surgical intervention to save lives and stabilize for further evacuation.

Priority II–Priority MEDEVAC category assigned to sick and wounded casualties requiring prompt medical care.

Priority III–Routine MEDEVAC category assigned to casualties requiring evacuation but whose condition is not expected to deteriorate significantly.

Priority IV–Convenience MEDEVAC category assigned to casualties for whom evacuation by medical vehicle is a matter of medical convenience rather than necessity.

pronation The act of turning the palm of the hand backward or downward, performed by internal rotation of the forearm.

protecting power An entity such as the International Committee of the Red Cross or a nation appointed to document compliance with the Geneva Conventions during conflict. The protecting power is recognized as empowered to represent the other country and protect its interests. Poland was the protecting power for the United States in Iraq after the first Gulf War.

protozoa Single-celled microscopic microorganisms.

pruritus Itching following the administration of a medication.

psychological dependence When the patient is convinced that he or she has a need for the medication.

psychosomatic disturbance An expression of an emotional conflict through physical symptoms.

pubis One of two bones that form the anterior portion of the pelvic ring.

pulmonary artery The major artery leading from the right ventricle of the heart to the lungs; it carries oxygen-poor blood.

pulmonary blast injuries Pulmonary trauma resulting from short-range exposure to the detonation of explosives.

pulmonary contusion Injury to the lung parenchyma that results in capillary hemorrhage into the tissue.

pulmonary veins The four veins that return oxygenated blood from the lungs to the left atrium of the heart.

pulse pressure The difference between the systolic and diastolic pressures.

puncture wound A stab injury from a pointed object, such as a nail or a knife.

pupil The circular opening in the center of the eye through which light passes to the lens.

pupils for equality and reactivity to light (PERL) An assessment tool which measures the casualty's level of consciousness.

pustules Superficial and elevated lesions < 1 cm containing pus that result from infection.

pyelonephritis Kidney infection.

pyriform fossae Two pockets of tissue on the lateral borders of the larynx.

quarters Restriction and rest in the patient's place of domicile with freedom of movement within the living space.

raccoon eyes Bruising under or around the orbits that is commonly seen following a basilar skull fracture; also called periorbital ecchymosis.

radial artery The artery pertaining to the wrist.

radiation Emission of heat from an object into surrounding, colder air.

radius The bone on the thumb side of the forearm.

rapid trauma survey A brief exam done to find all life-threatening injuries.

red blood cells (erythrocytes) Cells that carry oxygen to the body's tissues.

regurgitation When a vector vomits a pathogen into a host while it feeds on the host.

reservoir Any place where a microorganism can multiply or survive.

respiration The exchange of gases between a living organism and its environment.

respiratory rate The number of times a casualty breathes in 1 minute.

responsiveness The way in which a casualty responds to external stimuli, including verbal stimuli (sound), tactile stimuli (touch), and painful stimuli.

resuscitation device, individual chemical (RDIC) Used to ventilate an apneic patient while the patient is in MOPP-4.

retained person (RP) Enemy who is medical personnel, a chaplain, or is in a voluntary aid society.

retina A delicate 10-layered structure of nervous tissue located in the rear of the interior of the globe of the eye that receives light and generates nerve signals that are transmitted to the brain through the optic nerve.

retractions Movements in which the skin pulls in around the ribs during inspiration.

retroperitoneal abdomen Area that lies behind the thoracic and true abdomen and contains the kidneys, ureters, pancreas, posterior duodenum, ascending and descending colon, abdominal aorta, and inferior vena cava.

rhinitis Inflammation of the nasal membranes resulting in sneezing, itching, rhinorrhea, and nasal congestion.

rotation-flexion injury A type of injury typically resulting from high acceleration forces; can result in a stable unilateral facet dislocation in the cervical spine.

round bones The small bones that are found adjacent to joints that assist with motion.

rule of nines A system that assigns percentages to sections of the body, allowing calculation of the amount of skin surface involved in a burn area.

rule of palms A system that estimates total body surface area burned by comparing the affected area with the size of the patient's palm, which is roughly equal to 1% of the patient's total body surface area.

sacroiliac joints The points of attachment of the ilium to the sacrum.

saline lock A special type of IV, also called a buff cap or heparin cap.

SAMPLE history A key brief history of a casualty's condition to determine Signs and symptoms, Allergies, Medications, Pertinent past history, Last oral intake, and Events leading to injury.

sanguineous Drainage that contains blood.

sarin (GB) A nerve agent that is one of the G agents; a highly volatile colorless and odorless liquid that turns from liquid to gas within seconds to minutes at room temperature.

scaphoid Sunken appearance of the skin.

scapula A large, flat, triangular bone along the posterior thorax that articulates with the clavicle and humerus.

sclera The white part of the eye.

secondary blast injury Penetrating or nonpenetrating injuries caused by ordinance projectiles or secondary missiles.

secondary intention A strategy of allowing a wound to heal on its own without surgical closure.

second-degree burn A burn that involves the epidermis and part of the dermis, characterized by pain and blistering; previously called a partial-thickness burn.

selective permeability The ability of the cell membrane to selectively allow compounds into the cell based on the cell's current needs.

sensitization Developing sensitivity to a substance that initially caused no allergic reaction.

septic shock Shock caused by severe bacterial infection.

serosanguineous Drainage that contains serum and blood.

serous Clear, watery discharge that has been separated from its solid elements.

shock A condition in which the circulatory system fails to provide sufficient circulation to enable every body part to perform its function; also called hypoperfusion.

shock wave Waves of pressure from muzzle velocities above 2,000 fps that precede the bullet and compress the tissue ahead of and around the bullet. Shock waves can reach pressures above 200 atmospheres.

short bones The bones that are nearly as wide as they are long.

side effects Any effects of a medication other than the desired ones.

sinuses Cavities formed by the cranial bones that trap contaminants and keep them from entering the respiratory tract and act as tributaries for fluid to and from the eustachian tubes and tear ducts.

sinusitis A bacterial infection of one of the paranasal sinuses.

situational assessment Centers around an awareness of the tactical situation and current hostilities in order to safely and effectively render care to the casualty.

six Ps of musculoskeletal assessment Pain, Paralysis, Paresthesias, Pulselessness, Pallor, and Pressure.

skeletal muscle Muscle that is attached to bones and usually crosses at least one joint; striated or voluntary muscle.

skin lesion A term that describes any change in skin appearance.

skull The structure at the top of the axial skeleton that houses the brain and consists of 28 bones that comprise the auditory ossicles, the cranium, and the face.

small arms Individually carried weapons commonly carried by military personnel, including pistols, rifles, and machine guns; they shoot solid or hollow-point projectiles generally less than 20 mm in diameter.

small intestine The portion of the digestive tube between the stomach and the cecum, consisting of the duodenum, jejunum, and ileum.

smallpox A highly contagious biologic disease; it is most contagious when blisters begin to form.

snow blindness A burn to the eye from UV radiation.

sodium/potassium pump The mechanism by which the cell brings in two potassium ions and releases three sodium ions.

soman (GD) A nerve agent that is one of the G agents; twice as persistent as sarin and five times as lethal; it has a fruity odor, as a result of the type of alcohol used in the agent, and is both a contact and inhalation hazard that can enter the body through skin absorption and through the respiratory tract.

spall Fragments from the shell casing and/or target.

spalling Delaminating or breaking off into chips and pieces.

spinal cord The part of the central nervous system that extends downward from the brain through the foramen magnum and is protected by the spine.

spinal nerves Carry messages to and from the spinal cord.

spleen An organ of the lymphatic system that is located in the left upper quadrant of the abdomen and consists of two types of lymph tissue that are associated with drainage of the spleen.

sprain An injury, such as a stretch or a tear, to the ligaments of a joint that commonly leads to pain and swelling.

sterilization Destroys all microorganisms and spores by exposing articles to heat or to chemical disinfectants long enough to kill them all.

sternum Also known as the breastbone, this bony structure along the midline of the thorax provides a point of anterior attachment for the thoracic cage.

streptococcal (strep) pharyngitis A bacterial infection that usually presents with a sudden onset of severe sore throat, fever, tender neck glands, nausea, and malaise.

stress A load on the system; one of the body's processes for dealing with uncertain changes and danger.

stress behaviors Stress related actions that can be observed by others.

stressor An event or situation that creates personal conflict or poses a threat that requires the body to adapt or change

striated muscle Skeletal muscle that is under voluntary control.

subclavian artery The artery that travels from the aorta to each upper extremity.

subcutaneous Beneath the skin.

subcutaneous emphysema The presence of air in soft tissues, causing a characteristic crackling sensation on palpation.

subcutaneous (SC) injection Injection into the tissue between the skin and muscle; a medication delivery route.

subcutaneous layer Beneath the skin.

sulfur mustard (H) A vesicant chemical agent; it is a brownish-yellowish oily substance that is generally considered very persistent; it has the distinct smell of garlic or mustard and, when released, is quickly absorbed into the skin and/or mucous membranes and begins an irreversible process of damaging the cells.

superficial frostbite A type of frostbite characterized by altered sensation (numbness, tingling, or burning) and white, waxy skin that is firm to palpation, but the underlying tissues remain soft.

superior vena cava One of the two largest veins in the body; carries blood from the upper extremities, head, neck, and chest into the heart.

supination To turn the forearm laterally so that the palm faces forward (if standing) or upward (if lying supine).

suprasternal notch Found on the neck, where the sternum and clavicle meet.

surfactant A proteinaceous substance that lines the alveoli; decreases alveolar surface tension and keeps the alveoli expanded.

susceptible hosts Where the microorganism can reside.

syncopal episode Fainting; brief loss of consciousness caused by transiently inadequate blood flow to the brain.

synovial joints Joints that permit movement of the component bones.

synovial membrane The lining of a joint that secretes synovial fluid into the joint space.

systemic complications Moderate to severe allergic reaction affecting the systems of the body.

tabun (GA) A nerve agent that is one of the G agents; it is 36 times more persistent than sarin and approximately half as lethal; it has a fruity smell and is unique because the components used to manufacture the agent are easy to acquire and the agent is easy to manufacture.

tachycardia Rapid heart rhythm, more than 100 beats/min.

tachypnea Rapid respirations.

Tactical Combat Casualty Care (TC-3) Principles of care used when providing care to casualties in a tactical or combat environment.

Tactical Evacuation Phase of care when the casualty is being evacuated.

Tactical Field Care Phase of care that begins when the casualty and combat medic are no longer under hostile fire; the phase when most medical care is provided.

tarsals The ankle bones.

tendinitis Inflammation of a tendon that most commonly results from overuse.

tendon The fibrous portion of muscle that attaches to bone.

tension lines The pattern of tautness of the skin, which is arranged over body structures and affects how well wounds heal.

tension pneumothorax Accumulation of air under pressure in the chest cavity, usually secondary to a penetrating chest wound; can be rapidly fatal if not treated.

tertiary blast injury Injury from whole body displacement and subsequent traumatic impact with environmental objects.

testicular torsion A condition whereby a testicle essentially twists upon itself.

therapeutic effect The expected positive effect of the medication.

thermal burn An injury caused by radiation or direct contact with a heat source on the skin.

thermolysis The liberation of heat from the body.

thermoregulation The ability of the body to maintain temperature through a combination of heat gain by metabolic processes and muscular movement, and heat loss through respiration, evaporation, conduction, convection, and perspiration.

third-degree burn A burn that extends through the epidermis and dermis into the subcutaneous tissues beneath; previously called a full-thickness burn.

third spacing The shifting of fluid into the tissues, creating edema.

thoracic abdomen Area below the diaphragm but enclosed by the lower ribs.

thoracic inlet The superior aspect of the thoracic cavity, this ring-like opening is created by the first vertebra, the first rib, the clavicles, and the manubrium.

thorax The part of the body between the neck and the diaphragm, encased by the ribs.

thyroid cartilage The main supporting cartilage of the larynx; a shield-shaped structure formed by two plates that join in a V shape anteriorly to form the laryngeal prominence known as the Adam's apple.

tibia The shin bone.

TIC Mnemonic standing for Tenderness, Instability, and Crepitus.

tidal volume A measure of the depth of breathing; the volume of air that is inhaled or exhaled during a single respiratory cycle.

tincture of benzoin A liquid that, when applied to skin, becomes very sticky and helps hold bandages and dressings in place.

tinea capitis Fungal infection on the scalp.

tinea corporis Also called ringworm; an erythematous plaque with central clearing and well-defined and usually raised margins.

tinea cruris Also called jock itch; a ringed lesion that extends from the skin fold between the scrotum and upper thigh.

tinea pedis Also called athlete's foot; a common superficial fungal infection.

tinnitus Ringing in the ears.

tonicity The osmotic pressure of a solution, based on the relationship between sodium and water inside and outside the cell, that takes advantage of their chemical and osmotic properties to move water to areas of higher sodium concentration.

tonsils Lymphatic tissues located in the posterior pharynx; they help to trap bacteria.

total lung capacity The total volume of air that the lungs can hold; approximately 6 L in the average adult male.

toxic effect Caused by the intake of high doses of medications, ingestion of medications not intended for ingestion, or when a medication accumulates in the system.

trachea The conduit for all entry into the lungs; a tubular structure that is approximately 10 to 12 cm in length and is composed of a series of C-shaped cartilaginous rings; also called the windpipe.

tracheal shift A deviation of the trachea from its normal anatomic position; usually associated with tension pneumothorax.

trade name The brand name that a manufacturer gives a medication; capitalized.

traumatic brain injury (TBI) An injury to the brain from an event such as a blast, fall, direct impact, or motor vehicle accident which causes an alteration in mental status.

TRD-P Mnemonic standing for Tenderness, Rigidity, Distension, and Pulsating masses.

trending Process of determining, following several sets of baseline vital signs, whether a severely injured casualty's condition has stabilized or is deteriorating.

triage The medical sorting of casualties according to the type and seriousness of the injury, likelihood of survival, and establishment of priorities of treatment and evacuation.

true abdomen Area that contains the small intestine, bladder, and in females the uterus, fallopian tubes, and ovaries.

tubule A section of the kidney where the filtration of wastes, electrolytes, and water is controlled.

turbinates Three bony shelves that protrude from the lateral walls of the nasal cavity and extend into the nasal passageway, parallel to the nasal floor; serve to increase the surface area of the nasal mucosa, thereby improving the processes of warming, filtering, and humidification of inhaled air.

turgor Loss of elasticity in the skin.

tympanic membrane The eardrum; a thin, semitransparent membrane in the middle ear that transmits sound vibrations to the internal ear by means of the auditory ossicles.

ulna The larger bone of the forearm, on the side opposite the thumb.

ulnar artery The artery of the forearm that travels along its medial aspect.

upper airway All anatomic airway structures above the level of the vocal cords.

urticaria The formation of hives following the administration of a medication.

uvula A soft-tissue structure that resembles a punching bag; located in the posterior aspect of the oral cavity, at the base of the tongue.

V agent (VX) One of the G agents; it is a clear, oily agent that has no odor and looks like baby oil; it is over 100 times more lethal than sarin and is extremely persistent.

Vacutainer A device that connects to a catheter to assist with blood collection.

vallecula An anatomic space, or "pocket," located between the base of the tongue and the epiglottis; an important anatomic landmark for endotracheal intubation.

vasovagal reaction A reaction consisting of precordial distress, anxiety, nausea, and sometimes syncope.

vectors Objects used to transfer the agent from the point of release to the target.

vehicles Ways that microorganisms are transmitted.

veins The blood vessels that transport blood back to the heart.

velocity The rate of change of position or speed. Commonly measured in meters per second (m/s).

venipuncture The technique that permits access to a vein, usually to withdraw a blood specimen, initiate an intravenous infusion, or instill a medication.

venom A toxin produced by some animals.

ventilation The process of moving air into and out of the lungs.

venule The smallest branch of a vein.

vertebral body Anterior weight-bearing structure in the spine made of cancellous bone and surrounded by a layer of hard, compact bone that provides support and stability.

vertical compression A type of injury typically resulting from a direct blow to the crown of the skull or rapid deceleration from a fall through the feet, legs, and pelvis, possibly causing a burst fracture or disk herniation; forces are transmitted through vertebral bodies and directed either inferiorly through the skull or superiorly through the pelvis or feet.

vesicants Blister agents; the primary route of entry for vesicants is through the skin.

vesicle An elevated lesion containing serous fluid that is < 1 cm.

vials Small glass bottles for medications; may contain single or multiple doses.

virulence A pathogen's strength to cause disease.

visceral pleura The thin membrane that lines the lungs.

vocal cords White bands of tough tissue that are the lateral borders of the glottis.

voluntary muscle Muscle that can be controlled by a person.

wheals Also called hives; transient, elevated lesions caused by localized edema.

white blood cells (leukocytes) Blood cells that play a role in the body's immune defense mechanisms against infection.

xyphoid process An inferior segment of the sternum often used as a landmark for CPR.

Index

Credits

Chapter 1

Section Opener Courtesy of Sgt. Ezekiel R. Kitandwe/U.S. Navy; Chapter Opener Courtesy of Mr. Jerry Harben/U.S. Army; 1-6 © Shout Pictures/Custom Medical Stock Photo; 1-10A Courtesy of Z-Medica Corporation; 1-10B Courtesy of TraumaCure, Inc.; 1-11 Courtesy of North American Rescue, Inc.; 1-12 Courtesy of Staff Sgt. Cassandra Locke/U.S. Air Force; 1-13 Courtesy of North American Rescue, Inc.; 1-14A&B © Jones and Bartlett Publishers. Ready-Heat Blankets provided courtesy of TechTrade, LLC; 1-14C Courtesy of PerSys Medical, A Division of Performance Systems; 1-15 Used with permission of Smiths Medical; 1-17 Courtesy of Cephalon, Inc.

Chapter 2

Chapter Opener © Stephen Morton/AP Photos; 2-2 © John Radcliffe Hospital/Photo Researchers, Inc.; 2-3A&B © Charles Stewart & Associates

Chapter 4

Chapter Opener © Karel Prinsloo/AP Photos

Chapter 5

5-1 © Shout Pictures/Custom Medical Stock Photo

Chapter 6

Chapter Opener © Michael English, MD/Custom Medical Stock Photo; 6-4A © E.M. Singletary, MD. Used with permission; 6-4B, 6-5 © Charles Stewart & Associates

Chapter 8

8-9, 8-10 © Charles Stewart & Associates; 8-11 © E.M. Singletary, MD. Used with permission

Chapter 10

Chapter Opener © Stevie Grand/Photo Researchers, Inc.; 10-1 © Dr. P. Marazzi/Photo Researchers, Inc.; 10-4A&B © Charles Stewart & Associates; 10-5A © Amy Walters/ShutterStock, Inc.; 10-5B © E.M. Singletary, MD. Used with permission

Chapter 11

11-1 Courtesy of Staff Sgt. Osvaldo Sanchez/U.S. Army; 11-2 Courtesy of Beretta U.S.A. Corp. Used with permission; 11-3 Courtesy of Heckler & Koch. Used with permission; 11-4A&B Courtesy of O.F. Mossberg & Sons. Used with permission; 11-5 Courtesy of Colt Defense LLC. Used with permission; 11-6 Courtesy of Remington Arms Company, Inc. Used with permission; 11-7, 11-8 Courtesy of FNH USA; 11-9 © Brent Wong/ShutterStock, Inc.; 11-15 © E.M. Singletary, MD. Used with permission; 11-16 © Robi Kastro/AP Photos

Chapter 12

12-1 © ajt/ShutterStock, Inc.; 12-4 © pixelman/ShutterStock, Inc.; 12-6 © Photodisc; 12-11 Courtesy of Pyng Medical Corporation; 12-12 Courtesy of Glenmark Generics Inc. Used with permission; 12-13 Photo provided by private source; 12-14 Courtesy of Meridian Medical Technologies, Inc. (A subsidiary of King Pharmaceuticals, Inc.); 12-15 Courtesy of Cephalon, Inc.; 12-16 Courtesy of Baxter International, Inc. Used with permission

Chapter 14

Chapter Opener Courtesy of Staff Sgt. Shawn Weismiller/U.S. Air Force/U.S. Department of Defense

Chapter 16

Chapter Opener Courtesy of Staff Sgt. Jacob N. Bailey/U.S. Air Force; 16-15, 16-16, 16-17, 16-18, 16-19, 16-20, 16-21, 16-22, 16-23 Courtesy of Ferno Washington, Inc.; 16-24A Courtesy of Staff Sgt. Suzanne M. Jenkins/U.S. Air Force; 16-24B Courtesy of U.S. Air Force; 16-25 Courtesy of Lance Corporal Kelly R. Chase, U.S. Marine Corps/U.S. Department of Defense

Chapter 17

Section Opener Courtesy of SFC Milton H. Robinson/U.S. Department of Defense; 17-1, 17-2 Courtesy of U.S. Department of Defense; 17-3A © Laurin Rinder/Dreamstime.com; 17-3B © Charles Brutlag/Dreamstime.com

Chapter 18

18-1, 18-2 © AP Photos; 18-4 Courtesy of Peltor, part of Aearo Technologies, a 3M Company. Used with permission; 18-5 Courtesy of E-A-R Specialty Composites, part of Aearo Technologies, a 3M Company. Used with permission; 18-6 Courtesy of Staff Sgt. Aaron D. Allmon II/U.S. Air Force; 18-7 Courtesy of E-A-R Specialty Composites, part of Aearo Technologies, a 3M Company. Used with permission; 18-9, 18-10, 18-11 © Dr. P. Marazzi/Photo Researchers, Inc.

Chapter 19

19-1 © Custom Medical Stock Photo/Alamy Images; 19-7 Courtesy of 3M. Used with permission

Chapter 20

20-3 © Medical-on-Line/Alamy Images; 20-6A © E.M. Singletary, MD. Used with permission; 20-7 © Custom Medical Stock Photo; 20-9 © E.M. Singletary, MD. Used with permission; 20-10, 20-11, 20-12 Courtesy of 3M. Used with permission; 20-13, 20-14, 20-15 Courtesy of C.R. Bard, Inc. Used with permission; 20-16 Courtesy of Cardinal Health; 20-17 Courtesy of Zimmer, Inc.; 20-18 © M. English, MD/Custom Medical Stock Photo; 20-19 © Dr. P. Marazzi/Photo Researchers, Inc.; 20-20 © Hercules Robinson/Alamy Images; 20-21 © Charles Stewart & Associates; 20-22 © Medical-on-Line/Alamy Images; 20-23 © Phototake, Inc./Alamy Images; 20-24 © Dr. P. Marazzi/Photo Researchers, Inc.

Chapter 22

22-1 Courtesy of U.S. Department of Defense

Chapter 23

23-1 Courtesy and © Becton, Dickinson and Company

Chapter 24

24-4B © David M. Martin, MD/Photo Researchers, Inc.

Chapter 25

25-8 © Chet Childs/Custom Medical Stock Photo; 25-9 © Dr. P. Marazzi/Photo Researchers, Inc.; 25-10 Courtesy of John T. Halgren, MD, University of Nebraska Medical Center; 25-11 © Dr. M.A. Ansary/Photo Researchers, Inc.; 25-12 © Dr. P. Marazzi/Photo Researchers, Inc.

Chapter 26

26-4 © Medical-on-Line/Alamy Images

Chapter 28

Chapter Opener Courtesy of Megan T. Guffey; 28-2 Used with permission of The Knowledge and Skills Site of The Royal College of Surgeons of Edinburgh (www.edu.rcsed.ac.uk); 28-4 © Perov Stanislav/ShutterStock, Inc.; 28-5, 28-7 Courtesy of National Cancer Institute; 28-8 Courtesy of Adam Buchbinder; 28-9 Courtesy of John Pozniak; 28-10 Courtesy of James L. Horwitz, MD/Rainbow Pediatrics; 28-11 Courtesy of Dr. Heinz F. Eichenwald/CDC; 28-12 © Scott Camazine/Alamy Images; 28-13 Courtesy of Joe Miller/CDC; 28-15 Courtesy of Dr. Thomas F. Sellers, Emory University/CDC; 28-16 Courtesy of CDC; 28-17 Courtesy of Bruno Goignard, MD and Jeff Hageman, MHS/CDC; 28-18, 28-19, 28-20 Courtesy of Dr. Lucille K. Georg/CDC; 28-21 © Custom Medical Stock Photo/Alamy Images; 28-22 © Steven Kazlowski/Peter Arnold, Inc.

Chapter 29

29-2 Courtesy of Neil Malcom Winkelmann

Chapter 30

Chapter Opener Courtesy of Sgt. Monroe Seigle/U.S. Marines; 30-2 Courtesy of Megan T. Guffey; 30-4 Courtesy of Neil Malcom Winkelmann; 30-5 Courtesy of Dr. Jack Poland/CDC; 30-6 Courtesy of USGS; 30-7A © Frank B. Yuwono/ShutterStock, Inc.; 30-7B © Steve McWilliam/ShutterStock, Inc.; 30-8 Courtesy of James Gathany/CDC; 30-9 Courtesy of World Health Organization/CDC; 30-10 © Joao Estevao A. Freitas (jefras)/ShutterStock, Inc.; 30-11 Courtesy of James Gathany/CDC; 30-12 Courtesy of CDC; 30-13 © blickwinkel/Alamy Images; 30-14 © Visual&Written SL/Alamy Images; 30-15 Courtesy of Kenneth Cramer, Monmouth College; 30-16A&B Courtesy of Department of Entomology, University of Nebraska; 30-17 © Crystal Kirk/ShutterStock, Inc.; 30-18A © Photos.com; 30-18B Courtesy of Ray Rauch/U.S. Fish & Wildlife Service; 30-18C © SuperStock/Alamy Images; 30-18D Courtesy of Luther C. Goldman/U.S. Fish & Wildlife Service

Chapter 31

Section Opener Courtesy of Staff Sgt. Jeanette Copeland/U.S. Air Force; 31-2A © Drbouz/Dreamstime.com; 31-2B © Sugarfree.sk/Dreamstime.com; 31-2C © Ischneider/Dreamstime.com; 31-4 Courtesy of Dr. Saeed Keshavarz/RCCI, Research Center of Chemical Injuries/IRAN; 31-5 © Chikumo Chiaki/AP Photos; 31-6 Courtesy of James H. Steele/CDC; 31-7 Courtesy of CDC

Chapter 32

Chapter Opener Courtesy of Staff Sgt. Lakisha Croley/U.S. Air Force; 32-1 Courtesy of Mass Communication Specialist 3rd Class Ja'lon A. Rhinehart/U.S. Navy; 32-3 Courtesy of Quartermaster Supply (www.qm-supply.com); 32-4 Courtesy of Journalist 1st Class Dennis J. Herring/U.S. Navy; 32-5 Courtesy of Quartermaster Supply (www.qm-supply.com); 32-6 Photo courtesy of 3M © 2008. Used with permission; 32-7 Courtesy of U.S. Army; 32-8 Courtesy of U.S. Department of Defense; 32-9 Courtesy of Ferno Washington, Inc.

Chapter 33

Chapter Opener Courtesy of Dr. J. Noble, Jr./CDC; 33-2, 33-3, 33-4 Courtesy of Meridian Medical Technologies, Inc. (A subsidiary of King Pharmaceuticals, Inc.)

Chapter 35

Section Opener © ICRC; Chapter Opener © jan kranen-donk/ShutterStock, Inc.; 35-1 © National Library of Medicine; 35-2 © Andy Z/ShutterStock, Inc.; 35-3 © National Library of Medicine; 35-7A Courtesy of Master Sgt. Johan Charles Van Boers/U.S. Army; 35-7B Courtesy of Chief Mass Communication Specialist Edward G. Martens/U.S. Navy; 35-7C Courtesy of Mass Communication Specialist 2nd Class Kenneth W. Robinson/U.S. Navy; 35-8 Courtesy of SFC Johan Charles Van Boers, 55th Signal Company, Combat Camera, Ft. Meade, Maryland/U.S. Army; 35-9 Courtesy of National Archives [208-AA-288BB(2)]; 35-10 Courtesy of National Archives [238-NT-592)

Combat Medic in Action Courtesy of Senior Airman Steve R. Doty/U.S. Air Force